Bethesda Handbook
of Clinical Hematology

Bethesda Handbook of Clinical Hematology

Editors

Griffin P. Rodgers, M.D., F.A.C.P.
*Chief, Molecular and Clinical Hematology Branch,
Deputy Director, National Institute of Diabetes,
Digestive and Kidney Diseases
National Institutes of Health
Bethesda, Maryland*

Neal S. Young, M.D., F.A.C.P.
*Chief, Hematology Branch
National Heart, Lung, and Blood Institute
National Institutes of Health
Bethesda, Maryland*

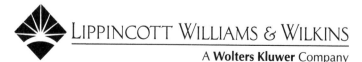

LIPPINCOTT WILLIAMS & WILKINS

A **Wolters Kluwer** Company

Philadelphia · Baltimore · New York · London
Buenos Aires · Hong Kong · Sydney · Tokyo

Acquisitions Editor: Jonathan Pine
Developmental Editor: Lisa Kairis
Project Manager: Nicole Walz
Senior Manufacturing Manager: Ben Rivera
Creative Director: Doug Smock
Senior Marketing Manager: Adam Glazer
Production Services: Maryland Composition
Printer: RR Donnelley-Crawfordsville

Library of Congress Cataloging-in-Publication Data

Bethesda handbook of clinical hematology / editors, Griffin P. Rodgers, Neal S. Young.
   p. ; cm.
   Includes bibliographical references and index.
   ISBN-13: 978-0-7817-4715-8
   ISBN-10: 0-7817-4715-5
1. Blood—Diseases—Handbooks, manuals, etc. 2. Hematology—Handbooks, manuals, etc.
I. Rodgers, Griffin P. II. Young, Neal S.
   [DNLM: 1. Hematologic Diseases. WH 120 B562 2005]
RC633.B49 2005
616.1'5—dc22

2004020888

Contents

Preface

Life is short, the art long.
-Hippocrates c460–357 BC

The accessibility of blood and bone marrow has made hematology, historically, the engine of basic research in internal medicine. Hematology has thrived at the National Institutes of Health because of this close relationship with the research laboratory. Investigators from the various institutes in Bethesda have contributed to the knowledge of blood diseases from the study of individual patients with sometimes rare diseases, and to the development of clinical protocols for the rigorous assessment of diagnostic criteria or treatments, both established and novel. Our hematology fellowship programs have fostered a scientific approach to hematology, not only to assess outcomes but also to advance the experimental basis of our understanding of blood diseases and the application of laboratory insights to their treatment in practice. The collegial relationships among local institutions and individuals in the greater Washington area who share training and patients have greatly furthered these efforts.

Handbooks are intended to be highly accessible, both literally and figuratively. Our Handbook has been designed to be carried in the white coat pocket of the student, resident, and fellow on a hematology or oncology service, and in the briefcase of the internist, hospitalist, family practitioner, and pediatrician, whose practice includes patients with blood diseases. We have purposely combined authors who are recognized experts in their fields with senior fellows who have had current experience learning hematology and caring daily for hematology patients, and encouraged a thoughtful approach to the presentation of the core knowledge using tables, algorithms, meaningful figures, and bulleted text structures. The Handbook is organized according to disease categories and hematological problems of importance to the consulting and treating hematologist, and additional chapters are provided to acquaint the reader with familiar and new laboratory methodologies that underlie modern clinical approaches to diagnosis and treatment.

We are indebted to our many colleagues for their scholarly contributions and their willingness to participate in this endeavor. We are also grateful for the skilled help of the staff at Lippincott Williams & Wilkins in bringing this Handbook to fruition.

Griffin P. Rodgers, M.D.
Neal S. Young, M.D.

Disclaimer: This work was not performed as official NIH duties.

Dedication

For our children, with love:
  Chris and Gregory Rodgers
  Andrea, Max, and Giorgio Young

Contributing Authors

Salah Abbasi, M.D. *Division of Hematology/Oncology, Lombardi Cancer Center, Georgetown University Medical Center, Washington, DC*

Jame Abraham, M.D., F.A.C.P. *Section of Hematology/Oncology, Mary Babb Randolph Cancer Center, West Virginia University, Morgantown, West Virginia*

Firoozeh Alvandi, M.D. *Department of Transfusion Medicine, Clinical Center, National Institutes of Health, Bethesda, Maryland*

Barbara Alving, M.D., M.A.C.P. *National Heart, Lung, and Blood Institute, National Institutes of Health, Bethesda, Maryland*

A. John Barrett, M.D., F.R.C.P., F.R.C.P. (Pathology) *Stem Cell Allotransplantation Section, Hematology Branch, National Institutes of Health, Bethesda, Maryland*

Minocher Battiwalla, M.D. *Transplant Section, Department of Medicine, Roswell Park Cancer Institute; State University of New York at Buffalo, Buffalo, New York*

Charles D. Bolan Jr., M.D., Colonel U.S. Army Medical Corps *Department of Medicine, Uniformed Services University of the Health Sciences, Bethesda, Maryland; Walter Reed Army Institute of Research; Department of Transfusion Medicine, Clinical Center, National Institutes of Health, Bethesda, Maryland*

Bruce D. Cheson, M.D. *Division of Hematology/Oncology, Georgetown University; Hematology, Lombardi Comprehensive Cancer Center, Washington, DC*

Richard Childs, M.D. *Hematology Branch, National Heart, Lung, and Blood Institute, National Institutes of Health, Bethesda, Maryland*

Sandeep S. Dave, M.D. *Stem Cell Allotransplantation Section, Hematology Branch, Warren Grant Magnuson Clinical Center, National Heart, Lung, and Blood Institute, National Institutes of Health, Bethesda, Maryland*

Cynthia E. Dunbar, M.D. *Molecular Hematopoiesis Section, Hematology Branch, National Heart, Lung, and Blood Institute, National Institutes of Health, Bethesda, Maryland*

Thomas A. Fleisher, M.D. *Department of Laboratory Medicine, Warren G. Magnuson Clinical Center, National Institutes of Health, Bethesda, Maryland*

Patrick F. Fogarty, M.D. *Hematology Service, Department of Laboratory Medicine, Clinical Center, Naitonal Institutes of Health, Bethesda, Maryland*

Martin Gutierrez, M.D. *Center for Cancer Research, National Cancer Institute, National Institutes of Health, Bethesda, Maryland*

Peiman Hematti, M.D. *Department of Medicine, University of Wisconsin-Madison Medical School, Madison, Wisconsin*

McDonald K. Horne, III, M.D. *Department of Laboratory Medicine, National Institutes of Health, Bethesda, Maryland*

Matthew M. Hsieh, M.D. *Hematology Branch, National Heart, Lung, and Blood Institute, National Institutes of Health, Bethesda, Maryland*

Elaine S. Jaffe, M.D. *Hematopathology Section, Center for Cancer Research, National Institutes of Health; Laboratory of Pathology, Center for Cancer Research, National Cancer Institute, Bethesda, Maryland*

Craig M. Kessler, M.D. *Division of Hematology and Oncology, Georgetown University Medical Center, Washington, DC*

Harvey G. Klein, M.D. *Department of Transfusion Medicine, National Institutes of Health, Bethesda, Maryland*

Pallavi P. Kumar, M.D. *HIV and AIDS Malignancy Branch, National Cancer Institute, National Institutes of Health, Bethesda, Maryland*

Roger Kurlander, M.D. *Department of Laboratory Medicine, Clinical Center, National Institutes of Health, Bethesda, Maryland*

Susan F. Leitman, M.D. *Blood Services Section, Department of Transfusion Medicine, National Institutes of Health, Bethesda, Maryland*

Steven J. Lemery, M.D. *Hematology Branch, National Heart, Lung, and Blood Institute, National Institutes of Health, Bethesda, Maryland*

Lawrence S. Lessin, M.D., M.A.C.P. *Washington Cancer Institute, Washington Hospital Center, Washington, DC*

Robert I. Liem, M.D.   *Division of Hematology, Oncology Stem Cell Transplant, Children's Memorial Hospital, Chicago, Illinois*

Richard. F. Little, M.D.   *HIV and AIDS Malignancy Branch, Center for Cancer Research, National Cancer Institute, National Institutes of Health, Bethesda, Maryland*

Johnson M. Liu, M.D.   *Department of Medicine, Mount Sinai School of Medicine, New York, New York*

Jaroslaw P. Maciejewski, M.D., Ph.D.   *Experimental Hematology and Hematopoiesis, Cleveland Clinic Lerner College of Medicine; Hematology/Oncology, Cleveland Clinic Foundation, Cleveland, Ohio*

Henry L. Malech, M.D.   *Laboratory of Host Defenses, National Institute of Allergy and Infectious Diseases, National Institutes of Health, Bethesda, Maryland*

Vera Malkovska, M.D., M.R.C.P., F.R.C. (Pathology)   *Hematology, Washington Cancer Institute, Washington Hospital Center, Washington, DC*

Jeffrey L. Miller, M.D.   *Laboratory of Chemical Biology, National Institute of Diabetes and Digestive and Kidney Diseases, National Institutes of Health, Bethesda, Maryland*

Pierre Noel, M.D.   *Department of Medicine, Uniformed Services, University of Health Sciences, Bethesda, Maryland; Hematology Service, Laboratory Medicine, Clinical Center, National Institutes of Health, Bethesda, Maryland*

Patricia Ann Oneal, M.D.   *Hematology Branch, National Heart, Lung, and Blood Institute, National Institutes of Health, Bethesda, Maryland*

Margaret E. Rick, M.D.   *Hematology Service, Department of Laboratory Medicine, National Institutes of Health, Bethesda, Maryland*

Antonio Risitano, M.D.   *Division of Hematology, Frederico II University of Naples, Naples, Italy*

Jamie Robyn, M.D., Ph.D.   *Laboratory of Allergic Diseases, National Institute of Allergy and Infectious Diseases, National Institutes of Health, Bethesda, Maryland*

Griffin P. Rodgers, M.D., F.A.C.P.   *Molecular and Clinical Hematology Branch, National Institutes of Health; National Institute of*

Diabetes, Digestive and Kidney Diseases, National Institutes of Health, Bethesda, Maryland

Geraldine P. Schechter, M.D.   *Hematology Department, Veterans Administration Hospital, Washington, DC*

Phillip Scheinberg, M.D.   *Hematology Branch, National Heart, Lung, and Blood Institute, National Institutes of Health, Bethesda, Maryland*

Carmine Selleri, M.D.   *Division of Hematology, Frederico II University of Naples, Naples, Italy*

Elaine Sloand, M.D.   *National Institutes of Health, Bethesda, Maryland*

Scott Solomon, M.D.   *Stem Cell Allotransplantation Section, Hematology Branch, National Heart, Lung, and Blood Institute, National Institutes of Health, Bethesda, Maryland*

Ramaprasad Srinivasan, M.D.   *Hematology Branch, National Heart, Lung, and Blood Institute, National Institutes of Health, Bethesda, Maryland*

Louis M. Staudt, M.D., Ph.D.   *Metabolism Branch, National Cancer Institute, National Institutes of Health, Bethesda, Maryland*

John F. Tisdale, M.D.   *Molecular and Clinical Hematology Branch, National Institute of Diabetes and Digestive and Kidney Diseases, National Institutes of Health, Bethesda, Maryland*

Alan S. Wayne, M.D.   *Pediatric Oncology Branch, National Cancer Institute, National Institutes of Health, Bethesda, Maryland; Department of Pediatrics, Johns Hopkins University School of Medicine, Baltimore, Maryland*

Adrian Wiestner, M.D., Ph.D.   *Hematology Branch, National Heart, Lung, and Blood Institute, National Cancer Institute, Bethesda, Maryland*

Wyndham Wilson, M.D.   *Medicine Branch, National Cancer Institute, National Institutes of Health, Bethesda, Maryland*

Neal S. Young, M.D.   *Hematology Branch, National Heart, Lung, and Blood Institute, National Institutes of Health, Bethesda, Maryland*

1

Iron Deficiency

McDonald K. Horne, III

Iron deficiency is the most common cause of anemia throughout the world. In the United States approximately 10% of women of childbearing age and young children are depleted of iron (1). Iron deficiency anemia is especially frequent among the elderly, among whom anemia resulting from inadequate utilization of iron stores is also prevalent (2).

PATHOPHYSIOLOGY

True versus Functional Iron Deficiency

Iron deficiency anemia is caused by:

- A lack of endogenous iron ("true" iron deficiency) or
- Inadequate utilization of endogenous iron ("functional" iron deficiency).

Functional iron deficiency anemia is associated with a variety of chronic diseases. It also occurs when iron is not supplied rapidly enough to support the level of erythropoiesis driven by erythropoietin.

Iron Balance

The bulk of total body iron is contained in the hemoglobin of the circulating red cells. Normally, this iron is recycled when senescent erythrocytes undergo phagocytosis in the reticuloendothelial system (RES), predominantly in the spleen (Fig. 1-1). The majority of phagocytosed iron is released into plasma and bound to transferrin, developing red cells endocytose transferrin-bound iron. Iron enters this cycle by absorption from the duodenum and exits in sloughed epithelial cells, in red cells lost in menses, and through a miniscule amount of normal gastrointestinal bleeding.

Dietary iron is present as inorganic salts in meat and vegetables and in heme in meat (3).

- Heme iron is the most bioavailable because it is soluble at the alkaline pH of the duodenum, where iron is absorbed.
- Inorganic iron in food is in the ferric form, which must be solubilized in the acidic stomach and bound to small ligands that allow it to remain in solution during passage into the duodenum.

Meat enhances the absorption of inorganic iron, whereas the tightly chelated inorganic iron in vegetables is much less available. Inorganic iron must be divalent to be absorbed by the duodenal epithelium. Thus, oral medicinal iron is always ferrous. Ferric iron is enzymatically reduced in the brush border of the duodenum before transport into enterocytes. From there enterocyte iron is transported into the bloodstream where it is oxidized back to the ferric state and bound to transferrin.

1

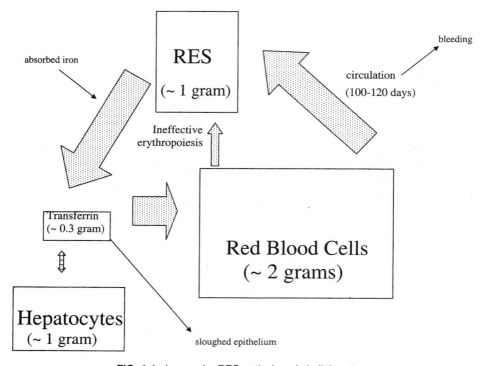

FIG. 1-1. Iron cycle. RES, reticuloendothelial system

- Adult males must absorb approximately 1 mg of iron each day to maintain neutral iron balance; menstruating females require approximately twice this amount.
- During pregnancy and periods of rapid growth, positive iron balance is needed to support increased production of hemoglobin and myoglobin.
- Negative iron balance results from increased loss of iron (nearly always because of bleeding), inadequate dietary intake, and increased utilization of iron (Table 1-1).

An average adult derives approximately 20 mg of transferrin-bound iron each day from approximately 20 mL of red cells reaching the end of their lifespan. This iron is recycled into new cells to replace senescent erythrocytes. If red cells exit this cycle prematurely because of bleeding, the iron to replace these cells must come from some other source, either RES stores or the diet. Stores are more important. At most only 3 to 4 mg of iron can be absorbed from the diet each day, only enough to produce 3 or 4 mL of red cells. However, approximately 40 to 60 mg of iron can be transferred from ferritin to transferrin per day to produce 40 to 60 mL of red cells but this is the physiologic maximum (4). No more red blood cells can be produced unless additional iron is provided in the form of dietary supplements.

Erythropoietin

Erythropoietin (EPO) is produced by interstitial fibroblasts in the kidneys in response to the prevailing tissue oxygen tension. Developing red cells consume EPO, and the rate of this consumption appears to influence the plasma EPO concentration. For a given degree of

TABLE 1-1. *Causes of true iron deficiency*

<u>Increased loss of iron</u>
 Bleeding
  Menorrhagia
  Gastrointestinal
  Surgery
  Trauma
  Childbirth
  Excessive phlebotomy
  Blood donations
  Factitious
 Chronic hemoglobinuria
  Mechanical heart valve hemolysis
  Paroxysmal nocturnal hemoglobinuria
<u>Decreased intake of iron</u>
 Dietary deficiency
  Limited meat
 Malabsorption
  Sprue
  Achlorhydria:
   Gastric atrophy
   Partial gastrectomy
   Proton pump inhibitors
   Inflammatory bowel disease
<u>Increased utilization of iron</u>
 Pregnancy
 Rapid growth

anemia, EPO levels tend to be inversely correlated with the degree of erythroid hyperplasia (5). With iron deficiency, which characteristically causes mild erythroid hyperplasia (although ineffective), the EPO concentration is typically 30 to 300 U/L (normal, 4 to 20 U/L) depending on the degree of anemia (Fig. 1-2). In contrast, in states of red cell aplasia, with virtually no EPO consumption by developing red cells, EPO levels may be several times higher.

PROGRESSIVE LABORATORY ABNORMALITIES OF IRON DEFICIENCY

- When more iron is lost than absorbed, *stainable marrow iron* (RES hemosiderin) and *serum ferritin* begin to decrease (Fig. 1-3). A bone marrow examination is rarely necessary in evaluating a patient for iron deficiency; the serum ferritin usually provides adequate information about body iron stores (6). However, serum ferritin is increased by inflammation, which stimulates ferritin synthesis independent of the amount of storage iron, and especially by damage to hepatocytes, which leak their intracellular contents.
- As storage iron becomes depleted and the iron supply to red cells becomes limiting, erythroblasts begin inserting more transferrin receptors into their membranes. Some transferrin receptors are shed into the circulation where they are measurable (7). Elevated *serum soluble transferrin receptor concentration* is not specific for iron deficiency and can be seen also in any state of erythroid hyperplasia, as well as in myelodysplasia.
- When storage iron has been depleted, *serum iron* and *transferrin saturation* decrease (Fig. 1-3), while the *transferrin concentration* usually increases.
- When transferrin saturation reaches approximately 16%, the supply of iron to developing red cells becomes rate limiting, and the *red cell count* decreases (8).

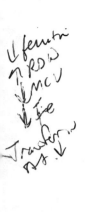

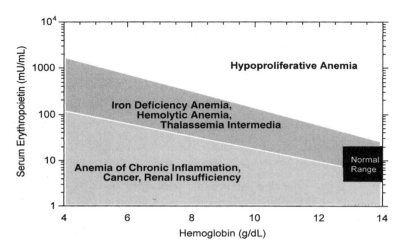

FIG. 1-2. Relationship of erythropoietin (EPO) level to hemoglobin concentration.

- Iron deficient red cells are smaller than normal, and therefore the *red cell distribution width* (RDW) increases.
- When microcytes become more numerous, the *mean cell volume* (MCV) decreases below normal, typically at a hemoglobin of approximately 10 g/dL.

ANEMIA OF CHRONIC DISEASE

Anemia of chronic disease (ACD) is characterized by *hypoferremia despite seemingly adequate or increased iron stores*. ACD develops in patients with chronic infectious, inflammatory, or neoplastic diseases (9).

In ACD, inflammatory cytokines:

- Directly suppress erythropoiesis;
- Blunt the response of EPO to the resulting anemia;
- Promote the sequestration of iron in the macrophage storage pool; and
- Limit the amount of transferrin-iron available for erythropoiesis (10).

Characteristically ACD is mild and asymptomatic. Although *usually normocytic, the MCV is often on the low end of normal and may be in the microcytic range. While serum iron concentration and transferrin saturation often suggest iron deficiency, the transferrin concentration is not elevated and may be low.* Furthermore, there is evidence of storage iron in the form of an elevated serum ferritin. Serum EPO levels in ACD are lower than in other anemias of the same degree (Fig. 1-2).

The diagnosis of true iron deficiency in a patient with a chronic disease can be particularly difficult because the underlying illness can cause hypoferremia despite the presence of storage iron and can elevate serum ferritin even in the absence of storage iron.

- The most reliable diagnostic parameter, at least for patients with infectious and other inflammatory diseases, is reported to be *the ratio of serum transferrin receptor concentration (milligrams per liter) to the log of the serum ferritin concentration* (7).

Because soluble transferrin receptor concentration and ferritin concentration change in opposite directions with iron deficiency, their ratio is especially sensitive to iron status and

Earliest   Causes of misleading results

Reduced RES iron

Marrow hemosiderin   .... Inadequate sample, poor staining

Serum ferritin .... Inflammation, liver disease

⬇

Reduced serum Fe,
        transferrin saturation   Inflammation
Elevated serum transferrin

⬇

Elevated serum transferrin receptor .... Erythroid hyperplasia
                                               (hemolysis,
                                               megaloblastosis)

⬇

Reduced red cell count, hemoglobin .... Polycythemia vera with iron
                                           deficiency

⬇

Elevated RDW
Reduced MCV   .... ACD, thalassemia, hemoglobin E,

                                           chronic lead poisoning, hereditary
                                           sideroblastic anemia

Latest

FIG. 1-3. Development of laboratory abnormalities during negative iron balance. RES, reticulo-endothelial system; Fe, iron; RDW, red cell distribution width; MCV, mean cell volume; ACD, anemia of chronic disease.

appears to distinguish ACD from true iron deficiency, with or without a chronic disease. However, the ratio is not useful in patients with renal disease on hemodialysis, in whom a transferrin iron saturation of less than 20% and/or a ferritin of less than 100 µg/L identifies the need for iron supplementation.

TREATMENT OF IRON-DEFICIENCY ANEMIA

Oral Iron Therapy

- A daily supplement of approximately 200 mg of elemental iron taken on an empty stomach provides the marrow with enough iron to raise the blood hemoglobin concentration approximately 0.25 g/dL per day (Table 1-2).

Oral iron can cause nausea or constipation in some patients. Because symptoms tend to correlate with the amount of iron ingested, the dose should be lowered until tolerable or the medication should be discontinued until the symptoms resolve and then restarted at a lower dose. Smaller amounts are therapeutic; the response is just slower. Patients should have a stool softener prescribed as needed. Often nausea can be avoided by taking iron with food.

TABLE 1–2. *Oral iron supplements (over-the-counter)*

	Tablet (mg)	Elemental iron (mg)	Maximum daily dose (tablets)	AWP of maximum dose per month*
Iron salts				
Ferrous sulfate	300	60	3	$2.55
Ferrous gluconate	300	35	3	$4.57
Ferrous fumarate	325	107	3	$3.00
Polysaccharide iron complex (Niferex)		150	1	$7.12

*Average wholesale price (2003 Drug Topics Redbook).

This practice reduces iron absorption but usually does not make patients refractory to iron. Ascorbic acid may improve absorption. Sometimes changing the type of iron salt relieves gastrointestinal symptoms, although this may just reflect a lower iron content of some preparations.

- Slow-release formulations of iron are said to cause fewer gastrointestinal side effects, but they also often contain less iron per dose and are considerably more expensive than the salts in Table 1-2. Furthermore, they may release their iron below the duodenum, where absorption is minimal.

A variety of medications can reduce oral iron absorption (Table 1-3) and should not be taken within several hours of iron tablets. Conversely, oral iron supplements can hinder the absorption of other drugs (Table 1-4).

- Another way to replenish iron is by increasing lean meat intake. Because the heme of meat is so readily absorbed and without gastrointestinal side effects, it is thus an excellent source of iron. The presence of heme in the diet also increases the absorption of inorganic iron. However, dietary alteration may not be realistic if the patient prefers vegetables or has a limited grocery budget.

Iron supplements should obviously be continued until the anemia resolves, which usually only requires a few weeks. To accumulate storage iron, supplements must be continued for several months because the rate of iron absorption slows in the absence of anemia. The serum ferritin can be used to determine when iron stores are sufficient.

TABLE 1–3. *Medications and foods that reduce iron absorption*

Antacids (alkaline liquids, H2-blockers, proton pump inhibitors)
Tetracyclines (especially doxycycline)
Pancreatic enzyme supplements
Biphosphonates
Cholestyramine
Calcium supplements
Tea
Dairy products
Phosphonates (vegetables)

TABLE 1–4. *Medications malabsorbed because of the coadministration of iron*

Quinolone antibiotics
Biphosphonates
Cefdinir
Levodopa, carbidopa, methyldopa
Thyroxine
Penicillamine
Mycohenolate mofetil
Zinc or copper salts

Intravenous Iron Therapy

Three formulations of parenteral iron are currently marketed in the United States: iron dextran (DexFerrum, INFeD), sodium ferric gluconate in sucrose (Ferrlecit), and iron sucrose (Venofer) (Table 1-5). All are primarily used to treat iron deficiency in patients undergoing long-term hemodialysis (11,12). Because these patients are often in negative iron balance and are frequently receiving EPO, they can rarely maintain an adequate supply of iron with oral supplements only. Iron dextran has been the traditional parenteral supplement for hemodialysis patients in the United States, but it has been associated with serious adverse reactions in 2% to 3% of patients, including deaths. Ferric gluconate has only been available in the United States since 1999 and iron sucrose since 2000, but a long experience in Europe has indicated that serious adverse reactions associated with these agents are rare, and no deaths have been reported to date. Therefore, the newer agents are clearly safer and therefore preferable. Dosing regimens approved by the US Food and Drug Administration are shown in Table 1-5. Although the package insert for ferric gluconate prescribes an initial test dose, many authorities feel this is unnecessary because of the safety record of this drug. A test dose is not prescribed for iron sucrose.

Apart from hemodialysis, negative iron balance is rarely so marked or so protracted that oral iron supplements are insufficient. However, when patients cannot tolerate an adequate

TABLE 1–5. *Intravenous iron supplements*

	FDA-approved dosing	AWP per dose*
Ferric gluconate complex in sucrose (Ferrlecit; 12.5 mg/mL iron)	125 mg iron in 10 mL over at least 10 minutes or Same dose plus 90 mL 0.9% sodium chloride over 1 hour	$86
Iron sucrose (Venofer: 20 mg/mL iron)	100 mg iron in 5 mL into dialysis line at 1 mL/min or Same dose plus 95 mL 0.9% sodium chloride over at least 15 minutes	$69

*Average wholesale price (2003 Drug Topics Redbook).

dose of oral iron, such as during pregnancy, or when they have severe and recurrent gastrointestinal or uterine hemorrhage, parenteral iron may be indicated.

- The dose in these circumstances is determined by the degree of anemia and can be estimated by assuming that a hemoglobin concentration of approximately 14 g/dL reflects a total body red cell mass of approximately 30 mL packed cells per kilogram and that some amount of storage iron is desirable. For example, if a patient's hemoglobin concentration is 10 g/dL, his deficit is 4 g/dL or 4/14 = 0.29 of his normal red cell mass. For a 70-kg individual this deficit represents 70 kg × 30 mL RBC/kg × 0.29 = 600 mL of packed red cells. Because each milliliter of packed red cells normally contains approximately 1 mg of iron, this patient needs approximately 600 mg of iron to restore his hemoglobin concentration to normal. To replete his iron stores, an additional 500 to 1,000 mg of iron is necessary. Therefore, the total dose should be approximately 1,100 to 1,600 mg of iron.

In the past, this whole dose was often given at once using iron dextran. However, this approach incurred a small risk of an anaphylactic reaction and frequently resulted in arthralgia and myalgia several days later. Today with alternatives to iron dextran and by limiting the dose to 100 to 125 mg of iron per day, adverse reactions are unusual. Infusions can be administered 3 or 4 times each week.

Response to Iron Therapy

Whether iron therapy is given orally or parenterally:

- Within *3 or 4 days,* peripheral blood *reticulocytes* increase in otherwise healthy individuals, and
- Within the *first week* of initiating iron, the *hemoglobin* should rise.

There is no significant difference in response to oral and parenteral iron if full doses of oral iron can be given. Failure to observe an increase in hemoglobin after 1 to 2 weeks suggests problems: an incorrect diagnosis of iron deficiency, continued bleeding (in which case reticulocytes will increase despite no improvement in the anemia), noncompliance with therapy, and/or iron malabsorption.

A patient can be tested for iron malabsorption by measuring serum iron concentration immediately before and then 2 to 4 hours after taking the usual dose of iron in the fasting or nonfasting state. Although this test is not standardized and can yield misleading results if the postsample is not drawn at the optimal time, it can be helpful when the serum iron clearly rises into the normal range.

ADMINISTRATION OF ERYTHROPOIETIN

- Subcutaneous administration of EPO is preferrable to intravenous because it requires approximately one-third less drug (Table 1-6).
- The prescribed dose should be rounded to the nearest vial size to avoid waste. EPO is formulated in 2,000, 3,000, 4,000, 10,000, 20,000, and 40,000 units per vial.

Patients undergoing hemodialysis typically receive EPO two or three times per week to coincide with their dialysis treatments (12). Although this schedule is often used in other settings, it may require otherwise unnecessary trips to a medical facility. Therefore, convenience drove the development of a weekly regimen of 40,000 to 60,000 units for patients with cancer with chemotherapy-related anemia (13,14). The anemia of chronic inflammatory disease is usually treated with two or three injections of EPO per week, although once-weekly injections of 40,000 units likely would be just as effective (13,15).

Darbepoietin alfa is a recently introduced recombinant EPO that is hyperglycosylated to

TABLE 1–6. *Erythropoietin regimens for iron-replete patients**

	Initial Dose	
	Epoetin alfa	Darbepoetin alfa
Cancer chemotherapy	40,000 units sc once weekly (13, 14)† or 150 U/kg sc 3 times per week	3–5 μg/kg sc every 2 weeks 16)† or 2.25 μg/kg sc once weekly (21)
Anemia of chronic disease	150 U/kg sc 2–3 times per week (13)	
HIV/zidovudine (if serum EPO <500 U/L)	100 units/kg sc 3 times per week	
Chronic hemodialysis	40 U/kg sc 2–3 times per week (12)	0.45 μg/kg sc once weekly (21)
Dose adjustment:	If hemoglobin rises 1 g/dL per 2 weeks, reduce dose by 50%. If hemoglobin rises <1 g/dL by 4 weeks, increase dose by 50% If hemoglobin rises <1 g/dL by 8 weeks, discontinue.	

*Transferrin saturation 20%, ferritin 100 μg/L.
† Average wholesale price $500–$600 per week for a 70 kg patient (2003 Drug Topics Redbook). sc, subcutaneously;

slow its clearance. Because its serum half-life is threefold longer than native EPO, it can be administered less frequently (16).

An adequate iron supply is required for an optimal response to EPO (15). Time and money are wasted by administration of EPO when there is evidence of absolute or functional iron deficiency. Even parenteral iron is much less expensive than EPO. In general the iron supply is adequate if the transferrin saturation is greater than 20% and the serum ferritin is greater than 100 μg/L.

TREATING ANEMIA OF CHRONIC DISEASE

The only truly satisfactory long-term solution to ACD is adequate treatment of the primary disorder. Fortunately, because it is typically mild, this anemia usually does not require specific therapy. However, it may be more severe, particularly if it is compounded by iron deficiency.
Patients with chronic diseases:

• Do not respond to oral iron unless they are also iron deficient, but
• They may respond to parenteral iron even when they have endogenous iron stores.

However, the benefit of parenteral iron is short-lived because the iron is poorly reutilized (17). If the injections are discontinued, the hemoglobin returns to its baseline value, and the administered iron becomes part of the storage pool.

The anemia is treated more effectively with pharmacologic doses of EPO, which can at least partially overcome the suppressive effect of cytokines and directly stimulate erythroid proliferation (18–20). The benefit of EPO may be limited by true or functional iron deficiency, which can be treated with oral iron. However, even with the combination of iron and EPO, the hemoglobin may only increase approximately 0.5 to 1 g/dL per month (an otherwise healthy iron-deficient individual can generate a hemoglobin increment of this magnitude in

2 to 4 days). Although the hemoglobin will increase, the effects of the inflammatory cytokines persist so that the iron from senescent red cells continues to be diverted to stores rather than reutilized in new red cell production. Therefore, although EPO and iron can eliminate the need for red cell transfusions, the effect of EPO and iron on the patient's distribution of iron is the same as that of red cell transfusions: more and more iron accumulates in the storage pool. The situation is different in patients with severe renal disease, who are chronically losing iron by intermittent bleeding or dialysis and do not become iron overloaded.

REFERENCES

1. Looker AC, Dallman PR, Carroll MD, et al. Prevalence of iron deficiency in the United States. *JAMA* 1997;277:973–976.
2. Ania BJ, Suman VJ, Fairbanks VF, et al. Incidence of anemia in older people: an epidemiologic study in a well defined population. *J Am Geriatr Soc* 1997;45:825–831.
3. Bothwell TH, Baynes RD, MacFarlane BJ, et al. Nutritional iron requirements and food iron absorption. *J Intern Med* 1989;226:357–365.
4. Hillman RS, Henderson PA. Control of marrow production by the level of iron supply. *J Clin Invest* 1969;48:454–460.
5. Cazzola M, Guarnone R, Cerani P, et al. Red blood cell precursor mass as an independent determinant of serum erythropoietin level. *Blood* 1998;91:2139–2145.
6. Lipschitz DA, Cook JD, Finch CA. A clinical evaluation of serum ferritin as an index of iron stores. *N Engl J Med* 1974;290:1212–1216.
7. Punnonen K, Irjala K, Rajamaki A. Serum transferrin receptor and its ratio to serum ferritin in the diagnosis of iron deficiency. *Blood* 1997;89:1052–1057.
8. Bainton DF, Finch CA. The diagnosis of iron deficiency anemia. *Am J Med* 1964;37:62–70.
9. Cash JM, Sears DA. The anemia of chronic disease: spectrum of associated diseases in a series of unselected hospitalized patients. *Am J Med* 1989;87:638–644.
10. Spivak JL. Iron and the anemia of chronic disease. *Oncology* 2002;16 (Suppl 10):25–39.
11. Michael B, Coyne DW, Fishbane S, et al. Sodium ferric gluconate complex in hemodialysis patients: adverse reactions compared to placebo and iron dextran. *Kidney Int* 2002;61:1830–1839.
12. NKF-DOQI Clinical practice guidelines for the treatment of anemia of chronic renal failure. *Am J Kidney Dis* 1997;30 (Suppl 3): S194–S195.
13. Gabrilove JL, Cleeland CS, Livingston RB, et al. Clinical evaluation of once-weekly dosing of epoetin alfa in chemotherapy patients: improvements in hemoglobin and quality of life are similar to three-times-weekly dosing. *J Clin Oncol* 2001;19:2875–2882.
14. Rizzo JD, Lichtin AE, Woolf SH, et al. Use of epoetin in patients with cancer: evidence-based clinical practice guidelines of the American Society of Clinical Oncology and the American Society of Hematology. *Blood* 2002;100:2303–2320.
15. Cazzola M, Mercuriali F, Brugnara C. Use of recombinant human erythropoietin outside the setting of uremia. *Blood* 1997;89:4248–4267.
16. Glaspy J, Tchekmedyian NS. Darbepoietin alfa administered every 2 weeks alleviates anemia in cancer patients receiving chemotherapy. *Oncology* 2002;16(Suppl 11):23–29.
17. Bentley DP, Williams P. Parenteral iron therapy in the anaemia of rheumatoid arthritis. *Rheumatol Rehabil* 1982;21:88–92.
18. Pincus T, Olsen NJ, Russell IJ, et al. Multicenter study of recombinant human erythropoietin in correction of anemia in rheumatoid arthritis. *Am J Med* 1990;89:161–168.
19. Schreiber S, Howaldt S, Schnoor M, et al. Recombinant erythropoietin for the treatment of anemia in inflammatory bowel disease. *N Engl J Med* 1996;334:619–623.
20. Kaltwaser JP, Kessler U, Gottschalk R, et al. Effect of recombinant human erythropoietin and intravenous iron on anemia and disease activity in rheumatoid arthritis. *J Rhematol* 2001;28:2430–2436.
21. Aranesp (darbepoietin alfa) [package insert]. Thousand Oaks, CA: Amgen, Inc., 2003.

2

Nutritional Deficiencies

McDonald K. Horne, III

Excluding extreme protein–calorie deprivation, nutritional causes of anemia are essentially limited to deficiencies of iron, folic acid, and vitamin B_{12}. Iron deficiency has been discussed in the previous chapter, and deficiencies of folic acid and vitamin B_{12} are discussed here. Both of these vitamins have different names that connote structural differences; we use "vitamin B_{12}" and "cobalamin" and "folic acid" and "folate" interchangeably and avoid more complex terminology.

VITAMIN REQUIREMENTS, SOURCES, STORES

The daily adult requirement for vitamin B_{12} is 1 to 3 μg and for folic acid approximately 200 μg (Table 2-1) (1).

Bacteria in the guts of herbivorous animals synthesize vitamin B_{12} and supply it to their hosts, who in turn provide it to humans in the form of meat. There is no vitamin B_{12} in plant products other than that attributable to bacterial contamination. Plants synthesize folic acid and provide it to humans directly in fruits and vegetables and indirectly in meat from herbivores.

The human body normally stores a 2- to 3-month supply of folic acid, although marginally nourished patients, such as chronic alcoholics, may have much smaller stores that can be depleted much sooner (2). In contrast, body stores of vitamin B_{12} are normally sufficient for 5 to 10 years (Table 2-1). Therefore, many years of malabsorption are required before cobalamin becomes depleted.

METABOLIC ROLES OF FOLATE AND VITAMIN B_{12}

The metabolic roles of folate and B_{12} are closely interrelated (Fig. 2-1). Folate derivatives are essential cofactors in thymidylate synthesis, which is a rate-limiting step in the synthesis of DNA. RNA synthesis is not dependent on folate. Therefore, deficiency of folate limits gene transcription but not RNA translation, retarding cell division but not cytoplasmic protein synthesis and *leading to the typical cytonuclear dissociation of maturation characteristic of megaloblastic hematopoiesis.* Because cobalamin supports the recycling of folate, vitamin B_{12} deficiency causes megaloblastic changes by restricting the folate supply. This restriction can at least be partially overcome by increasing dietary folate, *allowing the hematopoietic effects of cobalamin deficiency to be ameliorated by high doses of folic acid.* In contrast, the hematopoietic effects of folate deficiency cannot be overcome by treatment with vitamin B_{12}.

Cobalamin is also necessary in the pathway leading to the synthesis of S-adenosyl-methionine, which is the only donor of methyl groups for numerous reactions in the brain involving proteins, membrane phospholipids, and neurotransmitters (3). Presumably this function explains the frequent neuropsychiatric signs and symptoms associated with vitamin B_{12} deficiency (4). Folate is not involved in these reactions and cannot reverse the neuropsychiatric deficits caused by vitamin B_{12} deficiency. However, methyl-tetrahydrofolic acid is the methyl donor for the synthesis of methionine, the precursor of S-adenosyl-methionine. Therefore,

11

TABLE 2–1. *Vitamin B_{12} and folic acid: biology and dosing*

	Vitamin B_{12}	Folic acid
Source	Bacteria → Meat	Plants → Meat
Daily requirement	1–3 μg	~ 200 μg
Body store	2–5 mg	~ 20 mg
Time to deficiency	5–10 years	2–3 months
Oral dosing	1–2 mg/day	1 mg/day
Cost of dose	5–10 cents/day*	5–10 cents/day*

*Average wholesale price (2003 Drug Topics Redbook).

folate deficiency may restrict the synthesis of S-adenosyl-methionine and produce some neuropsychiatric effects as well (5).

DEVELOPMENT OF VITAMIN B_{12} DEFICIENCY: COBALAMIN MALABSORPTION

Cobalamin deficiency is rarely caused by inadequate intake or increased utilization of the vitamin (Table 2-2). Although strict vegetarians become depleted of vitamin B_{12}, vegetables

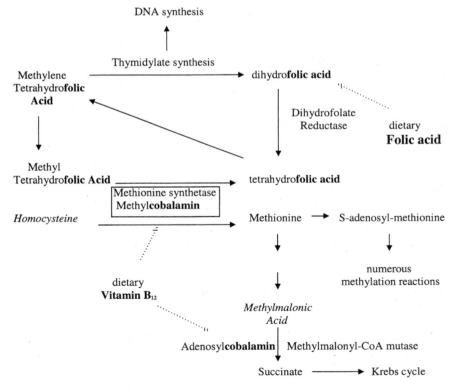

FIG. 2-1. Metabolic pathways involving folic acid and vitamin B_{12} (cobalamin).

TABLE 2–2. *Causes of vitamin B_{12} deficiency*

Gastrointestinal	Gastric atrophy: achlorhydria; achlorhydria + intrinsic factor deficiency
	Gastrectomy
	Terminal ileal resection
	Extensive celiac disease
	Crohn's disease of the stomach
	Bacterial overgrowth in the small bowel (achlorhydria, anatomical defects, impaired motility)
	Zollinger-Ellison syndrome
	Pancreatic insufficiency
	Human immunodeficiency virus
Medications	Megadoses of vitamin C, metformin, proton pump inhibitors
Increased utilization	Pregnancy
Toxin	Nitrous oxide
Dietary	Strict vegetarianism

often contain sufficient bacteria to provide a marginally adequate supply. A developing fetus shunts cobalamin from its mother, placing her at risk of deficiency, particularly if her baseline stores are low.

Defects in any of three levels of the gastrointestinal tract can lead to vitamin B_{12} malabsorption: the fundus of the stomach, the pancreas, or the small bowel. Obviously surgical removal or bypass of any of these regions leads to B_{12} malabsorption. Otherwise the etiology is inflammatory.

- *Stomach*: In the stomach, food (protein)-bound vitamin B_{12} must be freed by digestion with pepsin and bound to R-proteins, which is a generic term for proteins that bind B_{12} (1). The parietal cells in the fundus secrete both the acid necessary for this digestion and intrinsic factor, the protein to which cobalamin is later transferred in the alkaline duodenum. Therefore, any process that damages parietal cells can lead to vitamin B_{12} malabsorption and eventually its deficiency. The most common cause of B_{12} malabsorption is autoimmune atrophic gastritis, which increases in prevalence with age and may be associated with other autoimmune diseases, such as thyroiditis. *Helicobacter pylori,* which typically causes antral gastritis, can occasionally also infect the fundus (6). Proton pump inhibitors induce chronic hypochlorhydria but rarely cause clinically significant B_{12} malabsorption. Paradoxically, the hypersecretion of acid in the Zollinger-Ellison syndrome leads to B_{12} malabsorption by acidifying the small bowel, which must remain alkaline for the transfer of B_{12} from the R-binders to intrinsic factor.
- *Pancreas*: Deficiency of pancreatic enzymes retards the digestion of R-binders in the small bowel and therefore the release of B_{12} to intrinsic factor. Although pancreatic insufficiency causes cobalamin malabsorption, it rarely is significant enough to become clinically apparent.
- *Small bowel*: Vitamin B_{12}-intrinsic factor complexes undergo endocytosis by the mucosa of the terminal ileum. Inflammatory bowel disease or particularly extensive celiac or tropical sprue will interfere with this process (7). Bacterial overgrowth in the small bowel, especially common in the elderly, competes for B_{12} and makes it less available for absorption (8). Human immunodeficiency virus (HIV) is also sometimes associated with B_{12} malabsorption.

DEVELOPMENT OF FOLIC ACID DEFICIENCY

A diet poor in fresh vegetables is a major cause of folic acid deficiency (Table 2-3). Cooked vegetables and meat are less satisfactory sources because heating destroys much of the folate

TABLE 2–3. *Causes of folic acid deficiency*

Diet	Lack of fresh vegetables
Gastrointestinal disease	Celiac disease (gluten-sensitive enteropathy)
	Dermatitis herpetiformis
	Tropical sprue
	Small bowel resection
	Crohn's disease
	Enterohepatic diversion
Medications	Cytotoxic agents: methotrexate
	Antibiotics: pyrimethamine, cycloserine, trimethoprim
	Diuretics: triamterene
	Anticonvulsants: phenytoin, carbamazepine, phenobarbital, primidone
	Oral contraceptives
Ethanol	
Increased utilization/loss	Pregnancy
	Chronic hemolysis
	Exfoliative dermatitis
	Chronic hemodialysis

(less of a problem for vitamin B_{12}). Two other major causes are gastrointestinal diseases that affect the jejunum, where folic acid is absorbed, and conditions such as pregnancy, which increase folate consumption. Ethanol abuse and long-term use of certain medications lead to folate deficiency by interrupting folate metabolism or inhibiting its absorption.

PATIENT POPULATIONS AT RISK

- Vitamin B_{12} deficiency resulting from lack of intrinsic factor (pernicious anemia) is sometimes believed to be limited to elderly patients of European descent. In this population the median age at presentation is almost 70 years.
- Nevertheless, intrinsic factor deficiency may be almost as prevalent in African Americans and Latinos, who tend to present with vitamin B_{12} deficiency a decade earlier (9,10).
- Older patients are actually more likely to become B_{12} deficient from achlorhydria or small bowel bacteria overgrowth than because of lack of intrinsic factor (11).

Whereas cobalamin deficiency is generally found in older age groups, folic acid deficiency is likely to occur in any patient who has an inadequate diet or who has an increased need for the vitamin (Table 2-3).

CLINICAL PRESENTATION

The clinical presentation of vitamin B_{12} and folic acid deficiency covers a wide range of symptoms and signs (Table 2-4). The investigation of any new neuropsychiatric changes should include an evaluation of folate and vitamin B_{12} status, even in the absence of hematologic evidence of a deficiency (4).

LABORATORY EVALUATION

Hematologic Abnormalities

Macrocytosis develops before anemia when either folic acid or vitamin B_{12} is limiting (Table 2-5) (2, 12). With the advent of automated blood cell analyzers, isolated macrocytosis has become a typical presentation of deficiencies of either vitamin, although other causes of

TABLE 2–4. *Clinical and laboratory presentations of vitamin B_{12} or folic acid deficiency*

Hematologic
    Macrocytosis: Anemia, usually macrocytic but normocytic or microcytic if accompanied by iron deficiency or thalassemia
    Pancytopenia
Neuropsychiatric
    Peripheral neuropathy (paresthesias, hyporeflexia)
    Spinal cord degeneration (weakness, hyperreflexia, reduced vibratory and position sense)
    Memory loss, disorientation, depression
Gastrointestinal
    Malabsorption (weight loss, diarrhea, abdominal pain), glossitis
Reproductive
    Infertility, fetal loss

macrocytosis are more common (Table 2-6) (13). An unexplained rise in mean cell volume (MCV) of 5 fL or more, even within the normal range, should also attract suspicion. However, macrocytosis may be masked if the patient is also iron deficient or has a thalassemic trait. At hemoglobin concentrations below approximately 10 g/dL, serum lactate dehydrogenase (LDH) is usually elevated and can be quite high (2,12). LDH increases result from marked intramedullary death of developing red cells and a shortening of the circulating red cell life span and can mislead the clinician to suspect metastatic disease or a primary hemolytic anemia.

The earliest change in the peripheral blood caused by folate or vitamin B_{12} deficiency is hypersegmentation of the neutrophils, which can be easily overlooked unless a blood smear is carefully examined. Finding just 5% of neutrophils with five lobes or 1% with six lobes is highly suggestive of a deficiency (hypersegmentation can also be seen in myelodysplasia). In advanced deficiencies pancytopenia can develop.

There is rarely, if ever, a need to perform a bone marrow examination to evaluate vitamin

TABLE 2–5. *Progression of laboratory parameters*

	Normal	Negative balance	Depleted stores	Tissue deficiency	Anemia
		Folic acid deficiency			
Serum folic acid	5–20 (ng/mL)	<3	<3	<3	<3
RBC folic acid (ng/mL)	>200	>200	<200	<200	<200
Serum Hcy (μmol/L)	5–15	5–15	5–15	15–250	15–250
Hypersegmented neutrophils	0	0	0	+	++
MCV (fL)	80–95	80–95	80–95	90–110	100–130
Hemoglobin (g/dL)	12–15	12–15	12–15	12–15	<12
		Vitamin B12 Deficiency			
Serum cobalamin (pg/mL)	200–900	150–500	100–300	50–250	50–250
Serum MMA (μmol/L)	<0.4	<0.4	<0.4	0.4–20	1–20
Hypersegmented Neutrophils	0	0	0	+	++
MCV (fL)	80–95	80–95	80–95	90–110	100–130
Hemoglobin (g/dL)	12–15	12–15	12–15	12–15	<12

RBC, red blood cell; Hcy, homocysteine; MCV, mean cell volume; MMA, methylmalonic acid.

TABLE 2–6. *Causes of macrocytosis with or without anemia*

	Macrocytosis alone	Macrocytic anemia
Medications		
Cytotoxic chemotherapy (methotrexate, hydroxyurea cytosine arabinoside, azathioprine, others)	+	+
Anticonvulsants (phenytoin, carbamazepine primadone)	+	+
Antiretrovirals	+	+
Liver disease	+	+
Alcoholism with or without liver disease	+	+
Reticulocytosis	0	+
Folate deficiency	+	+
Vitamin B_{12} deficiency	+	+
Myelodysplasia	+	+
Hypothyroidism	+	+
>75 years old	+	+
Down's syndrome	+	0
Artifact (RBC agglutination)	+	0

RBC: red blood cell.

B_{12} and folic acid status. Megaloblastic changes in the marrow are identical in both deficiencies and are variable in intensity. A marrow examination cannot eliminate the diagnosis of myelodysplasia or even a smoldering leukemic process until cobalamin and folate deficiencies have first been excluded.

Vitamin Levels

A common starting point when vitamin B_{12} and folate deficiency is suspected is to measure the serum concentrations of the vitamins, with blood samples performed in the fasting state. The results, however, can be difficult to interpret (Table 2-7).

Serum folic acid does not reliably reflect the body's supply of the vitamin, unless it is consistently below approximately 3 ng/mL, and even at low levels does not distinguish between negative balance and actual tissue deficiency (14). Because *red cell folate* is packaged

TABLE 2–7. *Laboratory tests in folic acid and vitamin B_{12} deficiency*

	Folic Acid	Vitamin B_{12}
Serum folic acid	↓ →	→ ↑
Red cell folic acid	↓ →	→ ↓
Serum vitamin B_{12}	→ ↓	↓ →
Methylmalonic acid	→	↑
Homocysteine	↑	↑
Lactate dehydrogenase	↑	↑
Haptoglobin	→ ↓	→ ↓

at the time the cell is made and remains in the cell throughout its 3- to 4-month lifespan, the measured mean value may fail to indicate relatively recent reductions in dietary folate. Furthermore, the reproducibility of assays for red cell folate is relatively poor, so that border-line values can be misleading (14). To complicate matters further, red cell folate can be reduced by vitamin B_{12} deficiency and lead to an erroneous diagnosis (Table 2-7).

Interpreting *serum vitamin B_{12}* levels can also be problematic because serum B_{12} can actually be decreased in cases of folate deficiency (1). A more frequent problem, like that with folic acid, relates to uncertain physiologic levels of the vitamin. The normal range of serum cobalamin typically extends down to 200 pg/mL, because healthy, nonanemic donors occasionally have B_{12} concentrations this low. However, patients who are truly deficient in vitamin B_{12} can have serum cobalamin levels as high as or exceeding 300 pg/mL (14). The reason for this discrepancy is that the total cobalamin is measured, rather than just the vitamin B_{12} bound to transcobalamin, which is the metabolically available B_{12} but represents only approximately 20% of the total serum vitamin. Therefore, individuals who have relatively low concentrations of haptocorrin, which binds the other approximately 80% of the serum vitamin B_{12}, can have alarmingly low B_{12} levels (less than 100 pg/mL) without any harmful effect because they have adequate amounts of B_{12} bound to transcobalamin. Occasional com-pletely healthy patients have low haptocorrin levels, which unfortunately cannot be easily quantitated (15). Low haptocorrin levels also occur in patients with multiple myeloma (16).

Serum Methylmalonic Acid and Homocysteine

Measurements of methylmalonic acid (MMA) and homocysteine (Hcy), although they are more expensive than the vitamin assays, address vitamin deficiency more reliably. Although these metabolites can be elevated for other reasons (Table 2-8) (10,18), once these causes are excluded, the metabolites become highly specific reflections of vitamin B_{12} and folate depletion at the tissue level. Usually MMA and Hcy both become elevated when B_{12} is limiting, whereas only Hcy rises with folate deficiency. Normal levels of MMA and Hcy virtually exclude the possibility that B_{12} deficiency is affecting metabolism (10) (exceptions are rare and unexplained).

In 1% to 2% of cases of vitamin B_{12} deficiency only Hcy will be elevated, whereas this is true in approximately 90% of cases of folate deficiency. Therefore, elevated Hcy alone does not always differentiate B_{12} and folate deficiency but makes folate deficiency far more likely.

Therapeutic Trial

If the laboratory evaluation is impossible because resources are lacking or is inconclusive, a therapeutic trial can be diagnostic if a single vitamin is administered at a time. Vitamin

TABLE 2–8. *Causes of elevated methylmalonic acid and homocysteine*

	Methylmalonic Acid	Homocysteine
Vitamin deficiencies	Vitamin B_{12} deficiency	Folic acid deficiency
		Vitamin B_{12} deficiency
		Vitamine B6 (pyridoxine) deficiency
Genetic traits		Homozygous thermolabile tetrahydrofolate reductase
Renal disease	Renal insufficiency	Renal insufficiency
Endocrine	Pregnancy	Hypothyroidism
Drugs		Niacin, L-dopa
Metabolic	Volume contraction	Volume contraction

B_{12} should be prescribed first because it will do nothing for folic acid deficiency, whereas replacement with folic acid will improve the anemia secondary to B_{12} deficiency but not the neuropathic changes. The response to treatment can be judged by following the reticulocyte count and hemoglobin (see below). More expensive is measurement of Hcy or MMA levels 2 to 5 days after one or the other of the vitamins has been administered. The metabolites will fall only in response to replacement of the deficient vitamin (18).

DETERMINING THE CAUSE OF B_{12} OR FOLATE DEFICIENCY

- The *etiology of folate deficiency* must always be determined because virtually all causes are either preventable or treatable. If the diet is adequate, a gastrointestinal evaluation is indicated to search for the underlying causes (Table 2-3).
- In contrast, *if vitamin B_{12} is deficient* and the patient is not a vegan and there are no symptoms of gastrointestinal disease, an argument can be made to make no further evaluation and simply to treat with the vitamin.

If the patient and/or his physician feel compelled to confirm that the pathology lies in the stomach, a test for anti-intrinsic factor antibodies should be done (19). A positive test is diagnostic of pernicious anemia and is present in half the cases. Antiparietal cell antibodies are more common but are also found in a small percentage of normal individuals. Demonstrating an elevation in serum gastrin also strongly supports the diagnosis of gastric atrophy (20).

If the patient is unusually young to have achlorhydria or pernicious anemia (younger than 50 years old or younger if African American), a gastrointestinal evaluation is indicated (Table 2-2) (9). In the past, the Schilling test was used in an attempt to detect vitamin B_{12} malabsorption, but these tests are no longer performed because of lack of a commercial source for radiolabeled cobalamin and the realization that this test also often gives misleading results. The incidence of many malignancies, especially gastric cancer, is slightly higher in patients with pernicious anemia than in age- and gender-matched controls, and patients should be monitored for any signs of gastrointestinal blood loss, although more aggressive surveillance is not indicated (21).

TREATMENT/RESPONSE

There are two treatment goals:

- Replacement of the deficient vitamin and
- Correction of the cause of the deficiency.

The first goal is always achievable; the second may not be.

Vitamin B_{12} and folic acid can be given orally or parenterally. Diarrhea or other evidence of active malabsorption makes the parenteral route necessary. If the cause of the deficiency is dietary or gastric atrophy, oral replacement is sufficient.

In the past, in the United States vitamin B_{12} was always given intramuscularly, although the oral route was used in Europe. Recently, the effectiveness of oral B_{12} was demonstrated in a randomized, controlled clinical trial in this country, and now the oral route is preferred (22). Administration by mouth is reliable even in patients with pernicious anemia because approximately 1% of any oral dose of vitamin B_{12} is absorbed by simple diffusion across the mucosa. The recommended dose of 1 to 2 mg of vitamin B_{12} results in the absorption of approximately 10 to 20 μg, which is much more than the daily requirement. For most patients with vitamin B_{12} deficiency, lifelong treatment is required because the underlying cause is not reversible.

The usual dose of oral folic acid is 1 mg per day (Table 2-1), ample even during pregnancy or chronic hemolysis. If the deficiency is nutritional, replacement with folic acid should continue until the diet has become adequate. A month of daily folic acid should be sufficient to replenish body stores. If the etiology of the deficiency is small bowel dysfunction, higher doses for longer periods of time may be necessary.

The response to correction of vitamin B_{12} or folate deficiency is the same:

- Mental changes and tongue soreness improve almost immediately after starting to replace the deficient vitamin (1).
- After 4 to 5 days reticulocytosis appears and may elevate the MCV even further.
- Soon thereafter the hemoglobin concentration begins to rise.
- Neuropathic abnormalities, such as paresthesias, improve slowly over several months but may never disappear entirely if they have been long-standing.

If the hematologic response is blunted, additional etiologies for the anemia should be sought. It is not unusual for iron deficiency to accompany folate or vitamin B_{12} deficiency. An underlying anemia of chronic disease is always a possibility.

REFERENCES

1. Chanarin I. *The Megaloblastic Anaemias.* 3rd ed. Oxford: Blackwell Scientific, 1990.
2. Lindenbaum J, Allen RH. Clinical spectrum and diagnosis of folate deficiency. In: *Folate in Health and Disease.* New York: Marcel Dekker, 1995:43–74.
3. Reynolds EH, Carney MWP, Toone BK. Methylation and mood. *Lancet* 1984;2:196–198.
4. Lindenbaum J, Healton EB, Savage DG, et al. Neuropsychiatric disorders caused by cobalamin deficiency in the absence of anemia or macrocytosis. *N Engl J Med* 1988;318:1720–1728.
5. Shorvon SD, Carney MWP, Chanarin I, et al. The neuropsychiatry of megaloblastic anaemia. *Br Med J* 1980;281:1036–1038.
6. Kaptan K, Beyan C, Ural AU, et al. Helicobacter pylori—is it a novel causative agent in vitamin B12 deficiency? *Arch Intern Med* 2000;160:1349–1353.
7. Dahele A, Ghosh S. Vitamin B12 deficiency in untreated celiac disease. *Am J Gastroenterol* 2001; 96:745–750.
8. Haboubi NY, Montgomery RD. Small-bowel bacterial overgrowth in elderly people: clinical significance and response to treatment. *Age Aging* 1992;21:13–19.
9. Carmel R, Johnson CS. Racial patterns in pernicious anemia. *N Engl J Med* 1978;298:647–650.
10. Savage DG, Lindenbaum J, Stabler SP, et al. Sensitivity of serum methylmalonic acid and total homocysteine determinations for diagnosing cobalamin and folate deficiencies. *Am J Med* 1994;96: 239–246.
11. Dharmarajan TS, Adiga GU, Norkus EP. Vitamin B12 deficiency, recognizing subtle symptoms in older patients. *Geriatrics* 2003;58:30–38.
12. Stabler SP, Allen RH, Savage DG, et al. Clinical spectrum and diagnosis of cobalamin deficiency. *Blood* 1990;76:871–881.
13. Savage DG, Ogundipe A, Allen RH, et al. Etiology and diagnostic evaluation of macrocytosis. *Am J Med Sci* 2000;319:343–352.
14. Klee GG. Cobalamin and folate evaluation: measurement of methylmalonic acid and homocysteine vs vitamin B12 and folate. *Clin Chem* 2000;46:1277–1283.
15. Carmel R. A new case of deficiency of the R binder for cobalamin, with observations on minor cobalamin-binding proteins in serum and saliva. *Blood* 1982;59:152–156.
16. Hansen OP, Drivsholm A, Hippe E. Vitamin B12 metabolism in myelomatosis. *Scand J Haematol* 1977;18:395–402.
17. Allen RH, Stabler SP, Savage DG, et al. Diagnosis of cobalamin deficiency I: usefulness of serum methylmalonic acid and total homocysteine concentrations. *Am J Hematol* 1990;34:90–98.
18. Lindenbaum J, Savage DG, Stabler SP, et al. Diagnosis of cobalamin deficiency II: relative sensitivities of serum cobalamin, methylmalonic acid, and total homocysteine concentrations. *Am J Hematol* 1990;34:99–107.
19. Fairbanks VF, Lennon VA, Kokmen E, et al. Tests for pernicious anemia: serum intrinsic factor blocking antibody. *Mayo Clin Proc* 1983;58:203–204.
20. Lindgren A, Lindstedt G, Kilander AF. Advantages of serum pepsinogen A combined with gastrin

or pepsinogen C as first-line analytes in the evaluation of suspected cobalamin deficiency: a study in patients previously not subjected to gastrointestinal surgery. *J Intern Med* 1998;244:341–349.

21. Schafer LW, Larson DE, Melton LJ, et al. Risk of development of gastric carcinoma in patients with pernicious anemia: a population-based study in Rochester, Minnesota. *Mayo Clin Proc* 1985;60: 444–448.

22. Kuzminski AM, Giacco EJD, Allen RH, et al. Effective treatment of cobalamin deficiency with oral cobalamin. *Blood* 1998;92:1191–1198.

3

Hemolytic Anemia: General Overview with Special Consideration of Membrane and Enzyme Defects

Patricia A. Oneal, Geraldine P. Schechter, Griffin P. Rodgers, and Jeffery L. Miller

Hemolytic anemia is defined as decreased levels of erythrocytes in circulating blood (anemia) because of their accelerated destruction (hemolysis). All circulating erythrocytes are subject to physiologic stresses such as turbulence in blood flow, endothelial damage, and age-related catabolic changes. Normally, damaged red blood cells (RBC) are removed from the circulation by the reticuloendothelial system. In hemolytic syndromes, erythrocyte clearance by the reticuloendothelial system may be increased (extravascular hemolysis) or the cells may be lysed within the circulation (intravascular hemolysis). As a result, RBC survival is generally shortened to less than 100 days (normal is approximately 120 days). When sufficient numbers of erythrocytes are destroyed, oxygen delivery to tissues is impaired. Tissue hypoxia leads to increased release of erythropoietin, which signals the bone marrow to produce more red blood cells.

A hallmark of hemolytic anemia is an elevated number of immature erythrocytes (reticulocytes) in the peripheral blood. In low-level hemolysis, erythrocyte production may adequately compensate for blood cell destruction and minimize the anemia. Alternatively, patients with hemolysis and underlying defects in hematopoiesis may present with pronounced anemia without reticulocytosis. Hence, the evaluation of suspected hemolysis requires consideration of the hemolysis itself as well as the marrow's ability to compensate.

Dozens of genetic and acquired diseases manifest clinically as hemolytic anemia. Hemoglobinopathies and immune-mediated hemolysis are the most common; many of the other etiologies are quite rare. Of note, the precise cause for hemolysis in unusual hemolytic states often cannot be identified by standard clinical evaluation (1). Therefore, the diagnostic strategy usually begins with a search for common causes of hemolysis and proceeds toward rare etiologies. The extent of diagnostic studies should be guided by the magnitude of hemolysis and the available therapeutic options. With the information contained here, practicing clinicians should be able to develop a differential diagnosis, a clinical approach, and a therapeutic plan for patients with suspected hemolysis.

ETIOLOGY AND DIFFERENTIAL DIAGNOSIS

Grouping the various causes of the disease generates a differential diagnosis for hemolysis. As shown in Figure 3-1, hemolysis results from pathology intrinsic or extrinsic to the erythrocytes. Intrinsic hemolysis may then be categorized further according to hemoglobin, membrane, or enzyme-based factors. Alternatively, the patient's immune status or infectious agents can lead to hemolysis in the absence of intrinsic defects. Other chemical or physical features of the erythrocyte environment also cause hemolysis. A more complete differential that is organized according to these categories is shown in Table 3-1.

21

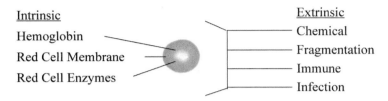

FIG. 3-1. Intrinsic and extrinsic causes of hemolysis.

TABLE 3–1. *Differential diagnosis of hemolytic anemia*

Intrinsic Causes of Hemolysis	Lecithin:cholesterol acyltransferase
Hemoglobin (see Chapter 4):	Phosphofructokinase
Hb SS	Phosphoglycerokinase
Thalassemias	Triose phosphate isomerase
Other hemoglobinopathies	*Extrinsic Causes of Hemolysis*
Heinz body hemolytic anemia	*Immune:*
Unstable hemoglobins	*Transfusion-based immunity*
Membrane:	*Hemolytic anemia of the newborn*
Hereditary spherocytosis	*Autoimmune syndromes*
Hereditary elliptocytosis	*Fragmentation/Physical Damage:*
Hereditary stomatocytosis	*Heart valves (mechanical and infected)*
Hereditary acanthocytosis	*Disseminated intravascular coagulapathy*
Hereditary pyropoikilocytosis	*Thrombotic thrombocytopenic purpura*
Hereditary xerocytosis	*Hemolytic uremic syndrome*
McLeod syndrome	*Hemodialysis*
*PNH	*Malignancy (metastatic disease)
Abnormal: Ankyrin	*Burns
Band 3	*Drowning
Band 4.1	*Marathon/March hemoglobinuria
Band 4.2	*Vasculitis
Band 4.5	*Malignant hypertension
Glycophorin C (Leach phenotype)	*Arteriovenous malformation
Spectrin	*Infections:*
Stomatin	*Malaria*
Enzymes:	*Babesiosis
Glucose-6-phosphate dehydrogenase	*Bartonellosis (Oroya fever)
Pyruvate kinase	*Clostridium perfringens
Glucose phosphate isomerase	*Chemical:*
Pyrimidine 5′ nucleotidase	*Oxidants in presence of glucose-6-
Adenosine deaminase	phosphate dehydrogenase deficiency
Aldolase	*Insect and snake venom
2,3 diphosphoglycerate mutase	Lead
Enolase	Chlorine (in hemodialysate fluid)
γ-glutamyl cysteine synthetase	Chloramine (in hemodialysate fluid)
Glutathione peroxidase	Arsine gas
Glutathione reductase	*Other Causes:*
Glutathione synthetase	*Liver disease*
Heme oxygenase-1	*Hypersplenism*
Hexokinase	

The more common causes are shown in italics, and the asterisks denote an association with intravascular hemolysis (3–6).

Most intrinsic causes for hemolysis are inherited, while the extrinsic causes of hemolysis are typically acquired. In some cases, such as paroxysmal nocturnal hemoglobinuria (PNH) or glucose-6-phosphate dehydrogenase (G6PD) deficiency, both intrinsic and extrinsic factors may contribute to the hemolytic picture. Consideration of the primary site of hemolysis (intravascular versus extravascular) may also be helpful in determining the origin of erythrocyte destruction (2).

To complete the differential diagnosis, diseases or events that may in part mimic a typical hemolytic episode should be considered. The laboratory evaluation may be normal with the exception of a single variable such as hemoglobin, absolute reticulocyte count, or unconjugated bilirubin. For instance, the compensatory reticulocytosis that occurs after an acute hemorrhagic event may be mistaken for evidence of hemolysis. In the absence of other clinical or laboratory abnormalities, artifactual reticulocytosis may be caused by a malfunction in the automated cell counter. While hypersplenism may be associated with increased red cell clearance and anemia, the abnormal red blood cell morphology seen in patients with asplenia is usually not associated with hemolysis. Finally, patients with chronic idiopathic unconjugated hyperbilirubinemia (Gilbert's disease) are not infrequently referred to a hematologist to rule out hemolysis (7).

CLINICAL APPROACH TO PATIENTS WITH SUSPECTED HEMOLYSIS

As with most diseases, the approach to hemolysis involves a combination of bedside and laboratory investigations directed by the judgment and skills of the clinician (Fig. 3-2).

Low-level or chronic hemolysis should be suspected in all patients with unexplained anemia. A detailed history and physical examination should be the cornerstone of each patient's evaluation.

History

Onset/duration (hereditary versus acquired)
History of fatigue
History of jaundice
Abdominal pain/cholelithiasis (chronic hemolysis)
Medications (may exacerbate enzyme deficiencies)
Travel (consider infection)
Infection
Vascular/cardiac surgery
Blood loss or sequestration (increases reticulocytes in the absence of hemolysis)
Discolored urine (intravascular hemolysis)
Complete family history (jaundice, gallbladder disease, splenectomy, hereditary anemia, or
   other inherited diseases)

Physical

Pallor
Increased temperature
Rapid pulse
Jaundice (chronic hemolysis)
Mechanical click from heart valves
Splenomegly

The laboratory evaluation is performed to confirm the suspected diagnosis, provide insight regarding the underlying mechanism, and gauge a therapeutic response. The complete blood count (CBC) usually confirms the diagnosis of anemia. Reticulocytosis increases the mean

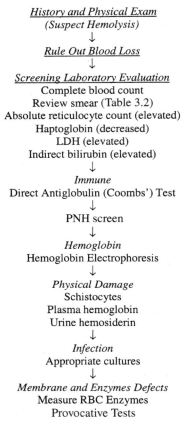

History and Physical Exam
(Suspect Hemolysis)
↓
Rule Out Blood Loss
↓
Screening Laboratory Evaluation
Complete blood count
Review smear (Table 3.2)
Absolute reticulocyte count (elevated)
Haptoglobin (decreased)
LDH (elevated)
Indirect bilirubin (elevated)
↓
Immune
Direct Antiglobulin (Coombs') Test
↓
PNH screen
↓
Hemoglobin
Hemoglobin Electrophoresis
↓
Physical Damage
Schistocytes
Plasma hemoglobin
Urine hemosiderin
↓
Infection
Appropriate cultures
↓
Membrane and Enzymes Defects
Measure RBC Enzymes
Provocative Tests

FIG. 3-2. A clinical approach to hemolytic anemia. LDH, lactate dehydrogenase; PNH, paroxysmal nocturnal hemoglubinura; RBC, red blood cell.

cell volume (MCV) and red cell distribution width (RDW). A critical test in the evaluation of all patients with suspected hemolysis is the reticulocyte count. An increased number of reticulocytes are present in hemolysis unless erythropoiesis is suppressed. Stressed erythropoiesis associated with hemolysis also causes the release of large polychromatic reticulocytes with a decreased area of central pallor into the circulation, called shift cells. They are easily identified on the peripheral smear (8). Reticulocytes are also identified in the laboratory by their RNA content. Reticulocytes comprise 0.5% to 1.5% of circulating erythrocytes in the absence of anemia, consistent with the normal turnover of 1% of normal red cell mass per day. Increased percentages are usually present in the setting of hemolysis. The uncorrected reticulocyte percentage may reflect increased erythropoiesis, prolonged survival of stress reticulocytes, and the lower total number of circulating RBC in the setting of anemia. Therefore, an absolute reticulocyte count more accurately measures the compensatory response than does the uncorrected reticulocyte percentage.

absolute reticulocyte count (ARC) = reticulocyte percentage/100 $\times$ erythrocyte count/mm^3 [1]

- Normal ARC 25,000–75,000/mm^3
- ARC >100,000/mm^3 after hemolysis (8a)

While a bone marrow examination is generally not required to determine the etiology of uncomplicated hemolysis, the peripheral blood smear should never be overlooked. This simple test is rapid, inexpensive, and may provide important clues regarding the mechanism of hemolysis (Table 3.2).

ACUTE INTRAVASCULAR HEMOLYSIS

The clinical syndrome associated with acute intravascular hemolysis deserves special attention. Its recognition may lead to rapid institution of specific therapies and prevent acute

TABLE 3.2 *Erythrocyte morphologies and associated pathology.*

Cell type	Intrinsic	Extrinsic
Acanthocyte	Glutathione peroxidase deficiency Hereditary choreo-acanthocytosis Abetalipoproteinemia McLeod syndrome LCAT deficiency	Liver disease Asplenia
Basophilic stippling	Hemoglobinopathies Ineffective erythropoiesis	Lead poisoning 5' nucleotidase deficiency
Elliptocyte	G6PD deficiency Hereditary elliptocytosis Protein band 4.1 Glycophorin C deficiency Pyropoikilocytosis	Malaria
Heinz bodies	G6PD deficiency Thalassemias Unstable hemoglobins	Drug-induced oxidant injury
Parasites		Malaria (shown) Babesiosis Bartonellosis
Pyropoikilocytes	Hereditary pyropoikilocytosis α-Spectrin mutation	Burns

(continued)

TABLE 3.2 *continued*

Cell Type	Intrinsic	Extrinsic
Schistocyte		Microangiopathic hemolytic anemia (see Table 3.1)
Sickle Cell	Hemoglobin SS Hemoglobin SC Hemoglobin S beta-thalassemia	
Spherocyte	Hereditary spherocytosis Ankyrin/Spectrin deficiency Hemoglobin C disease Band 3 defects Protein 4.2 defects	Immune-mediated hemolysis Infections Chemical Injuries
Stomatocyte	Hereditary stomatocytosis Rh null disease	Alcohol intoxication Liver disease
Target Cell	Thalassemias Hemoglobin C disease Unstable hemoglobins	Liver Disease

renal failure and even death. Diagnosis and treatment of *Clostridium perfringens* sepsis or thrombotic thrombocytopenia purpura may be triggered by a hemolysis workup. The causes of intravascular hemolysis are almost exclusively extrinsic (Table 3-1).

Examination of several key laboratory values may also be used to assess intravascular hemolysis. Small amounts of hemoglobin released into the circulation are metabolized in the liver after binding and clearance by haptoglobin. With robust intravascular hemolysis, a rapid decrease of serum haptoglobin to undetectable levels occurs. Free hemoglobin not bound to haptoglobin can be oxidized to methemoglobin or bound to transport proteins such as hemopexin or albumin, which the liver will then remove from the circulation. Free hemoglobin at levels of 100 to 200 mg/dL can be detected by visual examination of plasma or serum. The capacity of renal tubular cells to reabsorb free hemoglobin is limited to producing hemoglobin-uria. As tubular cells slough, iron staining can identify the tubular epithelium containing hemosiderin in the urine sediment. Cessation of hemolysis leads to a rapid recovery of the haptoglobin levels, but urine hemosiderin is detectable for longer periods (Fig. 3-3). Urine hemosiderin in the absence of urine hemoglobin provides clinical evidence for subacute or chronic intravascular hemolysis.

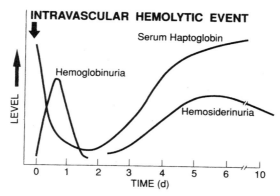

FIG. 3-3. Indicators of acute intravascular hemolysis. (From Hillman RS, Finch CA. Red Cell Manual 7th ed. Philadelphia: F.A.Davis Co., 1996, with permission.)

SPECIAL CONSIDERATION OF ENZYME AND MEMBRANE DEFECTS

Once the more obvious causes of hemolysis are ruled out, the clinician must consider those etiologies less frequently encountered in daily practice, including enzyme or membrane defects. The laboratory evaluation can be confusing because of the numerous etiologies and the diversity of tests available. Therefore, the extent of diagnostic testing is dictated by the magnitude of hemolysis and the impact of a specific diagnosis on therapy. Paroxysmal nocturnal hemoglobinuria is diagnosed by flow cytometry because of the associated absence of glycosylphosphatidylinositol-anchored proteins (e.g., CD59) on the plasma membranes of hematopoietic cells (see Chapter 6). General evaluation of the erythroid cytoskeleton is accomplished by fragility assays. In the case of enzymopathies, specific functional assays are available from reference laboratories. With the exception of G6PD, pyruvate kinase, and glucose phosphate isomerase, enzyme-based cases of hemolysis caused are rare.

ERYTHROID ENZYMOPATHIES

Enzyme deficiencies are most often associated with congenital nonspherocytic hemolytic anemia. Inheritance of G6PD and phosphoglycerate kinase deficiencies are chromosome X-linked; the other red cell enzyme abnormalities exhibit an autosomal recessive mode of inheritance. Based on their low incidence, laboratory evaluation of suspected enzymopathies requires the involvement of specialized or research laboratories (e.g., Mayo Medical Laboratories, Rochester, MN). Those assays measure the functional properties of each enzyme. In the setting of acute hemolysis, the magnitude of the functional deficit may be underestimated because of the generally higher levels of enzyme activity in reticulocytes and other "young" erythrocytes. As the clinical application of information contained in the human genome improves, genetic testing may become more practical for these enzymopathies. A genome-based profile of the known hemolysis-related enzymes is already available on the Internet (http://butler.cit.nih.gov/hembase/hembase.taf).

Enzyme deficiencies within two related metabolic pathways (Embden-Meyerhof and phosphogluconate) are most commonly associated with hemolysis. Glutathione reduction (phosphogluconate pathway; hexose monophosphate shunt) is necessary for the prevention of oxidative damage to other cellular proteins, including hemoglobin. Glucose metabolism (Embden-Meyerhof pathway) provides the sole source of energy to the cells once they lose their mitochondria. Below is a brief synopsis of the enzymopathies associated with hemolysis (organized according to the involved metabolic pathway).

Enzymes Involved in Glutathione Metabolism

Glucose-6-phosphate dehydrogenase (G6PD) deficiency is the most common RBC enzyme disorder associated with hemolysis. As an X-linked disorder, it is far more common in males. It has been estimated that this disorder affects millions of people throughout the world, the highest frequency occurring in the Mediterranean region, Africa, and China. Approximately 10% to 15% of African-American males are deficient in G6PD activity. G6PD catalyzes the conversion of glucose-6-phosphate to 6-phosphogluconate. When G6PD-deficient erythrocytes are exposed to oxidants, they become depleted of reduced glutathione (GSH). Once GSH is depleted, oxidation of other red blood cell sulfhydryl-containing proteins (including hemoglobin) occurs. Oxidation of hemoglobin leads to the formation of sulfhemoglobin and Heinz bodies. The World Health Organization has classified the known 400 G6PD variants according to the magnitude of the enzyme deficiency and the severity of hemolysis.

- Class I: Severe enzyme deficiency (less than 10% of normal enzyme activity). These rare patients have chronic active hemolysis.
- Class II: Severe enzyme deficiency but with only intermittent hemolysis (G6PD Mediterranean).
- Class III: Moderate enzyme deficiency (10% to 60% of normal) with intermittent hemolysis usually associated with infection or drugs (G6PD A-). (Commonly found in Africans and African Americans.)
- Class IV: No enzyme deficiency or hemolysis.
- Class V: Increased enzyme activity.

Classes IV and V are of no clinical significance. Among patients with classes I to III, four clinical presentations may be found:

  I. Congenital nonspherocytic hemolytic anemia
  II. Neonatal hyperbilirubinemia
  III. Acute hemolytic anemia
  IV. Favism

Patients with congenital nonspherocytic hemolytic anemia may demonstrate a lifelong hemolysis in the absence of infection or drug exposure. Those with class I G6PD variants appear to have genetic mutations that are central to the function of the G6PD protein. This functional defect is so severe that erythrocytes cannot withstand the normal stresses encountered in the circulation. The neonatal hyperbilirubinemia in G6PD-deficient infants is caused by increased bilirubin production from erythrocyte breakdown combined with the immaturity of the liver. Neonates with the class I variant are at greatest risk of developing neonatal hyperbilirubinemia; however, neonates with the Class II–III variants (i.e., Mediterranean and G6PD A-) may also be affected.

Patients with the most prevalent G6PD variants, Class II and III (G6PD A- and G6PD Mediterranean), are generally asymptomatic in the steady state. They are not anemic but their RBC survival is decreased. They present episodically with acute hemolytic anemia due to oxidative stress from infections (hepatitis, salmonellosis, and pneumonia) or drugs (Table 3-3). (A complete list of drugs and chemicals associated G6PD deficiency is available on the internet [http://www.uptodate.com/ or http://bnf.org/bnf/bnf/current/doc/4925.htm].) Favism is a term used to describe hemolysis associated with the ingestion of fava beans, which contain pyrimidine aglycones (divicine and isouramil). Favism is most commonly associated with the G6PD Mediterranean variant. Africans and African Americans with G6PD deficiency are less susceptible.

TABLE 3–3. *Drugs and chemicals to avoid in patients with glucose-6-phosphate dehydrogenase deficiency*

Dapsone
Methylene blue
Naphthalene
Nitrofurantoin
Phenzopyridine (Pyridium)
Phenylhydrazine
Primaquine
Sulfacetamide
Sulfamethoxazole (Bactrim, Septra)
Sulfanilamide
Sulfapyridine
Thiazosulfone
Toluidine blue
Trinitrotoluene
Quinolones

The definitive diagnosis of G6PD deficiency depends on quantitative enzyme assays. Heinz body inclusions are generated during acute, drug-induced hemolytic episodes. The spleen normally clears these inclusions (9). Treatment of a G6PD-deficient individual depends on the degree of hemolysis. Potentially harmful drugs should always be avoided and patients with infection should be carefully monitored for early signs of increased hemolysis. Blood transfusion may be life-saving during acute hemolytic episodes. Unfortunately, the potential benefit of splenectomy in these patients is not well defined (10).

γ-Glutamylcysteine synthetase is the rate-limiting enzyme in glutathione biosynthesis. Hemolytic anemia was first diagnosed in German siblings with low activity of this enzyme and normal glutathione synthetase. These siblings had a history of lifelong anemia and intermittent jaundice and later presented with spinocerebellar degeneration (11).

Glutathione peroxidase (GSH-Px) deficiency is an autosomal disorder affecting the redox reactions in erythrocytes. The enzyme is primarily responsible for the elimination of hydrogen peroxide from erythrocytes. Moderate deficiencies in GSH-Px activity may result in the formation of Heinz bodies and nonspherocytic hemolytic anemia in infants. Hemolysis usually disappears by 3 years of age despite ongoing deficiency of the enzyme. Oxidizing agents should be avoided in these patients (12).

Glutathione reductase is the enzyme that reduces oxidized GSH in the presence of flavin adenine dinucleotide. Reduction in glutathione reductase is believed to increase susceptibility to drug-induced hemolysis (13). Glutathione reductase activity increases with dietary supplementation of riboflavin, and a subset of these patients responds well to riboflavin dietary supplements.

Glutathione synthetase deficiency has been implicated in chronic hemolysis. This deficiency is characterized by hemolysis, metabolic acidosis, and mental deterioration. The disease is marked by accumulation of the metabolite oxyproline in the urine (14).

Enzymes Involved in Glucose Metabolism

Pyruvate kinase (PK) deficiency is the second most common enzymopathy associated with congenital nonspherocytic hemolytic anemia. Pyruvate kinase converts phosphoenolpyruvate to pyruvate, simultaneously generating adenosine triphosphate (ATP) from adenosine diphosphate (ADP). Pyruvate kinase activity decreases during RBC aging, as the enzyme is gradually denatured. The eventual result is failure of glycolysis as PK activity falls below a critical level. Because glycolysis is the sole source of ATP synthesis in the mature RBC, ATP depletion soon follows glycolytic failure.

This autosomal recessive disorder has been found in all major ethnic groups but is particularly common in northern Europeans. Most patients are compound-heterozygotes for the two most common mutant forms of the enzyme. True homozygotes exist in families where consanguinity is present. Approximately one-third of the cases present with jaundice during the newborn period, and one-third of those cases are severe enough to require transfusion. Death during the neonatal period is a result of severe anemia. The anemia is less severe in individuals with milder forms of the enzymopathy, and the diagnosis may not be established until later in childhood. Unfortunately, there is a poor correlation between PK activity and the severity of clinical hemolysis.

The beneficial effect of splenectomy in severe PK-deficient patients has been documented (15). However, no reliable way to predict success of splenectomy for individual cases currently exists. The results of splenectomy in other family members may be of major guidance in this matter. Concomitant splenectomy and cholecystectomy should be considered for a patient requiring surgery for removal of pigmented gallstones.

Glucose phosphate isomerase (GPI) deficiency is the third most common glycolytic enzyme associated with hemolytic anemia. GPI catalyzes the production of fructose-6-phosphate from glucose-6-phosphate. It is found in all ethnic groups, but is prevalent in individuals of northern European descent. In severe cases, anemia and hyperbilirubinemia are evident at birth. Acute hemolytic crises accompanying infections occurs with greater frequency in GPI deficiency than in other glycolytic enzymopathies (16).

Aldolase deficiency has been found to cause moderately severe lifelong hemolytic anemia, sometimes requiring transfusions during acute hemolytic crises. Aldolase catalyzes the conversion of fructose-1,6-diphosphate to dihydroxyacetone phosphate and glyceraldehydes-3-phosphate. Other congenital anomalies include short stature, mental retardation, delayed puberty, and a distinct facial appearance (17).

2,3-diphosphoglycerate mutase (DPGM) deficiencies of greater than 50% cause a compensated hemolytic anemia. DPGM converts 1,3-biphosphoglycerate to 2,3-diphosphoglycerate (2,3-DPG). Deficiencies of this enzyme may lead to a combination of hemolysis and polycythemia because of the resulting 2,3-DPG deficiency (18).

Enolase is the enzyme that converts 2-phosphoglycerate to phosphoenolpyruvate. Case studies have shown a decrease in the enzyme activity in patients with a mild spherocytic hemolytic anemia (19).

Hexokinase deficiency causes a rare congenital hemolytic anemia, predominantly in persons of northern European ancestry. Hexokinase acts at the initial enzymatic step in glycolysis, catalyzing the conversion of glucose to glucose-6-phosphate. Hexokinase activity in reticulocytes is considerably higher than in mature cells. Anemia is associated with a reduction of this enzyme activity to 25% that of normal erythrocytes (20).

Phosphofructokinase deficiency (also called Tarui disease) results in a glycogen storage disorder characterized by hemolysis and myopathy. Phosphofructokinase is an allosteric enzyme that catalyzes the irreversible conversion of fructose-6-phosphate to fructose-1, 6-diphosphate. Most affected individuals have exhibited exertional myopathy resulting in weakness, easy fatigability, muscle cramps on exercise, and myoglobinuria (21).

Phosphoglycerate kinase (PGK) deficiency results in a moderate-to-severe nonspherocytic hemolytic anemia. PGK converts 1,3 biphosphoglycerate to 3-phosphoglycerate. Because PGK deficiency is an X-linked disorder, severe hemolytic anemia and other clinical features are encountered in affected male subjects. Those patients with more severe enzyme deficiency are diagnosed during infancy. They may exhibit mild mental retardation, emotional lability, defects in speech, and or other neuropsychiatric abnormalities (22).

Triosephosphate isomerase (*TPI*) deficiency is a rare disorder characterized by severe hemolytic anemia, increased susceptibility to infection, and progressive neurologic deterioration. TPI promotes reversible conversion of dihydroxyacetone phosphate and glyceraldehyde-3-phosphate. Deficiencies usually become evident during infancy, with spasticity, motor retardation, hypotonia, weakness, and seizures (23).

Other Enzymopathies Associated with Hemolysis

Uridine 5' monophosphate hydrolase (pyrimidine 5' nucleotidase) is among the group of enzymes more commonly associated with hemolysis. It is an autosomal recessive disorder that is typically characterized by marked basophilic stippling and accumulation of high concentrations of pyrimidine nucleotides within the erythrocytes. This enzyme may be involved in the damaging effects of lead on red cells. Notably, patients with pyrimidine 5' nucleotidase deficiency may also have learning disabilities (24).

Adenosine deaminase (ADA) is a purine catabolic enzyme that converts adenosine to inosine. ADA deficiency causes inherited severe combined immunodeficiency. In contrast, elevations in ADA cause hemolytic anemia. Studies show that ADA amplification in reticulocytes results from increased translation of ADA mRNA (25).

Heme oxygenase-1 is an enzyme involved in the conversion of heme to bilirubin. Heme oxygenase-1 further provides protection against certain oxidative stresses. The first report of heme oxygenase-1 deficiency was noted in a 26-month-old child. By age 6, that child displayed severe growth retardation, asplenia, an abnormal coagulation/fibrinolysis system, and persistent hemolytic anemia. This enzyme deficiency may cause erythrocyte fragmentation and intravascular hemolysis (26).

Lecithin: cholesterol acyltransferase (LCAT) is an enzyme involved in lipoprotein metabolism. The production of that enzyme in the liver is reduced in patients with cirrhosis. Deficiencies of LCAT result in erythroid membrane defects caused by excess unesterfied cholesterol (27).

ERYTHROID MEMBRANE DEFECTS

The RBC membrane comprises integral and peripheral proteins distributed in the context of a lipid bilayer. Integral membrane proteins interact to form a lattice-like structure (cytoskeleton) at the cytoplasmic surface of the lipid bilayer that is responsible for the strength and deformability of the red blood cell. Band 3, a protein that functions as an anion exchanger (AE1), is the major protein that physically links the lipid bilayer to the underlying membrane cytoskeleton. The cytoskeleton proteins include spectrin, ankyrin, actin, band 3, band 4.1, and band 4.2. Other red cell membrane proteins serve roles in maintaining osmotic equilibrium or have adhesive properties. Interestingly, the exact function of several other erythroid membrane proteins remains vague.

Immune-mediated hemolysis is usually caused by antibodies directed toward erythrocyte membrane proteins. Approximately 24 proteins are largely responsible for transfusion-related alloimmunity (see Chapter 24). Nonimmune hemolysis may also be due to rare erythroid phenotypes involving those proteins. Nonimmune hemolysis due to the Rh-null phenotype is generally mild and well compensated with a reticulocyte count below 10%. The red cell morphology may be stomatocytic or spherocytic, and the osmotic fragility of their erythrocytes is increased (28). Weak expression of the Kell blood group results in the so-called "McLeod phenotype." This phenotype is X-linked and occurs with relatively high frequency in individuals who have chronic granulomatous disease (CGD). The McLeod phenotype is associated with acanthocytosis and mild hemolysis with slightly elevated reticulocyte counts (2% to 6%) (29). The first indication that a patient may have a membrane abnormality causing their hemolysis usually comes by examination of the peripheral blood smear. As shown in Table

3.2, the presence of spherocytes, elliptocytes, stomatocytes, acanthocytes or pyropoikilocytes may be the primary alert for an underlying membrane defects.

Hereditary spherocytosis (HS) is the most common hereditary anemia among people of northern European descent, occurring at a frequency of 1 in 5,000. The hereditary disease is commonly caused by mutations in the α- or β-spectrin and ankyrin genes. Spherocytes are identified by their small size and absence of the central pallor seen in normal erythrocytes. Splenectomy eliminates or minimizes the anemia in patients with moderate spherocytosis. Decisions regarding splenectomy must take into account the severity of hemolysis and the age of the patient (30).

The osmotic fragility test for HS has been used to detect hemolysis by measuring the fraction of total hemoglobin released from red cells at progressively more dilute salt concentrations. Hemolysis occurs in circulating HS spherocytes at salt concentrations that do not affect normal RBC. Preincubation for 24 hours accentuates the osmotic fragility of spherocytes and makes it easier to distinguish HS from other diseases. A cryohemolysis test may also be used to detect increased hemolysis in HS erythrocytes. Red cells are suspended in a hypertonic solution, briefly heated to 37°C, and then cooled to 4°C for 10 minutes. A widely separated degree of hemolysis between spherocytes and normal cells is seen with the cryohemolysis test, and asymptomatic disease carriers may also be identified (31). Although interesting, these tests are nonspecific and should be ordered conservatively.

Hereditary elliptocytosis (HE) is endemic in areas of Africa and Asia. Its prevalence is 2 to 5 per 10,000. In some patients, the inherited form is linked to the Rh gene on chromosome 1. The disease also results from mutations in the α-spectrin, β-spectrin, band 3, and band 4.1 genes. In the heterozygous state, people with HE have no clinical syndrome. Only a slight reticulocytosis and the characteristic abnormalities of the red blood cell morphology provide clues to the presence of HE. In the homozygous state, hemolysis may be lifelong and exacerbated by acute or chronic illnesses (32).

Hereditary stomatocytosis (xerocytosis) is identified by a pinched rather than circular area of central pallor in erythrocytes. The underlying defect involves the permeability of the red cell membrane to sodium and potassium. Most cases stem from high cell sodium content resulting in overhydration (33).

Acanthocytosis on the peripheral smear may be caused by acquired liver disease, other abnormalities in lipids or band 3. Abetalipoproteinemia is a rare genetic disorder resulting in hypolipidemia, acanthocytosis, malabsorption of fat, retinitis pigmentosa, and ataxia. Infants with this autosomal recessive disorder are normal at birth but soon develop steatorrhea, abdominal distension, and growth failure. Retinitis pigmentosa and ataxia appear between ages 5 to 10 years and are progressive. A separate syndrome characterized by chorea and acanthocytes in the absence of β-lipoprotein abnormalities also exists (34).

Hereditary pyropoikilocytosis is a severe type of HE resulting from a mutation in either protein 4.1 or α-spectrin. The usual presentation involves mild to moderate hemolytic anemia with evidences of poikilocytosis. The spectrin in these abnormal cells has an increased sensitivity to thermal denaturation (35).

TREATMENT OPTIONS FOR CONFIRMED HEMOLYSIS

Therapeutic strategies for hemolytic anemia are determined by the underlying etiology of red cell destruction. For an extrinsic cause, the treatment plan usually becomes obvious at the time of diagnosis. Immune-mediated hemolysis may require immunoglobulin infusion or immunosuppression. Infections are treated with antimicrobials. Erythrocyte fragmentation frequently can be reversed once identified. For thrombotic thrombocytopenic purpura or hemolytic-uremic syndrome, plasmapharesis is specifically indicated. Other extrinsic causes are treated with discontinuation of an erythrocyte-damaging drug or environment. Careful and frequent review of medications and diet is required, especially in patients with underlying G6PD deficiency.

Treatment modalities for intrinsic causes of hemolysis may be more difficult, as the hemolytic picture may change over time, and specific treatment may not exist. First ask if treatment is required. Chronic, compensated hemolysis that is currently unpreventable or untreatable may only require a yearly clinical evaluation with CBC, absolute reticulocyte count, and blood smear to determine whether the level of hemolysis is stable. For chronic hemolysis, folic acid should be used at an oral dose of 1 mg per day.

Treatments such as transfusion, splenectomy, or bone marrow transplantation should be reserved for marked hemolysis producing life-threatening anemia. In severe HP and HE, splenectomy is clearly beneficial and indicated. However, post-splenectomy complications of susceptibility to encapsulated bacteremia and sepsis along with the morbidity of this surgery need to be considered in less severe cases. Patients must be informed that the asplenic state carries a small risk of overwhelming and life-threatening infection. After splenectomy, special care must be taken to compensate for the loss of splenic function. The spleen is responsible for the clearance of encapsulated bacteria such as *Streptococcus pneumoniae, Haemophilus influenzae,* or *Neisseria meningitis.* The combined use of pneumococcal polysaccharide immunization and early empiric antibiotic therapy offer a high level of protection for postsplenectomy patients (36).

CONCLUSION

A broad range of genetic and acquired diseases is manifested by hemolysis. The differential diagnosis is useful in developing diagnostic and therapeutic strategies and should be thought of in terms of intrinsic or extrinsic causes of erythrocyte damage. A careful search for the cause of hemolysis should be pursued since specific treatments are so different. When a common cause of hemolysis is not found, an underlying enzyme or membrane defect should be sought.

Clinical severity in all cases of hemolysis is determined by the rate of red cell destruction, and the host's ability to compensate by producing fresh erythrocytes. Disease can vary from a subtle and clinically silent syndrome to hemolysis of sufficient intensity to dominate the clinical picture and even cause death if left untreated. Every therapeutic plan should be designed for both the severity of disease as well as the cause of hemolysis.

HELPFUL INTERNET SITES

http://www.ncbi.nlm.nih.gov:80/entrez/query.fcgi?db=OMIM
http://butler.cit.nih.gov/hembase/hembase.taf
http://bnf.org/bnf/bnf/current/doc/4925.htm.
http://www.uptodate.com/

REFERENCES

1. Handin RI, Lux SE, Stossel TP. *Blood: Principle and Practices of Hematology.* 3rd ed. New York: JB Lippincott Publishers, 2003.
2. Dacie JV. *The Haemolytic Anaemias: Secondary or Symptomatic Haemolytic Anaemias.* 3rd ed. Vol. 4. Edinburgh: Churchill Livingstone, 1995.
3. Nathan DG, Orkin SH, Oski FA. *Hematology of Infancy and Childhood.* 6th ed. Philadelphia: WB Saunders, 2003.
4. Foerster J, Lee RG, Wintrobe MM, eds. *Wintrobe's Clinical Hematology.* 10th ed. Philadelphia: Williams & Wilkins, 1999.
5. Beutler E, Stamatoyannopoulous G, eds. *The Molecular Basis of Blood Disease.* 3rd ed. Philadelphia: WB Saunders, 2001.

6. Dacie JV. The *Haemolytic Anaemias: The Hereditary Haemolytic Anemias.* 3rd ed. Vol. 3. Edinburgh: Churchill Livingstone, 1995.
7. Bunn HF, Forget BG. *Hemoglobin: Molecular, Genetic, and Clinical Aspects.* Philadelphia: WB Saunders, 1986.
8. Finch CA, Hillman RS. *Red Cell Manual.* 7th ed. Philadelphia: F.A. Davis, 1996.
8a. American Society of Hematology. www.hematology.org
9. Foerster J, Lee RG, Wintrobe MM, eds. *Wintrobe's Clinical Hematology.* 10th ed. Philadelphia: Williams & Wilkins, 1999.
10. Balinsky D, Gomperts E, Cayanis E, et al. Glucose-6-phosphate dehydrogenase Johannesburg: A new variant with reduced activity in a patients with cogenital non-spherocytic haemaolytic anemia. *Br J Haematol* 1973;25:385–390.
11. Richards F, Cooper MR, Pearce LA, et al. Familial spinocerebellar degeneration, hemolytic anemia and glutathione deficiency. *Arch Intern Med* 1974;134:534–537.
12. Necheles TF, Maldonado NI, Barquet-Chediak A, et al. Homozygous erythrocyte glutathione perioxidase deficiency: clinical and biochemical studies. *Blood* 1969;33:164–169.
13. Beutler E. Effects of flavin compounds on glutathione reductase activity: in vivo and in vitro studies. *J Clin Invest* 1969;48:1957–1966.
14. Mohler DN, Majerus PW, Minnich V, et al. Glutathione synthetase deficiency as a cause of hereditary hemolytic disease. *N Engl J Med* 1970;283:1253–1257.
15. Sandoval C, Stringel G, Weisberger J, et al. Failure of partial splenectomy to ameliorate the anemia of pyruvate kinase deficiency. *J Pediatr Surg* 1997;32:641–642.
16. Ravindranath Y, Paglia DE, Warrier I, et al. Glucose phosphate isomerase deficiency as cause of hydrops fetalis. *N Engl J Med* 1987;16:258–261.
17. Hurst JA, Baraitser M, Winter RM. A Syndrome of mental retardation, short stature, hemolytic anemia, delayed puberty and abnormal facial appearance. *Am J Med Genet* 1987;28:965–970.
18. Rosa R, Prehu MO, Beuzard Y, et al. The first case of complete deficiency of diphosphoglycerate mutase in human erythrocytes. *J Clin Invest* 1978;62:907–915.
19. Boulard-Heitzmann P, Boulard M, Tallineau C. Decreased red cell enolase in 40 year old woman with compensated haemolysis. *Scand J Haemotol* 1984;33:401–404.
20. Magnani M, Stoochi V, Cucchiarini L, et al. Hereditary nonspherocytic hemolytic anemia due to a new hexokinase variant with reduced stability. *Blood* 1985;66:690–697.
21. Tani K, Fujii H, Takegawa S, et al. Two cases of phosphofructokinase deficiency associated with cogenital hemolytic anemia. *Am J Hematol* 1983;14:165–167.
22. Guis MS, Karadsheh N, Mentzeer WC. Phosphoglycerate kinase San Francisco: a new variant associated with hemolytic anemia but not with neuromuscular manifestations. *Am J Hematol* 1987;25:175–182.
23. Clark AC, Szobolotzky MA. Triose phosphate isomerase deficiency: prenatal diagnosis. *J Pediatr* 1985;106:417–420.
24. Marinaki AM, Escuredo E, Duley JA, et al. Genetic basis of hemolytic anemia caused by pyrimidine 5'nucleotidase deficiency. *Blood* 2001;97:3327–3332.
25. Chottiner EG, Cloft, HJ, Tartaglia AP, et al. Elevated adenosine deaminase activity and hereditary hemolytic anemia: evidence for abnormal translational control of protein synthesis. *J Clin Invest* 1987;79:1001–1005.
26. Yachie A, Niida Y, Wada T, et al. Oxidative stress causes enhanced endothelial cell injury in human oxygenase-1 deficiency. *J Clin Invest* 1999;103:129–135.
27. Morse EE. Mechanisms of hemolysis in liver disease. *Ann Clin Lab Sci* 1990;20:169–174.
28. Nash R, Shojania AM. Hematological aspect of Rh deficiency: a case report and review of literature. *Am J Hematol* 1987;24:267–275.
29. Denson P, Wilkinson-Kroovand S, Mandell GL. Kx and its relationship to chronic granulomatous disease and genetic linkage to Kg. *Blood* 1981;58:34–37.
30. Duru F, Gurgey A, Ozturk G, et al. Homozygosity for the dominant form of hereditary spherocytosis. *Br J Heamatol* 1992;82:596–600.
31. Iglauer A, Reinhardt D, Schöter W, et al. Cryohemolysis test as a diagnostic tool for hereditary spherocytosis. *Ann Hematol* 1999;78:555–557.
32. Morle L, Pothier B, Alloisio N, et al. Red cell membrane alteration involving protein 4.1 and protein 3 in a case of recessive inherited haemolytic anemia. *Eur J Haematol* 1987;38:447–455.
33. Mentzer WC, Smith WB, Goldstone J. Hereditary stomatocytosis: membrane and metabolic studies. *Blood* 1975;46:659–669.

34. Vance JM, Pericak-Vance MA, Bowman MH, et al. Chorea-acanthocytosis: a report of three new families and implications for genetic counseling. *Am J Med Genet* 1987;28:403–410.
35. Liu SC, Palek J, Prchal J, et al. Altered spectrin dimer-dimer association and instability of erythrocyte membrane skeleton in hereditary pyropoikilocytosis. *J Clin Invest* 1981;68:597–605.
36. Eber SW, Langendorfer CM, Ditzig M, et al. Frequency of very late fatal sepsis after splenectomy for hereditary spherocytosis: impact of insufficient antibody response to pneumococcal infection. *Ann Hematol* 1999;78:524–530.

4

Hemolytic Anemia: Thalassemias and Sickle Cell Disease

Matthew M. Hsieh, John F. Tisdale, and Griffin P. Rodgers

Normal hemoglobin within red blood cells comprises two α- and two β-chains with an α to β synthesis ratio of 1:1. Thalassemias are a group of quantitative disorders with insufficient production of α- or β-chains, leading to an imbalanced accumulation of β- or α-chains, respectively. In contrast, hemoglobinopathies (or abnormal hemoglobin structural variants) are a separate group of qualitative disorders, with abnormal β- or α-chains in normal quantity, of which sickle cell disease (SCD) is best recognized. While these two disorders share features of variable degree of hemolytic anemia and transfusion-related complications, they differ in their pathophysiology, clinical manifestations, and management (Table 4-1).

The hemoglobinopathies and thalassemias are commonly encountered in areas where malaria is endemic, presumably because abnormal genes offer protection against malaria. However, there are observations that the malaria theory does not explain well. One is that thalassemia exists where there is little or no malaria, such as the Pacific; this may be explained in part by population migration and genetic drift. Another is why certain region contains only one type or pattern of hemoglobinopathy, such as hemoglobin (Hb) E in Southeast Asia, Hb C in West Africa, or only a few β-thalassemia mutations in a particular geographic location. Perhaps these regional differences are temporary, and over time, the different mutation patterns will be distributed globally.

PATHOPHYSIOLOGY

Thalassemias

Normally there are four copies of α-globin gene, two copies on each chromatid of chromosome 16 (Table 4-2) (1). α-Globin chains are essential in the synthesis of both fetal and adult hemoglobin. α-Thalassemia syndromes result from deletions of a large α-globin gene segment from unequal crossover or recombination, and less frequently from mutations. The deleted segments of DNA vary in size and can involve one ($\alpha-\alpha+$, or $\alpha+$) or both ($\alpha-\alpha-$, or $\alpha0$) alleles on the same chromatid. Deletion of one gene ($-+/++$) confers a silent carrier. Two-gene deletion ($--/++$ or $-+/-+$) is commonly referred as α-thalassemia minor or trait with microcytosis, hypochromia but little or no anemia. Deletion of three genes ($--/-+$) leads to Hb H ($\beta4$), which is an unstable form of hemoglobin. Hb H disease is manifested by hypochromia, moderately severe hemolytic anemia, and splenomegaly. Absence of all four genes leads to hydrops fetalis with Hb Bart's ($\gamma4$). Hb Bart's transport oxygen poorly, cause profound tissue hypoxia, lead to heart and liver failure, and are almost always incompatible with life (Fig. 4-1).

Both α-globin gene deletion haplotypes, ($-+$) and ($--$), occur equally in Southeast Asians, whereas the ($--$) haplotype is much less common in Mediterraneans and rare in Africans. Hence, all the α-thalassemic syndromes are seen in Southeast Asians, but hydrops

TABLE 4–1. *General features of thalassemia and sickle cell disease*

	α-Thalassemia	β-Thalassemia	Sickle cell disease
Geographic	Equatorial Africa, Mediterranean Middle East, Arabian peninsula, Caribbean India, Southeast Asia, South China		Africa
Pathophysiology	Quantitative Hb defect: Gene deletion(s) leading to reduced α-chain production and hemolytic anemia	Quantitative Hb defect: Mutations leading to reduced β chain production and hemolytic anemia	Qualitative Hb defect: Hb S polymerization leading to vaso-occlusion and hemolytic anemia
Therapy	Simple transfusions Iron chelation	Simple transfusions Iron chelation Hydroxyurea in selected individuals Transplantation	Simple and exchange transfusions Analgesia Hydroxyurea Transplantation

Hb, hemoglobin.

fetalis is uncommon to rare in Mediterraneans and Africans. There are α-globin structural variants that may occur alone or in combination with α-globin gene deletions, and lead to further reduction of α-globin synthesis: the best characterized is Hb Constant Spring.

Similar to α-thalassemia, β-thalassemia syndromes also arise from genetic alterations that significantly reduce β-globin chain production. In contrast to the α-globin genes, there are only two β-globin genes, one on each chromatid of chromosome 11. While there are almost 200 mutations described, only about 20 mutations account for the majority of β-thalassemic

TABLE 4–2. *Normal and variant hemoglobin*

Name	Designation	Molecular structure	Proportion in
Adult hemoglobin	A	$\alpha_2 \beta_2$	Adults: 97% Newborns: 20%–25%
Adult hemoglobin	A_2	$\alpha_2 \delta_2$	Adults: 2.5% Newborns: 0.5%
Fetal hemoglobin	F	$\alpha_2 \gamma_2$	Adults: <1% Newborns: 75%–80%
	Hb H	β_4	Adults: 0% Newborns: 15%–25% in Hb H disease
	Hb Bart's	γ_4	Adults: 0% Newborns: 15%–25% in Hb H disease, 100% in hydrops fetalis

Hb, hemoglobin.

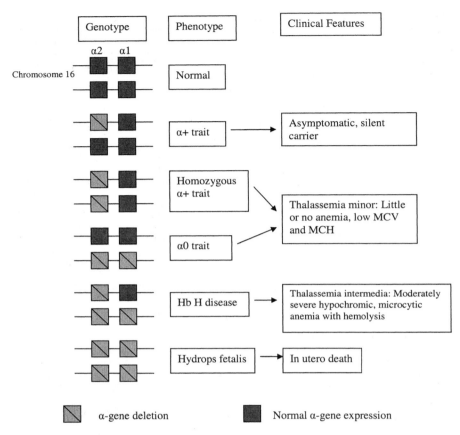

FIG. 4-1. α-thalassemia gene deletions and corresponding phenotypes.

individuals. Mutations are grouped by regional ethnic locations: Mediterranean basin, Southeast Asia, Africa, and Asian India. All disease-causing mutations alter β-globin gene mRNA transcription, processing, or translation. Some mutations decrease β-globin production by as little as 10%, and some by as much as 90%. Homozygosity or heterozygosity of mildly or severely affected alleles explains the wide range of clinical syndromes. Patients with one abnormal and one normal β allele have β-thalassemia minor or trait: the synthesis of β-chain is reduced by approximately one-half. Although normal hemoglobin A (α2β2) is mildly decreased, there is no accumulation of excess α-chains. There is hypochromia and microcytosis, but no clinically significant anemia, hemolysis, or ineffective erythropoiesis. The phenotype of two severe β-chain alleles is referred as β-thalassemia major or Cooley's anemia: β-chain synthesis and Hb A is virtually absent with α-chains in excess and consequently severe hemolytic anemia.

While the thalassemic syndromes are highly variable, severity is directly related to the imbalance of α- to β-chain ratio. A higher α- to β-chain ratio, 2–3:1, correlates with more severe β-thalassemia. In the severe thalassemic phenotype, excess unpaired α- or β-chains precipitate in erythrocyte precursors, resulting in their early death and ineffective erythropoiesis. Excess unpaired α- or β-chains also damage the red cell membrane and denature intracellular hemoglobin, promoting splenic sequestration and hemolysis, and eventually splenomegaly and anemia. Chronic hemolytic anemia and tissue hypoxia stimulate bone marrow expansion and produce skeletal and metabolic derangements: bony deformities, fractures, extramedullary hematopoiesis, and increased gastrointestinal iron absorption. In addition, red cell membrane damage, activation of platelets and endothelium, and abnormal levels of coagulation inhibitors (antithrombin III, proteins C and S) all contribute to increase the risk of thromboembolism.

In β-thalassemia, the compensatory increase in Hb A_2 and F is inadequate to offset the α- to β-chain imbalance. Genetic conditions that reduce α-chain excess (coinheritance of α-thalassemia, or increase in δ- or γ-chain production) or preserve some β-chain synthesis (a mild or silent β-thalassemic allele) ameliorate the severity of β-thalassemia. Thalassemia intermedia refers to patients with a lesser degree of hemolytic anemia, usually secondary to: compound heterozygosity of two mild β-thalassemia alleles, δ- and β-thalassemia, or Hb E and β-thalassemia; β-thalassemia with hereditary persistence of fetal hemoglobin (HPFH); or coexistence of α- and β-thalassemia.

Hemoglobinopathies: Hemoglobin Structural Variants

Hemoglobin variants of α- or β-chains, or the hemoglobinopathies, are caused by point mutations (most common), frameshift mutations, chain elongations, or chain fusions. The nomenclature of hemoglobinopathies employs alphabetic letters (S, C, or E), and sometimes locations of first discovery (O^{Arab} or D^{Punjab}) or name of the index case (Lepore or Constant Spring), then followed by the chain, location, and amino acid substitution (β6 Glu → Val).

Hemoglobin S

Sickle hemoglobin (Hb S) is the best characterized and the most important hemoglobinopathy. SCD is an inherited disorder in which normal glutamic acid is substituted by valine in the sixth codon of β-globin chain ($β^{6\,Glu→Val}$), which favors bonding of hemoglobin molecules. As a result, Hb S is less soluble when deoxygenated (in the normal oxygenation-deoxygenation cycle), precipitates and polymerizes quickly in red cells, and causes a morphologic change to a crescent shape. These rigid sickle cells lead to hemolytic anemia and vaso-occlusion, which together cause all the complications of SCD.

The lifespan of sickle cells is approximately 10 to 20 days, compared to 120 days for normal red cells. In the absence of clinically significant pain episodes, there is a chronic hemolytic anemia with mean hemoglobin of 7 to 8.5 g/dL, despite compensatory reticulocytosis of greater than 5% or 100 to 150 k/uL. Most sickle erythrocytes are removed in the spleen; some are destroyed intravascularly by mechanical forces or oxidative stress. Hemolysis has been implicated to activate inflammatory mediators, such as tumor necrosis factor-α (TNF-α), interleukin-2 (IL-2), thrombin, and platelet-activating factor (2). Leukocytosis is often associated with more frequent pain crises, stroke, and a shorter life expectancy in homozygous sickle disease (Hb SS) patients. Free hemoglobin, released by hemolysis, can consume nitric oxide and participate in endothelial dysfunction to promote vasoconstriction (3).

Vaso-occlusion begins with accumulation of sickle erythrocytes, and can occur in any vascular bed. Bone marrow and spleen are particularly susceptible because of their slow venous blood flow and high cell turnover rate. Pain crises in the long bones are the most common manifestation of SCD and repetitive vaso-occlusive episodes eventually lead to bone marrow and splenic infarction. Although normal lung oxygenates and potentially reverses polymerization, hypoxia or infection damage lung parenchyma activate pulmonary endothelium, and promote adherence of sickle erythrocytes. This process of vaso-occlusion in small and large pulmonary vessels can result in acute chest syndrome (4).

Other Hemoglobinopathies (E, C, Lepore, D, O^{Arab}, Constant Spring)

Hb E is a common hemoglobin variant, present in 15% to 30% of individuals in southern China and Southeast Asia. Hb E results from replacement of the normal glutamic acid to lysine in the twenty-sixth amino acid of the β-chain ($\beta^{26 \ Glu \rightarrow Lys}$) and leads to only 50% of mRNA's being spliced normally. Individuals with heterozygous and homozygous Hb E have mild anemia, hypochromia, and microcytosis. When Hb E is combined with β-thalassemia, the clinical features resemble those of β-thalassemia intermedia.

Hb C results from substitution of the normal glutamic acid to lysine in the sixth amino acid of β-chain ($\beta^{6 \ Glu \rightarrow Lys}$). Hb C is found mostly in individuals of African descent and is the second most common hemoglobinopathy in the United States and third most common worldwide. Carriers of Hb C are asymptomatic. Homozygous individuals (Hb CC) exhibit mild hemolytic anemia but are largely asymptomatic. Hb C combined with β-thalassemia produces mild to moderate hemolytic anemia with some features of β-thalassemia major. Compound heterozygosity with Hb C and Hb S (Hb SC) leads to milder anemia with fewer leg ulcers, pain crises, and osteonecrosis than with homozygous SCD (Hb SS); there is also a slightly lower risk of infection from encapsulated organisms. Retinal proliferative disease and splenomegaly, however, manifest earlier and more frequently in Hb SC disease.

Hb Lepore is a fused globin chain consists of N-terminal half of γ-chain and C-terminal half of β-chain. Similar to Hb Constant Spring, it produces low levels (2.5%) of normal β-chains. Although typically seen in Greeks or Italians, this variant can occur in a many ethnic groups of northern European descent. Hb Lepore can occur alone or in combination with other β-thalassemic mutations, leading to symptoms similar to β-thalassemia.

Hb D (same as Hb Los Angeles or Hb Punjab), another β-chain variant, is seen in Asian Indian population. When combined with β-thalassemia or SCD, the anemia is mild. Hb O^{Arab}, a rare β-chain variant, when combined with SCD (Hb SO^{Arab}), behaves similarly to full SCD. Hb Constant Spring, present in 5% to 10% of Southeast Asians, is caused by a point mutation in the stop codon of α-chain mRNA, leading to an elongated α-chain (α^{CS}). Because synthesis of β-globin is impeded (only approximately 1% is made), Hb Constant Spring behaves like an α-chain deletion. When α^{CS} is combined with a *cis* α-thalassemic defect ($\alpha^- \alpha^-$), it resembles Hb H disease. Fortunately α^{CS} is typically coupled with a normal α-chain gene ($\alpha^{CS} \alpha^+$) on the same allele, and hydrops fetalis has not been observed.

DIAGNOSIS

The diagnosis of SCD and thalassemias is now mostly accomplished by neonatal or prenatal testing (5,6). The goal of postnatal testing is to identify α- or β-thalassemia carriers, Hb S, C, E, and other clinically important hemoglobinopathies. The process typically begins with a complete blood count (CBC). When red indices are suggestive (Table 4-3), peripheral blood smear and high-performance liquid chromatography (HPLC) provide a provisional diagnosis (Fig. 4-2). HPLC has largely replaced traditional electrophoresis because it is able to reliably quantitate hemoglobin A_2, F, and S. Hemoglobinopathies are confirmed by isoelectric focusing or gel electrophoresis under alkaline (separates Hb S from Hb D/G) or acidic (separates Hb C, E, and O^{Arab}) conditions. Specific thalassemia mutations require polymerase chain reaction (PCR)-based DNA testing. Blood count indices vary widely and may deviate from typical values if there is concurrent iron deficiency or compound heterozygosity of other hemoglobinopathies. Any transfusion would also alter the hematologic parameters commonly found in each syndrome.

TABLE 4–3. *Hematologic characteristics of sickle cell disease and thalassemias*

Phenotype	RBC indices and hemoglobin composition
Normal	Total RBC: normal MCV >78 fl (or cubic microliter) or MCH >27 pg *Hb A >95%, F <1%, A$_2$ <3%
Thalassemia minor (trait)	MCV <78 fl or MCH <25 pg, elevated total RBC *Hb A, F 1%–7%†, †A$_2$ normal (in α-thalassemia trait); A$_2$ >3.5% (in β-thalassemia trait)
α-Thalassemia major (Hb H disease)	MCV <70 fl or MCH <25 pg, anemia *Hb A, F 1%–7%†, A$_2$ normal, Hb H 0.8%–40% Severe microcytosis, anisocytosis, hypochromia, and Hb H on peripheral smear
β-Thalassemia major	MCV <70 fl or MCH <25 pg, anemia *Hb A, F 1%–7%†, A$_2$ >3.5%†† Severe microcytosis, anisocytosis, hypochromia on peripheral smear
Sickle cell trait	*Hb A, S (S <50%)
Sickle cell disease	Hb SS: Hb S >50%, A$_2$ <4%; sickle cells in peripheral smear In SC disease: Hb S and C; less sickle cells but more target cells and spherocytes in peripheral smear
Hb S/β + thalassemia	*Hb A, S (S >50%)
Hb S/β0 thalassemia	*Hb S, faint band of A, A$_2$ >4%

* Screening hemoglobin electrophoresis or HPLC pattern.
† Hb F may be higher in individuals with concurrent δβ-thalassemia or hereditary persistence of fetal hemoglobin (HPFH)
†† Hb A$_2$ may be less than 3.5% with concurrent iron deficiency, some α-thalassemia, δβ-thalassemia, or certain β-chain mutations
RBC, red blood cell; MCV, mean cell volume; Hb, hemoglobin; MCH, mean corpuscular hemoglobin; SC, heterozygous for hemoglobin S and C.

α-Thalassemia Trait and Disease

Trans α-chain defect $(-+/-+)$ is more common in the Asian-Indian subcontinent, in Africa, and Afro-Caribbean regions, and less likely to produce clinically severe thalassemic phenotypes (Hb H or hydrops fetalis). *Cis* α-chain defect $(--/++)$, in contrast, can be seen in individuals from China, Southeast Asia, Greece, Turkey, or Cyprus. Screening is appropriate because the α-thalassemic phenotype may be moderate to severe. α-Thalassemia trait can been suspected with an elevated total red blood cell number, normal or borderline Hb A$_2$, mean cell volume (MCV) less than 78 μm, and mean corpuscular hemoglobin (MCH) less than 25 pg. The peripheral blood smear in Hb H disease can be stained with cresol blue to show Hb H precipitates within erythrocytes and reticulocytes.

β-Thalassemia Trait and Major

β-Thalassemia trait can be present in any ethnic group of northern European descent. Trait can be suspected from an elevated total red blood cell number, MCV less than 78 fl, MCH less than 27 pg, and normal or slightly low hemoglobin. On HPLC, there is a characteristic

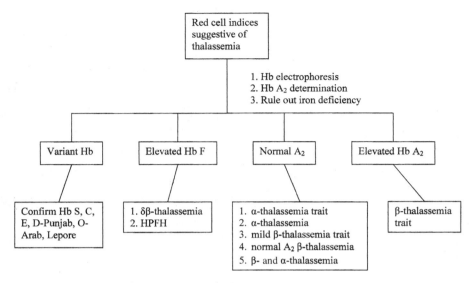

FIG. 4-2. Diagnostic schema for thalassemias.

elution pattern of variably elevated Hb F (higher in the Mediterranean variant, and lower in the African variant), normal Hb A, and greater than 3.5% Hb A_2. However, Hb A_2 may be normal (less than 3%) in individuals with concurrent iron deficiency or α-thalassemia; compound heterozygous δ- and β-thalassemia, or those with certain β-chain mutations. With β-thalassemia major, the MCV is usually less than 70 fl, MCH less than 25 pg, there is a variably low hemoglobin (5 to 9 g/dL), and no Hb A on HBLC.

Sickle Cell Trait and Disease

Sickle cell trait or disease can be diagnosed by the combination CBC, HPLC or hemoglobin electrophoresis, and the sickle solubility test. Sickle cell trait has near-normal red cell indices; hemoglobin may be slightly low to normal, and the MCH and red cell distribution width (RDW) may be slightly elevated. On screening HPLC or hemoglobin electrophoresis, Hb S comprises 35% to 50% of total hemoglobin, and Hb A_2 will be within the normal range. In contrast, in SCD Hb S comprises more than 50% (typically 70% to 90%) of total hemoglobin with slightly elevated Hb A_2 on HPLC and more sickle erythrocytes on peripheral blood smear. Trait or disease is then confirmed by sickle solubility test, and acidic or alkaline gel electrophoresis to screen for other concurrent hemoglobinopathies, such as Hb D or G. Sickle SC disease is easily distinguished by HPLC. Additionally, the peripheral smear in Hb SC disease shows fewer sickle cells, more spherocytes and target cells, and an uneven distribution of hemoglobin among red blood cells.

CLINICAL SYNDROMES AND TREATMENT OF SICKLE CELL DISEASE

Pain Episodes

Pain is the most frequent clinical manifestation of SCD (7). Many pain crises occur spontaneously, while some are precipitated by infection, stress, or dehydration. Frequent assessment and modification of therapy, involvement of a pain management service, and other consultations are important to address the complex etiology of pain in this disease. Evaluation begins by obtaining a full history of current and prior pain episodes. Physical examination and vital signs identify signs related to a pain episode. Acute pain can affect multiple sites: bones, joints, the cardiopulmonary system, central nervous system (CNS), or abdominal visceral organs. Chronic pain is typically confined to leg ulcers and the skeletal system.

Mild acute pain can often be managed in the outpatient setting with a combination of nonsteroidal anti-inflammatory drugs (NSAIDs), acetaminophen, and/or an oral opioid. Moderate to severe acute pain typically requires intervention in a day-hospital or emergency department, which begins with rapid assessment of the pain; hydration using 5% dextrose in half normal saline (D5 1/2 NS) and 20 mEq KCl, not exceeding 1 1/2 times maintenance; and an opioid analgesic (typically morphine, hydromorphone, or fentanyl). The choice, dose, and frequency of medication depend on the patient's outpatient drug regimen and prior responses. Severe pain is managed by bolus and continuous infusion of an opioid analgesic, often with patient-controlled delivery (PCA) pumps. In those with poor intravenous access, subcutaneous injection is an acceptable short-term alternative; however, intramuscular injection should be avoided because absorption varies. Parenteral meperidine should not be used as first-line treatment because its metabolite, normeperidine, has a long half-life and increases the risks of mood disturbances and seizures. Opioid agonists are metabolized by the liver and excreted variably by the kidney, and dose reduction may be necessary in those with hepatic impairment. Meperidine and morphine have active metabolites, should be used with great caution in patients with renal impairment, and avoided in patients with renal failure. Common side effects of all opioids—nausea, vomiting, pruritus, constipation, and respiratory depression—should be monitored and treated accordingly.

Nonopioid analgesics such as acetaminophen and NSAIDs have a ceiling effect and are often used with an oral opioid agonist. The total acetaminophen dose should not exceed 6 g daily in adults with normal hepatic function. Gastrointestinal, renal, and hematologic toxicities should be monitored. Benzodiazepines, antidepressants, antiemetics, and opioid agonist-antagonists such as pentazocine, nalbuphine, and butorphaol are useful adjuncts to opioid agonists and potentiate their analgesic effects. Gabapentin can be used for neuropathic pain.

In a recent review of chronic opioid therapy (8), failure to achieve desired analgesia resulted from (i) opioid tolerance, where the number of opioid receptors is reduced; (ii) opioid-induced hypersensitivity, where an individual experiences increased tenderness from known noxious stimuli; or (iii) worsening pain from progressive tissue damage. Prolonged, high-dose opioid therapy is associated with testosterone deficiency and suppression of immunity. Opioid dose escalation every 6 to 8 weeks or opioid rotation with a period of opioid abstinence may improve desired analgesia and minimize adverse effects in long-term analgesic therapy (Table 4-4).

Blood transfusions are not routinely administered during pain episodes. Transfusions become important for concurrent complications, such as acute chest syndrome, stroke, or other organ ischemia and damage (discussion following).

Infections

Because of functional asplenia, patients with SCD are at an increased risk of infection with encapsulated organisms: *Streptococcus pneumoniae, Hemophilus influenza,* and *Neisseria meningitides* (9). Several changes in patient management have reduced mortality rates. Neonatal diagnosis of SCD enables penicillin prophylaxis. In a placebo-controlled clinical trial (9), prophylactic penicillin in children prevented 84% of life-threatening infections caused

TABLE 4–4. *Comparative profiles of common opioid agonists for acute pain*

	Equivalent analgesic dosing	Site of metabolism and excretion*	Dose adjustment in hepatic impairment	Dose adjustment in renal impairment
Fentanyl	IV or transdermal: 25 μcg every hr	Liver: inactive metabolites Kidney: 75% of metabolites	No	GFR 10–50 mL/min: 75% of normal dosing GFR <10 mL/min: 50% of normal dosing
Hydro-morphone	Every 3–4 hrs IV: 1.5–2 mg PO: 6–7.5 mg IV:PO ratio 1:5	Liver: inactive metabolites Kidney: little excretion	Consider	Consider
Meperidine	Every 3–4 hrs IV: 100 mg PO: 250 mg IV:PO ratio 1:3	Liver: several active metabolites Kidney: >70% excretion	Yes	Use of meperidine with renal impairment should be avoided
Morphine	Every 3–4 hrs IV: 10 mg PO: 30 mg IV:PO ratio 1:3	Liver: active and inactive metabolites Kidney: >90% excretion	Yes	Use of morphine in renal impairment should use caution GFR 10–50 mL/min: 75% normal dosing GFR <10 mL/min: avoid morphine or 50% of normal dosing with caution
Oxycodone	Every 4 hrs IV: not available PO: 20–30 mg	Liver: active metabolites Kidney: variable excretion of metabolite	Yes, start one-third to one-half of normal dose	GFR 10–50 mL/min: 33% to 50% of normal dosing GFR <10 mL/min: 33% of normal dosing

* Opioid agonists are typically metabolized in the liver into active or inactive products, and are variably excreted by the kidneys.
IV, intravenous; GFR, Glomerulai filtration rate; PO, per oral.

by *S. pneumoniae.* Penicillin may be discontinued in those older than 5 years of age who have been vaccinated against *S. pneumoniae,* because there was no statistically significant benefit compared to placebo. Patients who are allergic to penicillin can receive erythromycin. Additionally, fever should be evaluated and managed promptly as a potential sepsis event, and empiric antibiotics administered while awaiting blood or urine culture and chest radiograph results. Finally, pneumococcal vaccination should begin in children and be renewed periodically. Influenza vaccinations should also be given yearly because viral infections can precipitate pain episodes and worsen anemia (Table 4-5).

Human parvovirus B19 is commonly spread among school-age children. B19 infects erythroid progenitors and causes transient red cell aplasia. While there is a wide range of clinical severity, influenza-like symptoms, fever, pain, and splenic sequestration can accompany an acute infection. Laboratory testing may reveal acute anemia, reticulocytopenia, and IgM antibody to parvovirus. Milder forms of SCD, e.g. Hb SC or Hb S/β + thalassemia, hydroxyurea treatment, or chronic transfusions, do not protect individuals with SCD from developing

TABLE 4–5. *Suggested penicillin prophylaxis and vaccination schedule for sickle cell patients (7)*

2 months to 2 years of age	2 to 3 years of age	3 to 5 years of age	Older than 5 years of age	Adults
Pen VK 125 mg BID or erythromycin 10 mg/kg BID		Pen VK 250 mg BID or erythromycin	May discontinue if vaccinated against *S. pneumoniae*	
Prevnar (7 valent) 2–4 doses q2 months	Pneumovax (23 valent) one dose		Repeat Pneumovax every 5 years	
	Yearly influenza vaccination			

severe complications (10). Parvovirus infection is also known as fifth disease, but in patients suffering transient aplastic crisis, the characteristic rash is absent. B19 can cross the placenta and cause hydrops fetalis and stillbirths; thus, pregnant staff should be strictly isolated.

Central Nervous System and Eye Disease

Stroke

Stroke is a major complication of SCD, more frequently in Hb SS than in Hb SC (11,12). Children tend to have more thrombotic strokes, adults more hemorrhagic strokes. General risk factors of thrombotic strokes are: age, prior transient ischemic attacks (TIAs), and systemic hypertension. Risk factors specific to SCD include a prior history of acute chest syndromes and low baseline hemoglobin in adults, dactylitis, severe anemia, and leukocytosis. For primary stroke prevention, the Stroke Prevention Trial (STOP) showed that children between 2 to 16 years of age who had transcranial Doppler (TCD) velocity greater than 200 cm/sec in the internal carotid or middle cerebral artery had a much lower incidence of brain infarction when managed with long-term transfusions to maintain Hb S less than 30% compared to supportive care (penicillin prophylaxis, vaccinations, folate supplementation, treatment of acute crises, and transfusions as needed) (11). Because the incidence of stroke is 11% up to 20 years of age, children with Hb SS should be screened with TCD ultrasonography every 6 to 12 months from age 2 to at least 18 years. Whether to continue ultrasonography beyond age 18 and the optimal timing of studies are uncertain.

Children with suspected stroke or TIAs are evaluated promptly, and hydration, therapy for hypoxia or hyperthermia, and blood pressure stabilization should follow immediately. Tissue plasminogen activator (t-PA) has not been extensively used in children and therefore is not recommended. The use of antiplatelet agents, aspirin or clopidogrel, is uncertain, but may be appropriate in selected circumstances. Computed tomography (CT) of the head without intravenous contrast, followed by magnetic resonance imaging and magnetic resonance arteriography (MRI/MRA), differentiate a hemorrhagic from thrombotic event. If a thrombotic stroke is present, exchange transfusions are initiated to reduce the Hb S level to less than 30% for a hemorrhagic stroke, treatment is based on the source and the extent of bleeding; exchange transfusion to reduce the Hb S level to less than 30% may be indicated. If imaging studies do not identify any abnormality, the next steps may involve observation, simple transfusions, and/or participation in clinical trials.

As the recurrence rate is high, long-term transfusion therapy to maintain Hb S less than 30% for a minimum of 3 to 5 years should be planned for children with thrombotic strokes. Long-term transfusions also can be considered in hemorrhagic stroke or vasculopathy (aneurysm or arterial stenosis). Some clinicians reduce the frequency of transfusions after 5 years.

Adults with acute strokes or TIAs are managed similarly to children; neurologic and neuro-surgical subspecialists are consulted when appropriate. However, there is no consensus on treatment guidelines (7). If a thrombotic stroke is identified, t-PA and antiplatelet therapy or exchange transfusions can be considered. If a hemorrhagic stroke is diagnosed, treatment is based on the source and the extent of bleeding; exchange transfusion to reduce the Hb S level to less than 30% may be indicated. For long-term therapy or secondary prophylaxis, antiplate-let therapy may be continued, with or without long-term transfusions to maintain the Hb S level less than 30%. Warfarin or dipyridamole may add to or substitute antiplatelet therapy for patients with recurrent strokes.

In managing patients with sickle cell anemia with strokes, several questions remain to be answered by clinical trials: (i) Should clinicians manage adults with SCD with stroke as children with SCD or as adults without SCD? (ii) Will long-term transfusions benefit those with nonocclusive hemorrhagic strokes, TIAs, or CNS vasculopathy? (iii) How long to con-tinue long-term transfusions once initiated for strokes in children? Some advocate until age of 18, while others suggest a minimum of 3 to 5 years from the date of stroke diagnosis. (iv) How often to screen asymptomatic children with TCD?

Eye Disease

Neovascularization within the eye results from repetitive vaso-occlusive episodes and leads to visual impairment. Proliferative changes are often asymptomatic early in the disease pro-cess: clinically detectable retinal changes are typically discovered between 15 to 30 years of age. Patients with Hb SC and sickle-thalassemia are disproportionately more prone to develop clinically significant ophthalmologic problems. Annual eye examinations starting in adoles-cence, carefully evaluating visual acuity, papillary reactivity, and anterior and posterior struc-tures, are important. In stage I eye disease, there is peripheral arteriolar occlusion; in stages II and III, vascular remodeling and neovascularization; in stage IV, vitreous hemorrhage; and in stage V, retinal detachment. These can be managed by observation, laser phototherapy or surgical correction.

In patients with SCD or sickle cell trait, direct eye trauma that causes bleeding into anterior chamber requires urgent evaluation. Sickle erythrocytes can occlude the trabecular channels, increase intraocular pressure, and cause acute glaucoma.

Cardiovascular Manifestations

Individuals with SCD have lower blood pressures compared to individuals with other types of chronic anemia. Renal sodium wasting is postulated as one possible cause although other mechanisms may be present. Blood pressures in SCD correlate with age, hemoglobin, and body–mass index. When systolic or diastolic blood pressures approach those of age-, gender-, and race-matched normal individuals, the risk of stroke and mortality increases.

There are other cardiac manifestations in SCD. Systolic flow murmurs, related to the degree of anemia, are frequent. On echocardiogram, pericardial effusions are found in approximately 10% of all studies; cardiac output, cardiac chamber size, and myocardial wall thickness are increased to improve the stroke volume without increasing the heart rate. With long-term and consistent increases in cardiac output, the ability to perform physical work is reduced by half in adults and by one-third in children. Given the larger heart chamber sizes, congestive heart failure is uncommon. For individuals receiving chronic transfusion therapy, there may be additional cardiac damage from iron overload, leading to more severe dilated cardiomyopathy and heart failure.

Myocardial infarction caused by large vessel occlusion (in the left anterior descending, circumflex, or right coronary artery) is rare, but cardiac damage from small vessel diseases may occur. Sudden death due to unexplained arrhythmia or autonomic dysfunction also has been described in adults with SCD.

Pulmonary Complications

Acute complications

Acute chest syndrome (ACS) is typically defined by temperature higher than 38.5°C, cough, a new pulmonary infiltrate on chest radiograph or rales on auscultation (often in multiple lobes), chest pain, and other respiratory symptoms (13–15). Children tend to have more respiratory symptoms (wheezing, cough, and fever), while adults manifest symptoms of musculoskeletal pain and dyspnea and have a more severe and sometimes fatal course. ACS is a frequent cause of death in both children and adults with SCD, the second most common cause of hospitalization, and the most typical complication following surgery and anesthesia. Frequent ACS episodes are associated with shortened survival. Risk factors for ACS are Hb SS, low fetal hemoglobin, high baseline hemoglobin (11 g/dL or greater) and high white blood cell count (greater than 15 k/uL), and prior episodes of ACS. ACS can take a mild, self-limited course, or progress rapidly to respiratory failure and multi-organ dysfunction. Complications for ACS include CNS injury (from anoxia, infarct, or hemorrhage), seizure, and respiratory failure.

While the etiology of ACS is often unknown (less than half of events had an identifiable cause), it can be triggered by pneumonia, pulmonary infarction from vaso-occlusion within the pulmonary vasculature, fat embolism from bone marrow infarction, or pulmonary thromboembolism. Microbiologic culture of sputum may reveal a variety of atypical organisms (chlamydia or mycoplasma), viruses (respiratory syncytial virus), and bacteria (*S. aureus, S. pneumoniae, or H. influenza*); up to 30% of microbiologic cultures are negative.

Evaluation of ACS includes vital signs, pulse oximetry or arterial blood gas, microbiologic culture of sputum and blood, nasopharyngeal swab for viral culture, chest radiograph, and complete blood count, liver, and renal function tests. Bronchoscopy may be indicated when patients do not respond to initial therapy.

Treatment for ACS includes oxygen, broad spectrum intravenous antibiotics (including for atypical organisms), simple and/or exchange transfusions as needed to improve oxygen saturation, bronchodilators (as airway hyperreactivity often accompanies ACS), and analgesia for pain. All of these efforts are aimed at reducing the percentage of sickle erythrocytes and minimizing sickle polymerization. Nitric oxide or acute pulmonary vasodilators are used for chronic pulmonary hypertension and may be beneficial in ACS. After an episode of ACS has been managed successfully, strategies to prevent future episodes include vaccinations (especially against pneumococcus), hydroxyurea, transfusions, or bone marrow transplantation.

Systemic fat embolism syndrome is a rare acute complication of SCD. Embolization occurs when there is a large bone marrow infarction and necrosis, and necrotic fat and marrow are released into the systemic circulation and lodge in the pulmonary vasculature. Fat embolization can precipitate or develop concurrently with ACS. Multiorgan failure may result. Risk factors for developing systemic fat embolism syndrome are Hb SC genotype, pregnancy, and prior corticosteroid treatment.

Chronic complications

Pulmonary hypertension from SCD is becoming more frequent as children with the disease survive into adulthood. The incidence of chronic pulmonary hypertension is estimated at approximately 20% of adult patients with SCD. While the exact cause is unknown, one or more of the following may contribute to its pathogenesis: sickle cell-related vasculopathy, pulmonary damage from recurrent ACS, high blood flow from anemia, and chronic hemolysis. Clinically, pulmonary hypertension can manifest as dyspnea, clubbing, loud second heart sound (P_2), an enlarged right side of the heart on chest radiograph, and abnormal oxygen saturation on room air at rest (95% or less). Pulmonary hypertension can be documented on echocardiogram by a tricuspid regurgitation jet velocity (TRV) of 2.5 m/sec or less or mean pulmonary arterial pressure (MPAP) of greater than 25 mm Hg. In one small series, where patients with SCD underwent right-side heart catheterization for clinical indications, pulmonary pressure was lower (MPAP 35 to 40 mm Hg), and cardiac output was higher (average 8.5 L/min) than in those with primary pulmonary hypertension (60 mm Hg and 3.0 L/min, respectively).

For pulmonary hypertension, there is currently no single preferred treatment, nor is one program beneficial to most patients. Simple transfusion to maintain the hemoglobin at approximately 9 g/dL can reduce pulmonary pressure in some, but the possible development of red cell antibodies limits the applicability of this approach. Hydroxyurea reduces the frequency and severity of vaso-occlusive crises and ACS, but may only delay the onset of pulmonary hypertension. Therapy for primary pulmonary hypertension such as calcium channel blockers (nifedipine or diltiazem), anticoagulation with warfarin (target international normalized ration [INR], 2 to 3), and continuous or nocturnal oxygen for hypoxemic patients can be considered. Prostacyclin, endothelin antagonist, and nitric oxide are important adjunctive agents that may benefit those with severe pulmonary pressure (TRV jet 2.9 m/sec or more).

Gallbladder, Hepatic, and Splenic Manifestations

SCD can affect the hepato-biliary and splenic systems in multiple ways (Table 4-6). Hyperbilirubinemia is common. Chronic hemolysis produces less than 4 mg/dL of unconjugated bilirubin. Other factors that increase total bilirubin level include: cholesterol intake, presence of Gilbert's syndrome, and cephalosporin antibiotic use. Biliary sludge and cholethiasis can occur as early as 2 to 4 years of age, have similar clinical manifestations, and are managed similarly to those without SCD.

Acute splenic sequestration (ASS) is caused by trapping of erythrocytes and presents with weakness, pallor, and an acute fall in hemoglobin, often by 2 g/dL or greater than 20% from baseline; tachypnea and abdominal fullness from acute splenomegaly (2-cm increase in palpated spleen size) may be present. ASS, similar to vaso-occlusive crises, can be precipitated by infections. The syndrome is seen in children under age 5 with Hb SS, older children with Hb SC, and in a few adults with Hb S/β^+ thalassemia. Children tend to have recurrent and

TABLE 4–6. *Sickle cell disease manifestations in gall bladder, liver, and spleen*

Gallbladder	1. Biliary sludge 2. Acute and chronic cholethiasis
Liver	1. Hemosiderosis: from iron overload 2. Hepatic crisis (RUQ syndrome): may occur with pain crisis. Clinically this syndrome consists of RUQ pain, transient elevation and improvement of AST/ALT (usually over days), fever, jaundice, and hepatic enlargement 3. Viral hepatitis: mostly from transfusions. AST and ALT typically increase slowly over months. 4. Hepatic sequestration: rare; typically with acute decrease in hemoglobin, elevated conjugated bilirubin (>20 mg/dL), alkaline phosphatase (2–3 times upper limit of normal), and hepatomegaly. Typically treated with simple transfusions.
Spleen	1. Splenic infarction: typically occurs over many years 2. Acute splenic sequestration: acute drop of >2 g/dL of hemoglobin, acute splenomegaly; more often in children. Treated with simple transfusions; chronic transfusions may be considered.

RUQ, Right upper quadrant; AST, aspartate transferase; ALT, alanine transferase.

severe episodes that require immediate attention with transfusion; a long-term plan of chronic transfusion therapy and/or splenectomy should be discussed. While ASS in children tends to be more severe, ASS in adults is typically self-limited, requiring only supportive care and observation.

Renal Abnormalities

There are several sickle cell-related manifestations in the kidneys. There is supranormal creatinine secretion in the proximal tubules, which explains lower serum creatinines (less than 0.5 mg/dL) observed in SCD. A serum creatinine approaching 0.9 to 1.0 mg/dL usually indicates subtle renal insufficiency. The renal medulla is composed of tubules and blood vessels, collectively called the vasa recta; this region is chronically acidic, hypoxic, and hypertonic, and is thus very susceptible to Hb S polymerization. Over time, gradual loss of vasa recta leads to an inability to concentrate urine. Hyposthenuria develops early in childhood and is frequently associated with nocturia, and is the chief reason individuals with SCD are so susceptible to dehydration. Hb S sickling also can lead to papillary necrosis and hematuria. Other renal manifestations include proteinuria from chronic glomerular damage, which in some individuals can progress to renal insufficiency or failure. Angiotensin-converting enzyme (ACE) inhibitors can ameliorate this progression, but electrolyte changes should be monitored carefully for hyperkalemia from chronic hemolysis. A decrease in hemoglobin from baseline due to renal insufficiency can be treated by erythropoietin injections and/or transfusions. Although erythropoietin levels are already elevated in renal failure, they are lower when corrected for the degree of anemia.

Priapism

Priapism is a sustained painful erection that can be classified as stuttering, if the duration is less than 3 hours and there is spontaneous resolution, or prolonged, if the duration is greater than 3 hours. Priapism begins early in puberty, and as many as 80% of men with SCD will have experienced at least one episode by 20 years of age. Priapism is caused by vaso-occlusion of the venous drainage of the penis, and physical examination will reveal a hard penis with a soft glans. At the onset of priapism, oral hydration and analgesia should be instituted. Prolonged priapism requires emergency department evaluation, intravenous hydration and analgesia—and represents urologic emergency. If not improved within 1 hour, blood aspiration and irrigation with dilute epinephrine from the corpus cavernosum under local anesthesia is needed (16). Simple or exchange transfusions are sometimes used.

Recurrent priapism can lead to impotence and fibrosis. None of the several treatments available has been well studied. Shunting procedures between the glans and distal corpus cavernosum (Winter's procedure) and medications to reduce the frequency of erection, such as pseudoephedrine, tricyclic antidepressants, β-blockers, or leuprolide, all have shown variable success. Simple or exchange transfusions have been employed.

Skeletal Complications and Leg Ulcers

Bone marrow hyperplasia from chronic anemia leads to osteopenia, increasing the risk of fractures in long bones and vertebra. Marrow hyperplasia also causes the characteristic deformation and growth disturbance such as "hair-on-end" appearance on skull x-ray, frontal bone "bossing," or protrusion of the maxilla. Repetitive vaso-occlusion in marrow sinusoids eventually causes bone infarction. When there is ischemic necrosis of juxta-articular bone, especially in the femur, humerus, or tibia, osteonecrosis ensues. In children prior to bone maturation, osteonecrosis is treated conservatively with analgesia, NSAIDs, and protected weight bearing. In adults, secondary degenerative arthritis can compound osteonecrosis, and the usual conservative treatment is ineffective. Core decompression and osteotomy with aggressive physical therapy have been reported to offer temporary relief of pain and increased joint mobility (17); joint replacement is reserved for those with severe symptoms or advanced disease.

Dactylitis or hand–foot syndrome in infants and young children presents with pain and swelling in one or more extremities (hands or feet). Plain radiograph may show periosteal elevation and a "moth-eaten" appearance. This syndrome usually requires hydration and analgesia, but transfusions or antibiotics are not necessary. There are no associated long term sequelae.

Bacteremia can lead to osteomyelitis or septic arthritis. Both present with warmth, tenderness, and edema caused by vaso-occlusion within bones; fever in the acute phase, increase in white blood cell count, and positive blood cultures help to distinguish infection from pain crisis. Positive microbial culture from aspiration of the bone or joint is diagnostic. Both of these infections are treated with surgical drainage and short-term (2 to 6 weeks) intravenous antibiotics. Additional temporary joint mobility exercises to improve the range of motion during the convalescent phase may be needed for septic arthritis.

Leg ulcers are seen in 10% to 20% of individuals with Hb SS, much less in patients with Hb SC or Hb S/β^+-thalassemic. Leg ulcers increase in frequency with age and are associated with lower mean hemoglobin (less than 6 g/dL) (18). Their exact etiology is unclear but trauma, chronic vaso-occlusion, edema, and hemolysis have all been implicated. Ulcers tend to locate in the ankles, tibia, or dorsum of the feet; other sites are rare. They begin as a small hyperpigmented area with edema, pain, and dysesthesia, subsequently appearing as denuded and "punched out" ulcers. Ulcers are typically infected locally, and osteomyelitis is rare (19). Two principles are important in promoting wound healing: reduction of local edema by elevation and/or pressure dressing, and debridement of ulcers by frequent wet-to-dry dressing changes to maximize granulation. There are many treatments available, but no single therapy works uniformly. Topical granulocyte macrophage-colony stimulating factor (GM-CSF), hydrocolloid occlusive dressings, zinc oxide-impregnated dressings, natural or synthetic dressings, L-arginine, oral zinc sulfate (200 mg three times per day), pentoxifylline, L-carnitine, and antithrombin III concentrates have all been used. Topical or systemic antibiotics are generally not helpful and eventually select for drug-resistant organisms. Ulcers smaller than 4 cm heal in weeks; larger ones may require consultation with a wound care service and plastic surgery for skin flaps. Transfusions can be considered for recurrent or persistent ulcers. The use of hydroxyurea in leg ulcer is controversial. There are reports of hydroxyurea causing leg ulcers in individuals with SCD and myeloproliferative disease, but in the Multicenter Study of Hydroxyurea (MSH) (20), hydroxyurea did not appear to change the incidence of leg ulcers. Other reports, however, suggest that fetal hemoglobin elevation is associated with reduced rates of leg ulcers (18).

THERAPY

Transfusions

Transfusions are an important therapy for SCD (Table 4-7). Transfusions are commonly used acutely, but also chronically for primary or secondary prevention of a specific complication. Transfusions can be separated into simple episodic, simple chronic, or exchange; it is important to notify the blood bank of the type (simple or exchange), indication, and expected duration (episodic or chronic) of therapy. A detailed transfusion history should be maintained that includes the total number of prior red cells units, presence of any red cell antibodies, percent Hb S, and the hemoglobin or hematocrit.

Of the potential complications that arise from multiple transfusions, the most significant is alloimmunization, or the development of red cells antibodies, leading to delayed hemolysis. When multiple antibodies are present, correctly matched blood units may be difficult to locate.

TABLE 4–7. *Indications for transfusions in sickle cell disease*

Indications for **simple episodic** transfusions
1. Acute chest syndrome (mild to moderate)
2. Severe anemia (Hb <5 g/dL) or a decrease of >20% from baseline
3. Preoperatively for major surgery with general anesthesia (target Hb 9–10 g/dL and Hb S ≤60%) (21)
4. Symptomatic patients with heart failure, dyspnea, hypotension, or other organ failure
5. Infection-related anemia (parvovirus B19) or hemolysis-related anemia (concomitant G-6-PD deficiency)
6. Hepatic sequestration
7. Splenic sequestration (more in children, drop in Hb by 2 g/dL, acute splenomegaly, with thrombocytopenia)

Consider in:
1. Prolonged priapism
2. Nonhealing leg ulcers

Usual indications for **simple chronic** transfusions
1. Primary or secondary stroke prevention (11)
2. Complicated pregnancy (by progressive anemia, preeclampsia, increased pain episodes, prior pregnancy loss, multiple gestations)—starting at 20 weeks (22)

Consider in:
1. In children following acute chest syndrome (14)
2. Pulmonary hypertension, moderate or severe
3. Silent, hemorrhagic, or vasculopathic stroke
4. Chronic heart failure
5. Splenic sequestration in children; transfuse until 5–6 years of age
6. Chronic debilitating pain
7. Renal failure related anemia
8. Recurrent priapism

Usual indications for **exchange** transfusions
1. Acute chest syndrome (moderate or severe)
2. Stroke (thrombotic, consider in hemorrhagic)
3. One or multiple organ failure
4. Hb SC patients with any of following:
   Preoperatively for major surgery requiring general anesthesia (23)
   Hepatic sequestration

Red cell antigen difference between sickle cell patients and blood donors (mostly Caucasians) is the major reason for the high rate of alloimmunization. Alloimmunization can be minimized by typing for Rh (D, E/e, and C/c) and Kell (K) antigens, in addition to the usual ABO-D typing. When a patient has a prior transfusion history, other minor antigens (Kidd, S, and Duffy) should also be typed. Prestorage leukocyte depletion can also be considered. Other potential complications include the usual transfusion reactions that can occur in patients with SCD: volume overload, acute hemolytic reactions, transfusion-transmitted infections (hepatitis B/C, HIV, West Nile virus, Creutzfeldt-Jacob disease), and iron overload (see below).

Fetal Hemoglobin Induction

The beneficial effect of fetal hemoglobin was first recognized from the observations that neonates with Hb SS do not develop SCD-related symptoms in the first 6 months of life, and patients with SCD with hereditary persistence of fetal hemoglobin (HPFH), such as in Saudi Arabia and India, have milder symptoms. *In vitro,* Hb F inhibits Hb S polymerization. Currently, hydroxyurea is the only Food and Drug Administration-approved drug for Hb F induction. Hydroxyurea is a cell cycle (S–phase)-specific agent that blocks the conversion of ribonucleotides to deoxyribonucleotides (Table 4-8). Its primary clinical effect is induction of fetal hemoglobin, but other benefits may include reduction of leukocyte and platelet counts, less hemolysis, decreased bone marrow cellularity, and generation of nitric oxide.

The MSH study was a randomized placebo-controlled clinical trial that confirmed the beneficial effects and the safety of hydroxyurea. The 150 hydroxyurea-treated patients had fewer episodes of pain and ACS, required less transfusion, and experienced minimal toxicity (20,24). Since the MSH, hydroxyurea has been used widely. Approximately 70% of SCD patients are likely hydroxyurea-responsive: the steady state Hb F should increase twofold from baseline or approximately 10% to 15%, and the total hemoglobin should rise by 1 to 2 g/dL. Whether hydroxyurea will ultimately prevent or reverse end-organ damage is unknown.

Hydroxyurea can be started at 10 to 15 mg/kg per day, and adjusted by increments of 5 mg/kg per day every 6 to 8 weeks, to a maximum of approximately 25 mg/kg per day. Compromised hepatic or renal function may require lower dosing. Within a few days of therapy, Hb F-containing reticulocytes will increase; at the end of 2 to 3 weeks, Hb F and total Hb F-containing red blood cells will rise. Other hematologic effects include increased MCV and decreased leukocytes (especially neutrophils), platelets, and reticulocytes. Two to 3 months are usually required before the effects on Hb F and blood counts are stabilized; a trial of 6 to 12 months is adequate to assess clinical benefit. Hydroxyurea in several cohorts of children has appeared safe (25), and adverse effects on growth and development have not been reported; the long-term effects of hydroxyurea in children, however, remain largely unknown.

TABLE 4–8. *Use of hydroxyurea*

Indications	Adults, adolescent, or children
	Hb SS or Hb S/β^0 thalassemia with frequent pain, history of ACS, severe vaso-occlusive events, severe anemia
Dosing	Start with 10–15 mg/kg per day
	Adjust by 5 mg/kg per day increment every 6–8 weeks; maximum of 25–35 mg/kg per day
	Duration: 6–12 months trial
Monitoring	CBC every 2 weeks, chemistry every 2–4 weeks, Hb F every 6–8 weeks
	At stable dose of hydroxyurea, CBC and chemistry every 4–8 weeks, Hb F every 8 weeks
	Keep ANC >2000/μL, reticulocytes >100 K/μL, and platelet >100 K/μL
	If marrow toxicity occurs, stop for 2 weeks, and start at a lower dose when blood counts recover
Treatment Endpoint	Less pain
	Increased Hb F to 10%–20% or 2–2.5-fold increase from baseline
	Increased hemoglobin if severely anemic
	Improved well-being, weight gain
Cautions	Dose reduction in hepatic or renal insufficiency
	Contraception for men and women

Hb, hemoglobin; ACS, acute chest syndrome; CBC, complete cell count; ANC, absolute neutrophil count.

Because hydroxyurea is an oral chemotherapeutic drug, contraception should be practiced in both men and women. Normal neonates have been delivered by women with SCD receiving hydroxyurea therapy but outcomes of any unplanned pregnancy should be discussed. The theoretical risk of developing a malignancy is another concern. While there are case reports of patients who have developed leukemia while receiving hydroxyurea, whether this rate is above that expected in the population is not known, and no definitive increase in the risk for leukemia has been documented with the use of hydroxyurea alone for individuals with myeloproliferative diseases or cyanotic heart disease.

While there are other inducers of fetal hemoglobin available in research protocols—5-azacytadine, decitabine, and butyrates—their nonoral formulation, the unknown long-term effects of DNA methylation (5-azacytadine and decitabine), unsustained increases in Hb F (arginine butyrates), and inconvenience (phenylbutyrates) make them less attractive (26).

Other Drugs

Agents that modify the pathophysiology of SCD are based on their ability to reduce Hb S polymerization *in vitro:* these include hemoglobin S modifiers (urea, organic compounds), inhibitors of the Gardos channel (clotrimazole, ICA 17403), chloride and cation channel blocker (dipyridamole, magnesium pidolate, NS-3623), antiadherence agents (Poloxamer 188, pentoxifylline), and nitric oxide. Many are in preclinical testing; some are in therapeutic trials. Erythropoietin, at doses 2 to 5 times those used in renal failure, in combination with hydroxyurea can increase total hemoglobin.

SPECIAL TOPICS

Contraception and Pregnancy

Hydroxyurea is a teratogen in animal models, and both men and women who are taking hydroxyurea should use contraception and discontinue the drug if pregnancy is planned. There is little published data on the effect of hydroxyurea on the developing fetus. In more than a dozen individuals who continued hydroxyurea throughout pregnancy, there were no fetal malformations. Hydroxyurea is also secreted into breast milk, and breast feeding should be avoided.

Pregnant women with SCD are at an increased risk of preeclampsia, sickle pain crises, acute anemia or hemolysis, and postpartum infections (endometritis or pyelonephritis) (27,28). Their miscarriage rate is at least 6%. Maternal mortality is low and the overall outcome of the pregnancies is favorable; more than 90% of infants have Apgar scores of 7 or greater. At least 20% of infants will be small for gestation age (less than tenth percentile), and at least 25% are born prematurely (average at 34 to 37 weeks). Hb SS women tend to have more frequent or severe complications than Hb SC women. Transfusions are usually reserved for pregnancies complicated by progressive anemia, increased pain episodes, preeclampsia, prior pregnancy loss, or multiple gestations; prophylactic transfusions are generally discouraged.

Anesthesia and Surgery

Surgery and anesthesia have higher morbidity and mortality in SCD compared to the general population; the risk is higher in those with Hb SS or Hb S/β^0 thalassemia than those with Hb SC or Hb S/β^+ thalassemia (21). Complications may be more frequent with regional anesthesia. Acute chest syndrome and postoperative infection are the most common, followed by pain crisis and stroke (Table 4-9).

SICKLE CELL TRAIT

Approximately 8% of African Americans have sickle cell trait (SCT) (7). Under physiologic conditions, vaso-occlusion does not occur. Carriers have normal life expectancy and many

TABLE 4–9. *Perioperative considerations for sickle cell patients*

Preoperative
1. Simple transfusions to achieve hemoglobin of 10 g/dL in Hb SS and Hb S/β^0 thalassemia. Individuals with Hb SC may require exchange transfusion, especially prior to abdominal surgery.
2. Blood typing for additional antigens, such as C, E, Kell, Kidd (Jk), S, and Duffy (Fy), to minimize alloimmunization.
3. Hydration

Postoperative
1. Hydration, oxygen, and monitoring respiration and peripheral perfusion.
2. Monitoring for acute chest syndrome, infection, pain crisis, or stroke.

Hb, hemoglobin.

participate successfully in competitive sports or rigorous military training. There are exercise-related mortalities reported in these individuals, which can be minimized by avoiding heat stress, dehydration, and sleep deprivation, and with gradual heat acclimation and exercise endurance.

Compared to the general population, persons with SCT have similar rates of developing heart disease, stroke, leg ulcers, or arthritis. They are also not more likely to develop complications from anesthetic agents. However, SCT is associated with increased risk for traumatic eye injury, hyposthenuria, hematuria, and splenic infarction. If traumatic eye injury occurs with hemorrhage into the anterior chamber, sickle erythrocytes may clog the trabecular outflow channels, increase intraocular pressure, and lead to acute glaucoma, requiring urgent evaluation and treatment. Microscopic medullary necrosis may lead to inability to maximally concentrate urine (hyposthenuria); renal papillary necrosis can cause hematuria. Changes in urinary frequency, pattern, and color should be closely evaluated. There have been occasional case reports of splenic infarction in SCT associated with hypoxemia or low or high altitude; this risk appears to be small, and there are athletes who have successfully competed in these geographic conditions. Pregnant women with SCT are at an increased risk for urinary tract infections, preeclampsia, and postpartum endometritis, their infants also tend to be smaller.

CLINICAL SYNDROMES AND TREATMENT OF THALASSEMIA

Anemia, Transfusions, and Splenomegaly

α-Thalassemia (mainly Hb H phenotype) and β-thalassemia are clinically characterized by chronic hemolytic anemia, hepato-splenomegaly, skeletal deformities, leg ulcers, gallstones, and folate deficiency. There are also two rare forms of α-thalassemia with mental retardation and developmental abnormalities, ATR 16 and ATR X syndromes. Transfusions and iron chelation are the mainstay of therapy and have improved the quality of life and extended life expectancy. After diagnosis in infancy or childhood, when to start transfusion depends on the impact which anemia has on the child: fatigue, reduced growth velocity, skeletal dysmorphism, poor weight gain, or organomegaly. Once initiated, the target hemoglobin in a transfusion regimen is 10 g/dL, but some have used a higher goal. Transfusions are administered every 2 to 4 weeks through adulthood. Improvements in clinical symptoms and signs can be seen in adequately transfused individuals. Red cell alloimmunization can be minimized as in SCD by typing for major and minor blood group antigens (ABO, Rh, Kell, Kidd, and Duffy) and prestorage leukocyte depletion.

Splenomegaly can be seen when transfusions are inadequate or in the presence of red cell alloimmunization, and is associated with worsening anemia, leukopenia, and thrombocytopenia. The hemoglobin will typically drop about 1.5 g/dL per week in nonsplenectomized individuals; in hypersplenism, this rate of decline will be higher and eventually there will be an inadequate rise in posttransfusion hemoglobin. Splenectomy will improve these hematologic parameters and transfusion effectiveness, but should be performed after vaccination for encapsulated organisms (*S. pneumoniae, H. influenza, and N. meningitidis*), and in children older than 5 years of age. Postsplenectomized transfusions should produce a 1 g/dL per week decrease in hemoglobin. Penicillin prophylaxis is appropriate. Postsplenectomy thrombocytosis can be variable but does not require antiplatelet therapy.

Iron Overload and Chelation

Early diagnosis and long-term transfusions have shifted the major complications of thalassemia from those secondary to the hemolytic anemia to the sequalae of iron overload. Excess iron from cumulative transfusions overwhelms the transferrin system and accumulates in the heart, liver, and various endocrine organs. The most serious result is heart failure and sudden unpredictable ventricular arrhythmia, which account for the majority of deaths in thalassemic individuals. Nonuniform deposition of iron in the cardiac myocytes leads to the loss of normal cardiac architecture and fibrosis, resulting in the dilated cardiomyopathy and life-threatening arrhythmia. Excess iron also accumulates in the liver, producing hepatic inflammation, dysfunction, and fibrosis. While CT or MRI imaging, superconducting susceptometry (SQUID), and serum ferritin are helpful in estimating the amount of iron in liver, biopsy remains standard. Furthermore, iron overload also affects various endocrine organs and can cause reduced growth velocity in children; hypothyroidism; hypogonadism with pubertal delay or arrest; hypoparathyroidism leading to hypocalcemia and osteoporosis, and diabetes. All are managed in collaboration with endocrinologists.

The toxic effects of excess iron can be minimized by iron chelation. Desferrioxamine (deferoxamine or Desferal) is the only Food and Drug Administration-approved drug in the United States for this purpose. Desferal binds to free iron in serum. The chelator can be administered as early as 2 1/2 years of age at 20 to 60 mg/kg (or 1.5 to 4 g per adult or adolescent) per day, and typically for at least 5 days a week. It is delivered by subcutaneous or intravenous injection over 8 to 12 or 24 hours (29,30). There is also evidence that twice per day subcutaneous bolus injection may also be efficacious (31). Side effects of desferrioxamine are infrequent; they include impaired vision or hearing, motor-sensory neuropathy, changes in renal or pulmonary function, joint pain, metaphyseal dysplasia, or growth retardation. Oral deferiprone was used in clinical trials and appeared promising, but enthusiasm has diminished because of common side effects of gastrointestinal discomfort, joint pain, and agranulocytosis, and controversy regarding effectiveness in iron removal and the possibility of hepatic fibrosis (32). There are other alternative chelators that currently under active preclinical (HBED) and clinical investigations (ICL 670A).

Fetal Hemoglobin Induction

The major endpoint for fetal hemoglobin induction in thalassemia is an increase in total hemoglobin. Unfortunately, hydroxyurea has not achieved this goal in most thalassemic major patients receiving chronic transfusions, possibly due to loss of Hb F response with transfusions or to certain mutations that are resistant to Hb F induction. Hydroxyurea, however, has had some effect in Hb Lepore/β-thalassemia, Hb E/β-thalassemia, and β-thalassemia intermedia (26). Erythropoietin also can be used with hydroxyurea but the response is variable. Other inducers of Hb F, such as butyrates, have increased Hb F but not total hemoglobin.

THERAPY WITH CURATIVE INTENT

Hematopoietic Stem Cell Transplantation

Myeloablative hematopoietic stem cell transplantation (HSCT) is currently the only cure for SCD and thalassemia (33). The lack of available human leukocyte antigen (HLA)-matched sibling donors and transplant-related complications have limited its wide applicability. For SCD, HSCT is generally reserved for patients less than 17 years of age, who are nonresponsive to hydroxyurea, and those with prior SCD-related organ damage (stroke, ACS, frequent pain crises, or multiple sites of osteonecrosis). For thalassemia, HSCT is also generally reserved for those less than 17 years of age with signs of liver dysfunction from iron damage (Pesaro class II and III). Encouraging animal and clinical data suggest reduced-intensity (nonmyeloablative) transplantations can achieve mixed donor and host hematopoiesis, and ameliorate disease complications. If confirmed, this approach may be a reasonable alternative for older individuals who otherwise meet criteria for a standard myeloablative HSCT. Related umbilical cord blood transplantation is also an alternative.

TABLE 4–10. *Clinical features of two common severe beta-globulin disorders*

Sickle cell disease and thalassemia syndromes
Common features related to pathophysiology:
1. Hemolytic anemia (variable degree)
2. Gallstones
3. Leg ulcers (less common in thalassemia)
4. Pulmonary hypertension (less common in thalassemia)
Common features related to chronic transfusions: (more common in thalassemia)
1. Red cell alloimmunization
2. Infections (HIV, hepatitis, WNV, CJD)
3. Iron overload
Dilated cardiomyopathy and arrhythmia
Endocrinopathy (hypothyroidism, hypogonadism, diabetes, osteoporosis)
Liver dysfunction and cirrhosis

SCD specific manifestations	Thalassemia specific manifestations
1. Vaso-occlusive pain	1. Splenomegaly
2. Stroke, retinal diseases	2. Thromboembolism
3. Acute chest syndrome	3. Infections: Yersinia spp.
4. Avascular necrosis (osteonecrosis), fat embolism, osteomyelitis	
5. Splenic sequestration and eventual infarct in Hb SS or Hb S/β^0 thalassemia; splenomegaly in Hb SC	
6. Priapism	
7. Hyposthenuria; renal damage by glomerular or tubular damage or papillary necrosis in some individuals	
8. Infections: Parvovirus B19, salmonella spp, *S. pneumoniae, H. influenza*	
9. Hepatic sequestration or crisis	

HIV, human immunodeficiency virus; WNV, West Nile virus; CJD, Creutzfeldt-Jacob disease; SCD, sickle cell disease; Hb, hemoglobin

Gene Therapy

Autologous transplantation following the insertion of a normal or therapeutic globin gene into hematopoietic stem cells is a rational approach to SCD and thalassemia (34). While problems in attaining reliable expression of globin constructs in erythroid progeny of hematopoietic stem cells proved seemingly insurmountable for a number of years, significant advances have been made toward this goal using lentiviral based upon the human immunodeficiency virus (HIV). Therapeutic correction of murine models of both β-thalassemia and SCD has been achieved using this approach. These advances, coupled with progress in the ability to achieve moderate levels of engraftment of genetically modified cells in large animals have set the stage for preclinical testing in the non-human primate autologous transplant model. These preclinical studies should allow better assessment of the recently documented risk for insertional mutagenesis as well as optimization of gene transfer techniques in order to increase the likelihood of ultimate clinical success while minimizing risks.

Summaries for SCD and thalassemia are provided in Tables 4-10 and 4-11.

TABLE 4–11. *Suggested health maintenance schedule (7)*

	Routine Health Maintenance	Supplement	Blood tests	Special Studies
Sickle Cell Disease				
Age 0–2 yr	Penicillin prophylaxis, Prevnar (7 valent), routine vaccinations	Folate, multivitamin, iron if appropriate	CBC every 3–6 months, Hb F q6 months	
Age 2–18 yr	Penicillin prophylaxis until age 5, Pneumovax (23 valent), routine vaccinations, yearly influenza vaccination, yearly eye exam,	Folate; iron if appropriate	CBC every 6 months, renal and hepatic function and iron studies yearly	TCD every 6–12 months, O_2 saturation every 6–12 months
Age >18 yr	Pneumovax, yearly influenza vaccination; yearly eye examination (especially in SC disease); hepatitis A and B vaccination	Folate; iron if appropriate	Every 6 months: UA for proteinuria, B_{12}, renal and hepatic function. Every 3–6 months: CBC, Hb F (if on hydroxyurea)	RUQ ultrasound every 1–2 years for biliary sludge; echo yearly; PFTs yearly
Thalassemia				
Age 0–2 yrs	Routine vaccinations, transfusion, possible iron chelation, growth velocity curve	Folate, multivitamin		
Age 2–18 yrs	Routine vaccinations; in those >5 yrs of age vaccinations for possible splenectomy; possible iron chelation; growth velocity curve	Folate, multivitamin	CBC, hepatic, renal functions, iron studies every 3–6 months.	Evaluate for iron overload; endocrine consultation every 6–12 months, echo yearly
Age >18 yrs	Vaccinations for possible splenectomy	Folate, multivitamin	CBC, hepatic, renal functions, iron studies every 6 months.	Evaluate for iron overload; endocrine consultation every 6–12 months; echo yearly

CBC, complete blood count; TCD, transcranial Doppler; RUQ, right upper quadrant; SC, heterozygous hemoglobin S and C; PFTs, pulmonary function tests.

REFERENCES

1. Rund D, Rachmilewitz E. Pathophysiology of alpha- and beta-thalassemia: therapeutic implications. *Semin Hematol* 2001;38:343–349.
2. Steinberg MH, Rodgers GP. Pathophysiology of sickle cell disease: role of cellular and genetic modifiers. *Semin Hematol* 2001;38:299–306.
3. Gladwin MT, Schechter AN. Nitric oxide therapy in sickle cell disease. *Semin Hematol* 2001;38: 333–342.
4. Platt OS. The acute chest syndrome of sickle cell disease. *N Engl J Med* 2000;342:1904–1947.
5. Cao A, Galanello R, Rosatelli MC. Prenatal diagnosis and screening of the haemoglobinopathies. *Baillieres Clin Haematol* 1998;11(1):215–38.
6. The laboratory diagnosis of haemoglobinopathies. *Br J Haematol* 1998;101:783–792.
7. *The Management of Sickle Cell Disease.* 4th ed. Bethesda, MD: National Institutes of Health: National Heart, Lung, and Blood Institute, 2002.
8. Ballantyne JC, Mao J. Opioid therapy for chronic pain. *N Engl J Med* 2003;349:1943–1953.
9. Gaston MH, Verter JI, Woods G, et al. Prophylaxis with oral penicillin in children with sickle cell anemia. A randomized trial. *N Engl J Med* 1986;314:1593–1599.
10. Smith-Whitley K, Zhao H, Hodinka RL, et al. Epidemiology of human parvovirus B19 in children with sickle cell disease. *Blood* 2004;103:422–427.
11. Adams RJ, McKie VC, Hsu L, et al. Prevention of a first stroke by transfusions in children with sickle cell anemia and abnormal results on transcranial Doppler ultrasonography. *N Engl J Med* 1998;339:5–11.
12. Ohene-Frempong K, Weiner SJ, Sleeper LA, et al. Cerebrovascular accidents in sickle cell disease: rates and risk factors. *Blood* 1998;91:288–294.
13. Vichinsky EP, Neumayr LD, Earles AN, et al. Causes and outcomes of the acute chest syndrome in sickle cell disease. *N Engl J Med* 2000;342:1855–1865.
14. Miller ST, Wright E, Abboud M, et al. Impact of chronic transfusion on incidence of pain and acute chest syndrome during the Stroke Prevention Trial (STOP) in sickle-cell anemia. *J Pediatr* 2001; 139:785–789.
15. Castro O, Brambilla DJ, Thorington B, et al. The acute chest syndrome in sickle cell disease: incidence and risk factors. The Cooperative Study of Sickle Cell Disease. *Blood* 1994;84:643–649.
16. Mantadakis E, Ewalt DH, Cavender JD, et al. Outpatient penile aspiration and epinephrine irrigation for young patients with sickle cell anemia and prolonged priapism. *Blood* 2000;95:78–82.
17. Styles LA, Vichinsky EP. Core decompression in avascular necrosis of the hip in sickle-cell disease. *Am J Hematol* 1996;52:103–107.
18. Koshy M, Entsuah R, Koranda A, et al. Leg ulcers in patients with sickle cell disease. *Blood* 1989; 74:1403–1408.
19. Eckman JR. Leg ulcers in sickle cell disease. *Hematol Oncol Clin North Am* 1996;10:1333–1344.
20. Charache S, Terrin ML, Moore RD, et al. Effect of hydroxyurea on the frequency of painful crises in sickle cell anemia. *N Engl J Med* 1995;332:1317–1322.
21. Vichinsky EP, Haberkern CM, Neumayr L, et al. A comparison of conservative and aggressive transfusion regimens in the perioperative management of sickle cell disease. The Preoperative Transfusion in Sickle Cell Disease Study Group. *N Engl J Med* 1995;333:206–213.
22. Koshy M, Burd L, Wallace D, et al. Prophylactic red-cell transfusions in pregnant patients with sickle cell disease. A randomized cooperative study. *N Engl J Med* 1988;319:1447–1452.
23. Neumayr L, Koshy M, Haberkern C, et al. Surgery in patients with hemoglobin SC disease. Preoperative Transfusion in Sickle Cell Disease Study Group. *Am J Hematol* 1998;57:101–108.
24. Steinberg MH, Barton F, Castro O, et al. Effect of hydroxyurea on mortality and morbidity in adult sickle cell anemia: risks and benefits up to 9 years of treatment. *JAMA* 2003;289:1645–1651.
25. Wang WC, Helms RW, Lynn HS, et al. Effect of hydroxyurea on growth in children with sickle cell anemia: results of the HUG-KIDS Study. *J Pediatr* 2002;140:225–229.
26. Atweh GF, Loukopoulos D. Pharmacological induction of fetal hemoglobin in sickle cell disease and beta-thalassemia. *Semin Hematol* 2001;38:367–373.
27. Smith JA, Espeland M, Bellevue R, et al. Pregnancy in sickle cell disease: experience of the Cooperative Study of Sickle Cell Disease. *Obstet Gynecol* 1996;87:199–204.
28. Sun PM, Wilburn W, Raynor BD, et al. Sickle cell disease in pregnancy: Twenty years of experience at Grady Memorial Hospital, Atlanta, Georgia. *Am J Obstet Gynecol* 2001;184:1127–1130.
29. Giardina PJ, Grady RW. Chelation therapy in beta-thalassemia: an optimistic update. *Semin Hematol* 2001;38:360–366.

30. Davis BA, Porter JB. Long-term outcome of continuous 24-hour deferoxamine infusion via indwelling intravenous catheters in high-risk beta -thalassemia. *Blood* 2000;95:1229–1236.
31. Franchini M, Gandini G, de Gironcoli M, et al. Safety and efficacy of subcutaneous bolus injection of deferoxamine in adult patients with iron overload. *Blood* 2000;95:2776–2779.
32. Olivieri NF, Brittenham GM, McLaren CE, et al. Long-term safety and effectiveness of iron-chelation therapy with deferiprone for thalassemia major. *N Engl J Med* 1998;339:417–423.
33. Sullivan KM, Parkman R, Walters MC. Bone marrow transplantation for non-malignant disease. *Hematology* 2000;319–338.
34. Tisdale J, Sadelain M. Toward gene therapy for disorders of globin synthesis. *Semin Hematol* 2001; 38:382–392.

5

Porphyrias

Peiman Hematti and Lawrence S. Lessin

The porphyrias are a diverse group of uncommon metabolic disorders caused by inherited deficiencies of the enzymes involved in the heme biosynthetic pathway. Mutations of the genes of all of these hemasynthetic enzymes have been identified. An exception is porphyria cutanea tarda, in which the enzyme deficiency in most cases is acquired. In all these ecogenic disorders, it is the interaction of genetic, physiologic, and environmental factors that cause disease in affected individuals. Each defective enzyme results in a characteristic clinical phenotype of porphyria, although disease mechanisms are not fully understood.

EPIDEMIOLOGY

Porphyria cutanea tarda is the most prevalent of porphyrias, both genetic and acquired combined, but acute intermittent porphyria is the most common of genetic porphyrias. Acute intermittent porphyria has an estimated incidence of 5 in 100,000 in the United States and northern European countries. Approximately 90% of patients with this inherited enzyme deficiency remain symptom free throughout their life. In contrast only rare cases of aminolevulinic acid dehydratase deficiency (ALAD) have been thus far reported.

PATHOPHYSIOLOGY

Heme is a complex of an iron atom and protoporphyrin IX. Heme is produced in a multistep biosynthetic pathway that functions mostly in the erythroid bone marrow and hepatocytes. Approximately 85% of the heme produced in the body is synthesized in erythroid cells to provide for hemoglobin formation. Most of the remainder is produced in the liver to provide heme for cytochrome P-450 and other enzymes. Eight enzymes are involved in this tightly regulated pathway that sequentially convert glycine and succinyl CoA into heme (Fig. 5-1). Sequences of the genes for all these enzymes and their molecular defects have been well characterized.

Mutations of the first enzyme, δ-aminolevulinic acid (ALA) synthase results in X-linked sideroblastic anemia. Mutations of the other seven enzymes result in porphyria syndromes because of overproduction of metabolic precursors and intermediates and/or their accumulation in tissues. All of these intermediate products are potentially toxic, and their overproduction causes the neurovisceral and/or photocutaneous symptoms characteristic of porphyria syndromes.

Despite the characterization of these disorders at the molecular level, the exact pathophysiologic mechanisms responsible for the specific organ manifestations are not fully understood.

Porphyrias are heterogeneous at the molecular level with numerous mutations found for each gene. There is a significant interaction between specific inherited genetic defects and acquired or environmental factors that result in a spectrum of clinical manifestations in affected patients. Patients with gene mutations for the acute hepatic forms of porphyrias may remain asymptomatic unless they are exposed to certain medications (Table 5-1) or hormones, or

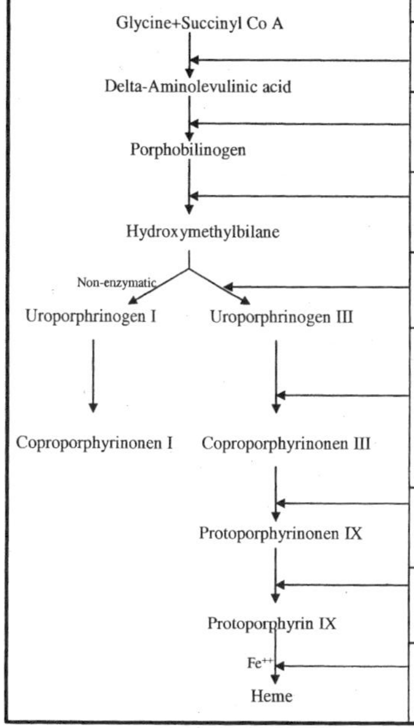

Enzyme Deficiency	Disease	Inheritance	Symptomatology	Hematological symptoms	Accumulated products
ALA synthase (ALAS)	Sideroblastic anemia (XLSA)	X-linked sideroblastic anemia	Hypochromic anemia	Hypochromic anemia	Ring Sideroblasts
ALA dehydratase (ALAD)	δ-Aminolevulinic acid dehydratase-deficient porphyria (ADP)	Autosomal recessive	Neurovisceral	None	Urinary ALA & coproporphyrin; RBC Zn protoporphyrin
Porphobilinogen Deaminase (PBGD)	Acute intermittent porphyria (AIP)	Autosomal dominant	Neurovisceral	None	Urinary ALA & PBG
Uroporphyrin-ogen III cosynthase (UCoS)	Congenital Erythropoietic porphyria (CEP)	Autosomal recessive	Photocutaneous	Hemolytic anemia, Splenomegaly	Urinary and RBC Uroporphyrin I and, Coprporphyrin I
Uroporphyrinogen Decarboxylase (UROD)	Porphyria cutanea tarda (PCT)	Acquired (type I) Autosomal dominant (type II & III)	Photocutaneous	None	Urinary uroporphyrin & 7-carboxylic porphyrin; Fecal isocoproporphyrin
	Hepatoerythropoietic porphyria (HEP)	Autosomal recessive	Photocutaneous	Hemolytic anemia, Splenomegaly	Urinary uroporphyrin; Fecal isocoproporphyrin, RBC Zn protoporphyrin
Coproporphyrinogen oxidase (CPO)	Hereditary coproporphyria (HCP)	Autosomal recessive	Neurovisceral & Photocutaneous	None	Urinary ALA & PBG; Fecal coproporphyrin
Protoporphyrinogen oxidase (PPO)	Variegate porphyria (VP)	Autosomal dominant	Neurovisceral & Photocutaneous	None	Urinary ALA &PBG; Urinary & fecal coproporphyrin
Ferrochelatase (FeC)	Erythropoietic protoporphyria (EPP)	Autosomal dominant	Photocutaneous	Anemia	RBC protoporphyrin; Fecal protoporphyrin

Glycine+Succinyl Co A

Delta-Aminolevulinic acid

Porphobilinogen

Hydroxymethylbilane

Uroporphyrinogen I   Uroporphyrinogen III (Non-enzymatic)

Coproporphyrinonen I   Coproporphyrinonen III

Protoporphyrinonen IX

Protoporphyrin IX

Fe⁺⁺ → Heme

FIG. 5-1. Classification of porphyrias based on their corresponding enzymatic deficiencies and their major symptoms. (Modified from Sassa S, Shibahara S. Disorders of heme production and Catabolism. In: Handin RI, Lux SE, Stossel, TP, eds. *Blood: Principles and Practice of Hematology.* 2nd ed. Philadelphia, Lippincott Williams and Wilkins, 2003, with permission.)

TABLE 5–1. *Drugs considered unsafe or safe in the acute porphyrias*

Unsafe drugs	Safe Drugs
Alcohol	Acetaminophen
Aluminum-containing antacids	Aspirin
Barbiturates	Atropine
Carbamazepine	Cimetidine
Danazol	Corticosteroids
Erythromycin	Gabapentin
Metoclopramide	Gentamycin
Isoniazid	Insulin
Nifedipine	Narcotic analgesics
Phenytoin	Peniciliin and derivatives
Rifampin	Phenothiazines
Sulfonamide antibiotics	Propanalol

are stressed by starvation, infection, surgery, or other intercurrent disorders. Under these environmental circumstances, affected patients develop characteristic neurologic disturbances.

Photocutaneous hypersensitivity and resultant skin damage occurs after exposure to ultraviolet light. When porphyrins absorb light of this wavelength, they produce free radicals that can induce oxidant tissue damage. Consequently, avoidance of precipitating factors is key in the therapy of porphyrias.

CLASSIFICATION AND CLINICAL MANIFESTATIONS: HEPATIC AND ERYTHROPOIETIC TYPES

For clinical purposes, porphyrias can be classified into hepatic and erythropoietic types depending on the major tissue site of production and accumulation of the heme precursors. The major manifestations of the hepatic porphyrias are neurovisceral symptoms, including abdominal pain, neurologic symptoms, and psychiatric disorders, whereas the erythropoietic porphyrias usually present primarily with cutaneous photosensitivity and hemolytic anemia. Porphyrias can be also classified as acute porphyrias presenting with life-threatening neurovisceral manifestations and nonacute porphyrias characterized by photosensitivity syndromes, but there can be some overlap in clinical manifestations.

Because the porphyrias are well characterized at the molecular genetic level, they should be specifically classified by their unique enzyme deficiencies.

DIAGNOSIS

Many symptoms of the porphyrias are nonspecific, and diagnosis requires a high index of suspicion. However, although the porphyrias are often suspected in a patient with vague and unexplained complaints, actual diagnosis is rare. A useful first step is to determine which one of the three major manifestations of the porphyrias: neurovisceral symptoms, photosensitivity, or hemolytic anemia is present.

- Neurovisceral symptoms are present in δ-aminolevulinic acid dehydratase-deficiency (ADP), acute intermittent porphyria (AIP), hereditary coproporphyria (HCP), and variegate porphyria (VP).
- Photosensitivity is present in congenital erythropoietic porphyria (CEP), porphyria cutanea tarda (PCT), hepatoerythropoietic porphyria (HEP), HCP, VP, and erythropoietic protoporphyria (EPP).

- Neurovisceral symptoms and photosensitivity are present in HCP and VP.
- Hemolytic anemia is present in CEP, HEP, and EPP.

Laboratory testing is then required to confirm or exclude the various types of porphyrias. The diagnosis is made initially by detection of the metabolite produced and/or excreted in excess in red cells, plasma, urine, and/or feces. Porphyrin precursors in urine and total porphyrins in plasma are the initial diagnostic tests for acute and cutaneous porphyrias, respectively. Today the diagnosis of many of porphyrias can be confirmed by measuring the enzymatic activity in the appropriate tissue directly or by specific molecular genetic testing.

SPECIFIC TYPES OF PORPHYRIAS

δ-Aminolevulinic Acid Dehydratase-Deficiency Porphyria (ADP)

ADP is a rare autosomal recessive porphyria caused by markedly deficient activity of ALAD, the second enzyme in the heme biosynthetic pathway. The diagnosis has been unequivocally confirmed only in a few cases. Clinical manifestations are primarily neurovisceral, and their treatment and prevention are the same as for other acute porphyrias. Lead poisoning should be excluded, since it also diminishes activity of ALAD, may present as a clinical phenocopy, and is far more common.

Acute Intermittent Porphyria (AIP)

AIP is inherited as autosomal dominant condition resulting from a partial deficiency of porphobilinogen deaminase (PBGD) activity (the third enzyme of the pathway). Approximately 90% of heterozygotes remain biochemically normal and clinically asymptomatic throughout life. Clinical expression of the disease is usually the result of exposure to factors such as endogenous and exogenous corticosteroid hormones, a low-calorie diet, certain drugs (barbiturates and sulfonamide antibiotics are most commonly implicated), alcohol ingestion, and stresses such as intercurrent illnesses, infection, and surgery. Symptoms usually develop after puberty and are more frequent in women. The pathophysiologic hallmark of the disease is neurologic dysfunction affecting peripheral, autonomic, and/or central nervous systems occurring as intermittent acute attacks. The most common symptom is acute abdominal pain (in 90% of cases) which may be generalized or localized, but tenderness, fever, and leukocytosis are absent because the symptoms are neurologic in origin, from the visceral autonomic nervous system involvement. Gastrointestinal manifestations also include abdominal distention, nausea, vomiting, diarrhea, or constipation. Peripheral sensory or motor neuropathy is another common feature of AIP. Psychiatric symptoms including hysteria, anxiety, apathy, depression, phobia, psychosis, agitation, disorientation, hallucinations, and schizophrenic-type behaviors can be the only manifestations of the disease. Acute attacks may be accompanied by seizures, either a manifestation of the porphyria itself or caused by hyponatremia (from inappropriate secretion of antidiuretic hormone), also commonly occur during attacks. Sympathetic hyperactivity results in tachycardia (in 80% of cases), hypertension, tremors, and sweating. Because of the nonspecific nature of symptoms and signs, use of highly sensitive and specific laboratory tests is essential to the diagnosis.

During acute attacks, symptomatic treatment may include narcotic analgesics, phenothiazines, and low-dose benzodiazepines. Although intravenous glucose (at least 300 g per day) can be effective in acute attacks of porphyria, intravenous heme is now considered the treatment of choice to reduce excretion of porphyria. Infusion of heme should be initiated as soon as possible after onset of an attack, but the rate of recovery depends on the degree of neuronal damage and may take days to months. Any intercurrent infection or disease should also be treated immediately. Identification and avoidance of precipitating factors is also essential for prevention. Cyclical attacks in some women associated with fluctuations in estrogen and progestins can be prevented with a long-acting gonadotropin-releasing hormone analogue.

Congenital Erythropoietic Porphyria (CEP)

CEP, an autosomal-recessive disorder also known as Gunther's disease, is caused by deficient activity of uroporphyrinogen III synthase (the fourth enzyme of the pathway) and is associated with hemolytic anemia and cutaneous lesions. Severe cutaneous photosensitivity usually begins in early infancy as blistering of sun-exposed areas of the skin. Recurrent vesicles, bullae, and secondary infection can lead to cutaneous scarring and deformities. Porphyrin deposition may also occur in bones, leading to brownish discoloration of teeth. Protecting skin from sunlight is essential.

Mild to severe hemolytic anemia and secondary splenomegaly are features of CEP and anemia can be severe. Transfusion is effective but results in iron overload if chronic. Splenectomy may reduce hemolysis and decrease the transfusion requirement. In transfusion-dependent children, allogenic stem cell transplantation can be considered.

Porphyria Cutanea Tarda (PCT)

Porphyria cutanea tarda, the most common of the porphyrias, is caused by acquired or inherited deficiency of uroporphyrinogen decarboxylase (the fifth enzyme of the pathway). The disease occurs worldwide but its exact incidence is not known. The disease can be *sporadic* (noninherited or type I, most common) or *familial* (types II and III), although these subtypes are not distinguishable clinically. The frequency of disease varies in relation to risk factors such as alcohol use, smoking, hepatitis C and human immunodeficiency virus (HIV) infection. The hallmark of PCT is cutaneous photosensitivity presenting as chronic blistering lesions on sun-exposed areas of skin without neurologic manifestations. Chronic changes including cutaneous thickening, scarring, and calcification can mimic systemic sclerosis. Also common are facial hypertrichosis and hyperpigmentation. PCT is almost always associated with abnormalities in liver function tests, and the risk of developing hepatocellular carcinoma is significantly increased in this disease.

Alcohol ingestion, estrogens, iron supplements, and, if possible, any drugs that may exacerbate the disease should be avoided. A complete response can usually be achieved by repeated phlebotomy to reduce hepatic iron and is still considered standard treatment. Low dose chloroquine or hydroxychloroquine are also effective, especially when phlebotomy is contraindicated. In contrast, similar skin lesions in VP, HCP, CEP, and HEP are unresponsive to these therapeutic interventions.

Hepatoerythropoietic Porphyria (HEP)

This rare form of porphyria has been recently described. HEP is clinically indistinguishable from CEP and is caused by homozygous defect of the same enzyme involved in porphyria cutanea tarda. Patients usually present after birth with blistering skin lesions and scarring. Hemolytic anemia is often present with splenomegaly. Avoiding sunlight is essential.

Hereditary Coproporphyria (HCP)

HCP is an autosomal dominant porphyria resulting from deficiency of coproporphyrinogen oxidase (the sixth enzyme of the pathway). The neurovisceral symptoms and other manifestations as well as the precipitating factors are virtually identical to those of AIP but photosensitivity similar to PCT may also occur in one-third of the patients. Avoidance of precipitating factors as in AIP is important. Neurologic symptoms are treated as in AIP but in contrast to PCT, phlebotomy or chloroquine is not effective for cutaneous lesions.

Variegate Porphyria (VP)

This hepatic porphyria, the result of a mutation of the protoporphyria oxidase gene, is transmitted as autosomal dominant disorder and is particularly common in South African whites (prevalence of 3 in 1,000) because of a genetic founder effect from a couple who emigrated from Holland to South Africa in late 1600s. The disease was termed variegate because it can present with either neurovisceral symptoms, cutaneous photosensitivity, or both. Neurovisceral symptoms are very similar to those of AIP and are provoked by the same precipitates. Acute attacks are treated with glucose and heme infusion as in AIP. Occurrence of skin manifestations is usually separate from the neurovisceral symptoms, and avoiding sun exposure is the only effective preventative measure for cutaneous photosensitivity.

Erythropoietic Protoporphyria

EPP, also known as protoporphyria, results from deficiency of ferrochelatase activity (the last enzyme in the heme biosynthetic pathway). EPP is the most common erythropoietic porphyria and third most common porphyria in general. Skin photosensitivity beginning in childhood is typical of the disease but the skin lesions are different from other porphyrias. Erythema, burning, and itching accompanied by swelling can develop within minutes of sun exposure, but sparse vesicles and bullae are seen in only a minority of the cases. Chronic skin changes may occur but severe scarring is rare. Oral β-carotene (120 to 180 mg per day) can be effective in many patients with EPP, in contrast to those with photosensitivity from other forms of porphyria. The mechanism of action of β-carotene is not clear but is attributed to its antioxidant effect. In some patients, accumulation of protoporphyrin causes chronic liver disease that can progress to hepatic failure and death. Neurovisceral symptoms are seen only in patients with severe hepatic complications. Protoporphyrin-rich gallstones may occur. Mild anemia is sometimes seen in patients with EPP but hemolysis is either infrequent or very mild. Splenectomy may be helpful when the disease is accompanied by hemolysis and significant splenomegaly. Caloric restriction, drugs, and exogenous sex hormones should be avoided. Intravenous heme therapy is sometimes beneficial. Liver transplantation has been performed but the protoporphyrin-induced damage can recur in the donor liver.

REFERENCES

1. Anderson KE, Sassa S, Bishop DF, et al. Disorders of heme biosynthesis: X-linked sideroblastic anemia and the porphyrias. In: Scriver CR, Beaudet AL, Sly WS, Valle D, eds. *The Metabolic and Molecular Bases of Inherited Disease.* 8th ed. Vol. 2. New York, McGraw-Hill, 2001;2991–3062.
2. Sassa S, Shibahara S. Disorders of heme production and catabolism. In: Handin RI, Lux SE, Stossel TP, eds. *Blood: Principles and Practice of Hematology.* 2nd ed. Philadelphia, Lippincott Williams and Wilkins, 2003;1435–1501.
3. Foran SE, Abel G. Guide to porphyrias. A historical and clinical perspective. *Am J Clin Pathol* 2003; 119(suppl):86–93.
4. Sassa S. The porphyrias. *Photodermatolo Photoimmunol Photomed* 2002;18:56–67.
5. Sassa S. Hematologic aspects of the porphyrias. *Int J Hematol* 2000;71:1–17.
6. Sassa S, Kappas A. Molecular aspects of the inherited porphyrias. *J Intern Med* 2000;247:169–168.
7. Schmid R, ed. The porphyrias. *Semin Liver Dis* 1998;18:1–101.
8. Elder GH, Hift RJ, Meissner PN. The acute porphyrias. *Lancet* 1997;349:1613–1617.

6

Bone Marrow Failure Syndromes: Aplastic Anemia, Acquired and Constitutional, Paroxysmal Nocturnal Hemoglobinuria, Pure Red Blood Cell Aplasia, and Agranulocytosis

Neal S. Young, Phillip Scheinberg, and Johnson M. Liu

The bone marrow failure syndromes are characterized by inadequate blood cell production leading to low red blood cell, white blood cell, and/or platelet counts in the peripheral blood. Marrow failure can be acquired or constitutional, and may affect all three blood cell lines, resulting in pancytopenia, or only a single lineage. In most, the bone marrow shows a simple deficiency of the related precursor cells but marrow failure can also occur with relatively cellular marrows, presumably as a result of ineffective hematopoiesis, and can be associated with cytogenetic abnormalities (see Chapter 7) or a genetically altered cell, as in paroxysmal nocturnal hemoglobinuria, discussed in this chapter because of its intimate relationship to aplastic anemia (AA) (1). Even the paradigmatic syndrome of AA clinically and pathophysiologically shows overlap with related diseases (Fig. 6-1A).

ACQUIRED APLASTIC ANEMIA

Acquired AA is characterized by pancytopenia with a hypocellular, often "empty," bone marrow.

AA is uncommon in the West: its incidence in Europe is approximately 2 new cases per 1 million. However, the disease is twofold to threefold more frequent in East Asia and probably elsewhere in the developing world. In most series, patients are young; the majority present between 15 and 25 years of age. Historically, chemicals (benzene) and drugs (chloramphenicol) were implicated as causative but without satisfactory mechanisms of pathogenesis. The most important current associations are with nonsteroidal anti-inflammatory drugs, antithyroid drugs, penicillamine, allopurinol, and gold (Table 6-1) (2). Nonetheless, most AA is idiopathic, or without a presumed environmental factor in an individual patient.

Etiology and Pathophysiology

- *Hematopoiesis* is severely reduced in all AA, as observed in bone marrow specimens, CD34 cell counts, magnetic resonance imaging, or in functional studies of progenitors.
- Clinical and laboratory studies suggest that most acquired AA is secondary to immunologically mediated destruction of hematopoietic cells by cytotoxic lymphocytes (CTL) and their cytokine products, especially interferon-γ (IFN-γ) and tumor necrosis factor-α (TNF-α).
- Marrow failure rarely can follow infectious mononucleosis (Epstein-Barr virus [EBV] infection) and is a component of the stereotypical posthepatitis AA syndrome, which is unasso-

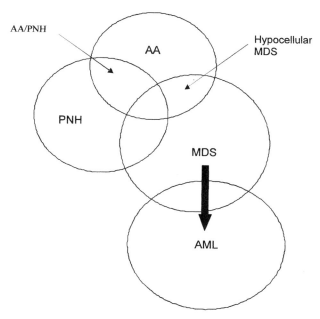

FIG. 6-1A. Venn diagram of the relationship among bone marrow failure syndromes. AA, aplastic anemia; PNH, paroxysmal nocturnal hemoglobinuria; MDS, myelodysplastic syndrome; AML, acute myeloid leukemia.

ciated with any known hepatitis virus. EBV and the putative agent of seronegative hepatitis behave as triggers for immune system activity. In contrast, parvovirus B19 directly infects and kills erythroid progenitor cells and causes pure red cell aplasia but not AA.
• Direct killing of marrow cells by cytotoxic agents occurs after cancer chemotherapy, producing transient marrow aplasia, but is probably unusual as a mechanism of idiosyncratic drug-associated AA.

Clinical Features

• Anemia leads to fatigue, weakness, lassitude, headaches, and in older patients dyspnea and chest pain; these symptoms are most commonly responsible for the clinical presentation.
• Thrombocytopenia produces mainly mucosal bleeding: petechiae of the skin and mucous membranes, epistaxis, and gum bleeding are frequent and early complaints. Bleeding is not brisk from low platelets unless in the presence of accompanying physical lesions, as in gastritis and fungal infection of the lungs. The most feared complication of thrombocytopenia is intracranial hemorrhage.
• Infection is unusual at presentation.
• Dark urine suggests paroxysmal nocturnal hemoglobinuria (PNH).

Occasionally moderate cytopenias are identified serendipitously by routine blood work or at preoperative evaluation.

• Constitutional symptoms (malaise, anorexia, and weight loss) should be absent.

TABLE 6–1. *Drugs associated with aplastic anemia in the International Aplastic Anemia and Agranulocytosis Study*

Drug
Nonsteroidal analgesics
Butazones
Indomethacin
Piroxicam
Diclofenac
Antibiotics
Sulfonamides*
Antithyroid drugs
Cardiovascular drugs
Furosemide
Psychotropic drugs
Phenothiazines
Corticosteroids
Penicillamine
Allopurinol
Gold

*Other than trimethoprim–sulfonamide combination.

Physical findings range from a patient who appears well with minimal findings to an acutely ill patient with signs of systemic toxicity. Cachexia, lymphadenopathy, and splenomegaly are not seen and suggest an alternative diagnosis.

- Thrombocytopenia results in petechiae, ecchymoses, gingival oozing, epistaxis, subconjunctival and retinal hemorrhage.
- Anemia is reflected in pallor of the skin mucous membranes, and nail beds.
- Constitutional AA is suggested by areas of hyperpigmentation or hypopigmentation of the skin, abnormal hands and thumbs, and short stature (Fanconi anemia), and nail dystrophy and oral leukoplakia (dyskeratosis congenita).

Diagnosis and Differential Diagnosis

At diagnosis:

- Marked pancytopenia or reduction in two of three or, less commonly, one of three cell lines.
- Peripheral blood smear shows reduced platelets and neutrophils, normal red cells.
- Microspherocytes and giant platelets suggestive of peripheral destruction are not present.
- Bone marrow markedly hypocellular on biopsy (1-cm core); residual lymphocytes, plasma cells, mast cells on aspirate smear can be seen.
- Overall marrow biopsy cellularity is low (less than 30%, excluding lymphocytes), but there may be pockets of cellularity, so-called hot-spots.
- Myeloblasts and megakaryocytes are almost always absent.
- Marrow cytogenetics should be normal.

In secondary marrow failure, the degree of pancytopenia is usually moderate and the underlying illness is usually obvious from history and physical examination (e.g., stigmata of alcohol liver disease, presence of other autoimmune disease or infection). However, pancytopenia has many causes, of which AA is not the most common (Table 6-2).

Most important is to distinguish among primary marrow diseases (Table 6-3, Fig. 6-1B):

- Constitutional AA presenting in adults. A family history is highly suggestive. There may be no or only subtle physical stigmata. Patients younger than 40 years of age (or older if the history or examination is suggestive) should be tested for Fanconi anemia. Although phenotypic abnormalities have been classically described in both Fanconi anemia and dyskeratosis congenita, patients with adult onset constitutional AA may have extremely subtle signs on routine physical examination, or no characteristic findings at all (3).
- Myelodysplasia is hypocellular in approximately 20% of cases. Dysplastic changes in AA when present are mild and limited to erythrocytes. In myelodysplasia, megaloblastic changes are more extreme; megakaryocytes are preserved and can be aberrantly small and mononuclear; and myeloid precursors may be increased and often poorly granulated. Chromosomal analysis of bone marrow cells is almost always normal in AA, while myelodysplasia is often associated with cytogenetic abnormalities. Nonetheless, the distinction may be so difficult that some patients are best labeled AA/myelodysplastic syndrome (MDS).

TABLE 6–2. *Differential diagnosis of pancytopenia*

Pancytopenia with hypocellular bone marrow
   Acquired aplastic anemia
   Inherited aplastic anemia
   Some myelodysplastic syndromes
   Rare aleukemic leukemia
   Some acute lymphoblastic leukemia
   Some lymphomas of the bone marrow
Pancytopenia with cellular bone marrow
   Primary bone marrow diseases
      Myelodysplasia syndromes
      Paroxysmal nocturnal hemoglobinuria
      Myelofibrosis
      Hairy cell leukemia
      Some aleukemic leukemia
      Myelophthisis
      Bone marrow lymphoma
   Secondary to systemic diseases
      Systemic lupus erythematosus, Sjögren's syndrome
      Hypersplenism
      Vitamin B_{12}, folate deficiency (familial defect)
      Overwhelming infection
      Alcoholism
      Brucellosis
      Ehrlichiosis
      Sarcoidosis
      Tuberculosis and atypical mycobacteria
Hypocellular bone marrow with or without cytopenia
   Q fever
   Legionnaire's disease
   Toxoplasmosis
   Mycobacteria
   Tuberculosis
   Anorexia nervosa, starvation
   Hypothyroidism

TABLE 6–3. *Diseases easily confused with aplastic anemia*

Disease	Distinguishing characteristics	Diagnostic test
Constitutional*		
Fanconi anemia	Younger patients; family history and physical anomalies (short stature, *café au lait spots*, anomalies of the upper limb or thumb)	Chromosome analysis of stressed blood lymphocyte cultures
Dyskeratosis congenita	Younger patients; family history and physical anomalies (nail changes, leukoplakia)	Short telomeres mutations in TERC, TERT, DKC1
Acquired		
Myelodysplasia	Older patients, insidious onset, marrow usually normocellular or hypercellular	Marrow morphology Marrow cytogenetics
Aleukemic leukemia	Very young or very old patients	Blasts in buffy coat and spicules
PNH	Hemolysis (high LDH, low haptoglobin, hemoglobinuria), venous thrombosis	Deficient GPI-anchored proteins on flow cytometry
Myelofibrosis	Hepatosplenomegaly Leukoerythroblastic blood smear	Fibrosis on marrow biopsy
Large granular lymphocytosis	Older age, insidious, neutropenia	Large granular lymphocytes in peripheral smear Flow cytometry T-cell receptor rearrangement

*Phenotypic abnormalities may be subtle or absent.
PNH, paroxysmal nocturnal hemoglobinuria; LDH, lactate dehydrogenase; GPI, glycosylphosphoinositol anchor (GPI).

- PNH/AA. Small PNH expanded clones are common—as many as 50% of cases at presentation—in the setting of marrow failure now that flow cytometry has replaced the Ham test. Growth of clone size over time may lead to clinical hemolysis. Thrombosis is rare.
- Acute lymphocytic leukemia in children and acute myelogenous leukemia in the elderly can occasionally present with pancytopenia and marrow hypocellularity.
- Myelofibrosis has a characteristic leukoerythroblastic blood picture, marrow is dry tap (rather than watery, as in AA), and hepatosplenomegaly is common.
- Large granular lymphocytosis is characterized by prolonged periods of neutropenia, less frequently anemia or thrombocytopenia, and increased numbers of large granular lymphocytes in the peripheral blood. Marrow is usually cellular; diagnosis rests on flow cytometry or molecular evidence of rearrangement of the T-cell receptor.

Severe AA is defined by two of the following three peripheral blood count criteria.

1. Absolute neutrophil count less than 500 per microliter.
2. Platelet count less than 20,000 per microliter.
3. Reticulocyte count (automated) less than 60,000 per microliter.

Definitive Treatments

Definitive therapy of AA consists of allogeneic hematopoietic stem cell transplantation (HSCT) or immunosuppression; both have dramatically changed the natural course of this

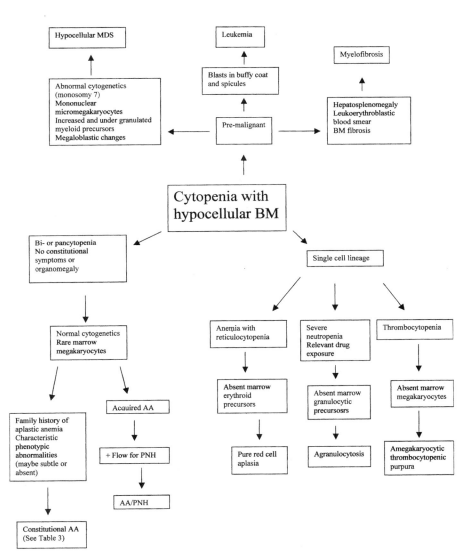

FIG. 6-1B. Differential diagnosis of cytopenias. MDS, myelodysplastic syndrome; BM, bone marrow; AA, aplastic anemia; PNH, paroxysmal nocturnal hemoglobinuria.

illness, with 5-year survival of 75% in patients undergoing either treatment (4). Support with growth factors alone or in combination with transfusion is used but are of uncertain long-term benefit and unlikely to change the natural history of the disease. The main distinctions between immunosuppression and HSCT are shown in Table 6-4.

- *HSCT* cures AA. Most transplants are performed using a histocompatible sibling donor and most recipients are young. Overall long-term survival is approximately 70% (5). HSCT is almost always preferred in children until approximately age 20 who have an appropriate donor. With current cyclophosphamide-based conditioning, major toxicities are related to graft-versus-host disease (GVHD) and infection (not always easily separable). GVHD risk increases with recipient age. Modest numbers of erythrocyte and platelet transfusions probably do not increase the risk of graft rejection, especially with leukocyte-depleted products. Because transplant success is correlated with time from diagnosis, laboratory studies of younger AA patients should include prompt human leukocyte antigen (HLA) typing of the potential recipient and sibling donors.
- Seventy percent of patients will lack a suitable matched sibling donor. Transplantation from matched unrelated donors (MUD) is now more feasible with the development of huge donor registries and an effective network. Results overall are about half as good as with HLA-matched family members but likely to improve with modifications of conditioning regimens and shorter times to transplant from diagnosis (6). Donor searches should be initiated early for younger patients who might be eligible later for a MUD. For unclear reasons umbilical cord blood transplantation has been associated with poor results in marrow failure states.
- *Immunosuppression* using regimens combining antithymocyte globulin (ATG) and cyclosporine is standard therapy. Approximately two-thirds of patients improve to transfusion-independence and, overall survival rates at 5 years are comparable to HSCT. Immunosuppression is almost always preferred in older patients, especially if the neutrophil count is not severely decreased. One frequently used protocol for horse ATG is 40 mg/kg per day for 4 days. Rabbit ATG is administered at 3.5 mg/kg per day for 5 days. (There is no evidence that one preparation is superior to the other.) Corticosteroids, such as methylprednisolone at 1 mg/kg, are usually administered during the first 2 weeks to ameliorate serum sickness.

Major toxicities of ATG include immediate allergic reaction, serum sickness, and transient blood count depression. Anaphylaxis is rare but has been fatal and may be predictable by skin testing. Treatment of ATG allergy is mainly symptomatic: intravenous hydration, antihis-

TABLE 6–4. *Bone marrow transplantation versus immunosuppression*

	HSCT	Immunosuppression
Applicability	HLA-matched sibling	All
Cost	High	Moderate
Age limits	Best in children Adults younger than 40	All ages
Outcome	65%–90% long-term survival	70% hematologic response
Short-term toxicity	10%–30% die of GVHD, infection, pneumonitis, venoocclusive hepatic disease or graft failure	Rare anaphylaxis
Long-term effects	Hematologic cure; modest increase in risk of solid tumors	Incomplete cure with possibility of development of PNH, MDS, AML

GVHD, graft-versus-host disease; PNH, paroxysmal nocturnal hemoglobinuria; MDS, myelodysplastic syndrome; AML, acute myeloid leukemia.

tamines (for urticaria) and meperidine (for rigors), and increased doses of corticosteroids (for symptomatic serum sickness). Cyclosporine is begun at 10 mg/kg in adults and 12 mg/kg in children, with dose adjustment to maintain blood levels at approximately 200 ng/mL. We administer cyclosporine for 6 months after ATG. Renal and liver function monitoring is required to avoid nephrotoxicity; hypertension, gingival hypertrophy, and tremulousness, which are common side effects.

Prognosis is strongly correlated to hematologic response at 3 months, especially the robustness of blood count recovery (7). Even after hematologic response to ATG, blood counts may decrease, especially on withdrawal of cyclosporine. Reinstitution of cyclosporine usually suffices but retreatment with ATG may be necessary and relapse is sometimes irreversible and fatal. Evolution to a clonal hematologic disease occurs in approximately 15% of patients over the decade after initial therapy, manifest as a dysplastic bone marrow or cytogenetic abnormalities, especially monosomy 7 and trisomy 8.

Other therapies that are occasionally successful include growth factor combinations (erythropoietin and granulocyte colony-stimulating factor [G-CSF]); androgens; high-dose cyclophosphamide (controversial because of prolonged neutropenia it induces) (8). Our approach to treatment is shown in Figure 6-2.

PAROXYSMAL NOCTURNAL HEMOGLOBINURIA

PNH is a rare clonal disease of the bone marrow, which can produce a clinical triad of (i) hemolysis, (ii) venous thrombosis, and (iii) AA (9).

Etiology and Pathophysiology

- A somatic mutation in a gene called *PIG-A* occurs in a hematopoietic stem cell.
- Leads to deficient synthesis of a glycolipid moiety called the glycosylphosphoinositol (GPI) anchor.
- Lack of cell surface presentation of a large family of GPI-linked proteins.
- Absence of one of these proteins, CD59, on the cell surface of erythrocytes leads to their susceptibility to complement and to intravascular hemolysis
- *PIG-A* mutant cells are probably present in normal adult marrow, but clonal expansion of these cells is unusual, except especially in AA (approximately 50% of cases) and in myelodysplasia, where they may range in size from small to large.
- Which GPI-anchored proteins are important in permitting clonal expansion in AA and MDS and in the thrombotic proclivity is unknown.

Clinical Features

- *Intravascular hemolysis,* classically as periodic bouts of dark urine in the morning but also as continuous red cell destruction and without evident hemoglobinuria.
- *Venous thrombosis in unusual sites,* especially hepatic, mesenteric, and portal veins and intracranial veins.
- *Marrow failure,* frank AA, or poor marrow function despite a relatively cellular histology.

Diagnosis

Intravascular hemolysis is unusual (see Chapter 3), and PNH should be considered in the setting of a suggestive history, hemoglobinuria, and elevated LDH (lactate dehydrogenase). There may be accompanying iron deficiency and neutropenia/thrombocytopenia.

Patients with PNH can present with symptoms of stroke or abdominal pain caused by Budd-Chiari syndrome. PNH clonal expansion should be sought in patients with AA and MDS.

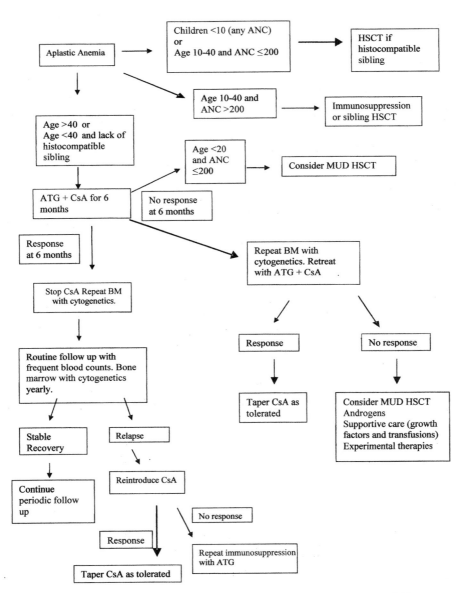

FIG. 6-2. Treatment of severe aplastic anemia. ANC, absolute neutrophil count; HSCT, hematopoietic stem cell transplantation; MUD, matched unrelated donors; BM, bone marrow; ATG, antithymocyte globulin; CsA, cyclosporine A.

Flow cytometry provides evidence of a PNH clonal expansion through quantitation of GPI-anchored proteins on erythrocytes and granulocytes (especially the latter in the transfused patient). However, severe hemolysis and thrombosis typically occur only in patients with large clones (more than 20% to 50% erythrocytes).

Treatment

The course is highly variable. AA patients postimmunosuppressive therapy with expanded clones may be asymptomatic; modest and intermittent hemolysis managed with transfusions alone is consistent with long survival; conversely, PNH can be associated with catastrophic thrombotic events. Clones may spontaneously disappear in some patients.

- Transfusion to maintain hemoglobin levels consistent with full activity. Use of washed erythrocytes is not necessary.
- Iron supplementation as required; loss of hemoglobin as a result of intravascular destruction prevents secondary hemochromatosis.
- Corticosteroids, usually in moderate doses (30 to 50 mg of prednisone on alternate days) have been frequently used to control hemolysis but never rigorously tested. A short trial in a patient with continuous red cell destruction may be warranted.
- Marrow failure as frank AA with associated PNH should be treated with stem cell transplantation (SCT) or immunosuppression (discussed earlier); a PNH clone appears to predict a higher rate of response to ATG and cyclosporine in both AA and MDS.
- Most patients in Western series die of thrombotic complications, and thromboses, once they occur, may be refractory to anticoagulation. At least one uncontrolled trial has suggested that coumadin prophylaxis is effective, but the relative risk of hemorrhage secondary to chronic anticoagulation for years, even decades, in this population remains unclear (10).
- SCT is the only curative therapy, but may carry a higher risk in PNH because of comorbid conditions; nonmyeloablative conditioning regimens may offer improved survival. Transplant should be considered in patients with severe marrow failure or thrombotic complications.
- A monoclonal antibody directed to the active component of C5 was successful in blocking hemolysis in one small series and will be tested in a larger American trial.

PURE RED CELL APLASIA

Pure red cell aplasia (PRCA) is defined as anemia with absent reticulocytes and marrow erythroid precursor cells (11). This rare aregenerative anemia has a number of interesting clinical associations and is also usually responsive to treatment.

Etiology and Pathophysiology

- Constitutional PRCA is Diamond-Blackfan anemia (DBA).
- Acquired PRCA often behaves as an immunologically mediated disease. Clinical associations include thymoma (but probably less than 10% of PRCA cases), collagen-vascular syndromes, myasthenia gravis, chronic lymphocytic leukemia, and large granular lymphocytic leukemia.
- PRCA may also be seen in MDS, especially with 5q-syndrome.
- Parvovirus B19 infection is often asymptomatic, but may cause erythema infectiosum (fifth disease) in children and transient aplastic crisis in patients with underlying hemolysis. Virus infection is ordinarily terminated by production of neutralizing antibodies. Persistence of parvovirus results from failure to mount a neutralizing antibody response, leading to chronic erythroid precursor destruction and anemia. Persistence of parvovirus B19 can occur in an immunodeficient host: in congenital immunodeficiencies (Nezelof's syndrome), iatrogenic

(immunosuppressive drugs and cytotoxic chemotherapy), and HIV infection-induced immunodeficiency.

Clinical Features and Diagnosis

Reticulocytes are severely depressed; erythroid precursor cells are usually absent but a few normoblasts may be present in the marrow. Giant pronormoblasts signal parvovirus; uninuclear micromegakaryocytes, 5q-syndrome. Other blood counts are normal, as are cytogenetics (except for PRCA associated with MDS). Thymoma should be excluded by computed tomography (CT) scan.

Parvovirus B19 antibodies are usually absent, or only IgM may be observed; virus can be detected in the blood by DNA hybridization.

Treatment

- For DBA, corticosteroids are standard; patients may be dependent on low doses, and relapse may not always be responsive to reinstitution of treatment. Despite transfusions and adequate iron chelation, patients may develop fatal late complications, including neutropenia and pulmonary hypertension.
- For acquired PRCA corticosteroids in moderate doses are usually first therapy, followed by either other immunosuppressives such as cyclosporine, ATG, and more recently (in a few case reports) monoclonal antibodies to CD20 (rituximab) or the interleukin-2 receptor (daclizumab), or cytotoxic drugs such as moderate doses of azathioprine or cyclosphosphamide administered orally.
- Thymomas should be excised because they are locally invasive; surgery does not necessarily resolve the anemia.
- Persistent parvovirus B19 infection responds to intravenous immunoglobulins at 0.4 g/kg daily for 5 to 10 days. Patients with large viral loads, especially in the acquired immunodeficiency syndrome, may relapse and require periodic re-treatment.

AGRANULOCYTOSIS

Severe neutropenia with either complete or partial absence of myeloid precursor cells is agranulocytosis.

Etiology and Pathophysiology

- Most agranulocytosis is drug-associated (Table 6-5). Idiopathic pure white cell aplasia (without exposure to a suspicious drug) is exceedingly rare, and similar to PRCA, may also be associated with thymoma (12).
- Mechanisms of drug destruction of granulocyte precursors include direct effects (as with thorazine) and immune (antibody)-mediated (as with dipyrone) (Table 6-6).

Diagnosis and Treatment

- The patient is usually older with a history of clear exposure to an incriminated agent, usually with introduction of the drug in the preceding 6 months. Absent neutrophils on smear should lead to a confirmatory bone marrow examination.
- Classic presentation is fever and sore throat.
- Recovery occurs spontaneously but over a highly variable time period, from a few days to several weeks. G-CSF or GM-CSF is almost always administered without clear evidence of efficacy.

TABLE 6–5. *Drugs associated with agranulocytosis*

Heavy metals
  Gold
  Arsenic compounds
Analgesics
  Aminopyrine, dipyrone
  Butazones
  Indomethacin
  Ibuprofen
  Acetaminophen
  Para-aminosalicylic acid
  Sulindac
Antipsychotics, sedatives, antidepressants
  Phenothiazines
  Tricyclics
  Chlorodiazepoxide
  Barbiturates
  Serotonin reuptake inhibitors
Anticonvulsants
  Phenytoin
  Ethosuximide
  Carbamazepine
Antithyroid drugs
  Propylthiouracil
  Methimazole
Cardiovascular drugs
  Procainamide
  Captopril
  Nifedipine
  Quinidine
  Propranolol
  Methyldopa
  Propafenone
  Aprinidine
Sulfa drugs
  Thiazide diuretics like spironolactone
    and acetazolomide
  Oral hypoglycemics
  Sulfasalazine
  Dapsone
  Sulfa antibiotics

Antibiotics
  Sulfa antibiotics
  Pyrimethamine
  Penicillins
  Cephalosporins
  Macrolides
  Vancomycin
  Clindamycin
  Aminoglycosides
  Antituberculosis agents
  Levamisole
Antimalarials
  Mebendazole
Antifungals
  Fluconazole
Antiviral
  Zidovudine
Antihistamines
  Cimetidine
  Ranitidine
  Chlorpheniramine
Miscellaneous
  Isoretinoin
  Omeprazole
  Colchicine
  Allopurinol
  Aminoglutethimide
  Metoclopramide
  Ticlopidine
  Tamoxifen
  Penicillamine
  Insecticides
  Hair dye
  Chinese herbal medicines

TABLE 6–6. *Immune versus toxic agranulocytosis*

	Immunologic	Toxic
Paradigm drug	Aminopyrine	Phenothiazine
Time to onset	Days to weeks	Weeks to months
Clinical	Acute, often explosive symptoms	Often asymptomatic or insidious onset
Rechallenge	Prompt recurrence with small test dose	Latent period, high dose required
Laboratory	Leucoagglutinins	Evidence of direct or metabolite mediated toxicity to cells

- Fever and signs of infection require prompt administration of broad-spectrum antibiotics by a parenteral route.
- Mortality remains substantial (approximately 10%) because of the combination of patient age, comorbid conditions, and lethal sepsis.

CONSTITUTIONAL BONE MARROW FAILURE SYNDROMES: MARROW FAILURE AFFECTS ALL THREE LINEAGES (ERYTHROCYTES, GRANULOCYTES, PLATELETS)

Among the constitutional disorders that present with AA, it is important to consider Fanconi anemia (FA) and dyskeratosis congenita (DC). Genes mutated in FA and in DC have been identified and are important in housekeeping functions in the cell; they have a key role in genomic stability and the maintenance of telomeres, respectively. An algorithm for laboratory testing to exclude FA and DC is presented next.

Fanconi Anemia

- Autosomal recessive inheritance; most common of the constitutional syndromes, seen in all races; diagnosed on the basis of positive chromosome breakage test (discussion following).
- Chief criteria of pancytopenia, hyperpigmentation, malformation of the skeleton, small stature, and hypogonadism.
- Malformations of the eye, ear, genitourinary and gastrointestinal tracts, cardiopulmonary and central nervous systems can occur.
- FA is notoriously heterogeneous in the degree and number of clinical manifestations, and patients presenting solely with either congenital malformations or hematologic abnormalities may either be misdiagnosed or go unrecognized entirely.

Clinical Features

- The diagnosis is suggested when a child presents with hyperpigmented or hypopigmented skin lesions; short stature (poor growth); anomalies of the upper limb or thumb; male hypogonadism; microcephaly; characteristic facial features, including a broadened nasal base, epicanthal folds, and micrognathia; and structural renal abnormalities. When this constellation of physical anomalies is accompanied by bone marrow failure (which may often trigger initial medical evaluation), confirmation of the diagnosis can then be made by standard diepoxybutane (DEB) or mitomycin C (MMC) chromosome breakage analysis (discussion following).
- The mean age at diagnosis is usually 8 or 9 years.

Diagnostic Tests

- Chromosome breakage test with DEB or MMC.
- Based solely on definition by the DEB test, nearly 40% of patients may be free of major physical anomalies. These patients with FA with normal appearances may go unrecognized unless there is a high index of suspicion for familial disease.
- Another challenge is the diagnosis of FA in older patients. Although the mean age of diagnosis is in the first decade of life, FA has been described recently in a 56-year-old woman.

Hematologic Presentations and Cancer Predisposition

- The symptoms and signs of FA typically relate to the hematologic presentation of cytopenias from marrow failure. Often thrombocytopenia or leukopenia is noted before full pancytope-

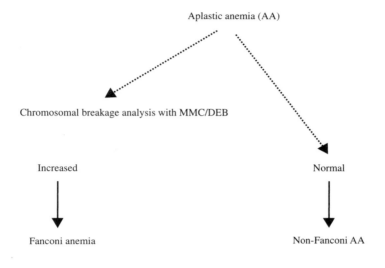

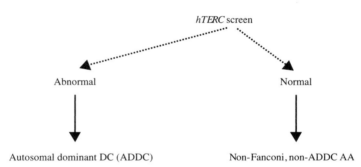

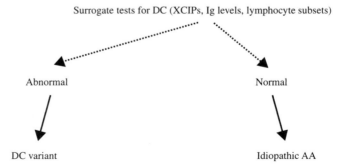

FIG. 6-3. Constitutional marrow failure. Figure courtesy of I. Dokal.

nia; furthermore, the pancytopenia typically worsens with time. Almost all patients with FA will develop hematologic abnormalities in their lifetime. Erythropoiesis is usually macrocytic.

- Classically, the bone marrow is hypocellular and fatty, indistinguishable from that seen in acquired AA. Microscopic examination of the marrow may show dyserythropoiesis and dysplasia. Some patients may develop or even present with a morphologically defined MDS or frank acute myeloid leukemia (AML).
- The crude risk of leukemia (exclusive of MDS) is approximately 5% to 10%, while the cumulative incidence of leukemia is approximately 10% by age 25. Less commonly recognized is the probability of developing MDS, approximately 5%, which appears also to correlate with a poor prognosis for patients with FA. Clonal karyotypic abnormalities, identical to those seen in non-FA MDS and secondary AML, are frequently found in patients with FA, whether or not they meet marrow morphologic criteria for a defined MDS. The prognostic significance of these clonal chromosomal abnormalities in patients with FA is not entirely clear, however, because cytogenetic changes can fluctuate over time. Certain clonal abnormalities may be associated with poor prognosis, such as gains of chromosome 3q.
- Solid organ malignancies have been noted, with a crude risk of 5% to 10% of patients overall (the risk increases with age, as those patients who have survived into adulthood develop solid tumors). Particularly common are vulvar, esophageal, and head and neck cancers. In addition to these (presumed) *de novo* tumors, a subset of long-term survivors of SCT will develop secondary malignancies, typically head and neck.

Stem Cell Transplantation and Supportive Care

- Allogeneic SCT from an HLA-matched sibling donor is the only curative therapy for the hematologic manifestations of FA (aplasia or myelodysplasia). Typically, decreased doses of cyclophosphamide and irradiation must be used in order to avoid severe toxicity because of the chemosensitivity and radio sensitivity of patients with FA. Transplantation centers, which generally adopted this modified conditioning regimen with or without thoraco-abdominal irradiation (TAI), have reported good results for patients with FA who did not present with leukemia or preleukemic transformation.
- Umbilical cord blood transplantation from related donors has also been successfully applied to a small number of patients with FA. A few patients with FA have also undergone successful SCT with cord blood from unrelated donors.
- Clearly, young patients with an HLA-compatible sibling should be treated by SCT at the earliest stages of marrow failure in preference to other therapies. However, most patients do not have an HLA-identical donor and are dependent on the identification of a suitably matched nonsibling relative or unrelated donor. A small number of FA patients have undergone bone marrow transplantation (BMT) from such alternative sources (matched unrelated and haploidentical family donors) to treat either aplasia or myelodysplasia, with or without clonal chromosomal abnormalities. The results from these alternative donor transplants have generally been inferior to those from matched sibling donor transplants, but are improving rapidly.

Patients lacking a suitable HLA-compatible donor (either sibling or matched unrelated) may benefit from chronic administration of androgens or hematopoietic growth factors (HGFs), which may serve as temporizing measures.

Androgens

- Androgens have been shown to induce hematologic responses in approximately 50% of patients although their effectiveness in raising blood counts may be neither durable nor complete in all lineages. Typically, androgen therapy is initiated when the platelet count is consistently below 30,000 per microliter and/or the hemoglobin less than 7 g/dL. Orally administered oxymetholone, at a dose of 2 to 5 mg/kg per day, is usually combined with prednisone, 5 to 10 mg every other day, in order to counterbalance the anabolic properties of oxymetholone with catabolic actions of corticosteroids.

- Androgen therapy is associated with liver toxicities including transaminase enzyme elevation, cholestasis, peliosis hepatitis, and hepatic tumors. Injectable androgens are associated with a decreased risk of hepatotoxicity, but pediatricians have sometimes objected to their use over concerns of pain and local bleeding: one standard formulation is nandrolone decanoate, administered by intramuscular injection at a dose of 1 to 2 mg/kg per week.

Hematopoietic Growth Factors

- Levels of most growth factors are markedly increased in FA as they are in acquired AA, likely as a compensatory physiologic response.
- One worrisome aspect of long-term growth factor administration is the theoretical risk of stimulating a leukemic clone, particularly in patients prone to developing MDS or AML, or speeding the process of stem cell exhaustion.
- Long-term administration of G-CSF may have transient beneficial effects on multiple hematopoietic lineages in some patients.

Dyskeratosis Congenita

- Classic DC is an inherited bone marrow (BM) failure syndrome characterized by the mucocutaneous triad of abnormal skin pigmentation, nail dystrophy, and mucosal leukoplakia.
- It has been observed in many races and estimated prevalence of DC is approximately 1 per 1,000,000 persons.
- X-linked–recessive, autosomal-dominant, and autosomal-recessive forms of the disease are recognized.
- A variety of other (dental, gastrointestinal, genitourinary, hair graying/loss, immunologic, neurologic, ophthalmic, pulmonary, and skeletal) abnormalities have also been reported.
- BM failure is the principal cause of early mortality with an additional predisposition to malignancy and fatal pulmonary complications.
- Clinical manifestations in DC often appear during childhood although there is a wide age range. The skin pigmentation and nail changes typically appear first, usually by the age of 10 years. BM failure usually develops below the age of 20 years; 80% to 90% of patients will have developed BM abnormalities by the age of 30 years. In some patients the BM abnormalities may appear before the mucocutaneous manifestations and can lead to an initial diagnosis of idiopathic AA.
- The clinical features of these disorders are heterogeneous and this makes diagnosis based on clinical criteria alone difficult and unreliable.
- Oxymetholone can produce durable hematological responses in more than more than 50% of patients with DC, but patients have to be monitored carefully for side effects.
- The current definitive treatment is allogeneic SCT. In patients with DC and FA low-intensity transplant protocols are producing prompt engraftment, reduced toxicity, and have the potential to reduce the risk of secondary malignancies.

Diagnostic Testing

Because the genes mutated in the X-linked recessive (*DKC1*) and autosomal dominant (*hTERC*) DC subtypes are now known, it is possible to substantiate the diagnosis in a significant proportion of patients. However, because these tests are complicated, it is necessary to be selective in screening. We suggest it is appropriate to screen for the *DKC1* gene if patients are male and have two of the following: abnormal skin pigmentation, nail dystrophy, leukoplakia, and/or BM failure. The situation regarding the *hTERC* screen is different for two reasons. First, we already know that a subgroup of patients with AA have mutations in *hTERC*. Second, screening for *hTERC* is relatively easy. Therefore it is reasonable to undertake analysis of the *hTERC* gene in all patients presenting with AA. There is as yet no easy universal functional test for DC. In patients with presenting with AA it is also important to undertake chromosomal breakage analysis for FA (Fig 6–1 and 6–3).

MARROW FAILURE USUALLY INVOLVES SINGLE LINEAGE

Diamond-Blackfan Anemia

- Probably the second most common constitutional marrow failure syndrome after FA.
- Most patients present with anemia in the neonatal period or in infancy.
- Approximately 30% of affected children present with a variety of associated physical anomalies. Thumb and upper limb malformations and craniofacial abnormalities are common. Other defects: atrial or ventricular septal defects, urogenital anomalies, and prenatal or postnatal growth retardation.
- A moderately increased risk of developing hematologic and solid organ malignancies.
- Most cases are sporadic, with an equal gender ratio, but 10% to 25% of patients have a positive family history for the disorder.
- Pathophysiology and basic molecular defect unclear. (RPS19 mutations in a subgroup of patients.)

Hematologic Findings

- Minimal diagnostic criteria for DBA: normochromic anemia in infancy (younger than 2 years), low reticulocyte counts, absent or decreased bone marrow red cell precursors (less than 5% of nucleated cells), and a normal chromosome breakage test (to rule out FA).
- Additional features: presence of malformations, macrocytosis, elevated fetal hemoglobin, and elevated erythrocyte adenosine deaminase (eADA) level.
- Some patients identified after the age of 2 years after a more severely affected family member first diagnosed.
- Anemia usually severe at the time of diagnosis (usually macrocytic).
- The bone marrow aspirate is usually normocellular, but erythroblasts are markedly decreased or absent. The other cell lines are normal, but mild to moderate neutropenia, thrombocytopenia, or both may occur later in the course.
- Progression of the single-lineage erythroid deficiency of DBA into pancytopenia and AA is rare but may occur.
- Differential diagnosis includes transient erythroblastopenia of childhood (TEC). Both TEC and DBA show similar marrow morphology, but TEC is self-limited, with a recovery within 5 to 10 weeks.

Treatment Modalities

- Initial treatment in DBA is transfusions, but long-term administration of red cells may cause secondary hemochromatosis.
- Corticosteroids are mainstay of treatment, and at least 50% of patients respond. There is no known predictor of steroid responsiveness, and later relapses occur. During treatment, some patients may recover sensitivity to corticosteroids or even proceed to a spontaneous remission.
- Allogeneic BMT is a treatment option for DBA in steroid-resistant patients.
- Hematopoietic growth factor (HGF) therapy with interleukin-3 (IL-3) or EPO has been

attempted for DBA. Only IL-3 has shown some effect in a subgroup of patients, and it has been suggested that IL-3 may play a role early in the treatment.

Shwachman-Diamond Syndrome

- Probably the third most common constitutional marrow failure syndrome after FA.
- Autosomal recessive disorder usually manifests in infancy and characterized by exocrine pancreatic insufficiency, short stature, and bone marrow dysfunction.
- Additional clinical features include: metaphyseal dysostosis, epiphyseal dysplasia, immune dysfunction, liver disease, growth failure, renal tubular defects, insulin-dependent diabetes mellitus, and psychomotor retardation.
- Hematologic manifestations: neutropenia, raised fetal hemoglobin (Hb F) levels, anemia, thrombocytopenia, impaired neutrophil chemotaxis.
- Predilection for malignant myeloid transformation and MDS.

Exocrine pancreatic dysfunction (at least one of the following):

1. Abnormal quantitative pancreatic stimulation test;
2. Serum cationic trypsinogen below normal range;
3. Abnormal 72-hour fecal fat analysis plus evidence of pancreatic lipomatosis by ultrasonogram or CT scan.

Hematologic abnormalities (at least one of the following):

1. Chronic (on two occasions at least 6 weeks apart) single lineage or multilineage cytopenia with bone marrow findings consistent with a defect in production.
a. Neutrophil counts less than 1.5×10^9 per liter.
b. Hemoglobin concentration less than 2 standard deviations below mean, adjusted for age.
c. Thrombocytopenia less than 150×10^9 per liter.
2. Myelodysplastic syndrome.

Supportive data: short stature, skeletal abnormalities, liver dysfunction. To be excluded: cystic fibrosis, Pearson syndrome, cartilage hair hypoplasia, celiac disease.

Kostmann Syndrome

- Autosomal-recessive disorder.
- Characterized by severe neutropenia and an early stage maturation arrest of myelopoiesis, leading to bacterial infections from early infancy.
- Also, autosomal dominant and sporadic forms, with different point mutations in the neutrophil elastase gene in a subgroup of patients
- More than 90% of these patients respond to G-CSF (filgrastim, lenograstim) with absolute neutrophil count (ANC) that can be maintained around 1.0×10^9 per liter. Adverse events include mild splenomegaly, moderate thrombocytopenia, osteoporosis and malignant transformation into myelodysplastic syndrome/leukemia. Development of additional genetic aberrations (G-CSF-receptor or RAS gene mutations, monosomy 7) during the course of the disease indicates an underlying genetic instability.
- Hematopoietic SCT is still the only available treatment for patients refractory to G-CSF.

Congenital Amegakaryocytic Thrombocytopenia

- Characterized by severe thrombocytopenia caused by a lack of megakaryocytes in the bone marrow from birth.

- Diagnosis based mainly on the exclusion of other forms of congenital thrombocytopenia with ineffective megakaryopoiesis such as FA.
- Molecular basis may be mutation in the *c-mpl* gene coding for the thrombopoietin receptor.
- At time of diagnosis, the bone marrow of patients with congenital amegakaryocytic thrombocytopenia (CAMT) is normocellular with a normal representation of all hematopoietic lines except for megakaryocytes. During the course of CAMT, the disease usually evolves into AA.
- SCT has been shown to be the only curative therapy.

REFERENCES

1. Young NS. Acquired aplastic anemia. *Ann Intern Med* 2002;136:534–546.
2. Kaufman DW, Kelly JP, Levy M, et al. *The Drug Etiology of Agranulocytosis and Aplastic Anemia.* New York, Oxford Univesrity Press, 1991.
3. Fogarty PF, Yamaguchi H, Wiestner A, et al. Late presentation of dyskeratosis congenita as apparently acquired aplastic anaemia due to mutations in telomerase RNA. *Lancet* 2003;362:1628–1630.
4. Bacigalupo A, Brand R, Oneto R, et al. Treatment of acquired severe aplastic anemia: bone marrow transplantation compared with immunosuppressive therapy. The European Group for Blood and Marrow Transplantation experience. *Semin Hematol* 2000;37:69–80.
5. Deeg HJ, Leisenring W, Storb R, et al. Long term outcome after marrow transplantation for severe aplastic anemia. *Blood* 1998;91:3637–3645.
6. Margolis DA, Casper JT. Alternative-donor hematopoietic stem-cell transplantation for severe aplastic anemia. *Semin Hematol* 2000;37:43–55.
7. Rosenfeld S, Follmann D, Nunez O, et al. Antithymocyte globulin and cyclosporine for severe aplastic anemia: association between hematologic response and long-term outcome. *JAMA* 2003; 289:1130–1135.
8. Tisdale JF, Dunn DE, Geller N, et al. High-dose cyclophosphamide in severe aplastic anaemia: a randomised trial. *Lancet* 2000;356:1554–1559.
9. Rosse WF, Nishimura J. Clinical manifestations of paroxysmal nocturnal hemoglobinuria: present state and future problems. *Int J Hematol* 2003;77:113–120.
10. Hall C, Richards S, Hillmen P. Primary prophylaxis with warfarin prevents thrombosis in paroxysmal nocturnal hemoglobinuria (PNH). *Blood* 2003;102:3587–3591.
11. Kang EM, Tisdale JF. Pure Red Cell Aplasia. In: Young NS. *Bone Marrow Failure Syndromes.* Philadelphia, Saunders, 2000;135–155.
12. Young NS. Agranulocytosis. In: Young NS. *Bone Marrow Failure Syndromes.* Philadelphia, Saunders, 2000;156–182.

7

Myelodysplastic Syndromes

Minoo Battiwalla and Neal S. Young

The myelodysplastic syndromes (MDS) are a heterogeneous group of clonal stem cell disorders characterized by ineffective hematopoiesis and a variable tendency to progress to acute myelogenous leukemia (AML). Increasingly, MDS is diagnosed incidentally when modestly abnormal blood counts trigger a bone marrow examination.

MDS is a disease of older adults; the median age is in the mid-60s. Estimates of its incidence range from 10 to 100 per million, and in the elderly the rate may be twofold to eightfold higher, making MDS a relatively common hematologic disease. Death as a result of MDS occurs from the complications of cytopenias and/or progression to AML, but many patients will succumb first to comorbidities of the elderly.

Myelodysplasia of the marrow can be seen in aplastic anemia, especially as a late event after immunosuppressive treatment, in the course of Fanconi anemia, and with paroxysmal nocturnal hemoglobinuria (PNH) and T-large granular lymphocyte lymphoproliferative states (T-LGL) disorders, and preceding AML (Fig. 7-1).

ETIOLOGY AND PATHOGENESIS

MDS is related to the accumulation of somatic mutations in an hematopoietic stem cell. In secondary MDS, prior chemotherapy (alkylating agents and toposisomerase inhibitors) and ionizing radiation are clearly etiologic; the latency period between exposure and the development of secondary MDS is typically 5 to 10 years. Radiation has been implicated in the marrow failure syndromes historically reported in occupationally and accidentally exposed individuals and in atomic bomb victims. For most MDS, age is the principal risk factor. However, MDS can occur in young persons: in treated aplastic anemia, as a consequence of Fanconi anemia, and *de novo*.

The bone marrow is typically hypercellular, implying that ineffective hematopoiesis rather than absence of stem cells results in the cytopenias. In general, early MDS (refractory anemia) is characterized by an increased susceptibility to apoptosis, while late MDS (in transition to leukemia) is associated with reduced apoptosis. Although the principal defect is in the hematopoietic stem cells, immunological factors and the bone marrow microenvironment contribute to the bone marrow failure (Fig. 7-2). There are significant abnormalities in apoptosis, cytokine profiles, angiogenesis and the T-cell repertoire. Specific mutations, in particular, abnormalities in chromosomes 7 and a complex karyotype, predispose to leukemic transformation. In contrast, 5q-, del 20q, and -Y are recurrent chromosomal abnormalities not associated with a high risk of transformation. *Ras* mutations and platelet-derived growth factor-β (PDGF-β)-receptor translocations are more common in chronic myelomacrocytic leukemia (CMML).

CLINICAL FEATURES

Patients present with symptoms caused by cytopenias, usually anemia. "Anemia of the elderly" may be unrecognized MDS. Lymphadenopathy and splenomegaly are absent. The

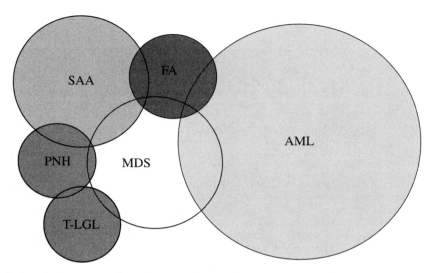

FIG. 7-1. AML, acute myelogenous leukemia; FA, Fanconi anemia; MDS, myelodysplastic syndrome; SAA, severe aplastic anemia; T-LGL, T-cell large granular lymphocytic leukemia.

clinical course is variable: patients may be aysmptomatic or have mild anemia progressing to transfusion-dependence over many years, others have an aggressive course with multilineage involvement and rapid evolution to acute leukemia.

DIAGNOSTIC STUDIES

- Peripheral blood smear typically shows macrocytosis, hypogranular neutrophils, sometimes with Pelger-Huet nuclei and other abnormal nuclear patterns, and circulating micromegakyarocytes. Significant numbers of large granular lymphocytes should raise suspicion of a T-cell large granular lymphocytic leukemia (T-LGL)/MDS overlap syndrome.
- Bone marrow biopsy is frequently hypercellular but is frankly hypocellular in approximately 20% of MDS. Abnormal localization of immature precursors (ALIPs) near boney trabeculae is characteristic. On the aspirate smear, look especially for an increase in myeloblasts and dysplastic morphology in the white cell and/or the megakaryocytic lineages. Mononuclear, small, or dysplastic megakarytocytes are evidence of MDS. Erythroid dysplasia alone is less specific, but large numbers of ringed sideroblasts identify a specific MDS subtype.
- Chromosome analysis of marrow cells is critical; abnormal cytogenetics strongly suggest MDS and influence prognosis. Karyotyping should be repeated as chromosome patterns can evolve. Fluorescent *in situ* hybridization (FISH), while not now routine, may provide more subtle information than karyotyping alone. A stress test for Fanconi anemia is recommended for younger patients even if physical examination is normal.
- Flow cytometry has limited utility; blasts enumeration, critical to prognosis, can be assessed by routine morphology. Nevertheless, expert flow cytometry can be highly specific in diagnosing MDS, and, in the future, may offer useful phenotypic information.
- Human leukocyte antigen (HLA) typing is needed for to evaluate younger patients for allotransplantation and may provide predictive information for responsiveness to immunosuppression.

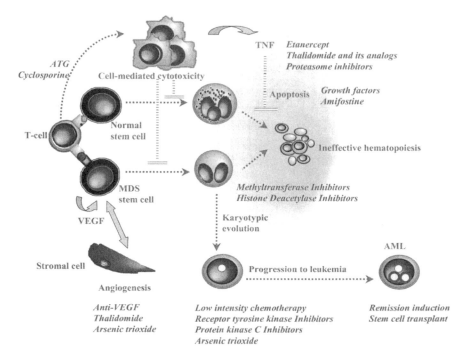

FIG. 7-2. Natural history and pathogenesis of bone marrow failure. AML, acute myelogenous leukemia; ATG, antithymocyte globulin; MDS, myelodyspolastic syndrome; TNF, tumor necrosis factor; VEGF, vascular endothelial growth factor.

CLASSIFICATIONS

- Accurate classification and prognosis for this highly heterogeneous disorder is necessary to individualize therapy.
- The first validated classification, the French-American-British (FAB; expanded in 1982) was based on morphology (Table 7-1) (1). This scheme, in use for the past 20 years,

TABLE 7–1. *French-American-British subtypes*

Type		BM blast %	Frequency (%)	Median survival
Refractory anemia	RA	<5	30–40	35 months
Refractory anemia with ring sideroblasts	RARS	<5	15–25	35 months
Chronic myelomonocytic leukaemia	CMMoL	<20	15	12 months
Refractory anemia with excess blasts	RAEB	5–20	15–25	18 months
Refractory anemia with excess blasts in transformation	RAEB-t	20–30	5–15	6 months

recognized that the risk of leukemic progression was proportional to the blast count in the marrow.

- The International Prognostic Scoring System (IPSS; Table 7-2), derived from analyses of outcomes in large series of patients, combined information from cytogenetics, cytopenias, and blast count to generate a prognostic score (2). These values separate median survivals for patients with low risk (5.7 years), intermediate-1 (3.5), intermediate-2 (1.2), and high-risk (0.4) MDS.
- The new World Health Organization (WHO) classification (Table 7-3) attempts to define risk better and separate individual syndromes (3,4).Some of the perceived deficiencies of the FAB are addressed by including the prognostic relevance of cytopenias and karyotypic information in addition to blast counts. (Table 7-3). RAEB-t is discarded and the threshold for defining AML is lowered to 20%.
- 5q-syndrome is one of several specific MDS syndromes. Deletion of 5q, between bands q31 and q33, is separate in the WHO classification. 5q-syndrome usually manifests as anemia, with or without mild neutropenia and platelet counts either preserved or elevated. The prognosis is relatively good. Several cytokines, growth factors and their receptors are found at the 5q locus, but their pathophysiologic importance is unknown. Early reports suggest that complete cytogenetic responses may be seen with Revlimid, a thalidomide analogue, in 5q-syndrome.
- Hypocellular MDS, while not categorized in any schema, may be easily confused with aplastic anemia, and patients may respond more favorably to immunosuppression with antithymocyte globulin (ATG).
- CMML is biologically distinct, now classified as a myeloproliferative disease by the WHO, although often associated with a dysplastic marrow. Angiogenesis, autocrine vascular endo-thelial growth factor stimulation, tyrosine kinase overactivity and *ras* mutations appear to figure in the pathogenesis of the proliferation. Standard therapy of CMML is hydroxyurea and transfusions; patients with the PDGF-β receptor associated mutations benefit from imatinib, and other agents with potential activity are toposisomerase I inhibitors (topotecan), farnesyl transferase inhibitors, antiangiogenic agents and demethylating agents.
- Therapy-related (or secondary) MDS is an important subtype, constituting approximately 15% of cases in most series. This subtype has the highest rate of progression (75%) to acute leukemia, almost always difficult to treat and rapidly fatal. Almost all patients have recurrent chromosomal abnormalities: deletions in chromosomes 5 and/or 7 occur at a mean interval of 4 to 5 years after exposure to alkylating agents, and 11q23 abnormalities follow in a shorter time period after topoisomerase II inhibitors. A very high frequency of therapy-related MDS is seen in patients who have undergone high-dose chemotherapy (up to 19% at 10 years), more likely the result of the cumulative prior therapy, especially alkylating agents, rather than the autotransplant. Overall, median survival is only 9 months.

TABLE 7–2. *International prognostic scoring system*

	0	0.5	1.0	1.5	2.0
Blasts %	<5	5–10		11–20	21–30
Karyotype*	Good	Intermediate	Poor		
Cytopenias	0 or 1	2 or 3			

* Good, normal, −Y, del(5q), del(20q); Poor, complex (>3 abnormalities) or chromosome 7 anomalies; Intermediate, other abnormalities.
Scores: Low, 0; INT-1, 0.5–1.0; INT-2, 1.5–2.0; and High, 2.5.
Patients with 21%–30% blasts may be consdered as MDS or AML.
MDS, myelodysplastic syndrome; AML, acute myelogenous leukemia.

TABLE 7–3. *World Health Organization Classification*

Category	MDS cases %	Peripheral blood	Bone marrow	Rate of AML progression %
RA	5–10	Anemia <1% blasts <1 × 10 e⁹ per liter monocytes	Erythroid dysplasia *only* <5% blasts <5% ringed sideroblasts	6
RARS	10–15	Anemia <1% blasts <1 × 10 e⁹ per liter monocytes	Erythroid dysplasia *only* 15% ringed sideroblasts <5% blasts	1–2
RCMD	24	Bicytopenia or pancytopenia <1% blasts No Auer rods <1 × 10 e⁹ per liter monocytes	Dysplasia in >10% of cells in = 2 cell lines <5% blasts in marrow No Auer rods <15% ringed sideroblasts	11
RCMD-RS	15	Bicytopenia or pancytopenia No or rare blasts No Auer rods <1 × 10 e⁹ per liter monocytes	Dysplasia in >10% of cells in = 2 cell lines >15% ringed sideroblasts <5% blasts No Auer rods	11
RAEB-1&2	40	Cytopenias <1 × 10 e⁹ per liter monocytes	Unilineage or multilineage dysplasia	
		RAEB-1: <5% blasts, no Auer rods	5–9% blasts, no Auer rods	25
		RAEB-2: 5–19% blasts, Auer rods ±	10–9% blasts, Auer rods ±	33
MDS-U		Cytopenias No or rare blasts No Auer rods	Unilineage dysplasia in granulocytes or <5% blasts No Auer rods	unknown
5q-syndrome		Anemia <5% blasts Platelets normal or increased	Normal to increased megakaryocytes <5% blasts No Auer rods Isolated del(5q)	uncommon

AML, acute myelogenous leukemia; BM, bone marrow; MDS, myelodysplastic syndrome; MDS-U, unclassified; RA, refractory anemia; RAEB, refractory anemia with excess blasts; RARS, refractory anemia with ringed sideroblasts; RCMD, refractory cytopenia with multilineage dysplasia.

From Komkroji R, Bennet JM. The myelodysplastic syndromes: classification and prognosis. *Curr Hemotol Rep Vol.* 2. 2003;2:179–185.

- MDS associated with large granular lymphocytosis (LGL). Significant numbers of circulating T-LGLs should prompt suspicion of this overlap syndrome; the diagnosis is confirmed by a clonal pattern of T-cell receptor gene rearrangement. Cases of T-LGL/MDS may have hematologic responses to therapy directed against the T-LGL component, such as cyclosporine; HLA-DR4 is a strong predictor of responsiveness.
- Pediatric MDS is unusual and should lead to evaluation for genetic syndromes, such as Fanconi anemia, Bloom syndrome, neurofibromatosis type 1, Schwachman syndrome, Pearson disease, Kostmann syndrome, familial monosomy 7, and constitutional chromosomal abnormalities.

THERAPY

Therapeutic strategies combine supportive care, suppression of the MDS clone and its leukemic progeny, efforts to improve bone marrow function, and curative attempts with allogeneic stem cell transplantation (Table 7-4). Optimum management often requires the application of some or all of these approaches, preferably in the context of a research protocol (Table 7-5). Evidence-based decisions may be constrained by the clinical heterogeneity of MDS and the paucity of adequate data from clinical trials.

Supportive Care

Supportive care in MDS is influenced by the irreversible nature of the underlying disease and recognition that cytopenias are the single most important contributor to mortality.

- Even moderate degrees of anemia may not be well tolerated by the elderly, especially in the presence of cardiopulmonary disease, and maintenance of higher hemoglobin levels

TABLE 7–4. *Therapeutic strategies for myelodysplastic syndrome*

Supportive care
  Transfusion
  Antimicrobials
  Iron chelation
Treatments aimed at improving bone marrow function
  Growth factors (erythropoietin, G-CSF, GM-CSF)
  Immunosuppression (ATG, cyclosporine)
  Anticytokine approaches (thalidomide and analogues)
  Antiapoptosis
Treatments directed at the abnormal clone
  Low-intensity chemotherapy (hydroxyurea, melphalan, low-dose ara-C, VP-16)
  Induction regimens (anthracycline/ara-C combinations, FLAG, ADE)
  DNA methyltransferase inhibitors (5-azacytidine, decitabine)
  Histone deacetylase inhibitors
  Farnesyl transferase Inhibitors
  Antiangiogenesis (arsenic trioxide, anti-VEGF, RTK-Is, thalidomide)
  Remission induction/autologous stem cell transplant
Curative attempts (stem cell transplantation)
  Myeloablative transplantation
  Reduced intensity conditioning

ADE, Ara-C, daunorubicin, etoposide; FLAG, Fludarabine, Ara-C, G-CSF; RTK-I, receptor tyrosine kinase inhibitor; G-CSF, granulocyte colony-stimulating factor; GM-CSF, granulocyte-macrophage colony-stimulating factor; ATG, antithymocyte globulin; VEGF, vascular endothelial growth factor; VP-16, etoposide

TABLE 7-5. *Risk-adjusted schema for management of myelodysplastic syndrome*

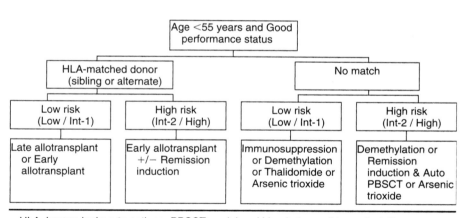

HLA, human leukocyte antigen; PBSCT, peripheral blood stem cell transplantation

(greater than 9 g/dL) can much improve the quality of life without altering transfusion frequency. Iron chelation should be instituted in patients who are younger, without serious comorbidities, and who are in favorable diagnostic categories.

- Leukodepletion of blood products and single-donor platelet transfusions reduce the risk of eventual alloimmunization to platelets. If a prophylactic regimen is adopted, 10,000 platelets per microliter is usually an adequate threshold.
- Neutrophils may be dysfunctional in MDS, lowering the threshold for instituting neutropenic

precautions. Infections in the setting of neutropenia must be treated aggressively, bearing in mind the combined effects of neutropenia and therapy.

Growth factors are typically used at the lowest doses which maintain a response (5).

- Combinations of erythropoietin and granulocyte colony-stimulating factor (G-CSF) are synergistic, even when they fail individually, with hematologic improvements in 40% of patients with low-grade MDS (6). Helpful algorithms suggest that patients with low erythropoietin serum levels and more modest degrees of anemia may be most responsive. However, growth factors do not appear to enhance survival or progression to leukemia and they are best considered a part of supportive care.

SPECIFIC THERAPIES

Allotransplant is the only curative therapy. Consequently, every effort must be made to offer this to eligible patients with a matched donor (sibling or unrelated). Patients who may not tolerate a traditional transplant (because of debilitation or older than 55 years of age) may be offered reduced intensity conditioning. Carefully selected patients in their seventh decade have undergone successful transplants using this approach. The IPSS score also predicts relapse and survival in transplant patients. While there has been a decrease in regimen-related toxicity with reduced conditioning intensity, there is a high rate of relapse in patients with advanced MDS. Consequently, standard allotransplant still remains the treatment of choice in younger patients. Three-year disease-free survivals as high as 75% have been reported for patients with low-risk MDS undergoing standard HLA-matched transplants. Conversely, allotransplantation is too aggressive for elderly patients with low-risk MDS. Patients who achieve a complete remission with chemotherapy and can be successfully mobilized, may benefit from an autologous transplantation but this strategy is still investigational.

5-Azacytidine is the first agent documented to be superior to supportive care alone in a randomized control trial with multiple end points: at 75 mg/m^2 per day subcutaneously for 7 days every 4 weeks, treated patients showed improvement in transfusions, slower progression to leukemia, and better quality of life (7). 5-Azacytidine and its active metabolite decitabine belong to the class of epigenetic modulators; at low doses they induce cellular differentiation by inhibiting DNA methyltransferase, while at higher doses they exert a direct cytostatic effect. Decitabine, the active metabolite of 5-azacytidine has shown promising activity.

ATG at 40 mg/kg per day for 4 days produces hematologic responses in approximately one-third of patients with low-risk MDS (8). Subjects who are younger than 50 years of age, with a lower duration of red cell transfusion dependence, and who are HLA-DR15-positive are the most likely to respond immunosuppression with ATG (9).

Thalidomide inhibits angiogenesis, interferes with cellular adhesion, alters inflammatory cytokine profiles, and is capable of producing hematological responses in approximately 20% of transfusion-dependent patients. However, cumulative toxicities limit its use. Nonteratogenic and nonneurotoxic analogues of thalidomide show far greater potency, superior safety and efficacy in early clinical trials. Among these, Revlimid has shown promise in low-grade MDS, and appears to be unique in inducing complete cytogenetic responses in the 5q-syndrome.

Arsenic trioxide, currently approved for acute promyelocytic leukemia, is capable of inducing hematologic responses in approximately one in four cases and could be a useful agent for high-risk myelodysplasia. The exact mechanism of action at the lower doses used in myelodysplasia is not known but it targets sulfhydryl groups and acts at multiple levels to induce apoptosis.

Cyclosporine (5 mg/kg per day for 3 months, tapered to a low maintenance dose thereafter) may be effective especially in patients with T-LGL/MDS who are HLA-DR4-positive.

The role of cytototoxic chemotherapy in the treatment of MDS remains an area of controversy. Many guidelines have suggested a role for standard chemotherapy to eliminate the neoplastic clone, and popular agents are cytosine arabinoside and topotecan. However, no prospective studies show long-term survival benefit. Unlike de novo AML, advanced MDS often demonstrates high response rates to induction chemotherapy, only to be followed by the virtual certainty of relapse (up to 90%). Likely futile efforts to eradicate an MDS clone have to be balanced against the risk of further reduction of the marrow reserve. Some chemotherapy (hydroxyurea or etoposide) may be useful for leukemia reduction with a palliative goal once MDS transforms, especially in the aged patient.

TARGETED THERAPIES

There is great interest in therapies directed against cytokine pathways (thalidomide and its analogues), antiapoptosis, antiangiogenesis, and signal transduction inhibitors (receptor tyrosine kinase inhibitors, arsenic trioxide and farnesyl transferase inhibitors). Promising developments in the field are the shift in emphasis from eliminating the MDS clone using chemotherapy to improving the cytopenias; treatments effective for distinct syndromes; practical utilization of good prognostic stratification schemes; the adoption of standardized response criteria; and the availability of newer pharmaceutical agents targeting relevant biologic pathways.

REFERENCES

1. Bennett JM, Catovsky D, Daniel MT, et al. C. (1982) Proposals for the classification of the myelodysplastic syndromes. *Br J Haematol* 1982;51:189–199.
2. Greenberg P, Cox C, LeBeau MM, et al. International scoring system for evaluating prognosis in myelodysplastic syndromes. *Blood* 1997;89:2079–2088.
3. Harris NL, Jaffe ES, Diebold J, et al. World Health Organization classification of neoplastic diseases of the hematopoietic and lymphoid tissues: report of the Clinical Advisory Committee meeting-Airlie House, Virginia, November 1997. *J Clin Oncol* 1999;17:3835–3849.
4. Vardiman JW, Harris NL, Brunning RD. The World Health Organization (WHO) classification of the myeloid neoplasms. *Blood* 2002;100:2292–2302.
5. Rizzo JD, Lichtin AE, Woolf SH, et al. Use of epoetin in patients with cancer: evidence-based clinical practice guidelines of the American Society of Clinical Oncology and the American Society of Hematology. *Blood* 2002;100:2303–2320.
6. Hellstrom-Lindberg E, Ahlgren T, Beguin Y, et al. Treatment of anemia in myelodysplastic syndromes with granulocyte colony-stimulating factor plus erythropoietin: results from a randomized phase II study and long-term follow-up of 71 patients. *Blood* 1998;92:68–75.
7. Silverman LR, Demakos EP, Peterson BL, et al. Randomized controlled trial of azacitidine in patients with the myelodysplastic syndrome: a study of the cancer and leukemia group B. *J Clin Oncol* 2002; 20:2429–2440.
8. Molldrem JJ, Leifer E, Bahceci E, et al. Antithymocyte globulin for treatment of the bone marrow failure associated with myelodysplastic syndromes. *Ann Intern Med* 2002;137:156–163.
9. Saunthararajah Y, Nakamura R, Wesley R, et al. A simple method to predict response to immunosuppressive therapy in patients with myelodysplastic syndrome. *Blood* 2003;102:3025–3027.

8

The Myeloproliferative Disorders: Polycythemia Vera, Thrombocythemia, and Myeloid Metaplasia

Jamie Robyn and Elaine M. Sloand

The chronic myeloproliferative disorders (MPD) are clonal hematopoetic stem cell diseases characterized by overproduction of one or more blood cell lines (Fig. 8-1). Unlike myelodysplasia, the MPD are associated with normal maturation and effective hematopoiesis. Organomegaly is common and often symptomatic. Varying degrees of extramedullary hematopoesis and leukemic transformation are also seen in those affected with MPD. Although algorithms have been devised for polycythemia vera, essential thrombocytosis and idiopathic myelofibrosis, diagnosis may be problematic in some instances because of significant overlap of clinical symptomatology and the absence of diagnostic markers (1,2). A recent retrospective study demonstrated that fatal thromboembolism was the most common cause of death in the MPD (3). This chapter focuses on polycythemia vera (PV), essential thrombocytosis (ET), and myelofibrosis with myeloid metaplasia (MMM). Chronic myelomonocytic leukemia (CMML) is included as well although it is placed in a separate disease category (myeloproliferative/ myelodysplastic disorders) by the World Health Organization (WHO) classification. Chronic myeloid leukemia, hypereosinophilic syndrome, and systemic mastocytosis are discussed in separate chapters.

POLYCYTHEMIA VERA

PV was first described by Vaquez in 1892. In the early 1900s, Osler recommended phlebotomy as treatment for PV. In 1951, Dameshek classified PV as a MPD. In 1967, Wasserman organized the Polycythemia Vera Sudy Group designed to define the natural history of PV and to determine optimal therapeutic management.

Epidemiology

The incidence of PV is 2 per 100,000. The etiology of the disease is unknown, but rare familial cases have been described (4).

The median age at presentation is 60 years and the male to female ratio is 1–2:1. The median survivals of untreated PV is 1.5 years, PV treated with phlebotomy, 3.5 years, and PV treated with myelosuppression, 7 to 12 years.

Pathophysiology

PV is a clonal stem cell disorder with trilineage myeloid involvement; some studies suggest that PV involves the B lymphocytes as well. PV is characterized by growth factor-independent erythroid proliferation producing an elevated red cell mass. While the blood and marrow are

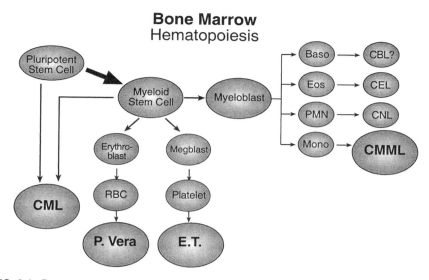

FIG. 8-1. Bone marrow hematopoiesis. Baso, basophil; CML, chronic myelogenous leukemia; CMML, chronic myelmonocytic leukemia; CNL, chronic neutrophil leukemia; Eos, eosinophil; ET, essential thrombocytosis; Mono, monocytes; PMN, polymorphonuclear leukocytes; P. vera polycythemia vera; RBC, red blood cells.

the major sites of disease involvement, extramedullary haematopoiesis may occur in the liver and spleen as well, especially in the spent phase of PV. While a few cases of congenital polycythemia caused by abnormal expression of a truncated form of the erythropoietin receptor have been described, there is no evidence that erythropoietin (EPO) receptor mutations are involved in the pathogenesis of PV. Splicing defects in EPO receptor RNA in some patients with PV are of unclear significance (5).

At diagnosis, 10% to 20% of patients with PV have abnormal cytogenetics including trisomy 8, trisomy 9, and deletion 20q. Loss of heterozygosity at chromosome 9p, undetectable on routine cytogenetics, is found in 33% of patients. The frequency of chromosomal abnormalities increases with disease progression (4).

Clinical Features

The elevated red cell mass in PV may result in a myriad of clinical signs and symptoms including:

- Hypertension
- Thrombosis, venous or arterial
- Pruritis
- Erythromelalgia
- Ulceration of fingers and toes
- Joint pain
- Epigastric pain
- Weight loss
- Headache
- Weakness
- Paraesthesias
- Visual disturbances

- Vertigo
- Tinnitus
- Ruddy cyanosis
- Conjunctival plethora

Pruritis aggravated by bathing is a distinctive feature of PV and is present in almost 50% of patients. PV is the most common cause of erythromelalgia. It is noteworthy that PV is one of the few disorders where digital ischemia occurs in the presence of palpable pulses (6). Increased cellular turnover in PV may result in gout or kidney stones. Palpable splenomegaly is found in 70% of patients.

The most frequent cause of death in PV is thrombosis. Sites of thrombosis in PV include:

- Venous thrombosis

Lower extremities
Pulmonary vessels
Mesenteric vessels
Hepatic vessels causing Budd-Chiari syndrome
Portal veins
Splenic veins

- Arterial thrombi

Coronary vessels leading to myocardial infarction
Cerebrovascular causing TIA and ischemic stroke

Ten percent of patients with Budd-Chiari syndrome have coexistent PV.

Less than 10% of patients experience major bleeding and hemorrhage is the cause of death in only 2% to 10% of patients with PV. A variety of platelet defects are detectable in patients with PV; acquired von Willebrand disease exists in 33% of patients and is associated with increased bleeding risk.

While erythrocytosis distinguishes PV from the other MPD, only 20% of patients with PV present with erythrocytosis alone while 40% have trilineage hyperplasia at the onset of disease. PV can also present with isolated leukocytosis or thrombocytosis. Typical bone marrow findings in PV include hypercellularity, atypical megakaryocyte hyperplasia and clustering, and decreased stainable iron. Laboratory abnormalities include elevated leukocyte alkaline phosphatase (70% of patients) and elevated serum B12 (40% of patients).

The risk of transformation to acute leukemia is 1.5% in patients treated with phlebotomy alone. Patients with PV have a 10% to 25% risk of transforming into the spent phase (postpoly-cythemic myeloid metaplasia) at 10 and 25 years of follow-up, respectively. The spent phase is characterized by normalization of the red cell mass associated with cytopenias, increasing splenomegaly because of extramedullary hematopoiesis, and collagen fibrosis of the bone marrow.

Diagnostic Criteria

The WHO criteria for the diagnosis of PV are shown in Table 8-1 (4). While erythrocytosis distinguishes PV from the other myeloproliferative disorders, not all patients with PV have elevated hematocrits and not all patients with elevated hematocrits have PV. Dehydration can cause spurious elevation of the hematocrit, resulting in apparent erythrocytosis. A hematocrit greater than 60% in men or 55% in women is usually caused by an elevated red cell mass. Direct determination of blood volume and red cell mass is usually required. On the other hand, erythrocytosis may be masked by expanded plasma volume secondary to spleno-megaly or by occult blood loss. Iron deficiency can also cause a decrease in the hematocrit in patients with PV. Secondary erythrocytosis caused by elevation of serum EPO must also be excluded. Conditions associated with physiologically appropriate production of EPO caused by hypoxemia as well as diseases associated with inappropriate EPO production that result in erythrocytosis are listed below:

TABLE 8–1. *WHO criteria for diagnosis of polycythermia vera*

A1. ~~Elevated RBC~~ mass >25% above mean normal predicted value, or Hb >18.5 g/dL in men, 16.5 g/dL in women*
A2. No cause of secondary erythrocytosis, including:
Absence of familial erythrocytosis
No elevation of EPO because of:
Hypoxia (arterial pO_2 92%)
High oxygen affinity hemoglobin.
Truncated EPO receptor
Inappropriate EPO production by tumor
A3. Splenomegaly
A4. Clonal genetic abnormality other than Ph chromosome or BCR/ABL fusion gene in marrow cells
A5. Endogenous erythroid colony formation *in vitro*
B1. Thrombocytosis >400 × 10⁹ / L
B2. WBC >12 × 10⁹ / L
B3. Bone marrow biopsy showing panmyelosis with prominent erythroid and megakaryocytic proliferation
B4. Low serum EPO levels

Diagnose PV when A1 + A2 and any other category A are present or when A1 + A2 and any two of category B are present.
* or >99th percentile of method-specific reference range for age, gender, altitude of residence. WHO, World Health Organization; RBC, red blood cell count; Hb, hemoglobin; EPO, erythropoietin.

EPO overproduction secondary to hypoxia

Lung disease
High altitude
Smoking (8-carboxyhemoglobin)
Cyanotic heart disease
Methemoglobinemia
High oxygen affinity hemoglobin
Cobalt

EPO overproduction

Tumors—renal, brain, hepatoma, uterine fibroids, pheochromocytoma
Renal artery stenosis
Neonatal
Inappropriate EPO secretion
Bartter's syndrome
Renal cysts, hydronephrosis

Other causes

EPO receptor hypersensitivity
Congenital erythrocytosis
Androgen therapy
Adrenal tumors
Autotransfusion (blood doping), self-injection of EPO
Polycythemia vera

Note that EPO levels in PV may be either low or normal; high EPO levels are not consistent with PV.

TABLE 8–2. *Features distinguishing PV from secondary polycythemia, and apparent polycythemia**

Findings	Polycythemia vera	Secondary Polycythemia	Apparent Polycythemia
Splenomegaly	+	−	−
Leukocytosis	+	−	−
Thrombocytosis	+	−	−
Red blood cell volume	↑	↑	Normal
Arterial oxygen saturation	Normal	↓	Normal
Serum vitamin B_{12} level	↑	Normal	Normal
Leukocyte alkaline phosphatase	↑	Normal	Normal
Marrow	Panhyperplasia	Erythroid hyperplasia	Normal
EPO level	↓	↑	Normal
Endogenous CFU-E growth	+	−	−

*The differences listed are not present in all patients. CFU-E, colony forming units-erythrocytes.
(From Ernest Beutler, et al. Williams hematology. New York: McGraw Hill, 2001, with permission.)

Laboratory studies which may be useful in evaluation of erythrocytosis are:

- Arterial blood gas measurement
- Iron studies
- Serum EPO level
- Liver and kidney function studies
- Abdominal ultrasound or computed tomography (CT) scan
- Bone marrow aspirate and biopsy
- Red cell mass

Table 8-2 shows clinical findings and assay results of testing distinguishing secondary polycythemia from PV. Specialized studies may be required in equivocal cases. For example a recently described polymerase chain reaction (PCR)-based assay for overexpression of PRV-1 (CD177) mRNA in peripheral granulocytes is positive in most patients with PV, but not in secondary erythrocytosis (7); large prospective trials are in progress to assess the role of PRV1 in clinical diagnosis. Also, reduced thrombopoietin (TPO) receptor (c-mpl) levels are found in PV megakaryocytes and platelets, but these also have been observed in some patients with ET and MMM. Production of endogenous erythroid colonies *in vitro* is seen in PV but not in secondary erythrocytosis (8). When it is impossible to make a definitive diagnosis, laboratory evaluation should be repeated in 3 months.

Staging and Prognostic Features

In untreated PV, median survival is only 6 to 18 months; death most frequently results from thrombosis. Other causes of mortality include transformation to acute leukemia or to spent phase (postpolycythemic myeloid metaplasia). Although thrombocytosis and qualitative platelet abnormalities often occur, elevation of the hematocrit over 45% confers the greatest risk of thrombosis, presumably due to hyperviscosity. Age over 70 and a previous history of thrombosis are also important predictors of recurrent thrombotic events.

Treatment

Efficacy of the various treatment options should translate to an individual agent's ability to reduce thrombotic risk and slow leukemic transformation, balanced against drug toxicities.

The Polycythemia Vera Study Group (PSVG) was an international study group that in 1967 organized a large series of randomized trials. PVSG-01 randomly assigned 431 patients to phlebotomy, chlorambucil, or P-32. The thrombosis rate for patients treated with phlebotomy alone was 37.3%, significantly higher than for those treated with chlorambucil or P-32. However, there were an excess of deaths secondary to leukemia in the chlorambucil and P-32 arms of the study. In the PVSG-05 study, aspirin added to phlebotomy did not decrease the thrombotic risk but instead increased bleeding complications. The PSVG-08 study showed hydroxyurea significantly lowered the risk of thrombosis compared with phlebotomy alone but exhibited a trend toward increase in the risk of leukemic transformation.

Therapy in PV is based on risk of thrombosis which depends on a number of factors. Risk stratification seen below:

Low-risk
Age, less than 60 years and
No history of thrombosis, and
Platelet count less than 1.5 million per microliter, and
No cardiovascular risk factors (smoking, obesity)

High-risk
Age older than 60 years, or
Previous history of thrombosis or
Cardiovascular risk factors (smoking, athrosclerosis, hyperlipidemia)

Intermediate-risk
Neither high-risk nor low-risk

Phlebotomy is the treatment of choice for most patients. The hematocrit should be maintained at less than 45% in men and less than 42% in women by this procedure. For patients over 69 years of age, phlebotomy is often supplemented with hydroxyurea to decrease the hematocrit to target levels. Additional treatment may be required in patients with thrombosis, hemorrhage, severe pruritis, painful splenomegaly, B symptoms or very high leukocyte or platelet counts (9,10). In the presence of these complicating features, hydroxyurea or interferon-α should be added. Because there is ongoing debate about the risk of leukemic transformation, some physicians are reluctant to use hydroxyurea in younger patients and prefer to use interferon-α instead for cytoreduction. Busulfan or P-32 may be used in the elderly who may be unable to tolerate hydroxyurea. Note that while the addition of myelosuppressive agents may reduce the incidence of thrombosis, they may also increase the risk of leukemia. Suggested treatment algorithm is seen in Table 8-3. See Table 8-4 for therapeutic agents and side effects.

Low-dose aspirin appears effective for alleviation of microvascular sequelae including headache, vertigo, visual disturbances, distal paraesthesias, and erythromelalgia. The safety and benefits of low-dose aspirin in PV have been investigated in a multicenter project (ECLAP) (5,11). Aspirin lowered the risk of cardiovascular death, nonfatal myocardial infarction, nonfatal stroke, and total mortality; treatment nonsignificantly increased major bleeding. Aspirin should not be used if there is a history of hemorrhage or with extreme thrombocytosis (more than 1 million per cubic millimeter). Anagrelide has been approved for use in all MPD to lower platelet counts, although cost and toxicity exclude this drug for many individuals (Table 8-4).

Pruritis is a problem in 40% to 50% of patients with PV. Variably effective measures include reduction of water temperature and use of antihistamines. Other agents of uncertain efficacy for these symptoms include cholestyramine, PUVA, and interferon-α. Recently the selective serotonin reuptake inhibitors paroxetine (20 mg every day) or fluoxetine (10 mg every day) have been shown to provide relief in many patients suffering from pruritis (12).

Patients with PV undergoing surgery are at high risk of postoperative complications. Elective procedures should be postponed until the hematocrit is less than 45% for more than 2 months.

TABLE 8–3. *Algorithm for management of patients with polycythemia vera*

Low-risk young patients (<40 years)	High-risk patients (≥40 years, ≤69 years)
↓	
Phlebotomy + low-dose aspirin (40 mg/day) to maintain hematocrit <45%. Aspirin should not be utilized in patients with history of a hemorrhagic episode or with extreme thrombocytosis (>1 × 10⁶/mm³) and acquired von Willebrand syndrome	• Previous thrombosis • High rate of phlebotomy
	↓

↓	• Low-dose aspirin therapy (40 mg/day)
	• Myelosuppression
	  – Interferon-α (3.0 × 10⁶ units three times a week; alter dose depending on response and toxicity)
	  – If disease is not controlled or cannot tolerate Interferon-α, hydroxyurea 30 mg/kg for 1 week then 15 mg/kg
	  – If disease is not controlled or cannot tolerate hydroxyurea busulfan 4–6 mg/day PO for 4–8 weeks. Stop when blood counts are normalized or platelet count is <300,000/mm³.
	  – Occasional supplemental phlebotomy if hematocrit >47%; when patient relapses (phlebotomy more often than once every 2–3 months or patient is symptomatic) initiate therapy again at same dose

• Thrombosis or hemorrhage • Systemic symptoms • Severe pruritus refractory to histamine antagonists • Painful splenomegaly	
↓	
Interferon-α (3.0 × 10⁶ units three times a week; alter dose depending on response and toxicity)	
↓	↓
If hematocrit control is inadequate or patient cannot tolerate interferon, start hydroxyurea: 30 mg/kg PO for 1 week, then 15–20 mg/kg – supplemental phlebotomy if hematocrit is >47%	No response
	↓
↓	• ³²P: 2.3 mCi/m² IV every 12 weeks as needed (limit 5 mCi per dose) • Phlebotomize for hematocrit >47% • Increase dose by 25% if no response
If hematocrit control is still inadequate, start busulfan: 4–6 mg/day PO for 4–8 weeks; stop when blood counts are normalized or platelet count is <300,000/mm³ – supplemental phlebotomy if hematocrit is >47%. When patient relapses, initiate therapy again at same dose	
	↓
	Persistent thrombosis and thrombocytosis in face of adequate hematocrit control
	↓
	Anagrelide
	Patient age > 69 years
↓	↓
Persistent thrombocytosis with repeated episodes of thrombosis in face of adequate hematocrit control	Phlebotomy + low-dose aspirin + hydroxyurea
	↓
↓	No response or poor compliance
Anagrelide	↓
	Busulfan 4–6 mg/day PO for 4–8 weeks. Stop when blood counts are normalized or platelet count is <300,000/mm³.
↓	
Painful splenomegaly or repeated episodes of thrombosis	↓
	No response
↓	↓
³²P	³²P
↓	↓
Persistent painful splenomegaly	Persistent thrombosis and thrombocytosis in face of adequate hematocrit control
↓	↓
Splenectomy + continued systemic therapy	Anagrelide

From Hoffman R. Polycythemia vera. In: Hoffman R, Benz EJ Jr, Shattil SJ, et al., eds. *Hematology: Basic Principles and Practice.* New York: Churchill-Livingstone, 2000:1146.

TABLE. 8-4. *Properties of Agents used to Treat PV and/or ET*

	Hydroxyurea	Anagrelide	Interferon alfa	Phosphorus-32
Drug class Mechanism of action	Antimetabolite Not genotoxic, impairs DNA repair by inhibiting ribonucleotide reductase	Imidazoquinazolin Interferes with terminal differentiation of megakaryocytes	Biologic response modifier Myelosuppressive	Radionuclide β-particle emitter, myelosuppressive
Specificity	Affects all cell lines	Affects platelet production, primarily	Affects all cell lines	Affects all cell lines
Pharmacology	Half-life approx. 4 hours, renal excretion	Half-life approx. 1.5 hours, renal excretion	Kidney is main site of metabolism	Half-life approx, 14 days
Starting dose	500 mg orally 2 or 3 times daily	0.5 mg orally 3 or 4 times daily	3–5 million units sc 3–5 days/wk	2.3 mCi/m^2, may be repeated in 3–6 mo
Onset of action	Approx. 3–5 days	Approx 6–10 days	3–26 wk to obtain remission	4–8 wk
Side effects observed in >10% of patients	Neutropenia anemia, oral ulcers, hyperpigmentation, rash, nail changes	Headache, forceful heartbeats, palpitations diarrhea, fluid retention	Flulike syndrome, fatigue, anorexia, weight loss lack of ambition, alopecia	Transient mild cytopenia(s)
Side effects observed in <10% of patients	Leg ulcers, lichen planuslike lesions of the mouth and skin, nausea, diarrhea	Congestive heart failure, anhythmias, anemia, light-headedness, nausea	Confusion, depression, autoimmune thyroiditis or arthritis, pruritus, myalgia	Prolonged pancytopenia in elderly patients
Rare side effects	Fever, liver function test abnormalities	Pulmonary hypertension, pulmonary fibrosis	Pruritus, hypedipidemia, transaminasemia	Delayed development of acute leukemia
Contraindications	Pregnancy, childbearing potential, breast-feeding	Congestive heart failure, pregnancy, childbearing potential	Anecdotal reports suggest safety during pregnancy	Pregnancy, childbearing potential
Annual cost	$1,700, for 500 mg 3 times daily	$6,300, for 0.5 mg 4 times daily	$17,000 for 5 million units sc 5 days/wk	Approximately $1,000 per treatment

From Tefferi A. Recent progress in the pathogenesis and management of essential thrombocythemia. *Leuk Res* 2001;25(5):373. Reproduced with permission from Elsevier Ltd.

Transformation to spent phase occurs on average 10 years after the initial diagnosis and is heralded by the development of cytopenias and splenomegaly. Hydroxyurea and interferon alpha may alleviate cytopenias due to splenomegaly. Splenectomy may appear necessary but can be followed by hepatomegaly secondary to extramedullary hematopoiesis. Low-dose splenic irradiation usually provides only short-term relief.

Stem cell transplantation remains an option for advanced PV and can be curative. Outcomes are more favorable in those transplanted in spent phase than in after evolution to acute leukemia (13).

ESSENTIAL THROMBOCYTOSIS

Essential thrombocytosis was first described by Epstein and Goedel in 1934 and called hemorrhagic thrombocythemia. Dameshek classified it as one of the MPD in 1951.

Epidemiology

The annual incidence of ET is estimated at 1 to 2.5 per 100,000. Most patients are between age 50 and 60 at presentation and there is no gender predilection A second peak occurs around age 30 when females are more often affected. The median survival of ET is more than 10 years (4). The etiology of the disease is unknown. Familial cases associated with molecular abnormalities of the thrombopoietin gene have been reported. The rate of clonal cytogenetic abnormalities in ET is approximately 5%.

Pathophysiology

Although ET has been traditionally described as a clonal disorder, X-chromosome inactivation studies suggest polyclonal hematopoiesis in some patients (14). ET remains a diagnosis of exclusion, because there are no defining cytogenetic or morphologic features.

Clinical Features

As many as half of patients are asymptomatic at presentation. Vasomotor symptoms occur in approximately 40% of patients and include visual disturbances, lightheadedness, headaches, palpitations, atypical chest pain, erythromelalgia, livedo reticularis, and acral paraesthesias. Thrombosis occurs in 15% of cases at presentation and in 10% to 20% during the course of the disease. Associated thrombotic events include deep vein thromboses (DVTs) and pulmonary embolism, digital ischemia, portal vein thrombosis, and cerebrovascular and coronary ischemia. Major hemorrhage occurs in 5% to 10% of patients during the disease course. Other disease associations include recurrent first-trimester abortions and palpable splenomegaly, which is present in less than 50% of patients. The risk of leukemic transformation is less than for other MPD.

Transformation to spent phase occurs in less than 5% of patients after 20 years and is heralded by the development of cytopenias and splenomegaly.

Diagnostic Testing

ET is characterized by persistent nonreactive thrombocytosis. WHO diagnostic criteria are shown in Table 8-5. The differential diagnosis includes reactive thrombocytosis and other MPD, as well as chronic myeloid disorders. Causes of thrombocytosis other than ET are listed below:

• Asplenia
• Acute hemorrhage

TABLE 8–5. *WHO diagnostic criteria for essential thrombocythemia*

Positive criteria
- Sustained platelet count $\geq 600 \times 10^9$ / L
- Bone marrow biopsy specimen showing proliferation mainly of the megakaryocytic lineage with increased numbers of enlarged, mature megakaryocytes

Exclusion criteria
- No evidence of PV
  Normal red cell mass or Hb <18.5 g/dL in men, 16.5 g/dL in women
  Stainable iron in marrow, normal serum ferritin or normal MCV
  If the former condition is not met, failure of iron trial to increase red cell mass or Hb levels to the PV range
- No evidence of CML
  No Philadelphia chromosome and no BCR/ABL fusion gene
- No evidence of chronic idiopathic myelofibrosis
  Collagen fibrosis absent
  Reticulin fibrosis minimal or absent
- No evidence of myelodysplastic syndrome
- No evidence that thrombocytosis is reactive because of:
  Underlying inflammation or infection
  Underlying neoplasm
  Prior splenectomy

WHO, World Health Organization; PV, polycythamemia vera; Hb, hemoglobin; MCV, mean cell volume; CML, chronic myelomonocytic leukemia.

- Infections
- Hemolysis
- Postthrombocytopenic rebound
- Cancer
- Inflammatory states (infection, collagen vascular disorders)
- Iron deficiency
- Pregnancy
- MPD (Note that most of the MPD may present with isolated thrombocytosis.)

Often a careful patient history will exclude reactive thrombocytosis. Laboratory testing to assist in diagnosis includes:

- Iron studies to exclude iron deficiency.
- C-reactive protein (CRP) and erythrocyte sedimentation rate (ESR), and fibrinogen to rule out an occult inflammatory or malignant process.
- Blood smear: Howell-Jolly bodies indicate anatomic or functional asplenia.
- Bone marrow morphology.
- Cytogenetics including FISH or PCR for BCR/ABL to exclude chronic myelomid leukemia (CML).

Decreased megakaryocyte c-mpl expression, increased granulocyte PRV-1 and endogenous erythroid colony formation can be seen in both PV and ET and do not distinguish between them (2). When a definitive diagnosis is not initially possible, later periodic evaluation may be revealing.

Treatment

The decision to treat must be based on risk-based management because life expectancy in this disease is nearly normal. High-risk patients are those over 60 years of age, or those who have a history of thrombosis. Low-risk patients are younger than 40 years old, with no history of thrombosis and without cardiovascular risk factors whose platelet counts are less than 1.5 million. Intermediate-risk patients are those who do not fall into either the high- or low-risk categories.

Choice of therapy is based on efficacy and toxicity (15). Therapeutic options include mechanical reduction of counts using plateletpheresis (in acute situations), myelosuppressive agents (alkylating agents, hydroxyurea, or radiophosphorus), maturation modulators (interferon-α or anagrelide) or antiplatelet agents (Table 8-4). Treatment should be focused on a platelet count goal of less than 400,000 per cubic millimeter.

Treatment Algorithm

Age: younger than 60
Low risk: No treatment*
Intermediate risk: No treatment*
High risk: Hydroxyruea or anagrelide*

Age: older than 60
Low risk: All are high risk
Intermediate risk: All are high risk
High risk: Hyroxyurea*

*Low-dose aspirin may be used but is not evidence based. Aspirin should not be used if platelet count is greater than 1.5 million per microliter. Women of childbearing age not using birth control should be treated with interferon-α based on anectodal evidence of safety in pregnancy.

Low- and intermediate-risk patients should be observed and not treated with cytoreductive therapy unless they develop extreme thrombocytosis in excess of 1.5 million. Cytoreductive therapy should be administered to high-risk patients. Hydroxyurea is usually the agent of first choice in high-risk patients with anagrelide and interferon-α used as the second line. Intermediate-risk patients are generally not given cytoreductive therapy unless they develop extreme thrombocytosis associated with bleeding or vasomotor symptoms unresponsive to aspirin.

Alkylating agents are generally not used because they are associated with an increased risk of leukemia. However, they are occasionally useful in the very elderly whose comorbidities make them intolerant to other therapies.

Hydroxyurea is effective in lowering platelet counts but causes bone marrow suppression. Questions remain about its leukemogenic potential, because no controlled randomized clinical trials have been conducted. Hydroxyurea should not be used in women of childbearing age.

Interferon-α is effective in reducing platelet count but is associated with significant side effects including flu-like symptoms and depression. Anagrelide acts by interfering with platelet maturation but is associated with toxicities including fluid retention, headache, and palpitations. Most abate within 2 to 4 weeks after initiation of therapy, so it is prudent to slowly titrate the dose. Anagrelide should be avoided in patients with cardiovascular comorbidities because of its side effect profile. Aspirin is efficacious in preventing recurrent thrombosis in patients with ET and especially useful for vasomotor symptoms. Aspirin is contraindicated in patients who have experienced bleeding episodes or if the platelet count exceeds 1.5 million.

Plateletpheresis is used in emergent situations accompanying thrombosis where abrupt decrease in platelet count is mandated.

All patients with ET should be instructed to avoid smoking and to avoid nonsteroidal anti-inflammatory drugs.

MYELOFIBROSIS WITH MYELOID METAPLASIA

Myelofibrosis was first described in 1879 by G. Hueck and was first included as one of the MPD in 1951.

Epidemiology

The annual incidence of MMM is 0.5 to 1.5 per 100,000. The median age at presentation is 65 years. The male to female ratio is 1:1. Median survival is only 3 to 5 years, so MMM has the worst outcome of all the MPD. The etiology of the disease is unknown but a familial occurrence has been reported in rare kindreds (4). A high incidence of MMM has been noted in individuals exposed to radiation at Hiroshima.

MMM that develops in late stage PV or ET is referred to as postpolycythemic metaplasia (PPMM) or postthrombocythemic myeloid metaplasia (PTMM), respectively. *De novo* MMM is often referred to as agnogenic myeloid metaplasia (AMM) or idiopathic myelofibrosis.

Pathophysiology

The marrow fibroblasts in MMM are not themselves derived from the abnormal clone. Increased levels of PDGF, transforming growth factor (TGF)-β, and other cytokines produced by megakaryocyes are thought to be responsible for the marrow fibrosis. Cytogenetic abnormalities are seen in approximately 50% of patients and include 13q-, 20q-, 12p-, trisomy 8, and trisomy 9. High levels of $CD34^+$ cells have been noted in the circulation of patients with MMM and appear to correlate with the extent of myeloproliferation (16).

Clinical Features

Approximately one-third of patients are asymptomatic at diagnosis. Presenting complaints include profound fatigue, symptoms of anemia, abdominal discomfort, early satiety, or diarrhea caused by splenomegaly, bleeding, weight loss, and peripheral edema. Constitutional symptoms including fever and night sweats occur in most patients during the course of the disease. Splenomegaly is common in MMM and may be marked. Episodic left upper quadrant pain can occur secondary to splenic infarction. Palpable hepatomegaly is found in the majority of cases. Extramedullary hematopoiesis may occur in almost any organ.

Laboratory abnormalities in patients with MMM may include leukocytosis or leukopenia, and thrombocytosis or thrombocytopenia. The classic blood smear shows leukoerythroblastosis. However bone marrow morphologic findings vary from mild to marked fibrosis (17). Osteosclerosis and periostitis can cause severe bone pain. Elevations of lactate dehydrogenase, serum B12, and alkaline phosphatase are commonly seen. Transformation to acute leukemia occurs in approximately 20% of patients during the first decade after diagnosis.

Diagnostic Testing

There is no standard for the diagnosis of MMM. The bone marrow is often inaspirable leading to a "dry tap." The classic peripheral smear shows teardrop-shaped red cells, nucleated red cells and granulocyte precursors (leukoerythroblastosis). However, other marrow infiltrative processes can cause a similar picture and must be excluded (Table 8-6). The absence of splenomegaly makes a diagnosis of MMM suspect. Many benign and malignant conditions may mimic MMM, including metastatic cancer, granulomatous disease, connective tissue disease, lymphoma, systemic mast cell disease, hypereosinophilic syndrome, and other myeloid disorders. Both ET and PV can transform to MMM. Cytogenetics and FISH or PCR for BCR/ABL should be performed to exclude fibrotic CML.

Staging and Prognostic Features

MMM often progresses to marrow failure. Features associated with decreased survival include the following:

- Advanced age
- Hypercatabolic symptoms*

TABLE 8–6. *Causes of Marrow Fibrosis*

Nonhematologic	Hematologic
Infections	Myeloproliferative disorders
TB	ET, PV, MMM
Leishmaniasis	Hypereosinophilic syndrome
Histoplasmosis	Systemic mastocytosis
HIV	CML
Connective tissue disease	AML-M7
Renal osteodystrophy	MDS
Metastatic cancer	Multiple myeloma
Vitamin D deficiency	Hairy cell leukemia
Hypothyroidism	Lymphoma
Hyperthyroidism	ALL
Paget disease	Grey platelet syndrome
Gaucher's disease	

TB, tuberculosis; HIV, human immunodeficiency virus; ET, essential thrombocytosis; CML, chronic myelomonocytic anemia; MDS, myelodyplastic syndrome; ALL, acute lymphocytic anemia; PV, polycythemia vera; MMM, myelofibrosis with myeloid metaplasia; AML-M7, acute megakaryoblastic leukemia.

- Anemia (hemoglobin less than 10 g/dL)**
- Leukopenia (white cell count less than 4,000 per cubic millimeter)**
- Leukocytosis (white cell count higher than 30,000 per cubic millimeter)
- Abnormal cytogenetics or the presence of circulating granulocyte precursors or blasts*
- (*May be an indication for splenectomy or **transplantation. Splenic irradiation may provide short-term improvement in patients with symptoms referable to organomegaly who are not surgical candidates.)

Median survival in high-risk patients is less than 2 years while patients with low-risk features have median survivals of over 10 years.

Treatment

Treatment in MMM is largely palliative. Approximately 30% of patients with anemia will show improvement with a combination of androgen (oxymethalone 50 mg four times per day or fluoxymesterone 10 mg three times per day) and prednisone (30 mg/day) therapy. Responses are usually brief in duration. EPO is most often ineffective. In low-risk patients requiring transfusion support for symptomatic anemia, timely initiation of chelation therapy is warranted.

Hydroxyurea, busulfan, interferon, or melphalan may be used to control thrombocytosis, leukocytosis or organomegaly. Lower doses of hydroxyurea are used in MMM than in ET or PV (start at 20 to 30 mg/kg two or three times per week). None of these agents is effective in preventing disease progression or improving survival. Anagrelide and imatinib have not been successful and ongoing studies assess the efficacy of thalidomide in MMM.

Allogeneic stem cell transplantation for patients with poor prognosis remains the only treatment with curative potential (18). Debate continues as to the value of splenectomy prior to transplantation. Concerns about graft failure because of marrow fibrosis have proven unwarranted and, in fact, successful transplantation is associated with resolution of marrow fibrosis. In both the European bone marrow transplant and Seattle trials, the overall survival after myeloablative transplantation was 60%. Reduced intensity conditioning is being explored for older patients and for those who are not candidates for myeloablative protocols (13).

CHRONIC MYELOMONOCYTIC LEUKEMIA

Epidemiology

The annual incidence of CMML is estimated at 4 cases per 100,000. There is a male predominance of 1.5–3:1. The median age at presentation is 70 years. Median survival is estimated at 12 to 18 months. The etiology of the disease is unknown.

Pathophysiology

The WHO classification places CMML in the category labeled myelodysplastic/myeloproliferative, which is appropriate because the marrow cells in this disease show dysplastic features and there are many characteristics of myeloproliferation as well. The spleen, liver, and lymph nodes are the most common sites of extramedullary involvement. Clonal cytogenetic abnormalities are present in 20% to 40% of CMML and include trisomy 8, deletion 7q, and translocations involving 5q31–35; the latter activate the PDGFR-β and are associated with eosinophilia (4,19,20).

Clinical Features

CMML frequently presents with fatigue, fever, weight loss, or night sweats. There is risk of infection because of neutropenia and of bleeding secondary to thrombocytopenia. In approximately 50% of patients the white count at presentation may be normal or decreased while in the remainder it is elevated. In all cases there is persistent peripheral blood monocytosis, the defining feature of the disease. Progression to acute leukemia occurs in 15% to 30% of cases (21).

Diagnostic Testing

WHO diagnostic criteria include the following:

- Persistent peripheral blood monocytosis (greater than 1×10^9 per liter for more than 3 months).
- Absence of the Philadelphia chromosome or BCR/ABL fusion gene.
- Less than 20% blasts in the blood or bone marrow.
- Dysplasia of one or more myeloid lineages.
- Clonal cytogenetic abnormality.

If dysplasia is absent, the diagnosis can be made if there is a clonal abnormality and no other causes of monocytosis.

Staging and Prognostic Features

Based on peripheral blood leukocyte counts the FAB group proposed dividing CMML into a dysplastic and a proliferative form with a white count over 13,000 per cubic millimeter. Attempts to evaluate the prognostic value of these distinctions have yielded disparate results. Recent analysis of CMML patients diagnosed with CMML based on FAB classification identified the following factors as independently associated with shorter survival: hemoglobin less than 12 g/dL; lymphocyte count greater than 2,500 per cubic millimeter; medullary blast count 10% or more, and presence of circulating immature myeloid cells. Median survival was 12 months (22).

Treatment

Treatment approaches are all experimental and none has proven effective in modifying the natural course of the disease. Evaluation of treatment responses of CMML patients specifically is difficult, because they have historically been grouped under the myelodysplastic syndromes. Growth factors have been used to attempt to treat cytopenias and low-dose chemotherapy during the preleukemic phase of the disease. Hydroxyurea may be used to control cell counts in the proliferative phase. Although many patients respond initially to chemotherapy, complete responses are rare and remissions generally short-lived (23). A variety of low-dose chemotherapeutic agents including cytarabine, topotecan, fludarabine, oral idarubicin, and oral etoposide have showed little success in altering long-term survival rates. Imatinib mesylate is effective in the rare CMML patients who have PDGFRβ-translocations (24,25). Stem cell transplantation has proved successful in a small number of cases.

REFERENCES

1. Spivak JL. Diagnosis of the myeloproliferative disorders: resolving phenotypic mimicry. *Semin Hematol* 2003;40:1–5.
2. Kralovics R, Buser AS, Teo SS, et al. Comparison of molecular markers in a cohort of patients with chronic myeloproliferative disorders. *Blood* 2003;102:1869–1871.
3. Brodmann S, Passweg JR, Gratwohl A, et al. Myeloproliferative disorders: complications, survival and causes of death. *Ann Hematol* 2000;79:312–318.
4. Jaffe E, Harris LH, Stein H, et al. *Tumours of Hematopoietic and Lymphoid Tissues*. Lyon, France: IARC Press, 2001:49–55.
5. Spivak JL, Barosi G, Tognoni G, et al. Chronic Myeloproliferative disorders. *Hematology (Am Soc Hematol Educ Program)* 2003;200–224.
6. Spivak JL. Polycythemia vera: myths, mechanisms, and management. *Blood* 2002;100:4272–4290.
7. Klippel S, Strunck E, Temerinac S, et al. Quantification of PRV-1 mRNA distinguishes polycythemia vera from secondary erythrocytosis. *Blood* 2003;102:3569–3574.
8. Streiff MB, Smith B, Spivak JL. The diagnosis and management of polycythemia vera in the era since the Polycythemia Vera Study Group: a survey of American Society of Hematology members' practice patterns. *Blood* 2002;99:1144–1149.
9. Tefferi A. Polycythemia vera: a comprehensive review and clinical recommendations. *Mayo Clin Proc* 2003;78:174–194.
10. Spivak JL. The optimal management of polycythaemia vera. *Br J Haematol* 2002;116:243–254.
11. Landolfi R, Marchioli R, Kutti J, et al. Efficacy and safety of low-dose aspirin in polycythemia vera. *N Engl J Med* 2004;350:114–124.
12. Diehn F, Tefferi A. Pruritus in polycythaemia vera: prevalence, laboratory correlates and management. *Br J Haematol* 2001;115:619–621.
13. Fruchtman SM. Transplant decision-making strategies in the myeloproliferative disorders. *Semin Hematol* 2003;40:30–33.
14. Harrison CN, Gale RE, Machin SJ, et al. A large proportion of patients with a diagnosis of essential thrombocythemia do not have a clonal disorder and may be at lower risk of thrombotic complications. *Blood* 1999;93:417–424.
15. Tefferi A. Recent progress in the pathogenesis and management of essential thrombocythemia. *Leuk Res* 2001;25:369–377.
16. Barosi G. Myelofibrosis with myeloid metaplasia. *Hematol Oncol Clin North Am* 2003;17: 1211–1226.
17. Tefferi A. Myelofibrosis with myeloid metaplasia. *N Engl J Med* 2000;342:1255–1265.
18. Guardiola P, Anderson JE, Bandini G, et al. Allogeneic stem cell transplantation for agnogenic myeloid metaplasia: a European Group for Blood and Marrow Transplantation, Societe Francaise de Greffe de Moelle, Gruppo Italiano per il Trapianto del Midollo Osseo, and Fred Hutchinson Cancer Research Center Collaborative Study. *Blood* 1999;93:2831–2838.
19. Gunby RH, Cazzaniga G, Tassi E et al. Sensitivity to imatinib but low frequency of the TEL/PDGFRb fusion protein in chronic myelomonocytic leukemia. Haematologica. 2003;88:408–415.
20. Magnusson MK, Meade KE, Brown KE, et al. Rabaptin-5 is a novel fusion partner to platelet-derived growth factor beta receptor in chronic myelomonocytic leukemia. *Blood* 2001;98:2518–2525.
21. Cortes J. CMML: a biologically distinct myeloproliferative disease. *Curr Hematol Rep* 2003;2: 202–208.
22. Onida F, Kantarjian HM, Smith TL, et al. Prognostic factors and scoring systems in chronic myelomonocytic leukemia: a retrospective analysis of 213 patients. *Blood* 2002;99:840–849.

23. Bennett JM. Chronic myelomonocytic leukemia. *Curr Treat Options Oncol* 2002;3:221–223.
24. Apperley JF, Gardembas M, Melo JV, et al. Response to imatinib mesylate in patients with chronic myeloproliferative diseases with rearrangements of the platelet-derived growth factor receptor beta. *N Engl J Med* 2002;347:481–487.
25. Magnusson MK, Meade KE, Nakamura R, et al. Activity of STI571 in chronic myelomonocytic leukemia with a platelet-derived growth factor beta receptor fusion oncogene. *Blood* 2002;100: 1088–1091

9

Neutrophil Disorders and Neutropenias

Matthew M. Hsieh and Harry L. Malech

Neutrophil or polymorphonuclear cells (PMN) are 5 μm in diameter with a distinctive multilobed nucleus and many small granules. Neutrophil maturation begins with myeloblasts in the bone marrow. Myeloblasts differentiate into promyelocytes characterized by the appearance of primary (azurophil) granules containing myeloperoxidase, followed by myelocytes characterized by the formation of secondary granules containing lactoferrin and gelatinase, and progress through metamyelocytes, band form, and finally mature neutrophils. This normal process typically occurs over 10 to 14 days but may be accelerated in the setting of infection, leading to more mature cells retaining excessive numbers of large azurophil granules (toxic granulation). Once mature neutrophils exit bone marrow, they remain in circulation for 6 to 12 hours. At sites of infection or inflammation, neutrophils adhere to and migrate between postvenule endothelial cells to exit blood vessels into the tissues, where they persist for 1 to 3 days (1). Absent from overt infection, most neutrophils in the circulation progress to apoptosis and are inserted by macrophages in the spleen. Even without infection, baseline neutrophil migration into the mouth and gastrointestinal tract contributes to the barrier function of the mucosa, by preventing entry of bacteria into tissues at those sites. In severe neutropenia, the gastrointestinal tract is often the first site of invasive bacterial infection.

Neutrophils in the circulation are metabolically quiescent. When stimulated by inflammation-/infection-related cytokines or chemotactic factors, they exit the circulation by adherence to endothelial cells and migrate to sites of inflammation where they represent the first line of defense against bacteria. Neutrophils internalize microbial particles by phagocytosis via Fc receptors and complement C3, and granule contents and reactive oxidants are released into phagosomes to kill infecting organisms. Increased numbers of life-threatening bacterial and function infections occur in association with inherited or acquired disorders characterized by abnormal granule formation, poor neutrophil adherence, failure to produce microbicidal oxidants, or where there is very low production or increased destruction of neutrophils (1,2).

QUALITATIVE NEUTROPHIL DISORDERS

Leukocyte Adhesion Deficiency

The β_2 integrins in neutrophils are important for normal neutrophil egress from blood postcapillary venules, for migration through tissues, and for complement-mediated phagocytosis (Table 9-1). Three leukocyte β_2 integrins adhesion molecules share the CD18 protein antigen as a common subunit: CD11a/CD18 (lymphocyte function associated antigen-1); CD11b/CD18 (macrophage 1 antigen); and CD11c/CD18 (also known as p150/95). Mutations in the gene encoding CD18 are responsible for the leukocyte adhesion deficiency 1 (LAD1) disease (3). (LAD-2 has been described in only two individuals and relates to an abnormality of fucose glycosylation. In general, LAD used without the numerical identification refers to LAD-1.) LAD has an autosomal recessive inheritance pattern, affecting only a few individuals per million. LAD is associated with recurrent life-threatening infections and other characteristic clinical manifestations. Diagnosis is made by flow cytometry measurement of the amount

TABLE 9–1. *Outline of neutrophil disorders and neutropenials*

Disease	Molecular or genetic defect	Pathogenic organisms and sites affected	Clinical presentation
LAD	CD18	Gram-negative enteric bacteria, *S aureus*, candida species, aspergillus species	Recurrent infections of skin, soft tissue, respiratory and gastrointestinal tract; periodontal disease; delayed separation of umbilical cord
MPO deficiency	Reduced MPO from multiple defects	Candida species in those with diabetes	Typically with no or mild clinical disease
CGD	Defective NADPH oxidases	Catalse-positive organisms: *S. aureus*, *B. cepacia*, aspergillus species, nocardia species, *S. marcescens*	Cellulitis, lymphadenitis, pneumonia; abscess formation in lungs, liver, brain, and bone; granuloma in gastrointestinal or genitourinary tract
CHS	LYST mutation → giant granules	*S. aureus*, oropharyngeal organisms	Albinism, peripheral neuropathy, recurrent bacterial infections, periodontitis, easy bruising
SGD	C/EBPε	*S. aureus*, *S. epidermidis*, enteric bacteria	Recurrent skin and lung infections
Drug-induced neutropenia	Immune clearance or marrow suppression		Infection severity dependent on degree of neutropenia
Infection-related neutropenia	Immune clearance or marrow suppression		
Severe congenital neutropenia	Unknown, some with ELA2 mutation	*S. aureus*, *B. aeruginosa*, cellulitis, stomatitis, meningitis, perirectal abscess	Recurrent infections starting at 3–6 months of age; responsive to G–CSF injections; increased risk of MDS/AML
Cyclic neutropenia	Unknown, some with ELA2 19p13.3 mutation	Aphthous ulcers, gingivitis, stomatitis, cellulitis	21-day pattern of neutropenia; some may require G-CSF; no risk of MDS/AML
Autoimmune neutropenia	Antineutrophil antibodies		Coexisting autoimmune disorders
Idiopathic neutropenia	Unknown	Skin and oropharynx	Usually mild infections; rare severe infections; negative antineutrophil antibodies
Benign ethnic neutropenia	Unknown	Asymptomatic	Seen mostly in those of African descent, neutrophil count may range from 1,000–2,000 per microliter

From Lekstrom-Himes JA et al, NEJM, Dec 7 2000, p. 1704; Klempner MS et al, p. 24, with permission.
LAD, leukocyte adhesion deficiency; MPO, myeloperoxidase; CGD, chronic granulomatous disease; CHS, Chediak-Higashi syndrome; SGD, specific granule deficiency; G-CSF, granulocyte colony-stimulating factor; MDS, myelodyplastic syndrome; AML, acute myelogenous leukemia.

of CD11b or CD18 on the surface of neutrophils using specific antibodies. The severity of disease manifestations, including risk of early death from infection, correlates with the amount of β_2 integrins present. The moderate phenotype has 1% to 10%, while the severe phenotype has less than 1% detectable β_2 integrins. On the cellular level, there is poor neutrophil adhesion to endothelial and other immune cells, and neutrophils do not egress from the vasculature and migrate to sites of inflammation. The baseline peripheral neutrophil count, even in the absence of infection, is approximately 2 to 3 times normal; when infections are present, neutrophil numbers can exceed 60,000 μL. Sometimes this is mistaken for a leukemic condition. Despite high circulating levels of neutrophils, there may be only mild erythema or pain at sites of infection, and patients fail to form pus, a condition that has been termed tissue neutropenia. A hallmark of severe LAD is delayed separation of the umbilical cord, indicating a role for neutrophils in providing proteases and hyaluronidases required for that event. Other manifestations associated with severe LAD include recurrent infections of the skin (ulcers), oral cavity (gingivitis, peridontitis with early loss of primary and secondary teeth), respiratory tract (sinusitis, otitis media, pneumonia), gastrointestinal tract, and genital mucosa. Infection of the wall of the small bowel or colon complicated by perforation is a particular risk that often leads to a fatal outcome. Infections are commonly caused by *Staphylococcus aureus,* enteric organisms, candida and aspergillus species. In patients with milder forms of LAD who do not undergo transplantation and survive past the first decade, chronic large nonhealing ulcers of the lower extremities and groin are characteristic and difficult to control or treat. Therapies include bacterial prophylaxis with trimethoprim/sulfamethoxazole, supportive antibiotics during acute infections, surgical debridement when necessary, and skin grafting. There is a high mortality rate (approximately 75%) of severe LAD in the first year of life; successful bone marrow transplant is curative and should be considered for all patients.

Myeloperoxidase Deficiency

Myeloperoxidase (MPO) is the most abundant protein in neutrophil granules. MPO resides in the primary (azurophilic) granules and has antimicrobial functions (it catalyzes the production of hypochlorous acid from chloride and the hydrogen peroxide product of the phagocyte nicotinamide adenine dinucleotide phosphate [NADPH] oxidase). MPO deficiency (4) is the most common neutrophil abnormality, with an incidence of approximately 1 per 2,000 for partial deficiency and 1 per 4,000 for complete deficiency. Most individuals with MPO deficiency do not manifest any clinical problems although *ex vivo* assays of bacterial and fungal killing demonstrate a defect. MPO deficiency is inherited in an autosomal recessive pattern, but also can manifest as an acquired abnormality associated with leukemia or myelodysplasia. Identified mutations in the MPO gene may affect transcription, translation, and/or insertion of the heme group. Neutrophils with MPO deficiency mature, migrate, and phagocytose normally but are defective in microbial killing. Some individuals have a mildly increased frequency in bacterial infections, and with cofactors such as diabetes may have particular difficulty in clearing infection by Candida species (*Candida albicans, C. tropicalis, C. stelatoidea, and C. krusei*). Diagnosis of MPO deficiency may be made by measurement of peroxidase activity using flow cytometry or with certain automated blood counters that use peroxidase activity to distinguish subpopulations of circulating leukocytes. Because most disease is mild, antimicrobial and supportive therapy is sufficient. Prophylactic antibiotics should be limited to patients with recurrent infections or with another disorder predisposing to infections.

Chronic Granulomatous Disease

The chronic granulomatous diseases are a group of closely related inherited disorders characterized by defective phagocyte NADPH oxidase, manifested by a failure of stimulated neutrophils, monocytes, eosinophils, and macrophages to produce superoxide and hydrogen peroxide (1). Chronic granulomatous disease (CGD) affects approximately 5 individuals per 1 million, equally affecting all ethnic groups. CGDs are caused by mutations in any of four subunit components of the phagocyte NADPH oxidase. The clinically most severe is the X-linked, gp91phox subunit-deficient form, usually associated with total absence of any oxidant production and affecting almost 70% of patients with CGD. The other three types of CGD are inherited in an autosomal recessive pattern and consist mostly of p47phox-deficient CGD patients (25% of CGD patients) with the remainder comprising the much less common p67phox- or p22phox-deficient CGDs. Clinical manifestations of CGDs involve both recurrent infections and formation of inflammatory granulomas; severity and individual manifestations vary widely. The average age of diagnosis of X-linked CGD is before 3 years of age; females with the p47phox form of CGD are on average 9 years of age at diagnosis. Some patients with no family history may reach young adulthood before the disease is recognized.

Unlike patients with severe neutropenia or LAD who are infected primarily with commensal organisms (such as enteric bacterial normally found in the gastrointestinal tract), CGD patients are generally not susceptible to bacteria such as *Escherichia coli*. Instead, they are peculiarly susceptible to a defined group of environmental organisms that generally have the characteristic of being catalase-positive. The usual bacterial pathogens are *S. aureus*, nocardia, *Burkholderia cepacia* (and other Burkholderia species), and *Serratia marcescens*. Fungal pneumonia and other fungal infections aspergillus species are a particular problem, as well as infections with paecilomyces, and other fungi. Patients with CGD do not seem to be particularly susceptible to *C. albicans* infections (though candida species such as glabrata may be problematic). Infections are usually recurrent and prolonged, but episodic, and patients with CGD receiving effective prophylaxis may have many months or years between severe infection. The most common life-threatening infections in CGD are bacterial or fungal pneumonias, although local soft tissue infections and lymph node infections are more common. All other tissues can be involved including processes as diverse as osteomyelitis or brain abscess. Following pneumonia, the most common severe infections are liver abscesses. In patients with CGD receiving trimethoprim-sulfamethoxazole daily prophylaxis, severe staphylococcal deep-tissue infections are relatively uncommon, while almost 90% of liver abscesses appear to be caused by *S. aureus*. Liver abscesses are generally not easily drained pustular lesions, most often consisting of a solid granulomatous mass with microabcesses that requires surgical extirpation and prolonged antibiotic therapy.

In some individuals with CGD, granuloma formation may predominate over infection; in other cases, granulomatous inflammation can cause gastroesophageal junction or gastric outlet obstructions, bladder outlet obstruction, or chronic abdominal pain with diarrhea. Gastrointestinal granulomata may be indistinguishable from Crohn's disease and appear to respond to similar treatments. CGD granulomas are distinguished from granulomas of autoimmune diseases when they respond to treatment with a tapering dose of corticosteroids and controllable long-term on low-dose alternate-day prednisone.

CGD should be suspected where there is a family history of unexplained deaths in infant or young boys, in patients infected by suspected organisms (e.g., serratia osteomyelitis in an infant is almost diagnostic of CGD), and in children with pneumonia that does not rapidly resolve with conventional therapy. Diagnosis is made by a dihydrorhodamine flow cytometry measurement demonstrating defective oxidase activity in neutrophils, and is confirmed by quantitative assays of superoxide production. Acute infections are managed with antibiotics and supportive therapy. Because of the propensity of patients with CGD to become infected by unusual organisms such as nocardia or aspergillus, aggressive efforts to identify a pathogenic organism are essential to direct antimicrobial therapy. When infections resolve, a prophylactic regimen includes good oral hygiene with chlorhexidine and/or peroxide-based mouthwash, daily oral trimethoprim and sulfamethoxazole (TMP/SMX; 5 to 6 mg/kg per day TMP equivalent), daily oral itraconazole (4 to 5 mg/kg per day), and three-times-weekly subcutaneous injections of recombinant interferon-γ (0.05 mg/m^2). Surgical intervention may be necessary to identify pathogens, debride devitalized tissues, and accelerate recovery and response to therapy.

Granulomatous process can occur with or without infections; thus, appropriate microbial cultures are an important part of their evaluation. Gastrointestinal or genitourinary granulomata not associated with pathogen can be treated with 0.5 to 1 mg/kg of prednisone for 2 weeks, followed by gradual taper, although some patients require 0.1 to 0.25 mg/kg prednisone on a long-term basis for control of granuloma gastrointestinal and/or genitourinary problems. Hematopoietic stem cell transplant may be considered for some patients with severe disease and/or many recurrent infections who have an human leukocyte antigen (HLA)-matched sibling donor.

Chédiak-Higashi Syndrome

Chédiak-Higashi syndrome (CHS) (5) is a rare autosomal recessive disorder caused by *LYST* gene mutations, leading to abnormal intracytoplasmic protein transport and vacuole formation. This results in fusion of intracellular granules and uneven distribution of giant granules in the cytoplasm of neutrophils and many other cells, such as platelets, melanocytes, renal tubular cells, Schwann cells, thyroid follicular cells, and mast cells. Cells containing giant granules have impaired function, which can manifest as recurrent bacterial infections; bleeding or easy bruising; hypopigmentation of skin, eyes, and hair; recurrent infections; a peripheral nerve defect (neuropathy, nystagmus); and abnormal natural killer cell functions. The diagnosis is made by detecting large granules in neutrophils on the peripheral blood smear. Treatment includes supportive therapy and bacterial prophylaxis with TMP/SMX. Not all patients have recurrent infections, and some instead suffer progressive peripheral neuropathy that manifests during the third decade of life. A fatal, lymphoma-like condition can develop in CHS. Vitamin C was shown to partially reverse some of the cellular defects observed *in vitro,* but vitamin C treatment has not clearly been shown to reduce infection or alter the course of the disease. Stem cell transplantation can be considered for those who develop an accelerated phase with lympho-proliferative lymphoma-like syndrome.

Specific Granule Deficiency

The secondary (or specific) granules of neutrophils contain a variety of proteases and other antimicrobial molecules. These proteins perform important normal functions in infection control and possibly also wound healing. Specific granule deficiency (SGD) (6) occurs as a rare inherited disorder or more commonly appears associated with leukemia or myelodysplasia. Acute burn injury has also been noted to result in neutrophils deficient in specific granules, although their approval could be secondary to degranulation. Inherited specific granule deficiency can result from a mutation in the gene encoding a key regulatory factor required for late events during myeloid differentiation (CCAAT/enhancer binding protein ε). Failure of function of this DNA binding differentiation factor protein results in inability to produce the specific granule itself, the contents of the specific granule, as well as failure to produce some late myeloid phase proteins. Patients with SGD have recurrent bacterial infections in early childhood; common sites are skin (cellulitis) and respiratory tract (sinusitis, pneumonia, otitis media). Similar to LAD, there is no erythema or pus at the site of infections, and recurrent large nonhealing ulcers are a chronic problem. The presence of nonhealing ulcers in both specific granule deficiency and in LAD probably points to an important role of neutrophils not only for infection control but possibly also in wound healing. Treatment of SGD includes antibiotics for acute infections, and prophylaxis with daily TMP/SMX and itraconazole.

NEUTROPENIAS

Neutropenia is usually defined by an absolute neutrophil count (ANC) less than 1.5×10^9 per liter (or less than 1,500 per cubic millimeter). Neutropenia is present in some hereditary

TABLE 9–2. *Definitions of severity of neutropenia*

Degree of neutropenia and ANC	Neutrophil reserve	Duration of neutropenia
Normal: >1500 /mm³ Mild: 1,000–1,500 /mm³ Moderate: 500–1,000 /mm³ Some increased risk for infections Severe: <500 /mm³ Significant risk for infections	Normal if: No prior cytotoxic therapy Appropriate ANC increases in response to infection or stress Normal bone marrow biopsy	Periodic or episodic (e.g. after chemotherapy) Chronic

ANC, absolute neutrophil count.

syndromes, and can also result from infections, drugs or toxins, or autoimmune disorders. The risk of infection from neutropenia depends on three factors: the ANC, the neutrophil reserve in bone marrow, and the duration of neutropenia. Risk is increased with neutrophil count of 0.5 to 1.0 $\times$ 10^9 per liter (500 to 1,000 per cubic millimeter) and is greatest with less than 0.5 $\times$ 10^9 per liter (less than 500 per cubic millimeter). A falling neutrophil count or a significant decrease over steady-state levels, with a failure to increase neutrophil counts in the setting of bone marrow stress carries a higher risk of complication than a stable, chronically low neutrophil count over many months or years that rises significantly in response to infection (Table 9–2).

ACQUIRED NEUTROPENIAS

Drug-Induced Neutropenia

Drugs can cause mild neutropenia or agranulocytosis (ANC less than 500 per cubic millimeter) in one of two manners: either by direct cytotoxic effect to rapidly dividing bone marrow cells or by binding as haptens, leading to immune-mediated destruction of myeloid precursor cells. Most chemotherapy agents and many antimicrobials cause neutropenia by the first mechanism; neutropenia typically develops in 7 to 14 days, is dose related, and is dependent on continued administration of the drug. Sulfa and penicillin-like drugs cause neutropenia by the second mechanism; neutropenia can appear as early as 7 days after exposure to a drug, sometimes with associated fever or eosinophilia. The degree of neutropenia can be severe but resolution of the low white blood cell (WBC) count usually requires only that the sensitizing drug be discontinued. Cytokines such as granulocyte colony-stimulating factor (G-CSF) and granulocyte-macrophage colony-stimulating factor (GM-CSF) are commonly administered in agranulocytosis but are of unproven benefit. Neutrophil counts usually begin to recover 5 to 10 days after drug cessation. Readministration of the sensitizing drug may decrease neutrophil counts abruptly. While some drugs (Table 9–3) have more often been cited as a cause of drug-related neutropenia, severe immune-mediated drug-induced neutropenia can be associated with any drug including such unlikely agents as aspirin or Tylenol.

Infection-Related Neutropenia

Neutropenia after infections is common, and can result from neutrophil destruction, margination, sequestration, or marrow suppression. Neutropenia from viral infections can be seen as early as a few days, and can persist for the duration of viremia. The degree and duration is usually mild and short, but neutropenia from Epstein-Barr virus, hepatitis, and human

TABLE 9–3. *Abbreviated list of common drugs causing neutropenia (7)*

Sulfa-containing drugs
Antimicrobials: penicillin, cephalosporin
NSAIDs
Tricyclic antidepressants
Cardiac medications: antiarrhythmic agents, digoxin, diuretics, ACE inhibitors
Reflux/ulcer agents: cimetidine, ranitidine
Antipsychotic agents: clozapine
Antiviral agents (against HIV, HSV, CMV)
Rheumatoid arthritis agents: penicillamine, gold compounds
Antithyroid agents
Chemotherapy

NSAIDs, nonsteroidal anti-inflammatory drugs; ACE, angiotensin-converting enzyme; HIV, human immunodeficiency virus; HSV, herpes simplex virus; CMV, cytomegalovirus.

immunodeficiency virus (HIV) can be severe and protracted. Gram-negative bacterial infections can cause neutropenia in those with impaired marrow neutrophil reserve, such as neonates, the elderly, and the chronically immunosuppressed. Protozoal (Leishmania) and rickettsial (RMSF and Ehrlichia) infections also produce neutropenia, often with accompanying anemia and/or thrombocytopenia.

Immune-Related Neutropenia

This form of neutropenia is typically associated with specific antibodies directed to neutrophil antigens (not to be confused with antinuclear antibodies). These antibodies occur with or without autoimmune disorders. Many syndromes are clinically similar and are briefly discussed below.

In *alloimmune (or isoimmune) neonatal neutropenia* (8), maternal immunoglobulin G (IgG) antibodies are directed to fetal neutrophils causing moderate neutropenia that is self-limiting, lasting only a few weeks to a few months. These neonates have increased risk of infections and can develop pulmonary, skin or urinary tract infections from gram-positive or -negative organisms. Treatment is supportive with antibiotics, intravenous immunoglobulin (IVIg) and sometimes G-CSF.

Autoimmune neutropenia of infancy/childhood (8) is typically seen in children younger than 2 years of age. The degree of neutropenia varies, and infections in the oropharynx, ear, sinus, and upper respiratory tract can occur. The neutropenia may resolve spontaneously over many months or years and typically does not require treatment. Antibiotics and G-CSF are administered during acute infections, and TMP/SMX is often prescribed for prophylaxis.

Autoimmune neutropenia (8) in adults is best described in systemic lupus erythematosus, rheumatoid arthritis, or collagen vascular disease. Felty syndrome is manifested by the triad of neutropenia, rheumatoid arthritis, and splenomegaly. The degree of these neutropenias is variable, and treatment of the underlying autoimmune disorder will generally (but not invariably) improve neutropenia. While autoimmune neutropenia can occur without concurrent autoimmune disorders, the clinical syndromes are less well described.

Large granular lymphocytosis (LGL) (9) is caused by abnormally expanded T or natural killer (NK) cells infiltrating the bone marrow, spleen, and liver, resulting in variable degree of single lineage cytopenia, bicytopenia, or pancytopenia and splenomegaly. This may be an oligoclonal or monoclonal disease, and in its more aggressive form is considered a form of leukemia. LGL is typically described in individuals older than 55 years. Laboratory evaluation will reveal multiple abnormalities: 60% of affected individuals will have lymphocytosis greater than 5×10^9 per cubic millimeter, 80% with ANC less than 1.5×10^9 per cubic millimeter, 50% with hemoglobin less than 11 g/dL, 20% with platelets less 150 per cubic millimeter; 40% will have LGL count of 1 to 4×10^9 per cubic millimeter, and 40% with LGL count of 4 to 10×10^9 per cubic millimeter. LGL is also associated with autoimmune disorders, myeloid and B cell malignancies, or solid tumors. Bone marrow examinations are variable, but most show a hypercellular marrow. Treatment is not necessary until there are recurrent infections (or symptomatic anemia). Corticosteroids, methotrexate, and cyclosporine have been used with generally good response rates. However, aggressive monoclonal LGL disease requires specific chemotherapies appropriate to control leukemia.

CONGENITAL NEUTROPENIAS

Severe Congenital Neutropenia (Kostmann Syndrome)

In 1956, Kostmann described severe neutropenia associated with recurrent bacterial infections in several families in northern Sweden. This syndrome was later observed in other geographic locations (10). It is a rare clinical entity with an incidence rate of approximately 1 to 2 per million and a variable inheritance pattern. Neutrophil elastase (ELA 2) mutations have been identified in some affected individuals, and these mutations have been hypothesized to cause defective signal transduction and cause programmed cell death (apoptosis) at the myelocyte level. Additional genetic abnormalities can be acquired and may lead to myelodysplasia and/or acute myeloid leukemia: G-CSF receptor mutation, RAS oncogene mutation, or chromosome 7 monosomy.

Clinically, patients are infected at as early as 2 to 3 months of age by gram-positive or gram-negative bacteria in one or more of the following sites: skin, ears, oral or gastrointestinal mucosa, upper or lower respiratory tract, urinary tract, or blood. Blood counts usually reveal neutrophil count less than 500 per microliter (less than 0.5×10^9 per liter) with compensatory monocytosis and eosinophilia. Bone marrow biopsies show maturation arrest at the promyelocyte-myelocyte level, and absent band forms or mature neutrophils. Treatment includes supportive care and antibiotics for acute infections. G-CSF between 3 and 10 μg/kg has been successful in increasing neutrophil counts and reducing the frequency of infections. A minority of patients will require in excess of 30 μg/kg per day. Longer duration or high cumulative doses of G-CSF are not currently believed to be associated with acquisition of G-CSF mutations or a cause of the leukemias associated with this disorder. Toxicities of long-term G-CSF administration include bone pain from marrow expansion, osteopenia or osteoporosis, and splenomegaly. Bone marrow transplant is a curative option for patients with HLA-matched sibling donors.

Cyclic Neutropenia

The incidence of inherited cyclic neutropenia is not known (11). The cause is not completely understood, although neutrophil elastase 19p13.3 mutations are associated with this disorder and are hypothesized to cause neutrophil apoptosis and thus to initiate the cycling. Clinically, neutrophil counts oscillate predictably between low or agranulocytic to the low-normal range; the average cycle length is 21 days with neutropenic duration of 3 to 6 days. The nadir neutrophil count can be zero or as low as 200 per microliter (0.2×10^9 per liter). Platelet, reticulocytes, lymphocyte, and monocytes counts may also cycle or countercycle from a normal to a high range, coinciding or not with the neutrophil cycles. Serial bone marrow examinations will appear normal with normal neutrophil count and show decreased myeloid precursors in the neutropenic phase. Individuals with cyclic neutropenia are typically asymptomatic with normal neutrophil counts, but have fever, lymphadenopathy, mild skin infections, and/or oral mucosal ulcers during periods of neutropenia. Mild skin infections and/or mouth ulcers are treated symptomatically. In some individuals, G-CSF eliminates the cycling, while in others it shortens the cycles while increasing the levels of neutrophils at both the peak and the nadir, thus reducing infections. GM-CSF does not effectively treat inherited cyclic neutropenia.

OTHER NEUTROPENIAS

Idiopathic Neutropenia

Idiopathic or chronic idiopathic neutropenia affects approximately 2 to 4 individuals per million, and can be seen in both children and adults (10,12). The clinical behavior is similar to autoimmune neutropenia, except that antineutrophil antibodies are not detected and other studies are not diagnostic. Most individuals have moderate neutropenia with mild symptoms, if any. A small subset of patients have severe neutropenia, recurrent fever, oropharyngeal infections (mucosal ulcers, gingivitis), or severe systemic infections. Treatments are largely tailored for symptomatic relief and antibiotics dictated by sites of infection. G-CSF, 1 to 3 μg/kg per dose weekly or on alternate days, is used for the more severe clinical syndrome. Development of myelodysplastic syndrome or leukemias have not been observed. In general, patients whose neutrophil count increases with infection or stress have a benign clinical course.

Benign Ethnic Neutropenia

Benign ethnic neutropenia (BEN) is a condition seen mostly in individuals of African descent, including African Americans, Yemenite Jews, and certain populations in the Caribbean and Middle East (13,14). As many as 25% of normal African Americans will have lower WBC counts than age-matched Caucasians, although only a subset will have neutrophil counts less than 1.5×10^9 per liter. A stem cell disorder, excessive margination, and differentiation defects have been excluded as etiologic, suggesting that this is a normal population-based variant. The physiologic mechanisms controlling the normal set point for circulating levels of neutrophils are unknown. The CXCR4 chemokine receptor for the SDF-1 chemokine may play a role in egress of neutrophils from the marrow, and at least theoretically differences in expression or function of this cytokine/cytokine receptor could affect homeostatic blood counts. Perhaps normal variants in this or other receptors are responsible for population differences observed in average circulating neutrophil counts. Individuals with ethnic neutropenia are asymptomatic, without infections. When they acquire typical viral or bacterial infections, these infections are not more severe and do not need longer period of treatment. Laboratory evaluations show many blood counts that are abnormal for many years, and bone marrow examinations will be normal. Symptomatic treatment and antibiotics should be provided as needed (for a normal healthy adult) and no additional therapy is required, but it is important to note this variant to avoid unnecessary medical evaluation.

REFERENCES

1. Klempner M, Malech HL. Phagocytes: normal and abnormal neutrophil host defenses. In: Gorbach SL, Bartlett JG, Blacklow NR, eds. *Infectious Diseases*. 3rd ed. Philadelphia: Lippincott Williams & Wilkins, 2003:14–39.
2. Lekstrom-Himes JA, Gallin JI. Immunodeficiency diseases caused by defects in phagocytes. *N Engl J Med* 2000;343:1703–1714.
3. Bunting M, Harris ES, McIntyre TM, et al. Leukocyte adhesion deficiency syndromes: adhesion and tethering defects involving beta 2 integrins and selectin ligands. *Curr Opin Hematol* 2002;9:30–35.
4. Lanza F. Clinical manifestation of myeloperoxidase deficiency. *J Mol Med* 1998;76:676–681.
5. Ward DM, Shiflett SL, Kaplan J. Chediak-Higashi syndrome: a clinical and molecular view of a rare lysosomal storage disorder. *Curr Mol Med* 2002;2:469–477.

6. Gombart AF, Koeffler HP. Neutrophil specific granule deficiency and mutations in the gene encoding transcription factor C/EBP(epsilon). *Curr Opin Hematol* 2002;9:36–42.
7. Kaufman DW, Kelly JP, Jurgelon JM, et al. Drugs in the aetiology of agranulocytosis and aplastic anaemia. *Eur J Haematol Suppl* 1996;60:23–30.
8. Palmblad JE, von dem Borne AE. Idiopathic, immune, infectious, and idiosyncratic neutropenias. *Semin Hematol* 2002;39:113–120.
9. Lamy T, Loughran TP, Jr. Clinical features of large granular lymphocyte leukemia. *Semin Hematol.* 2003;40:185–195.
10. Dale DC, Cottle TE, Fier CJ, et al. Severe chronic neutropenia: treatment and follow-up of patients in the Severe Chronic Neutropenia International Registry. *Am J Hematol* 2003;72:82–93.
11. Dale DC, Bolyard AA, Aprikyan A. Cyclic neutropenia. *Semin Hematol* 2002;39:89–94.
12. Dale DC. Immune and idiopathic neutropenia. *Curr Opin Hematol* 1998;5:33–36.
13. Mason BA, Lessin L, Schechter GP. Marrow granulocyte reserves in black Americans. Hydrocortisone-induced granulocytosis in the "benign" neutropenia of the black. *Am J Med* 1979;67:201–205.
14. Haddy TB, Rana SR, Castro O. Benign ethnic neutropenia: what is a normal absolute neutrophil count? *J Lab Clin Med* 1999;133:15–22.

10

Childhood Hematologic Diseases

Robert I. Liem and Alan S. Wayne

Despite some overlap with disorders encountered in adults, many congenital and acquired hematologic diseases manifest primarily during childhood. In addition, pediatric hematology is distinguished by developmental differences in normal physiology and blood parameters. The purpose of this chapter is to highlight unique features in the evaluation, diagnosis and treatment of common pediatric hematologic conditions (1). The reader is referred to other chapters in this edition for additional details of the management of specific disorders.

ANEMIA

Normal red blood cell (RBC) values vary with age and are affected by such factors as race, sex and altitude (Table 10-1). The RBC count is highest at birth and continues to decrease gradually to a physiologic nadir at 2 to 4 months, at which point erythropoiesis is stimulated. Anemia is defined as an overall reduction in red cell mass or hemoglobin (Hb) concentration, usually set at 2 standard deviations below the mean normal value for the specific population.

Pediatric anemia is commonly classified according to RBC size (Table 10-2). Microcytic anemias account for the majority of cases of anemia in early childhood (Table 10-3). Screening for anemia in the first year of life is recommended for at-risk populations.

The initial diagnostic evaluation of a child with anemia should consist of a detailed history and physical examination and the following minimal laboratory testing: complete blood count (CBC), reticulocyte count, and examination of the peripheral smear (2). Consideration of the physiologic basis for anemia can be helpful in guiding further investigation (Table 10-4).

Microcytic Anemias

Iron deficiency is the most common cause of anemia during childhood and may result from a combination of low stores at birth, high requirements because of growth and blood volume expansion, inadequate nutrition, and poor bioavailability of dietary iron. Iron deficiency due to blood loss is most commonly a result of gastrointestinal tract irritation and occult hemorrhage associated with introduction of cow's milk before the first year of life or menstruation during adolescence. On history, additional risk factors for iron deficiency may include prematurity, limited or prolonged breast-feeding, non-iron–fortified formula or excessive intake of whole milk (generally more than 1 quart per day). Early iron deficiency may result only in a low ferritin. This is followed by a decrease in serum iron and transferrin saturation and an increase in total iron-binding capacity (TIBC) and free erythrocyte protoporphyrin (FEP). With frank deficiency, there is hypochromia, microcytosis, and anisocytosis on the blood smear. The platelet count also may be increased. A response to a trial of elemental iron (3 mg/kg per day) is often helpful in differentiating iron deficiency from thalassemia

TABLE 10–1. *Normal hematologic parameters in children*

| Age | Hemoglobin (g/dL) | | Hematocrit (%) | | MCV (fL) | | Neutrophils (10³/μL) | |
	Mean	−2 SD	Mean	−2 SD	Mean	−2 SD	Mean	Range
Birth	16.5	13.5	51	42	108	98	11	6–26
1 mo	14	10	43	31	104	85	3.8	1–9
3–6 mo	11.5	9.5	35	29	91	74	3.8	1–8.5
0.5–2 yr	12	10.5	36	33	78	70	3.5	1.5–8.5
2–6 yr	12.5	11.5	37	34	81	75	4.3	1.5–8
6–12 yr	13.5	11.5	40	35	86	77	4.4	1.8–8
12–18 yr								
Male	14	12	41	36	90	78	4.4	1.8–8
Female	14.5	13	43	37	88	78	4.4	1.8–8

Modified from Dallman PR: In Rudolph A, ed. *Pediatrics.* 16th ed. New York, Appleton-Century-Crofts, 1977:1111,1178.
MCV, mean cell volume; SD, standard deviation; mo, month; yr, year.

trait: an Hb increase of more than 1 g/dL at 1 month and reticulocyte peak at 10 to 14 days is diagnostic. Iron supplementation should be provided for 3 to 6 months.

Lead toxicity (3) often coexists with iron deficiency in at-risk populations and may further inhibit gastrointestinal absorption of iron. Lead poisoning should be suspected if there is a history of pica or exposure to lead-based paint. An elevated FEP and basophilic stippling on peripheral smear may be seen. Therapy should include oral treatment with succimer or, in severe cases, parenteral treatment with dimercaprol (BAL) or calcium-sodium ethylenedi-aminetetraacetic acid (EDTA).

Thalassemia syndromes are common causes of microcytic anemia in childhood. The α-thalassemias present in utero or at birth, whereas β-thalassemias are not evident until 6 months of age, when β-globin synthesis becomes predominant. Thalassemia trait is often mistaken for iron deficiency (4). In contrast to iron deficiency, β-thalassemia trait is associated with a normal red cell distribution width (RDW), basophilic stippling and targeting on the

TABLE 10–2. *Classification of childhood anemia*

Microcytic	Normocytic	Macrocytic
• Iron deficiency	• Chronic inflammation,	• Reticulocytosis
• Lead poisoning	Infection, Bone marrow	• Vitamin B_{12}, folate deficiency
• Thalassemia syndromes	suppression or infiltration	• Congenital pure red cell
• Sideroblastic anemias	• Congenital hemolytic	aplasia (Diamond-Blackfan)
• Chronic inflammation	anemias	• Bone marrow failure (aplastic
	• Acquired hemolytic anemia	anemia, Fanconi)
	(auto or alloimmune,	• Liver disease
	microangiopathic)	• Hypothyroidism
	• Acute or subacute blood loss	• Drug-related
	• Splenic sequestration	
	• Transient erythroblastopenia	
	of childhood (TEC)	

TABLE 10–3. *Evaluation of microcytic anemia*

	Iron deficiency	Thalassemia trait	Thalassemia major	Lead toxicity	Chronic cisease
RDW	↑	NL	↑↑	NL	NL
MCV	↓	↓	↓	↓	↓
RBC #	↓	NL	↓	↓	↓
FEP	↑	NL	NL	↑↑	↑
Iron	↓	NL	↑	NL	↓
TIBC	NL↑	NL	NL ↑	NL	NL ↓
% Sat	↓	NL	↑	NL	↓
Ferritin	↓	NL	↑	NL	NL ↑
Hgb A₂	↓	β >3.5% α <3.5%	β >3.5% α <3.5%	NL	NL

RDW, red cell distribution width; MCV, mean cell volume; RBC, red blood cells; FEP, free erythrocyte protoporphyrin TIBC, total iron binding capacity.

blood smear, and an elevated Hb A2 on electrophoresis. α-thalassemia trait is associated a normal Hb electrophoresis outside of the newborn period, although Hb Bart's (γ4) is present on newborn screening samples. In the evaluation of thalassemias, ethnic heritage is often suggestive and microcytosis should be seen in at least one parent. Thalassemia trait (heterozygous β- and 1 and 2 gene deletion α-thalassemias) requires no therapy. In contrast, in thalassemia major, aggressive packed RBC transfusion should be initiated early in life to eliminate the increased erythropoietic drive and allow normal linear growth and bone development. In utero transfusion has been used to prevent hydrops fetalis in 4-gene–deletion α-thalassemia (Hb Bart's disease). Care should be given to address iron overload and chelation therapy in transfusion-dependent children to prevent end organ damage later in life. As an alternative to life-long transfusion and chelation therapy, allogeneic bone marrow transplantation (BMT) is a curative approach for children with thalassemia major who have human leukocyte antigen (HLA)-matched sibling donors.

TABLE 10–4. *Characteristics of anemia based on pathophysiology*

Decreased production	Increased destruction	Blood loss	Mixed pathophysiology
• ↓ Reticulocytes • +/− ↓ WBC, platelets • Erythroid hypoplasia on marrow	• ↑ Reticulocytes • ↑ Indirect bilirubin, LDH • ↓ Haptoglobin • Hemoglobinuria • Abnormal morphology on smear • May have splenomegaly	• Acute or subacute blood loss (may be occult) • ↑ Reticulocytes • Evolving iron deficiency	• ↓ Reticulocytes in setting of increased destruction (as in parvovirus B19 associated aplastic crisis in sickle cell disease or other congenital hemolytic anemia)

WBC, white blood cells; LDH, lactate dehydrogenase

Normocytic Anemias

Anemia is a common manifestation of numerous systemic conditions in pediatrics. The anemia of acute inflammation and chronic disease is frequently mild and usually normocytic, although the mean cell volume (MCV) is occasionally low. Transferrin is frequently diminished. Treatment is aimed at the primary condition. Viral infection is the most common cause of transient bone marrow suppression in children and may result in both anemia and leukopenia. The hallmark of viral suppression is failure of the reticulocyte count to increase in the face of anemia. Usually, only close observation is required because the bone marrow suppression is self-limited.

Transient erythroblastopenia of childhood (TEC) is an acquired pure red cell aplasia that can also follow viral illness in previously healthy children (5). The median age for presentation is 2 years, in contrast to congenital pure red cell aplasia, which commonly presents in infancy. Reticulocytopenia and, occasionally, leukopenia and thrombocytopenia are seen. Most children with TEC recover in 1 to 2 months. Observation alone is usually sufficient, although short-term transfusion therapy may be required for cardiovascular compromise associated with severe anemia.

Hemolysis usually results in normocytic anemia. There are a large number of congenital and acquired hemolytic conditions of childhood. Immune-mediated hemolysis, either isoimmune or alloimmune, may present in neonates; autoimmune hemolytic anemia is seen in older children. Hemoglobinopathies such as sickle cell disease, enzyme deficiencies such as glucose-6-phosphate dehydrogenase deficiency, and membrane disorders such as hereditary spherocytosis (HS) should be considered in the differential diagnosis of hemolysis. Microangiopathic hemolysis may be seen in hemolytic uremic syndrome (HUS) and disseminated intravascular coagulation (DIC). Laboratory features consistent with hemolysis include reticulocytosis, elevated lactate dehydrogenase (LDH), indirect hyperbilirubinemia, decreased serum haptoglobin, and, in severe cases, hemoglobinuria. A direct Coomb's test indicates immune-mediated hemolysis. Examination of the peripheral smear may reveal characteristic red cell morphology. Thrombocytopenia and renal impairment are additional features of HUS. Treatment of hemolysis should be directed toward the underlying cause, with transfusions reserved for severe anemia and cardiovascular compromise. Immune hemolysis often requires corticosteroids and/or other immunosuppressive medications.

Macrocytic Anemias

Vitamin B_{12} deficiency is associated with megaloblastic changes in the bone marrow (6). In infants, B_{12} deficiency may be the result of maternal depletion and decreased stores at birth. In older children and adolescents, causes include pernicious anemia, malabsorption, dietary deficiency, and inborn errors of metabolism. Unrecognized, severe deficiency early in life may cause failure to thrive and even permanent neurologic damage. Symptoms in older children may include anorexia, weight loss, diarrhea, constipation, weakness, glossitis, peripheral neuropathy, ataxia, and dementia. Anemia is commonly accompanied by neutropenia, hypersegmented neutrophils, and thrombocytopenia. A low serum B_{12} level and a response to replacement therapy are confirmatory.

Folate deficiency is also associated with a megaloblastic bone marrow (6). The newborn infant has increased demands for folate. Risk factors for early deficiency include prematurity, low levels in maternal breast milk, and a predominance of goat's milk intake. In older children, folate deficiency is usually the result of malnutrition, although it may also be caused by certain medications, chronic hemolysis, malabsorption, and inborn errors of metabolism. Serum and erythrocyte folate levels will be low and the anemia should respond to small replacement doses of folic acid.

Diamond-Blackfan anemia (DBA) or congenital pure red cell aplasia is usually noted soon after birth or during the first year of life. The main other entity in the differential diagnosis is TEC, which more commonly presents after the first year of life. Twenty-five percent of patients with DBA have associated anomalies, such as short stature and/or abnormalities of the head, face, and upper limbs. Laboratory features include reticulocytopenia, high MCV (often only mildly elevated), increased Hb F, normal or decreased white blood cell (WBC) count, and normal or increased platelet count. The bone marrow shows erythroid hypoplasia. In considering the differential diagnosis, a normal CBC in the past supports TEC and an abnormal chromosomal breakage study confirms Fanconi anemia (FA). The majority of children with DBA respond to corticosteroids. Prednisone is begun at a dosage of 2 mg/kg per day, with a response usually seen within 1 month. Once the Hb has reached a satisfactory level, steroids should be tapered to the lowest possible dose (ideally on an alternate day schedule). Although spontaneous remissions have occurred, corticosteroid dependence is the rule and chronic transfusion and chelation therapy should be considered for those with associated toxicity. Allogeneic BMT may be curative (7).

Fanconi anemia can often be differentiated from acquired aplastic anemia by characteristics such as impaired growth and/or anomalies of the thumbs, radii, kidneys, head, eyes, ears, skin and/or genitourinary system. Inheritance is autosomal recessive and the family history may be positive for marrow failure and leukemia. There is a 10% to 35% risk of developing leukemia or myelodysplastic syndrome (8). The first hematologic signs of FA may develop in infancy and often includes macrocytosis, elevated Hb F and/or mild cytopenia(s). Severe pancytopenia usually develops later in life. The differential includes other familial or acquired bone marrow failure syndromes. Abnormal chromosomal breakage analysis or FA genotyping confirms the diagnosis. Anemia is commonly androgen-responsive. Only stem cell transplant is curative for the hematologic manifestations of FA, but modified pretransplant conditioning is required to avoid severe toxicity caused by chemotherapy and radiation sensitivity.

BLEEDING

Many congenital and acquired disorders of hemostasis, including platelet abnormalities, present in infancy and childhood. Importantly, normal ranges for coagulation assays are age-dependent and differ greatly from the neonatal period to infancy and later childhood (Table 10-5). Most coagulation proteins increase in parallel with gestational age. Because physiologic levels of many clotting factors are low at birth, it is often difficult to diagnose disorders of hemostasis in newborns.

Acquired Factor Deficiencies

Hemorrhagic disease of the newborn (HDN) is a complication of physiologic low levels of vitamin K-dependent factors in the newborn (9). Classic HDN presents on days 2 to 7 of life in otherwise healthy, full-term infants. Risk factors include poor placental transfer of vitamin K, marginal levels in breast milk, inadequate milk intake, and the sterile newborn gut. Although rarely necessary, diagnosis can be confirmed by screening coagulation tests and vitamin K-dependent factor levels. Determination of decarboxylated forms of vitamin K-dependent factors or protein induced by vitamin K antagonists may also be helpful. HDN should be prevented in all newborns by prophylactic administration of vitamin K at birth with a single dose of 0.5 to 1 mg intramuscularly or an oral dose of 2 to 4 mg, followed by continued supplementation in breast-fed infants.

Vitamin K deficiency can also be seen in children with liver disease, chronic antibiotic use, inadequate intake or disorders that interfere with vitamin K absorption, such as chronic diarrhea, cystic fibrosis, or other fat malabsorption syndromes. Therapy should include vitamin K administration as well as disease-specific measures.

DIC can be differentiated from vitamin K deficiency and liver disease by assaying coagulation factor levels. DIC results in a decrease in all clotting factors due to consumption. In contrast, factor VIII, the only clotting protein not synthesized solely in the liver, is normal

TABLE 10–5. *Normal age specific coagulation values*

Coagulation test	30–36 wk gestation at birth	Term infant at birth	1–5 yr	6–10 yr	11–16 yr	Adult
PT (sec)	13 (10.6–16.2)	13 (10.14–15.9)	11 (10.6–11.4)	11.1 (10.1–12.1)	11.2 (10.2–12)	12 (11–14)
aPTT (sec)	53.6 (27.5–79.4)	42.9 (31.3–54.5)	30 (24–36)	31 (26–36)	32 (26–37)	33 (27–40)
Fibrinogen (g/L)	2.43 (1.5–3.73)	2.83 (1.67–3.99)	2.76 (1.7–4.05)	2.79 (1.57–4)	3 (1.54–4.48)	2.78 (1.56–4)
II (U/mL)	0.45 (0.2–0.77)	0.48 (0.26–0.7)	0.94 (0.71–1.16)	0.88 (0.67–1.07)	0.83 (0.61–1.04)	1.08 (0.7–1.46)
V (U/mL)	0.88 (0.41–1.44)	0.72 (0.36–1.08)	1.03 (0.79–1.27)	0.9 (0.63–1.16)	0.77 (0.55–0.99)	1.06 (0.62–1.5)
VII (U/ml)	0.67 (0.21–1.13)	0.66 (0.28–1.04)	0.82 (0.55–1.16)	0.85 (0.52–1.2)	0.83 (0.58–1.15)	1.05 (0.67–1.43)
VIII (U/mL)	1.11 (0.5–2.13)	1.0 (0.22–1.78)	0.9 (0.59–1.42)	0.95 (0.58–1.32)	0.92 (0.53–1.31)	0.99 (0.5–1.49)
IX (U/mL)	0.35 (0.19–0.65)	0.53 (0.15–0.91)	0.73 (0.47–1.04)	0.75 (0.63–0.89)	0.82 (0.59–1.22)	1.09 (0.55–1.63)
X (U/mL)	0.41 (0.11–0.71)	0.4 (0.12–0.68)	0.88 (0.58–1.16)	0.75 (0.55–1.01)	0.79 (0.5–1.17)	1.06 (0.7–1.52)
XI (U/mL)	0.3 (0.08–0.52)	0.38 (0.1–0.66)	0.97 (0.56–1.5)	0.86 (0.52–1.2)	0.74 (0.5–0.97)	0.97 (0.67–1.27)
XII (U/mL)	0.38 (0.1–0.66)	0.53 (0.13–0.93)	0.93 (0.64–1.29)	0.92 (0.6–1.4)	0.81 (0.34–1.37)	1.08 (0.52–1.64)
XIIIa (U/mL)	0.7 (0.32–1.08)	0.79 (0.27–1.31)	1.08 (0.72–1.43)	1.09 (0.65–1.51)	0.99 (0.57–1.4)	1.05 (0.55–1.55)
vWF (U/mL)	1.36 (0.78–2.1)	1.53 (019–2.87)	0.82 (0.6–1.2)	0.95 (0.44–1.44)	1 (0.46–1.53)	0.92 (0.5–1.58)
ATIII (U/mL)	0.38 (0.14–0.62)	0.63 (0.39–0.87)	1.11 (0.82–1.39)	1.11 (0.9–1.31)	1.05 (0.77–1.32)	1.0 (0.74–1.26)
Protein C (U/mL)	0.28 (0.12–0.44)	0.35 (0.17–0.53)	0.66 (0.4–0.92)	0.69 (0.45–0.93)	0.83 (0.55–1.11)	0.96 (0.64–1.28)
Protein S, Total (U/mL)	0.26 (0.14–0.38)	0.36 (0.12–0.6)	0.86 (0.54–1.18)	0.78 (0.41–1.14)	0.72 (0.52–0.92)	0.81 (0.6–1.13)
Protein S, Free (U/mL)	N/A	N/A	0.45 (0.21–0.69)	0.42 (0.22–0.62)	0.38 (0.26–0.55)	0.45 (0.27–0.61)

Values expressed in units per milliliter are compared to pooled plasma, which contains 1.0 U/mL. However, pooled plasma contains 0.4 U/mL of free protein S.
Modified from Andrew M. Vegh P. Johnston M. et al. Maturation of the hemostatic system in childhood. *Blood* 1992:80 : 1998–2005; Andrew M, Paes B, Milner R, et al. Development of the coagulation system in the healthy premature infant. *Blood* 1988;72 : 1651–1657; Andrew M, Paes B, Milner R,et al. The development of the human coagulation system in the full-term infant. *Blood* 1987:70 : 165–170.
    PT, prothrombin time; aPTT, activated partial thromboplastin time; vWF, von Willebrand factor; wk, week; yr, year

or elevated in liver disease. Therapy should be directed at the underlying cause, although supportive measures may include treatment with fresh-frozen plasma (FFP).

Inherited Factor Deficiencies

Hemophilia A and B often present in early childhood. Hemophiliac newborns bleed with circumcision and rarely manifest intracranial hemorrhage after delivery. In the absence of a family history, the diagnosis of hemophilia is most often made when a child with moderate to severe factor deficiency begins to crawl or walk. Common symptoms include easy bruising, hemarthrosis in weight-bearing joints, and deep intramuscular hemorrhage. Central nervous system (CNS) bleeding is the most common cause of early mortality. Laboratory evidence for hemophilia includes a prolonged partial thromboplastin time (PTT), which corrects on mixing studies. An abnormally low factor VIII or IX level confirms the diagnosis. Care should be taken to evaluate and treat hemarthroses aggressively in children to prevent later development of chronic arthropathy. The treatment of hemophilia in children is similar to that in adults and includes factor replacement dosed according to the site, type, and severity of hemorrhage. The availability of recombinant factor VIII concentrates has increased the safety and feasibility of prophylaxis in children with frequent hemorrhagic episodes (10). In patients with mild hemophilia A, desmopressin is often effective for short-term management of mild bleeding. As in adults, routine screening for inhibitors should be used.

Von Willebrand disease (vWD) usually presents with less severe bleeding, primarily mucocutaneous, compared to hemophilia. Because recurrent bruising and epistaxis are common complaints in children, history should be directed toward the presence of prolonged, unusual, or severe bleeding. A careful family history may reveal similar symptoms in parents or siblings. The diagnosis is confirmed by abnormal assays for factor VIII, von Willebrand factor (vWF) antigen and activity, and multimer analysis. Factor VIII and vWF are acute phase reactants and, in children, falsely elevated levels caused by interval illnesses may obscure the diagnosis. Thus, repeat testing should be considered if the diagnosis of vWD is suspected. Therapy is as in adults.

Platelet Disorders

Neonatal alloimmune thrombocytopenia (NAIT) results from the placental transfer of maternal alloantibodies against paternally inherited antigens (most commonly HPA-1a) on fetal platelets. Newborns present with transient, isolated but severe thrombocytopenia that must be distinguished from other causes, including maternal immune thrombocytopenic purpura (ITP), severe infection, DIC, hypersplenism, and Kasabach-Merrit syndrome. Approximately 15% of affected neonates experience intracranial hemorrhage, either in utero or in the immediate postnatal period. Unlike Rh disease of the newborn, prior sensitization is not required and thus NAIT may occur with the first pregnancy. A normal platelet count in the mother helps to differentiate NAIT from maternal ITP. Immunophenotyping of maternal and paternal platelets is useful to confirm the diagnosis. The treatment of choice in severe NAIT is transfusion of maternal platelets. When they are not readily available, platelets obtained from a known HPA-1a–negative donor or from random donors may be used for active bleeding. Intravenous immunoglobulin (IVIG) or corticosteroids may also be used as a temporary measure either in the antenatal or postnatal periods, with dosing as in ITP.

Immune thrombocytopenic purpura affects approximately 1 in 10,000 children annually in the United States (11). In contrast to adults, ITP in childhood is usually a self-limited, benign condition. Children typically present under the age of 10. Eighty percent have spontaneous resolution within 6 months. Infants and older children are more likely to have prolonged thrombocytopenia. The typical presentation in acute ITP is the abrupt onset of mucosal bleeding, petechiae, and bruising in healthy children, often preceded by a viral illness. Most children present with severe thrombocytopenia (platelet counts less than 10,000 to 20,000 per micro-

TABLE 10–6. *Treatment regimens for childhood immune thrombocytopenic purpura*

IVIG: 1 g/kg × 1 day or 2 g/kg over 2–5 days
OR
Anti-D: 50–75 μg/kg × 1 day (Rh-positive patients only)
OR
Prednisone: 4–8 mg/kg per day × 7–21 days with taper
OR
Methylprednisolone: 30 mg/kg per day × 3 days

IVIG, intravenous immunoglobulin; Anti-D, anti-Rh(D) immune globulin.

liter) and an otherwise normal CBC. Large platelets are commonly seen on peripheral blood smear. Although acute ITP is a diagnosis of exclusion, healthy children with no other significant medical history or findings on physical examination rarely require extensive laboratory testing. Human immunodeficiency virus (HIV) assay should be considered. The diagnostic utility of bone marrow examination for a child with suspected ITP is low. Evaluation for chronic ITP should include bone marrow studies and testing for immunodeficiency and autoimmune disease. The need for treatment in acute ITP is often debated; current guidelines recommend therapy for significant bleeding or a platelet below 10,000 per microliter (12). Although the risk of intracranial hemorrhage is small, precautions should be taken to prevent head trauma and helmets are recommended for toddlers just learning to walk. There are several standard first-line therapeutic options (Table 10-6).

Inherited platelet disorders may be qualitative or quantitative; they are a rare cause of thrombocytopenia in infancy and childhood. The variety of qualitative disorders includes Glanzmann thrombasthenia (GT), Bernard-Soulier syndrome (BSS), platelet-type pseudo-vWD, and platelet storage granule defects. Quantitative defects are seen in congenital amegakaryocytic thrombocytopenia, thrombocytopenia-absent radii (TAR), X-linked thrombocytopenia, Wiskott-Aldrich syndrome (WAS), and May-Hegglin anomaly. Children with these disorders commonly present with petechiae, easy bruising, or mucocutaneous bleeding. Rarely, gastrointestinal or intracranial bleeding may occur. Screening for qualitative disorders requires platelet aggregation studies. Characteristic features of specific disorders should be sought (forearm deformities in TAR, immunodeficiency in WAS, macrothrombocytes in May-Hegglin anomaly). Treatment for bleeding is usually supportive. Platelet transfusions should be avoided if possible in patients with BSS and GT, because of the risk of developing alloantibodies to the missing platelet antigens GPIb-IX and αIIb-β3, respectively.

THROMBOSIS

As with coagulation factor levels, normal ranges for endogenous antithrombotic proteins are age- and gestation-dependent (Table 10-5). Notably, venous thromboembolic events (TEE) are less common in children compared to adults, with the exception of specific at-risk patient populations (very low-birth-weight or extremely ill neonates) (13). Unless specific risk factors are identified, arterial thrombosis is extremely infrequent.

Anticoagulant and thrombolytic therapy should be dosed according to age and weight (Table 10-7). The duration, monitoring, efficacy, and long-term effects of anticoagulation in the management of TEE in children require further study. The treatment of children with oral anticoagulants is complicated by an increased risk of bleeding complications. As in adults, caution is required when instituting coumarin therapy. To avoid paradoxical thrombosis, heparinization should be continued until the international normalized ratio (INR) is therapeutic.

TABLE 10–7A. *Heparin therapy in children*

Age	Heparin bolus (U/kg)	Heparin* infusion (U/kg/hr)	Enoxaparin† (treatment)	Enoxaparin (prophylaxis)
Infants	75–100	28	<2 mos 1.5 mg/kg q12 h	<2 mos 0.75 mg/kg q12 h
Children	75–100	20	≥2 mos 1 mg/kg q12 h	≥2 mos 0.5 mg/kg q12 h
Adults	80	18	1 mg/kg q12 hr	30 mg q12 hr

Modified from Monagle P, Michelson AD, Bovill E, et al. Antithrombotic therapy in children. *Chest* 2001;119:344–370.
* Goal is aPTT of 1.5–2.5× control (60–85 sec).
† Goal is anti-factor Xa level of 0.5–1.0 U/mL 2–6 hours after injection.
mos, months of age; hr, hours

TABLE 10–7B. *Coumarin therapy in children**

Day 1	Days 2–4 INR	Days 2–4 Action	Maintenance INR	Maintenance Action
Load 0.2 mg/kg po if baseline INR 1.0–1.3	1.1–1.3	Repeat initial loading dose	1.1–1.4	Increase by 20% of dose
	1.4–1.9	50% of loading dose	1.5–1.9	Increase by 10% of dose
	2.0–3.0	50% of loading dose	2.0–3.0	No change
	3.1–3.5	25% of loading dose	3.1–3.5	Decrease by 10% of dose
	>3.5	Hold until INR <3.5, restart at 50% less than previous dose	>3.5	Hold until INR <3.5, restart at 20% less than previous dose

* Do not initiate coumarin until therapeutic heparinization. Heparin should not be discontinued until INR is therapeutic.
Reproduced with permission from Michelson AD, Bovill E, Andrew M. Antithrombotic therapy in children. *Chest* 1995;108:506–522.
po, orally; INR, international normalized ratio.

Congenital Prothrombotic Disorders

Children who are homozygous or compound heterozygous for deficiencies of anticoagulant proteins usually present in the neonatal or early childhood period. In the absence of additional risk factors, however, individuals who are heterozygous for thrombophilic conditions infrequently experience their first TEE early in life but they may present during adolescence. In general, evaluation for possible inherited deficiency is recommended for children with a family history of congenital thrombophilia, and if thromboses are unexplained, occur in unusual sites, are particularly severe, and/or are recurrent.

Protein C and S deficiency, in the homozygous state, classically presents as purpura fulminans within hours or days of birth. Purpura fulminans is more common with protein C deficiency and is characterized by acute DIC with rapidly progressive hemorrhagic necrosis of the skin and other thrombotic/hemorrhagic complications, including death. Homozygous infants usually have undetectable levels of protein C or S and their parents have heterozygous deficiency. Both functional and immunologic assays for protein C and S should be utilized. Acquired causes of protein C and S deficiency, such as liver disease and sepsis, should be excluded. Purpura fulminans should be treated with FFP and, if available, purified protein C concentrate. Warfarin-induced skin necrosis has been described in children with heterozygous protein C and S deficiency, and extreme caution is required when converting such individuals from heparin to warfarin anticoagulation.

Other inherited thrombophilic states including antithrombin III deficiency, factor V Leiden, prothrombin G20210A mutations, and homocysteinemia also have been associated with recurrent thromboembolism in children and adolescents. The incidence of deep vein thrombosis related to those conditions is low and the value of an extensive evaluation of the first TEE has been questioned.

Acquired Prothrombotic Disorders

As in adult patients, thromboembolism in children is usually secondary; central venous catheters are the most common cause. Neonates are at particularly high risk, and the use of umbilical lines may be associated with portal system thrombosis. Other risk factors include malignancy, surgery, trauma, pregnancy, congenital heart disease, Kawasaki disease, nephrotic syndrome, and systemic lupus erythematosus. Complete evaluation for possible underlying conditions should be undertaken. The laboratory examination should be guided by clinical findings and risk factors, and in most cases should include lupus anticoagulant or antiphospholipid antibody assay.

NEUTROPENIA

Normal neutrophil counts vary with age and are affected by race and other factors (Table 10-1). For example, the lower limit of normal in blacks may be 200 to 600 per microliter less than in whites.

Neutropenia is commonly encountered in pediatrics, most often caused by viral suppression. Children, like adults, are at increased risk for life-threatening bacterial infection when the absolute neutrophil count (ANC) falls below 500 per microliter. Common pyogenic infections seen in association with neutropenia include cellulitis, superficial or deep abscesses, pneumonia, sepsis, and recurrent or chronic otitis media and sinusitis.

General management recommendations include aggressive monitoring for and treatment of infection, judicious use of antibiotics, rapid institution of empiric broad-spectrum parenteral antibiotics for fever, and maintenance of good skin and oral hygiene. Granulocyte colony stimulating factor (G-CSF, filgrastim) is often effective in increasing the rate of ANC recovery in certain disorders.

Viral infections are the most common cause of transient neutropenia in childhood. Neutropenia usually develops during the first 24 to 48 hours of illness and commonly lasts up to a week or longer. Neutropenia may also occur with serious bacterial infections, especially in neonates.

Autoimmune neutropenia of childhood is the most common cause of chronic neutropenia in pediatrics, primarily affecting children younger than 3 years of age. The ANC at presentation is usually below 250 per microliter. Associated monocytosis is common and antineutrophil antibodies can be detected in most patients (14). Other causes of neutropenia should be excluded, such as immunodeficiency, drug-related, transient postinfectious, and congenital neutrophil disorders. Although the ANC is often extremely low or absent, most children experience only minor infections and thus, this condition is sometimes referred to as chronic benign neutropenia of childhood. Nonetheless, empiric, broad-spectrum parenteral antibiotics should be employed for the first few episodes of fever. If a child appears to have a benign course, subsequent febrile episodes might be managed more routinely unless there is documented infection or signs of sepsis. Daily trimethoprim/sulfamethoxasole may be useful in preventing recurrent minor bacterial infections. G-CSF is usually effective in low doses (1 to 2 μg/kg per day) and should be considered for children with recurrent, severe neutropenic complications. Spontaneous remission within the first few years of diagnosis is common, especially in young children.

Other extrinsic causes of neutropenia include drug therapy, splenic sequestration, inborn errors of metabolism, nutritional deficiency or bone marrow infiltration. Treatment should be directed at the underlying cause.

Cyclic neutropenia is characterized by periodic oscillations in the ANC. Cycles commonly occur every 3 to 4 weeks and the nadir is usually below 200 per microliter. Symptoms typically begin in the first year of life and commonly include recurrent fever, gingivitis, stomatitis with oral aphthous ulcers and pharyngitis. Diagnosis is confirmed by monitoring serial CBCs twice per week for 6 to 8 weeks to establish the periodicity of the neutropenia, which may also be accompanied by oscillations in other blood counts. Cyclic neutropenia is often an autosomal dominant condition, so parental history and/or CBCs may be helpful. Although cyclic neutropenia is a benign condition in most cases, serious infectious complications may occur. G-CSF in low doses (2 to 3 μg/kg per dose) daily or every other day should be titrated to raise neutrophil levels.

Severe congenital neutropenia (Kostmann disease) is an autosomal recessive disorder associated with severe (usually less than 200 per microliter), chronic neutropenia from birth. Recurrent bacterial infections include those commonly seen in more benign neutropenic conditions, as well as life-threatening sepsis, meningitis, and gastrointestinal tract infection. Neonates commonly present with omphalitis. Bone marrow examination reveals neutrophil developmental arrest. Standard therapy consists of daily G-CSF, but high doses may be required and patients undergoing long-term therapy are at high risk for myelodysplastic syndrome and acute myelogenous leukemia (15). BMT should be considered as a curative approach.

Shwachman-Diamond syndrome and Chédiak-Higashi syndrome are both autosomal recessive disorders that are associated with neutropenia. Shwachman-Diamond is characterized by progressive marrow failure, pancreatic exocrine insufficiency, short stature, and skeletal deformities. Two-thirds of patients have a moderate neutropenia that can be intermittent and responsive to G-CSF. Chédiak-Higashi is also a multiorgan disease that includes oculocutaneous albinism, recurrent bacterial infection, a mild bleeding disorder, and neuropathy. The accumulation of giant granules in neutrophils leads to premature destruction. Therapy is usually supportive and BMT is the only known cure.

LEUKOCYTOSIS

Leukocytosis refers to an increase in total WBC count for age. Neutrophilia is an increase in the ANC above 7,500 per microliter, although the upper limit of normal may be higher in newborns and infants. Neutrophilia may result from increased production, mobilization from the bone marrow, or peripheral demargination. In children, neutrophilia in the acute setting is most often due to bacterial or viral infection. Absolute lymphocytosis usually indicates an acute or chronic viral process. The evaluation of leukocytosis should include a detailed history and physical examination, looking closely for symptoms and signs of infection and for lymphadenopathy and hepatosplenomegaly. Examination of the peripheral blood smear is essential to distinguish normal from atypical and malignant white blood cells.

Leukocyte adhesion deficiency type I (LAD I) is a disorder of impaired phagocyte adhesion, chemotaxis, and ingestion, caused by partial or total deficiency of CD18-related surface glycoproteins. Its hallmark is the occurrence of repeated, severe bacterial or fungal infections in the absence of pus accumulation and despite persistent neutrophilia. Infants typically present in the newborn period with omphalitis or delayed umbilical cord separation. The diagnosis of LAD can be confirmed by flow cytometry. LAD type II, which is caused by defective fucose metabolism, produces a less severe phenotype. The treatment for both LAD I and II should be directed at the underlying infection. BMT may be curative.

Infectious mononucleosis (IM) is classically associated with atypical lymphocytosis and is caused by infection with Epstein-Barr virus (EBV) (16). In adolescents and young adults, a prodrome of fatigue and anorexia usually precedes development of fever, lymphadenopathy, exudative pharyngitis and hepatosplenomegaly. Young children commonly present with a mild respiratory illness only. Rash can occur, especially after treatment with penicillin or ampicillin. Hematologic complications, including immune-mediated hemolytic anemia, thrombocytopenia, aplastic anemia and hemophagocytosis can be seen, as can other rare complications such as CNS involvement, myocarditis, orchitis, and splenic rupture. Children with congenital immunodeficiency or taking immunosuppressive medications can develop lymphoproliferation, which can evolve into frank lymphoma. EBV in boys with Duncan syndrome (X-linked lymphoproliferative syndrome) results in fatal IM in the majority of cases.

Atypical lymphocytosis and early immunologic evidence of EBV infection, either by heterophil or EBV-specific antibody testing, are the most consistent laboratory findings. Nonspecific heterophil antibody tests are often negative in children younger than 4 years of age. Other infections, such as cytomegalovirus (CMV), pertussis, and cat-scratch disease should be excluded in the setting of EBV-negative IM. Therapy of IM is supportive. Rarely, short course corticosteroids are used to manage life-threatening manifestations, such as upper airway obstruction from tonsillar/adenoidal hypertrophy. To avoid splenic rupture, contact sports should be avoided until splenomegaly resolves.

HEMATOLOGIC MANIFESTATIONS OF SYSTEMIC CONDITIONS

Many systemic conditions can result in secondary hematologic abnormalities. Evaluation of the CBC and peripheral smear may also provide important clues during the evaluation of a diagnostic dilemma. A number of systemic disorders that have prominent hematologic findings and present predominantly in childhood are detailed below.

Lysosomal storage diseases are caused by a deficiency in specific enzymes of the lysosomal metabolic pathway and result in pathologic accumulation of normal substrate. Dramatic changes in the central nervous and hematologic systems as well as enlargement of organs that comprise the reticuloendothelial system, including liver and spleen result. Vacuolated lymphocytes and hypergranulated neutrophils in the peripheral blood and lipid-laden macrophages ("foam" or "storage" cells) in the bone marrow are commonly observed. Other characteristic cell types include the sea-blue histiocyte in Niemann-Pick disease and the Gaucher cell. Although specific enzyme replacement therapy has proven successful for some of these disorders, therapy is only supportive for others (17). BMT has proven curative in a limited number of the storage conditions.

Autoimmune lymphoproliferative syndrome (ALPS) is a rare disorder of early childhood caused by defective lymphocyte apoptosis (18). Symptoms include lymphadenopathy, splenomegaly, autoimmunity and risk of lymphoid malignancy. Autoimmune cytopenias are common. The presence of increased numbers of double negative (CD4 − /CD8 −) T-cells on flow cytometry supports the diagnosis, which can be confirmed by the demonstration of diminished lymphocyte apoptosis. A number of molecular defects have been identified, most commonly mutations in Fas (*TNFRSF6*, CD95). Therapy is mainly supportive, although immunosuppressive medications may be needed to manage complications of autoimmunity and lymphoproliferation.

Collagen vascular diseases commonly have hematologic manifestations, most often anemia of chronic illness and/or autoimmune-mediated cytopenias. Aplastic anemia has been described in systemic lupus erythematosus (SLE). Patients with autoimmune disorders are at increased risk for developing antiphospholipid antibodies, although such lupus anticoagulants result in prolongation of prothrombin time (PT) and PTT, they predispose to thromboembolism rather than bleeding.

TRANSFUSION SUPPORT

The indications for transfusion in infants and children are similar to that in adults. Patient size, blood volume, and underlying condition mandate special precautions in regard to dosing and risks. In all cases, careful consideration should be given to the indication for, appropriate dose of, and potential toxicities of the specific blood product. Formulas to calculate pediatric transfusion requirements are detailed in Table 10-8.

Packed red blood cells (PRBCs) should be transfused in children according to age-specific blood volumes and target hemoglobin levels. Unless rapid replacement is required for shock or rapid loss, the recommended infusion rate is 2 to 4 mL/kg per hour or 10 to 15 mL/kg aliquot over 4 hours. With volume intolerance, gradual correction can be achieved by infusing small aliquots (5 to 10 mL/kg) over 4 to 6 hours. Diuretics may be helpful. When rapid correction is required but is limited by fluid intolerance, partial exchange transfusion should be performed: whole blood is removed in small aliquots and replaced with equal volumes of PRBCs.

Platelets transfused at a dose of 0.1 U/kg are expected to increase the platelet count by 30,000 to 50,000 per microliter in most infants and children. The target posttransfusion platelet count varies with the clinical situation. In general, the aim should be to raise the count to a

---

TABLE 10–8. *Transfusion dosing in pediatrics*

TBV estimate
    Newborn 100 mL/kg
    Child   80 mL/kg
    Adult   65 mL/kg

PRBC
    PRBC volume (mL) = $\dfrac{(HCT_d - HCT_i) \times TBV}{HCT_{prbc}}$
    Manual partial RBC exchange*
    Exchange volume (mL) = $\dfrac{(HCT_d - HCT_i) \times TBV}{HCT_{prbc} - \dfrac{(HCT_i + HCT_d)}{2}}$

Platelets
    0.1 unit/kg should increase the platelet count by approximately 50,000/μL
FFP
    10 ml/kg should increase the factor activity level by approximately 20%
Cryoprecipitate
    0.3 U/kg should increase the fibrinogen level by approximately 200 mg/dL

---

* Adapted from Neiburg PI, Stockman JA. Rapid correction of anemia with partial exchange transfusion. *Am J Dis Child* 1977;131:60–61.

HCT should be in fractions (e.g., 40% = 0.4); HCT$_i$ initial; HCT$_d$ desired; HCT$_{prbc}$ usually 0.65–0.8; TBV, total blood volume; PRBC, packed red blood cells; RBC, red blood cells; FFP, fresh-frozen plasma.

level where bleeding stops. Values of around 50,000 per microliter usually suffice, although normal counts should be maintained for life-threatening situations, such as CNS, vascular, or surgical hemorrhage. In the setting of myelosuppression, prophylactic platelet transfusion is recommended at a level of 10,000 per microliter for patients without additional risk factors for severe bleeding. To minimize the risk of bleeding in newborns, counts should be maintained above 30,000 per microliter of platelets for full-term and 50,000 per microliter for premature infants. Prophylactic transfusions are not indicated in the setting of ITP and other antibody-mediated forms of platelet destruction, where no transfusion-related increment is expected; rather, transfusions should be reserved for life-threatening bleeding. To decrease the risk of alloimmunization in children who require multiple transfusions, single-donor (apheresis) and leucocyte-depleted platelets should be used whenever possible.

Fresh-frozen plasma (FFP) is recommended for children with coagulopathy as evidenced by prolonged PT and/or PTT who have active bleeding or to prevent hemorrhage in those at high risk (preoperatively). FFP should be used to replace clotting factors for which specific concentrates are not available, and a dose of 10 to 15 mL/kg usually raises the clotting activity by approximately 20%. Multiple doses may be required if there is ongoing consumption. The rate of transfusion is limited by citrate toxicity, and vital signs and ionized calcium levels should be monitored closely when large or rapid infusions are used.

Cryoprecipitate is used primarily to combat bleeding with hypofibrinogenemia. A dose of 0.3 U/kg will increase the fibrinogen level by approximately 200 mg/dL.

Specialized Blood Products to Prevent Toxicities

WBC removal by leukofiltration should be performed for those who require multiple transfusions to decrease the risk of sensitization to leukocyte antigens. Leukodepletion also decreases the risks of febrile reactions and CMV transmission.

Irradiation of cellular blood products with 2500 cGy should be used to prevent transfusion-associated graft-versus-host disease in the following situations: (i) potential immunocompromised host, including very low birth weight infants, immunodeficiency, malignancy, marrow or organ transplantation; (ii) blood from first-degree family members or HLA-matched donors; (iii) all granulocyte transfusions.

REFERENCES

1. Nathan DG, Oski FA. *Hematology of Infancy and Childhood.* 6th ed. Philadelphia: W.B. Saunders Company, 2003.
2. Hermiston ML, Mentzer WC. A practical approach to the evaluation of the anemic child. *Pediatr Clin North Am* 2002;49:877–891.
3. Canfield RL, Henderson CR, Cory-Slechta DA, et al. Intellectual impairment in children with blood lead concentrations below 10 micrograms per deciliter. *N Engl J Med* 2003;348:1517–1526.
4. Earley A, Valman HB, Altman DG, et al. Microcytosis, iron deficiency, and thalassaemia in preschool children. *Arch Dis Child* 1990;65:610–614.
5. Cherrick I, Karayalcin G, Lanzkowsky P. Transient erythroblastopenia of childhood. Prospective study of fifty patients. *Am J Pediatr Hematol Oncol* 1994;16:320–324.
6. Rosenblatt DS, Whitehead VM. Cobalamin and folate deficiency: acquired and hereditary disorders in children. *Semin Hematol* 1999;36:19–34.
7. Vlachos A, Federman N, Reyes-Haley C, et al. Hematopoietic stem cell transplantation for Diamond Blackfan anemia: a report from the Diamond Blackfan Anemia Registry. *Bone Marrow Transplant* 2001;27:381–386.
8. Rosenberg PS, Greene MH, Alter BP. Cancer incidence in persons with Fanconi anemia. *Blood* 2003;101:822–826.
9. Sutor AH, von Kries R, Cornelissen EA, et al. Vitamin K deficiency bleeding (VKDB) in infancy. ISTH Pediatric/Perinatal Subcommittee. International Society on Thrombosis and Haemostasis. *Thromb Haemos* 1999;81:456–461.

10. Liesner RJ, Khair K, Hann IM. The impact of prophylactic treatment on children with severe haemophilia. *Br J Haematol* 1996;92:973–978.
11. Kuhne T, Imbach P, Bolton-Maggs PH, et al. Newly diagnosed idiopathic thrombocytopenic purpura in childhood: an observational study. *Lancet* 2001;358:2122–2125.
12. Medeiros M, Buchanan GR. Idiopathic thrombocytopenic purpura: beyond consensus. *Curr Opin Pediatr* 2000;12:4–9.
13. Monagle P, Adams M, Mahoney M, et al. Outcome of pediatric thromboembolic disease: a report from the Canadian Childhood Thrombophilia Registry. *Pediatr Res* 2000;47:763–766.
14. Kobayashi M, Nakamura K, Kawaguchi H, et al. Significance of the detection of antineutrophil antibodies in children with chronic neutropenia. *Blood* 2002;99:3468–3471.
15. Freedman MH, Bonilla MA, Fier C, et al. Myelodysplasia syndrome and acute myeloid leukemia in patients with congenital neutropenia receiving G-CSF therapy. *Blood* 2000;96:429–436.
16. Krabbe S, Hesse J, Uldall P. Primary Epstein-Barr virus infection in early childhood. *Arch Dis Child* 1981;56:49–52.
17. Schiffmann R, Brady RO. New prospects for the treatment of lysosomal storage diseases. *Drugs* 2002;62:733–742.
18. Carter LB, Procter JL, Dale JK, et al. Description of serologic features in autoimmune lymphoproliferative syndrome. *Transfusion* 2000;40:943–948.

11

Acute Myelogenous Leukemia

Scott Solomon and Vera Malkovska

Acute myelogenous leukemia (AML) is a heterogeneous group of diseases characterized by uncontrolled proliferation of myeloid progenitor cells. Leukemic myeloid cells gradually replace normal hematopoiesis in the bone marrow. The genetic changes arising in the neoplastic clone lead to cascades of molecular events that cause abnormal proliferation, aberrant differentiation and inhibition of normal hematopoiesis by the malignant cells.

Characterization of transforming genetic events is becoming increasingly important in establishing diagnosis, defining prognosis, and planning therapy in AML. Untreated AML kills patients usually within weeks to months of diagnosis. Advances in chemotherapy and supportive management have improved the survival of younger patients with AML, but the majority of older patients die of the leukemia. The current challenge is to improve understanding of the molecular mechanisms of AML and to design leukemia-specific treatments that would be applicable to older patients.

EPIDEMIOLOGY

The annual mortality rate from AML in the United States is 2.2 per 100,000, resulting in approximately 10,000 deaths per year. AML accounts for approximately 15% to 20% of acute leukemias in children and adolescents and 90% in adults. The incidence of AML increases with age, and most patients are over 60 years at presentation (Fig. 11-1).

ETIOLOGY

The precise molecular origins of AML are unknown. The pathophysiologic mechanisms are multiple, act in concert, and probably are distinct in different types of AML. Inherited genetic predisposition and environmental mutagens such as radiation, drugs, and other toxins all play a role in the development of AML. Genetic causes are suggested by the increased incidence of AML in identical twins, as well as the known association of AML with a variety of congenital disorders. AML arising from preexisting hematologic disorders, most commonly the myelodysplastic syndromes, have inferior prognosis. Resistance to treatment and short survival is characteristic of AML after exposure to chemotherapy and radiation.

Known risks factors for AML include:

1. Environmental exposures
   - Benzene and its derivatives, ethylene oxides and herbicides
   - Ionizing radiation

2. Genetic disorders
   - Down's syndrome
   - Bloom syndrome

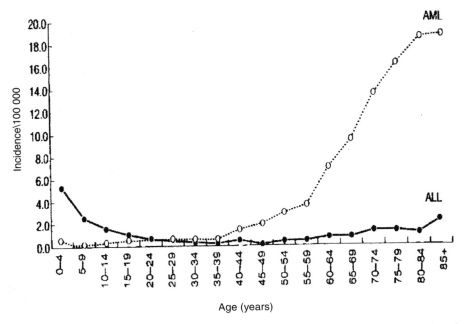

FIG. 11-1. The age-related incidence of acute myelogenous leukemia (AML) in the United States.

- Fanconi anemia
- Ataxia telangiectasia
- Kostmann syndrome
- Klinefelter syndrome

3. Preexisting hematologic disorders
   - Myelodysplastic syndromes (MDS)
   - Myeloproliferative disorders
   - Paroxysmal nocturnal hemoglobinuria

4. Treatment-associated
   - Alkylating agents: AML usually arises from MDS, after a 3- to 10-year latency period and is associated with characteristic chromosomal abnormalities, mainly deletions involving chromosomes 5 or 7.
   - Topoisomerase II inhibitors: lack preceding myelodysplasia, have a shorter latency, exhibit monocytic morphology, and are associated with characteristic cytogenetic changes involving the long arm of chromosome 11 (11q).
   - Radiotherapy alone or in combination with chemotherapy.

At the molecular level, AML is a multistep process that requires at least two different genetic events. The first causes a block in cellular differentiation, and the second increases cellular proliferation. A failure of myeloid differentiation is also seen in MDS, while abnormalities in myeloid proliferation occur in chronic myeloid leukemia (CML). The transformation of chronic-phase CML into blast crisis is associated with new mutations that cause maturation arrest. This process is believed to further support the "two-hit" hypothesis first generated by

TABLE 11–1. *Common genetic mutations in acute myelogenous leukemia*

Mutations that impair differentiation	Proliferation/survival mutations
1. Typified by balanced translocations • t(8;21): AML-1-ETO: • inv 16 or t(16;16): CBFb-SMMHC • t(15;17); PML-RARα • 11q23 (multiple partners); MLL 2. Point mutations in transcription factors • Core binding factor (CBF) • CCAAT/enhancer binding proteinα (c/EBP) • Wilms tumor-1 (WT1)	1. Proto-oncogene mutations • Ras (G-binding protein) point mutations in 5%–20% • FLT3 (tyrosine kinase receptor) activating mutations in 30%–35% • C-kit (tyrosine kinase receptor) activating mutations 2. Tumor suppressor gene mutations • p53, Rb

Knudson. The two classes of mutations found in AML that are thought to cooperate in the malignant transformation are shown in Table 11- 1.

CLINICAL FEATURES

Patients with AML usually present with bone marrow failure that causes symptoms of anemia, bleeding from thrombocytopenia, and neutropenic infections. Tissue infiltration with leukemic blasts involving gums, skin, meninges, and other organs is most commonly associated with monocytic morphology. Striking bruising and life-threatening hemorrhage should raise suspicion of disseminated intravascular coagulation (DIC), frequently in acute promyelocytic leukemia. However, DIC can occur in any type of AML. Leukostasis and hyperviscosity causing organ dysfunction usually occurs with blast cell counts over 100,000. Often manifested by confusion, visual impairment and shortness of breath, leukostasis can also lead to hemorrhage in the retina, brain, lungs, and other organs. Rare but striking manifestations of AML include the Sweet syndrome, a skin rash with neutrophilic infiltrates in the dermis, and chloromas, tumors of myeloid blasts. Extramedullary leukemia portends a worse prognosis.

Symptoms and signs on presentation include:

- Marrow failure
  - Fatigue
  - Shortness of breath
  - Fever
  - Focal infections
  - Petechiae
  - Bruising
  - Bleeding (if severe, suspect promyelocytic leukemia)

- Tissue involvement
  - Bone pain, tenderness
  - Mild splenomegaly
  - Gingival hyperplasia
  - Central nervous system (CNS) and cranial nerve dysfunction
  - Visual changes (retinal involvement, hemorrhage, papilledema)

- Rare manifestations
  - Sweet syndrome
  - Chloromas

LABORATORY FINDINGS

The most common laboratory findings in AML include anemia, thrombocytopenia, neutropenia and myeloid blasts on the blood smear. In aleukemic leukemia, blasts are seen only in the bone marrow. Coagulopathy resulting from DIC is common in promyelocytic leukemia. Hyperuricemia from high cell turnover is often seen on presentation and worsens during chemotherapy. Rapidly rising serum levels of uric acid, potassium and phosphate with decreasing calcium herald a tumor lysis syndrome that can result in acute renal failure. Renal tubular dysfunction caused by muramidase released from leukemic blasts can add to the electrolyte abnormalities commonly seen in AML. Lactic acidosis tends to occur with leukostasis while high lactate dehydrogenase (LDH) is associated with CNS involvement. High numbers of leukemic blasts in blood samples can lead to spurious hypoglycemia, hypoxemia, and other abnormalities resulting from cellular metabolic activity in vitro. Rapid processing of anticoagulated blood samples avoids this artifact.

In addition to routine chest x-rays, imaging studies including computed tomography (CT) and magnetic resonance imaging (MRI) scans directed according to symptoms can reveal leukemic infiltrates, hemorrhage or infection.

Laboratory findings in AML include:

- Hematology
  - Increased white blood cell count with blasts in peripheral blood
  - Anemia
  - Granulocytopenia
  - Thrombocytopenia
  - DIC
- Chemistry
  - Hyperuricemia
  - Elevated blood-urea nitrogen (BUN) and creatinine (urate nephropathy)
  - High LDH
  - Hypokalemia (tubular dysfunction)
  - Lactic acidosis (leukostasis)
  - Hypercalcemia, rarely hypocalcemia
  - Spurious hypoxemia, hypoglycemia, hyperkalemia, or hypokalemia
- Imaging studies
  - Intracranial hemorrhage (often with hyperviscosity)
  - Thickened nerve sheets (MRI)
  - Lung infiltrates (CT)

CLASSIFICATION

The French-American-British (FAB) classification divides AML into eight subtypes (M0 to M7), based on morphology:

M0: Minimally differentiated AML: negative peroxidase reaction, ≥two or more myeloid markers by flow cytometry, frequently has complex cytogenetic abnormalities associated with poor prognosis.

M1: AML without maturation: less than 10% promyelocytes or more mature myeloid forms.

M2: AML with maturation: subset of patients have the t(8;21) translocation associated with favorable prognosis.

M3: Acute promyelocytic leukemia: in most cases heavy granulation and bilobed nuclear contour; rarely microgranular variant with inconspicuous granules. Most cases have t(15;17) translocation and favorable prognosis.

M4: Acute myelomonocytic leukemia: monocytes and promonocytes in the marrow exceed

20%. M4Eo variant contains more than 5% abnormal eosinophils; associated with the inv(16) cytogenetic abnormality and favorable prognosis.

M5: Acute monocytic leukemia: 80% or more of nonerythroid cells are monoblasts, monocytes, or promonocytes. Nonspecific esterase stain is positive. Associated with extramedullary disease and abnormalities of the long arm of chromosome 11 (11q).

M6: Acute erythroleukemia: more than 50% nucleated marrow cells are erythroid, often severely dyserythropoietic. Erythroblasts are strongly periodic acid-Schiff (PAS)-positive and glycophorin A positive.

M7: Acute megakaryocytic leukemia: may have micromegakaryoblasts. Diagnosis confirmed by immunophenotyping (CD41) or electron microscopy (platelet peroxidase).

The new proposed World Health Organization (WHO) classification also takes into account molecular genetics, therapy-related leukemias, and biphenotypic leukemias:

AML with recurrent cytogeneticAML not otherwise categorized translocations
• AML with t(8;21)(q22;q22)• AML minimally differentiated
• AML with t(15;17)(q22;q11) +• AML with maturation variants = APL (M3)
• AML with abnormal marrow eosinophils• AML wihtout maturation inv(16)(p13q22) or t(16;16)(p13;q11)
• AML with 11q23 (MLL) abnormalities• Acute myelomonocytic leukemia
AML with multilineage dysplasia
• With prior MDS• Acute monocytic leukemia
• Without prior MDS• Acute erythroid leukemia
AML and MDS; therapy-related
• Alkylating agent-related• Acute megakaryocytic leukemia
• Epipodophyllotoxin-related• Acute panmyelosis with myelofibrosis
• Other• Acute biphenotypic leukemias

DIAGNOSTIC EVALUATION

Leukemic myeloblasts are usually seen on the blood smear and are always found in the bone marrow biopsy. According to WHO consensus, the diagnosis of AML requires at least 20% myeloid blasts in he peripheral blood or bone marrow. The diagnostic evaluation of a patient with AML includes:

• Blood count and blood smear review
• Bone marrow aspirate and biopsy
  · Morphology with Wright-Giemsa stain
  · Immunophenotyping by flow cytometry
  · Cytogenetics
  · Gene analysis (for clinical research studies only)
• Lumbar puncture: if CNS symptoms, monocytic morphology or high blast count (after blasts cleared from blood)

The morphologic diagnosis of AML can be supported by the presence of Auer rods in the cytoplasm, positive cytochemistry with Sudan black, and staining for myeloperoxidase and esterases (Table 11-2). Immunophenotyping with a panel of monoclonal antibodies is particularly useful for distinguishing AML from acute lymphocytic leukemia (ALL) and for identification of the subtypes, including AML with minimal differentiation, erythroleukemia, and megakaryoblastic leukemia (Table 11-2). Cytogenetic abnormalities associated with morphologic subtypes can further support the diagnosis (Table 11-2).

TABLE 11–2. *Diagnostic markers of acute myelogenous leukemia*

| FAB class | Cytochemistry | | | Monoclonals for precursor cells | | | Myeloid markers | | | Monocyte markers | | | Common cytogenetic abnormalities |
	MPO	PAS	Esterase	Tdt	HLA-DR	CD34 (My10)	CD13 (My7)	CD 33 (My9)	CD15 (Leu MI)	CD11ᵇ (MO1)	Cd14 (My4)	Other	
M0 (undifferentiated)	<3% +	–	–	±!	+	+	+	±!	±!	–	–		11q13
M1 (myeloid)	<3% +	–	–	±!	+	+	+	+	–	±!	–		–5,–7,–17 del 3p +21,+8
M2 (myeloid with differentiation)	>10% +	–	–	–	+	–	+	+	+	±!	–		t(8;21) del 3p or inv3 –5,–7 (6;9),+8
M3 (promyelocytic APL)	++	–	–	–	–	–	+	+	±!	–	–		t (15;17)
M4 (myelomococytic)	+	–	+	–	+	–	+	+	+	+	+		inv(16) or –16q t(16;16) occ t(8;2),–5,–7 t(6;9)
M5 (monocytic)	–	+ block	++	–	+	–	±!	+	+	+	+		t(9:11) (p21;p23) +8
M6 (erythroid)	–	++	–	–	±!	–	±!	±!	–	±!	–	Glycophorin A	–5q,–5,–7,–3,+8
M7 (megakaryocytic)	–	±!	–	–	+	+	–	±!	–	–	–	Platelet glycorprotein	inv or del 3 pl8, +21

CD, cluster of differentiation; HLA-DR, human leukocyte antigen D-related; MPO, myeloperoxidase; PAS, periodic acid-Schiff; Tdt, terminal deoxynucleotidyl transferase.

PROGNOSTIC FACTORS

The most powerful prognostic factors that have been established over many decades, including age, cytogenetics, prior MDS, and treatment-related AML, are recently supplemented by molecular and genetic factors (1). A variety of characteristics have been suggested to be predictive for treatment outcome in AML:

• Age
• Cytogenetics
• AML arising from preexisting disease
• Treatment-related AML
• Performance status
• White blood cell count higher than 20,000 per microliter
• Features of multidrug resistance
• FLT3 internal tandem duplication
• CD34-positive blasts
• Delayed treatment response

Cytogenetic and molecular markers have superseded morphology as the most important prognostic indicators for survival (Table 11-3). Although cytogenetic analysis is an important predictor of outcome, most patients fall into the intermediate prognostic category and thus require further stratification. Studies of molecular genetic changes in AML can provide additional prognostic information and identify targets for therapy. The single most common genetic abnormality in AML identified to date is the FLT3 internal tandem duplication (FLT3-ITD). FLT3-ITD is associated with an increased relapse rate and reduced survival. Other molecular markers suggested to have prognostic significance include mutations of p53, c-KIT, and C/EBP, and high mRNA expression of EVI1, BCL2, and WT1.

The outcome of younger patients with AML has markedly improved over the last three decades because of advances in both chemotherapy and better supportive care (Fig. 11-2A). Approximately 40% of patients under the age of 55 can be cured with current treatments. Unfortunately, little progress has been made in improving the long-term survival of older adults with AML (Fig. 11-2B). These patients have more unfavorable disease characteristics, higher frequency of comorbid conditions, and poor tolerance of toxic therapy. Because the median age of AML patients is above 60 years, novel treatment strategies are needed for the older majority.

TABLE 11–3. *Impact of acute myelogenous leukemia karyotype on clinical outcome*

Karyotype	%	% CR	% EFS
Favorable			
t(8;21)	5–10	90	50–70
inv (16)	5–10	90	50–70
t(15; 17)	5–10	80–90	70
Intermediate			
Normal diploid, -Y	40–50	70–80	20–40
Unfavorable			
−5 / −7	20–30	40	5–10
+8	10	60	10–20
11q23, 20q-, other	10	60	10

CR, complete remission; EFS, event-free survival.

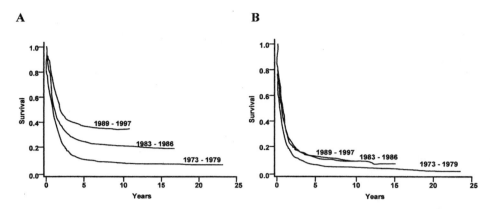

FIG. 11-2. Survival of patients with acute myelogenous leukemia (AML) treated on Eastern Cooperative Oncology Group (ECOG) studies over the last three decades. **(A)** Patients 55 years old or younger. **(B)** Patients older than 55 years old.

TREATMENT

Because AML is so strikingly heterogeneous, treatments must be individualized. Aside from age, the most important prognostic factors in determining the outcome of therapy are acquired genetic changes in leukemia cells as detected by conventional cytogenetics and alternative techniques such as fluorescent in situ hybridization (FISH) and polymerase chain reaction (PCR). AML can be divided into three prognostic categories based on cytogenetics: favorable, intermediate and unfavorable (Table 11-3). Recent studies have incorporated these prognostic groups into the treatment algorithms. In the future, a better understanding of distinct molecular entities within AML will lead to more refined and targeted treatment approaches. The first example of such specific treatment is the successful use of all-trans-retinoic acid (ATRA) for acute promyelocytic leukemia.

The treatment for AML is generally divided into two phases: remission induction and postremission therapy. The goal of the former is to achieve a complete remission (CR) defined by the following criteria: less than 5% blasts in a bone marrow that is 20% or more cellular, absent extramedullary leukemia, a neutrophil count greater than 1,000 per microliter, and a platelet count greater than 100,000 per microliter. The achievement of CR as defined by these simple criteria translates into improved survival. Disappearance of karyotypic or molecular abnormalities is not required for the definition of CR. Once a patient has entered CR, long-term survival requires postremission treatment. Clinical trials confirm an almost 100% risk of relapse when patients receive only induction chemotherapy. Intensive chemotherapy given after achievement of CR (similar to that given during induction) is termed consolidation therapy.

Initial Management

The initial care of AML patients needs to be well organized and executed by an experienced team.

The initial evaluation should include:

- History and physical examination
- Complete blood count with differential
- Examination of the peripheral blood smear
- Coagulation studies (prothrombin time [PT], activated partial thromboplastin time [aPTT], fibrinogen, D-dimer)

- Serum chemistries with uric acid, calcium, and phosphorus
- Renal and liver function tests
- Hepatitis B and C, herpes simplex virus (HSV), cytomegalovirus (CMV), varicella, and human immunodeficiency virus (HIV) serologies
- Bone marrow aspirate for morphology, cytochemistry, cytogenetics, and flow cytometry
- Bone marrow biopsy
- Human leukocyte antigen (HLA) typing of patient and siblings if patient younger than age 55 years
- Lumbar puncture, delayed until blasts cleared from blood, in patients at high risk for CNS involvement (CNS symptoms/signs, elevated leukocyte count, extramedullary disease, and monocytic morphology- FAB M4 or M5)
- Chest radiograph and electrocardiogram
- Evaluation of cardiac function (echocardiogram or multigated acquisition scan [MUGA]) in selected patients
- Central venous access catheter placement
- Parenteral hydration and allopurinol to prevent the tumor lysis syndrome

The initial evaluation is typically followed by an unhurried discussion with the patient about the diagnosis, prognosis, therapy toxicities, probable impact on lifestyle, and anticipated requirements for support by family and friends. In frail elderly patients, a decision to give only supportive treatment without chemotherapy may be reached jointly by the patient and the physician.

The final outcome depends not only on the choice of chemotherapy but also on close monitoring, preventive measures, and meticulous management of complications. Many events associated with AML therapy and their timing are predictable. For example, hyperleuko-cytosis, tumor lysis, and DIC tend to occur early, and marrow aplasia with resulting complications can be expected from the second week of chemotherapy. Patients should be monitored for side effects such as cardiotoxicity caused by anthracyclines or neurotoxicity from high doses of cytosine arabinoside. Infection prophylaxis includes meticulous care of indwelling central venous catheters and prevention of mucositis. Broad-spectrum intravenous antibiotics should be administered immediately if the patient becomes febrile during neutropenia. A treatment algorithm for febrile neutropenia based on local microbial sensitivity should be utilized. Prompt treatment of oral and perianal herpetic ulcerations prevents discomfort and bacterial superinfection. Consideration should be given to prophylactic antifungal therapy to decrease invasive fungal infections and colonization.

Induction Therapy

The most commonly used chemotherapy regimen consists of a combination of conventional doses of cytarabine, 100 to 200 mg/m^2 given by continuous intravenous (IV) infusion over 7 days, and 3 days of an anthracycline, generally daunorubicin, at 45 to 60 mg/m^2 per day given as an IV bolus (2). This "3 + 7" regimen results in CR rates of approximately 60% to 80% in patients younger than 55 to 60 years of age. If leukemia persists in the bone marrow at day 14 to 21, a second course of chemotherapy identical to the first course or using high-dose cytarabine (HDAC), is usually administered.

Although intensifying the induction regimen through the use of HDAC or the addition of etoposide does not increase the CR rate, it does improve CR duration and disease-free survival in younger patients (3,4). It remains unclear whether these benefits outweigh the increased toxicity and myelosuppression that accompanies the intensified regimens, especially as similar intensification could be delivered during postremission therapy.

Three randomized trials suggest that idarubicin at 12 to 13 mg/m^2 is a superior anthracycline to daunorubicin at 45 to 50 mg/m^2, particularly in younger patients (5–7). The CR rates are higher and fewer patients require two courses of induction to achieve CR. However, critics argue that the daunorubicin dose used in these studies is relatively low and a benefit in overall survival is not clear.

Postremission Treatment

Virtually all patients in CR after induction therapy have residual disease that without further treatment would lead to relapse. Multiple strategies have been explored to prevent relapse: low-dose maintenance chemotherapy, intensive consolidation chemotherapy, marrow ablative therapy with autologous stem cell rescue, and allogeneic stem cell transplantation. Low-dose maintenance therapy is generally not helpful and has shown minimal benefit only in patients who received suboptimal induction and consolidation (8).

Intensive consolidation treatment improves survival in younger patients with AML. A dose-dependent response to cytarabine has been shown in randomized controlled trials (9) (Table 11-4). Consolidation with HDAC-based therapy using daily doses of 1 to 6 g/m^2 (e.g., 2 to 3 g/m^2 twice daily on days 1, 3, and 5 or twice daily for 6 days) is now standard for patents younger than 60 years. The optimal number of courses of HDAC-based consolidation has not been determined, but current evidence suggests that two to four courses are reasonable (10). HDAC seems to be most beneficial to young patients and those with favorable cytogenetics (Table 11-4).

Hematopoietic Stem Cell Transplantation

High doses of marrow ablative chemotherapy and total body radiation followed by autologous or allogeneic stem cell rescue have been widely used in AML. Autologous stem cell transplantation (SCT) requires stem cell collection from the patient in CR. Allogenic stem cells are usually obtained from HLA-matched siblings or unrelated donors. Allogenic SCT confers an additional immune-mediated antileukemic activity, the so-called graft-versus-leukemia (GVL) effect. Multiple prospective randomized trials comparing standard consolidation chemotherapy with SCT have demonstrated that allogeneic SCT provides the best antileuke-

TABLE 11–4. *Role of high-dose Ara-C in consolidation*

	Ara-C dose		4-yr DFS	OS
Age <60	100 mg/m²	(n 203)	24%	35%
	400 mg/m²	(n 206)	29%	40%
	3 g/m²	(n 87)	44%	52%
Age >60	100 mg/m²	(n 48)	<16%	|
	400 mg/m²	(n 50)	<16%	9%
	3 g/m²	(n 31)	<16%	|
Favorable cytogenetics (n 57)	100 mg/m²		16%	
	400 mg/m²		57%	
	3 g/m²		78%	
Normal karyotype (n 140)	100 mg/m²		20%	
	400 mg/m²		37%	
	3 g/m²		40%	
Other cytogenetics (n 88)	100 mg/m²		<21%	
	400 mg/m²		<21%	
	3 g/m²		<21%	

DFS, disease-free survival; OS, overall survival.

TABLE 11–5. *Relapse rates following allogenic stem cell transplantation, antologous stem cell transplantation, and chemotherapy*

Study	Allo	Auto	Chemo
GIMEMA (11)	24	40	57
MRC 10 (12)	—	37	58
ECOG/SWOG (13)	29	48	61

Allo, allogenic; Auto, autologous; Chemo, chemotherapy.

mic therapy (lowest recurrence risk), followed by autologous SCT, which is in turn superior to conventional chemotherapy (Table 11-5).

The excellent antileukemic activity of allogeneic SCT has not always translated into better survival in prospective randomized trials analyzed on an intention-to-treat basis (Table 11-6). The significantly higher treatment-related mortality (TRM) rate of SCT makes this form of therapy most appropriate for younger patients with less favorable cytogenetic abnormalities (Table 11-7).

In patients lacking an available HLA-matched sibling donor, autologous SCT offers a theoretical benefit over conventional consolidation chemotherapy because of its associated lower relapse risk. Older randomized studies do not support a clear benefit for autologous SCT because of high procedural mortality (14% in the ECOG/SWOG study and 18% in the MRC AML 10 study). However, the use of peripheral blood as the source of stem cells has decreased TRM to approximately 5%, raising questions as to the relevance of the earlier studies to current practice. As both transplantation technology and chemotherapy continue to improve, the best treatment approach remains uncertain. Moreover, because AML is a heterogenous malignancy, the most appropriate therapy will be ultimately correlated with the cytogenetic and molecular characteristics of the disease.

Risk-Based Approach to Acute Myelogenous Leukemia Treatment (patients younger than 55 to 60 years of age)

Favorable-risk Cytogenetics

Patients with a favorable karyotype [t(8;21) or inv(16)] do well with either multiple rounds of intensive consolidation chemotherapy or autologous SCT. Long-term disease-free survivals

TABLE 11–6. *Recent trials evaluating allogenic stem cell transplantation on an intent-to-treat (donor vs. no donor) basis*

Trial	DFS (%)		OS (%)	
	Donor	No donor	Donor	No donor
EORTC/GIMEMA AML 8 (11)	46	33	48	40
GOELAM (14)	44	38	53	53
MRC AML 10 (12)	50	42	55	50
ECOG/SWOG (13)	43	35	46	52
EORTC/GIMEMA AML 10 (15)	51	41	58	49

DFS, disease-free survival; OS, overall survival.

TABLE 11–7. Outcome of EORTC/GIMEMA AML 10 study stratified by cytogenetic risk group

	DFS (%)		OS (%)		Relapse (%)	
Cytogenetic risk category	Donor	No donor	Donor	No donor	Donor	No donor
Good t(8;21), inv(16)	62	66	68	74	22	28
Intermediate (normal or -Y)	45	48	53	54	35	47
Poor (all other)	43	18	50	29	38	76

DFS, disease-free survival; OS, overall suvival.

of 60% to 70% can be achieved with either approach in younger patients. Allogenic SCT, with its higher TRM, is not appropriate for this subset.

Unfavorable-Risk Cytogenetics

If an HLA-matched family donor is available, patients should be evaluated for SCT as soon as possible after induction therapy. Although the CR rate in this group of patients is approximately 50%, the long-term survival rate with chemotherapy or autologous SCT has been disappointingly low. In younger, healthier patients without an HLA-matched family donor, consideration should be given to allogeneic SCT from a matched unrelated donor, haploidentical family member, or using umbilical cord blood.

Intermediate-Risk Cytogenetics

If an HLA-matched family donor is available, allogeneic SCT should be offered to patients younger than 55 to 60 years of age who have a good performance status, given the superior antileukemic activity of this therapy. Autologous SCT, following intensive consolidation for *in vivo* purging, should be considered for patients without an HLA-matched sibling donor. However, a clear benefit of allogeneic over autologous SCT has not been consistently demonstrated in the literature; studies have been limited by low numbers and heterogeneity of patients, outdated TRM, and large numbers of patients who did not receive the intended treatment. In general, the benefit of allogeneic SCT over autologous SCT will be seen in subgroups of younger healthier patients, in whom improvement in relapse risk outweighs the higher procedural mortality. In future, further risk stratification using newly defined molecular markers such as activating FLT3 mutations may help treatment decisions.

Treatment of Acute Promyelocytic Leukemia

Acute promyeloctic leukemia (APL) is the first example of leukemia in which therapy directed against the leukemogenic event (the t(15;17) resulting in the PML-RARα fusion transcript) leads to improved outcome. With better management of the associated coagulopathy and the introduction of the differentiating agents, ATRA and arsenic trioxide, APL now represents the most curable subtype of AML.

A frequently used treatment strategy consists of a combination of ATRA and anthracycline-based conditioning for induction therapy, two courses of anthracycline-based chemotherapy for consolidation, and maintenance therapy with intermittent ATRA alone (15 days every 3 months) or combined with chemotherapy (mercaptopurine (6-MP) and methotrexate). Using ATRA and an anthracycline for induction therapy, and ATRA-based maintenance therapy,

CR rates of 80% to 90% and cure rates of 70% to 80% can be expected. Recent data suggest that with more intensive induction or consolidation, maintenance chemotherapy may not be necessary.

The goal of induction and consolidation therapy should be the attainment of polymerase chain reaction (PCR) negativity for the PML-RARα rearrangement, as the persistence of such minimal residual disease predicts relapse. For patients who develop ATRA-resistant disease, arsenic trioxide has emerged as effective salvage therapy. Its role in the treatment of newly diagnosed APL is a subject of current study.

The incidence of coagulopathy and bleeding has diminished significantly with ATRA therapy, but hemorrhage does remain an important cause of death during the induction phase. The retinoic acid syndrome has emerged as a new major toxicity associated with ATRA; it is characterized by pleural and pericardial effusions, weight gain, edema, dyspnea, fever, episodic hypotension, and pulmonary infiltrates. The syndrome can be effectively treated with early administration of dexamethasone (10 mg three times a day for 3 to 5 days). The incidence of this complication is reduced in patients receiving concomitant chemotherapy during induction.

Treatment of Relapsed Acute Myelogenous Leukemia

Unfortunately, AML will recur in the majority of patients. If a suitable HLA-matched donor is available, the first option should be allogeneic SCT either at relapse or in second CR. In the absence of a suitable donor, management should be guided by the duration of the first CR. For patients with a CR duration of longer than 12 months, reinduction with the initial regimen or HDAC-containing regimen is reasonable, since it can achieve a CR rate of 50% to 60% and a 5% to 10% long-term disease-free state (DFS). For patients with shorter CR durations, the priority should be treatment on a clinical research trial. Novel agents currently being investigated include gemtuzumab ozogamicin (Mylotarg), a calicheamicin-conjugated anti-CD33 monoclonal antibody: farnesyltransferase inhibitors; FLT3 gene inhibitors; and other agents.

Hematopoietic Growth Factors

Colony-stimulating factors (CSFs) can shorten the duration of neutropenia during AML treatment and potentially improve outcomes. Both granulocyte macrophage-colony stimulating factor (GM-CSF) and granulocyte-colony stimulating factor (G-CSF) have been shown to accelerate neutrophil recovery after induction chemotherapy. Briefer periods of neutropenia translated into reduced infectious death and improved survival in older AML patients in one large randomized study (16), but not in another (17). G-CSF and GM-CSF also have been used to sensitize blasts to chemotherapy by recruiting cells into the cell cycle, however, numerous clinical trials have failed to show a reproducible benefit of such an approach. In general, CSFs given during induction chemotherapy shorten the period of neutropenia by 2 to 7 days, reduce infections in some patients, but have no consistent beneficial effect on survival or CR rate.

Acute Myelogenous Leukemia in Older Patients

Older adults have a dismal prognosis, which has not changed significantly over the last few decades (Fig. 11-2B). Care of these patients is challenging because of the higher rates of unfavorable prognostic features including comorbidity, high-risk cytogenetics and multidrug resistance of leukemic blasts. Older adults who do not have significant comorbidities should be treated with standard "3 + 7" induction therapy, for which an approximately 50% CR rate can be expected. Choice of postremission therapy for older patients remains problematic. In contrast to younger patients, no studies with HDAC-based therapy have demonstrated a survival advantage in patients older than 60 years of age. Because this population represents a majority of patients with AML, new strategies are needed to improve their outcomes.

Acute Myelogenous Leukemia in Pregnancy

The management of pregnant patients with AML is challenging. Delaying chemotherapy until delivery may be detrimental to the mother, whereas chemotherapy, particularly during the first trimester, poses serious risk to the developing fetus. In one single institution study, there were no congenital malformations in 17 live births after exposure to chemotherapy in the second and third trimester. CR rates were no different than that those seen in nonpregnant patients. In contrast, three of four mothers who delayed treatment until after delivery died shortly after the start of chemotherapy (18). Therefore, induction chemotherapy should be delivered once the patient is beyond the first trimester.

Evaluation of Minimal Residual Disease

Several studies suggest that the detection of minimal residual disease (MRD) predicts outcome in some patients with AML. Accurate quantitation of residual AML cells could allow individualization of therapy and thereby increase the likelihood of cure. A major goal of MRD detection is to identify patients at higher risk for relapse, which can lead to risk-adapted therapeutic approaches. Laboratory assays such as PCR and multicolor flow cytometry, which are sensitive enough to detect one leukemic cell in up to 10^4 to 10^5 normal cells, have been used to monitor MRD.

The significance of a positive MRD in AML varies depending on the type of leukemia, therapy employed, and the time of detection. The levels of residual disease that have predictive value need to be determined in specific types of AML, at defined time points during therapy. For example, the achievement of molecular remission in APL patients is critical to obtaining long-term disease-free survival, whereas persistence of the PML-RARα rearrangement after consolidation predicts relapse. In contrast, a positive molecular result in patients with t(8;21) AML is not necessarily associated with impending relapse. Although promising in APL, the clinical significance and utility of evaluating MRD remains unproven, and caution should be taken in applying these techniques to clinical practice outside prospective clinical trials.

Novel Therapeutic Targets in Acute Myelogenous Leukemia

The major goal of current AML treatment is to deliver aggressive cytotoxic chemotherapy in repetitive cycles in order to achieve disease eradication. Despite incremental improvements, less than half of young adults with AML are cured of their disease and outcomes in older patients are clearly poor. A major goal has been to identify new therapeutic targets, and agents with different modes of action and better toxicity profiles. With improved understanding of the mechanisms underlying leukemogenesis, several novel classes of drugs have entered clinical trials. These include antibody-based therapies, farnesyltransferase inhibitors (FTIs), FLT3 kinase inhibitors and other tyrosine kinase inhibitors, and inhibitors of methylation and angiogenesis. Based on the two-hit hypothesis for leukemogenesis, these drugs should ultimately be used in combination.

Gemtuzumab Ozagamicin (Mylotarg) consists of a humanized anti-CD33 monoclonal antibody covalently linked to a semisynthetic derivative of the potent cytotoxic agent calicheamicin (19). The antibody conjugate was approved by the U.S. Food and Drug Administration in May 2000 as single-agent therapy for first relapse AML in a subset of older patients. Future studies will address its role in induction (with chemotherapy) or maintenance therapy. Although nonhematologic toxicities are limited, its association with hepatic veno-occlusive disease may limit its clinical applicability, especially in patients who are transplant candidates.

FTIs represent a new class of small-molecule inhibitors that selectively inhibit farnesylation of a number of intracellular proteins such as Ras. Results of initial phase I testing with one such agent, R115777 (Zarnestra), have shown promising results in relapsed/refractory AML patients. Nonhematolgoic toxicity was limited, and clinical responses occurred in 10 (29%) of 34 evaluable patients, including 2 CRs (20).

FLT3 kinase inhibitors have generated interest because of the high frequency and poor prognosis of patients with AML with activating FLT3 mutations. One such agent, CEP-701, has shown significant activity in a single-agent phase II study in patients with relapsed/refractory AML and FLT3 mutations. Toxicity was very mild and clinical activity was seen in 5 of 14 heavily pretreated patients (21). However, response duration was less than three months, suggesting that it will probably be necessary to combine these agents with other drugs for substantial clinical benefit.

CONCLUSIONS

AML represents a genetically, morphologically, and clinically heterogeneous group of hematopoietic malignancies characterized by an uncontrolled proliferation of myeloid blasts. Although the precise cause of AML is unknown, many genetic and environmental risk factors have been identified. Mutations in at least two genes are probably necessary for the development of leukemia. The nature of the transforming genetic events determines the type of AML, response to therapy, and, to some extent, the final outcome. The most widely used classification of AML still remains the morphologically based FAB classification. Well-established prognostic factors including age, cytogenetics and preexisting disease; predictive molecular and genetic characteristics are now being identified. Advances in chemotherapy and supportive management have resulted in high remission rates. Unfortunately, less than half of younger patients and only 10% to 15% of patients over 60 years of age are cured of their disease. The poor outcome in the older majority of patients with AML reflects differences in biology of the leukemic cells and their decreased tolerance of cytotoxic drugs. The longest disease-free survival can be currently achieved with repeated cycles of intensive chemotherapy containing anthracyclines and cytosine arabinoside. Postremission consolidation therapy is crucial while maintenance is not necessary, perhaps with the exception of APL. Although questions remain about the optimal drugs for induction and about the length of consolidation, it is unlikely that refining standard chemotherapy will result in dramatic improvement in survival. Allogenic SCT decreases relapse rates for the price of higher treatment-related mortality. It is most widely used in younger patients with poor prognosis disease. Improvements in allotransplantation including nonmyeloablative transplants will benefit the minority of patients with HLA-matched donors. Future studies will better define the molecular events causing drug resistance, decreased apoptosis, and adhesion and increased proliferation of AML cells. These aberrant pathways could be targeted by specific therapies. Promising new treatments for AML include antibody-based therapies, tyrosine kinase inhibitors, and other drugs targeting signal transduction, inhibitors of drug resistance, immunomodulatory approaches, and vaccines. These treatments have the potential to be more selective, less toxic, and ultimately curative of AML.

REFERENCES

1. Giles FJ, Keating A, Goldstone AH, et al. Acute myeloid leukemia. *Hematology (Am Soc Hematol Educ Program)* 2002;73–110.
2. Yates J, Glidewell O, Wiernik P, et al. Cytosine arabinoside with daunorubicin or adriamycin for therapy of acute myelocytic leukemia: a CALGB study. *Blood* 1982;60:454–462.
3. Bishop JF, Lowenthal RM, Joshua D, et al. Etoposide in acute nonlymphocytic leukemia. Australian Leukemia Study Group. *Blood* 1990;75:27–32.
4. Bishop JF, Matthews JP, Young GA. A randomized trial of high-dose cytarabine in induction in acute myeloid leukemia. *Blood* 1996; 87:1710–1717.

5. Berman E, Heller G, Santorsa J, et al. Results of a randomized trial comparing idarubicin and cytosine arabinoside with daunorubicin and cytosine arabinoside in adult patients with newly diagnosed acute myelogenous leukemia. *Blood* 1991;77:1666–1674.

6. Vogler WR, Velez-Garcia E, Weiner RS, et al. Phase III trial comparing idarubicin and daunorubicin in combination with cytarabine in acute myelogenous leukemia: a Southeastern Cancer Study Group Study. *J Clin Oncol* 1992;10:1103–1111.

7. Wiernik PH, Banks PL, Case DC, et al. Cytarabine plus idarubicin or daunorubicin as induction and consolidation therapy for previously untreated adult patients with acute myeloid leukemia. *Blood* 1992;79:313–319

8. Cassileth PA, Harrington DP, Hines JD, et al. Maintenance chemotherapy prolongs remission duration in adult acute nonlymphocytic leukemia. *J Clin Oncol* 1988;6:583–587.

9. Mayer RJ, Davis RB, Schiffer CA, et al. Intensive postremission chemotherapy in adults with acute myeloid leukemia. Cancer and Leukemia Group B. *N Engl J Med* 1994;331:896–903

10. Elonen E, Almqvist A, Hanninen A, et al. Comparison between four and eight cycles of intensive chemotherapy in adult acute myeloid leukemia: a randomized trial of the Finnish Leukemia Group. *Leukemia* 1998;12:1041–1048.

11. Zittoun RA, Mandelli F, Willemze R, et al. Autologous or allogeneic bone marrow transplantation compared with intensive chemotherapy in acute myelogenous leukemia. European Organization for Research and Treatment of Cancer (EORTC) and the Gruppo Italiano Malattie Ematologiche Maligne dell' Adulto (GIMEMA) Leukemia Cooperative Groups. *N Engl J Med* 1995;332:217–223.

12. Burnett AK, Goldstone AH, Stevens RM, et al. Randomised comparison of addition of autologous bone marrow transplantation to intensive chemotherapy for acute myeloid leukemia in first remission: results of MRC AML 10 trial. UK Medical Research Council Adult and Children's Leukemia Working Parties. *Lancet* 1998;351:700–708.

13. Cassileth PA, Harrington DP, Appelbaum FR, et al. Chemotherapy compared with autologous or allogenic bone marrow transplantation in the management of acute myeloid leukemia in first remission. *N Engl J Med* 1998;339:1649–1656.

14. Harousseau JL, Cahn JY, Pignon B, et al. Comparison of autologous bone marrow transplantation and intensive chemotherapy as postremission therapy in adult acute myeloid leukemia. The Groupe Ouest Est Leucemies Aigues Myeloblastiques (Goelam). *Blood* 1997;90:2978–2986.

15. Sucia S, Mandelli F, de Witte, et al. Allogeneic compared with autologous stem cell transplantation in the treatment of patients younger than 46 years with acute myeloid leukemia (AML) in first complete remission (CR1): An intention-to-treat analysis of the EORTC/GIMEMA AML-10 trial. *Blood* 2003;102:1232–40.

16. Rowe JM, Andersen JW, Mazza JJ, et al. A randomized placebo-controlled phase III study of granulo-cyte-macrophage colony-stimulating factor in adult patients (> 55 to 70 years of age) with acute myelogenous leukemia: a study of the Eastern Cooperative Oncology Group (E1490). *Blood* 1995; 86:457–462.

17. Stone RM, Berg DT, George SL, et al. Granulocyte-macrophage colony-stimulating factor after initial chemotherapy for elderly patients with primary acute myelogenous leukemia. Cancer and Leukemia Group B. *N Engl J Med* 1995;332:1671–1677.

18. Greenlund LJ, Letendre L, Tefferi A. Acute leukemia during pregnancy: a single institutional experience with 17 cases. *Leuk Lymphoma* 2001;41:571–577.

19. Giles F, Estey E, O'Brien S. Gemtuzumab Ozogamicin in the treatment of acute myeloid leukemia. *Cancer* 2003;98:2095–2104.

20. Karp JE, Lancet JE, Kaufmann SH, et al. Clinical and biologic activity of the farnesyltransferase inhibitor R115777 in adults with refractory and relapsed acute leukemias: a phase I clinical-laboratory correlative trial. *Blood* 2001;97:3361–3369.

21. Smith BD, Levis M, Beran M, et al. Single agent CEP-701, a novel FLT3 inhibitor, shows biologic and clinical activity in patients with relapsed or refractory acute myeloid leukemia. *Blood* 2004;103: 3669–3676.

12

Acute Lymphoblastic Leukemia

Alan S. Wayne

Approximately 5,000 new cases of acute lymphoblastic leukemia (ALL) are diagnosed each year in the United States, more than half of these in children. ALL represents the most common pediatric malignancy, accounting for approximately 25% of childhood cancer. The peak prevalence of ALL is between the ages of 2 and 9 years. There is a slight male predominance and Caucasians have a twofold increased risk compared to African Americans.

ETIOLOGY AND RISK FACTORS

There are a variety of conditions that predispose to ALL, most notably trisomy 21 (Down's syndrome) where the relative risk is increased 20–fold. Other predisposing conditions include immunodeficiency and chromosomal breakage syndromes, but most often no such underlying disorder is found. Epstein-Barr virus (EBV) infection is implicated in a minority of cases of mature B-cell ALL. Environmental exposure risks have been suggested, but few (radiation) have been shown to be causal. Acquired chromosomal abnormalities confined to the lymphoblasts are found in more than 90% of cases, including aneuploidy (most commonly hyperdiploidy) and/or translocations that in some cases have been shown to be prenatal in origin. The genes involved in leukemogenesis are frequently transcription factors expressed in hematopoietic tissues.

CLINICAL FEATURES

Presenting signs and symptoms are almost always caused by blast infiltration of the bone marrow with resultant blood count abnormalities (Table 12-1). Other organs may also be involved. T-cell ALL frequently presents with bulky adenopathy, mediastinal mass, pleural effusion, and/or hyperleukocytosis. Gastrointestinal presentation due to Peyer's patch involvement, usually ileocecal intussusception, is almost always confined to mature B-cell ALL. There are a number of life- or organ-threatening presentations that require emergent intervention (Table 12-2).

LABORATORY FEATURES

Diagnosis is readily confirmed by the demonstration of lymphoblasts in the blood and/or bone marrow. Blast morphology can be classified into three categories (L1, L2, L3) according to the French-American-British (FAB) system (Table 12-3). Only the latter is of clinical and prognostic significance, because L3 morphology is indicative of mature B-cell or Burkitt-type ALL. Routine hematopathologic staining, immunohistochemistry, flow cytometry, and cytogenetics are used to define the subtype and further identify prognostic factors. The majority of ALL is of precursor B-cell (pre-B) phenotype (CD10, CD19, HLA-DR, TDT +), 10% to 20% is T-cell (CD2, CD7 +), and less than 5% is mature B-cell or Burkitt-type (CD20, surface-IgM κ or λ +). Certain cytogenetic abnormalities are not apparent on routine karyo-

TABLE 12–1. *Presenting features*

Common presenting signs and symptoms	Sites of involvement
70% Hepatosplenomegaly	100% Bone marrow
60% Fever	10% Anterior mediastinal mass
50% Fatigue	5% Central nervous system (CNS)
50% Lymphadenopathy	2% Testicular
40% Bleeding	<5% Other (eye, skin, pericardium,
40% Bone or joint pain	pleura, kidney, breast, ovary,
20% Anorexia	priapism, appendix)
10% Abdominal pain	

TABLE 12–2. *Emergency presentations*

Emergent presentation	Intervention
Leukostasis	Oxygen, leukapheresis
Neutropenia with fever or infection	Broad spectrum IV antibiotics
Thrombocytopenia	Platelet transfusion
Disseminated intravascular coagulation	Fresh frozen plasma, cryoprecipitate
Tumor lysis syndrome	IV hydration, allopurinol, alkalinization, dialysis
Airway obstruction	Oxygen, corticosteroids and/or radiation
Superior vena cava syndrome	Corticosteroids and/or radiation
Pericardial tamponade	Pericardiocentesis, corticosteroids
Intussusception	Surgical decompression
CNS manifestations	Corticosteroids and/or radiation
Ocular involvement	Radiation
Spinal cord compression	Corticosteroids and/or radiation

IV, intravenous; CNS, central nervous system.

TABLE 12–3. *Classification*

FAB morphology
    L1: homogeneous blasts, minimal cytoplasm
    L2: increased nuclear heterogeneity, prominent nucleoli
    L3: basophilic cytoplasm with prominent vacuolization
Bone marrow
    M1: <5% blasts
    M2: 5% to 25% blasts
    M3: >25% blasts
Cerebrospinal fluid cytology
    CNS-1: no blasts
    CNS-2: WBC $<5/\mu L$, + blasts
    CNS-3: WBC $\geq 5/\mu L$, + blasts (*or* symptomatic CNS
       involvement, e.g., cranial nerve palsy)

WBC, white blood cell count; CNS, central nervous system.

TABLE 12–4. *Common chromosomal translocations*

t(12;21): *TEL/AML1* (25% childhood ALL)
t(1;19): *E2A/PBX1*
t(9;22): *BCR/ABL* p190 fusion (25% adult ALL)
11q23: *MLL*, >25 fusion partners (70% infant ALL)
14q11 or 7q35: *TCR*, T-cell phenotype
t(8;14), t(8;22), t(2;8): c-*myc/Ig*, mature B-cell (Burkitt) phenotype

ALL, acute lymphoblastic leukemia.

typing and thus molecular testing may be required, most notably for t(12;21) in children (Table 12-4). Lumbar puncture is required to evaluate for the possibility of meningeal leukemia.

PROGNOSTIC FACTORS

Disease-free-survival (DFS) rates have improved steadily for children with ALL and currently, approximately 80% will achieve cure. Results are inferior in infants and adolescents. In adults, cure rates decline with advancing age, with overall DFS rates of approximately 40%. T-cell and mature B-cell disease have historically faired poorer than pre-B phenotype, however, stratified treatment has minimized this difference. A number of clinical and biologic features are used to stratify risk-directed treatment for individuals with pre-B ALL (Table 12-5) (1). Recently, cDNA microarray gene expression analysis has been shown to allow further discrimination in regard to diagnostic subtype, risk classification, and treatment response prediction (2).

TREATMENT

Many chemotherapy regimens have been shown to be effective for children and adults with ALL. Therapy should be stratified based on clinicopathologic features, and patients should be treated by physicians familiar with subtype-specific regimens. The following core recommendations are based on results of large cooperative group clinical trials (3–11).

- Therapy should be instituted as soon as possible for all patients.
- Treatment phases: Standard treatment, which is stratified based on phenotype and prognostic factors, includes induction, consolidation, central nervous system (CNS) sterilization,

TABLE 12–5. *Risk group assignment in B-precursor acute lymphoblastic leukemia*

	Standard risk	High risk	Very-high risk	Ultra-high risk
Age (years)	1–9	10–35	>35	<1
WBC (/μL)	<50,000	≥50,000		
CNS	Negative	Positive		
Chromosomes	t(12;21), Triple Trisomy 4/10/17	11q23, t(1;19)		t(9;22)
DNA Index	≥1.16	<1.16		
Treatment Response	RER		SER	Induction failure

RER, rapid early responder; SER, slow early responder; WBC, white blood cell count; CNS, central nervous system.

and maintenance for a total of 2 to 3 years (Table 12-6). Initial induction therapy often consists of 3 to 5 drugs given as a 28-day cycle, although there are alternative approaches (12). There are a variety of consolidation and intensification regimens in common use, some of which are detailed below. Multiple consolidation/intensification blocks are often used for high-risk patients. A late reinduction phase, also known as delayed intensification, improves DFS for children who are slow early responders (SER) (13). Randomized trials of various intensification blocks for adults have had mixed results (14,15). Prolonged maintenance with total treatment duration of 24 to 36 months improves DFS for both adults and children.

- Allogeneic stem cell transplantation (SCT): Although relapse rates are lower after allogeneic SCT compared to chemotherapy, treatment-related mortality rates are higher after transplantation (16). Thus, SCT is rarely used for children in first remission (CR1). Given the relatively poor results of chemotherapy in older individuals, some groups recommend allogeneic SCT in CR1 for adults with human leukocyte antigen (HLA)-matched sibling donors.
- Autologous stem cell rescue: High-dose therapy followed by stem cell rescue can be used as consolidation therapy in ALL, but multiple randomized trials have shown no significant DFS advantage compared to chemotherapy. Because of the increased risks associated with autologous transplant, this approach is not frequently used.
- Risk group assignment for B-precursor ALL: Although there is some variability in the approach to risk-adapted therapy, the aforementioned designations are suggested based on published pediatric cooperative group data (Table 12-5). Age, white blood cell (WBC) count, central nervous system (CNS) involvement, DNA index, and phenotype are used for the initial risk group assignment (1). Subsequently, the risk group may be elevated based on cytogenetics and response to induction, that latter of which is defined by morphologic blast reduction (in peripheral blood on day 7 or bone marrow on day 7 or 14) and/or minimal residual disease determination (by flow cytometry or polymerase chain reaction amplification). Prognostic factors are similar in adults, although the strong adverse influence of older age has limited further refinements in treatment stratification. Patients with ultra-

TABLE 12–6. *Common treatment regimens for pre-B acute lymphoblastic leukemia and T- acute lymphoblastic leukemia*

A: Induction (weeks 1–4)
  3-Drug (Standard Risk)
    - Prednisone 40–60 mg/m^2 per day *or* dexamethasone 6 mg/m^2 per day in divided doses orally × 21–28 days (day 0–)
    - Vincristine 1.5 mg/m^2 per dose (maximum dose 2 mg) IV weekly × 4 doses (days 0, 7, 14, 21)
    - *Escherichia coli* L-Asparaginase 6,000–10,000 IU/m^2 per dose IM × 6–9 doses, QOD, 3 days per week × 2–3 weeks
    - IT methotrexate:
      ○ CNS-1: Every 2 weeks × 2 doses (days 0, 14).
      ○ CNS-2 or CNS-3: Weekly × at least 4 doses and until 2 successive CNS-1 (days 0, 7, 14, 21).
  4-Drug (High Risk): Add the following to above
    - Doxorubicin 25–30 mg/m^2 per dose *or* Daunorubicin 25–45 mg/m^2 per dose IV weekly × 4 doses (Days 0, 7, 14, 21) *or* IV daily × 2–3 doses (Days 0, 1, +/− 2)
  5-Drug (Higher risk groups): Add the following to above
    - Cyclophosphamide 800–1,200 mg/m^2 per dose IV × 1 dose (day 0)
  Response evaluation
    - Day 14 Bone Marrow: M1 = rapid early responder; M2 or M3 = slow early responder
    - Day 28 Bone Marrow: M1 = remission, continue as below; M2 or M3 = induction failure, salvage re-induction required.

TABLE 12–6B. *Post-induction regimens*

Pretreatment criteria
- ANC ≥750 per microliter, platelets ≥75,000 per microliter
- ALT <20× the upper limit of normal, Direct bilirubin normal for age
- Serum creatinine normal for age
- No active infection or life-threatening organ dysfunction

Consolidation (week 5)
Standard Berlin-Frankfurt-Munster Study Group (BFM)
- Cyclophosphamide 1000 mg/m^2 per dose IV × 2 doses (days 0, 14)
- Mercaptopurine (6-MP) 60 mg/m^2 per dose orally once daily (administer at bedtime on an empty stomach to improve absorption) × 28 days (days 0–27)
- Vincristine 1.5 mg/m^2 per dose (maximum dose 2 mg) IV × 4 doses (days 14, 21, 42, 49)
- Cytarabine 75 mg/m^2 per dose IV or SQ (days 1–4, 8–11, 15–18, 22–25)
- IT Methotrexate weekly × 4 doses (days 1, 8, 15, 22)

Augmented BFM
- Cyclophosphamide 1000 mg/m^2 per dose IV × 2 doses (days 0, 28)
- Mercaptopurine (6-MP) 60 mg/m^2 per dose PO once daily (administer at bedtime on an empty stomach to improve absorption) × 28 days (days 0–13, 28–41)
- Vincristine 1.5 mg/m^2 per dose (maximum dose 2 mg) IV × 4 doses (days 14, 21, 42, 49)
- Cytarabine 75 mg/m^2 per dose IV or SQ (Days 1–4, 8–11, 29–32, 36–39)
- *E. coli* L-Asparaginase 6,000 IU/m^2 per dose IM × 12 doses, every other day 3 doses per week (days 14, 16, 18, 21, 23, 25, 42, 44, 46, 49, 51, 53)
- IT Methotrexate weekly × 4 doses (days 1, 8, 15, 22)

High-Dose Methotrexate with Leucovorin Rescue
- Refer to protocol-specific dosing, administration, and leucovorin rescue guidelines

Capizzi
- Cytarabine (Ara-C) 3,000 mg/m^2 per dose IV over 3 hours every 12 hours × 4 doses, weekly × 2 (days 0, 1 and Days 7, 8).
- *E. coli* L-Asparaginase 6,000 IU/m^2 per dose IM at hour 42 following Ara-C (3 hours after the completion of the fourth Ara-C infusion on days 1 and 8).

Ifosfamide/Etoposide
- Etoposide (VP-16): 100 mg/m^2 per dose IV × 5 doses (days 1–5).
- Ifosfamide: 1.8 g/m^2 per dose IV × 5 doses (days 1–5). Begin immediately upon completion of VP-16 infusion.
- Mesna: 360 mg/m^2 per dose IV prior to ifosfamide and every 3 hours × 8 doses/day (days 1–5).

Interim Maintenance
- Commonly usd between Consolidation and Delayed Intensification/Reinduction courses

Delayed Instensification/Reinduction
- Dexamethasone 10 mg/m^2 per day in divided doses orally × 14–28 days (day 0–)
- Vincristine 1.5 mg/m^2 per dose (maximum dose 2 mg) IV weekly × 5 doses (days 0, 14, 21, 42, 49)
- Doxorubicin 25–30 mg/m^2 per dose IV weekly × 3 doses (days 0, 7, 14)
- Cyclophosphamide 1,000 mg/m^2 per dose IV (day 28)
- 6-Thioguanine (6-TG) 60 mg/m^2 per dose orally once daily × 14 days (days 28–41)
- Cytarabine 75 mg/m^2 per dose IV or SQ (days 29–32, 36–39)
- IT Methotrexate × 2 doses (days 29, 36)

With or Without:
- *E. coli* L-Asparaginase 6,000 IU/ m^2 per dose IM × 6–12 doses (days 3, 5, 7, 10, 12, 14 +/− 42, 44, 46, 49, 51, 53)

TABLE 12–6C. *Maintenance/Continuation regimen*

Repeat cycles to complete 24–36 months of total treatment.
- Prednisone 40–60 mg/m^2 per day *or* dexamethasone 6 mg/m^2 per day in divided doses orally × 5 days every 28 days
- Vincristine 1.5 mg/m^2 per day (maximum dose 2 mg) IV every 4 weeks
- Mercaptopurine (6-MP) 75 mg/m^2 per dose* orally once daily (administer at bedtime on an empty stomach to improve absorption)
- Methotrexate 20 mg/m^2 per dose* orally once weekly.
- IT Methotrexate every 4–12 weeks for 1–2 years of treatment

*6-MP and methotrexate doses should be adjusted to maintain the absolute neutrophil count (ANC) between 750 and 1,500 per microliter and the platelet count greater than 75,000 per microliter.

IV, intravenous; IT, intrathecal; SQ, subcutaneous; IM, intramuscular.

high–risk features require more intensive treatment, and allogeneic SCT in CR1 is commonly considered for those with HLA-matched siblings.

- Infant ALL: Children younger than 1 year of age at diagnosis should be treated on age-specific protocols with certain agents dosed on a per-kilogram basis to decrease the risk of severe toxicity.
- T-ALL: Patients with T-cell phenotype are treated similarly to higher risk group pre-B ALL. Improved outcome has been associated with the use of intensified therapy that commonly includes high-dose methotrexate and intensified L-asparaginase (17).
- Mature B-ALL: Patients with mature B-cell phenotype ALL should be treated with Burkitt's lymphoma regimens: most commonly dose and sequence intensive, short course chemotherapy regimens that include hyperfractionated cyclophosphamide, high-dose methotrexate, and high-dose cytarabine (18,19).
- CNS-directed therapy: All patients require CNS sterilization. Intensive intrathecal chemotherapy in combination with systemic agents that have good CNS penetration, most notably dexamethasone and high-dose methotrexate, provides excellent prophylaxis (Table 12-7). To minimize neurotoxicity, radiation is usually reserved for those with active meningeal leukemia or at high risk of CNS relapse (T-cell phenotype with hyperleukocytosis) (Table 12-8).
- Testicular leukemia: Males with testicular involvement should receive radiation to both testes (Table 12-8).

DOSE MODIFICATION

Improved outcome is associated with greater drug exposure, thus attempts should be made to deliver protocol-specified doses unless toxicity prevents such. Importantly, 6-MP and methotrexate doses should be increased during maintenance to achieve a targeted degree of myelosuppression (Table 12-6C). In the event of significant chemotherapy-related toxicity, individual agents should be dose-reduced or discontinued as clinically indicated. Specific agents may require dose adjustment for renal or hepatic dysfunction. Patients with thiopurine S-methyltransferase deficiency (approximately 1:300 incidence) require significant dose reduction of 6-MP. Individuals with Down's syndrome tolerate methotrexate poorly.

EXTRAMEDULLARY LEUKEMIA

Radiation should be used to treat overt CNS or testicular leukemia (Table 12-8). Current chemotherapy regimens are associated with low rates of extramedullary relapse in both the

TABLE 12–7. *Intrathecal chemotherapy*

- Intrathecal chemotherapy delivered by lumbar puncture is part of all phases of treatment (unless full dose CNS radiation is required).
- Single agent intrathecal methotrexate is the standard treatment.
- Triple agent intrathecal chemotherapy is sometimes employed for those with CNS leukemia, especially in the management of meningeal relapse.
- To minimize the risk of meningeal contamination caused by traumatic lumbar puncture, spinal taps should be performed by clinicians experienced in the procedure. In addition, intrathecal chemotherapy should always be administered at the time of the first (i.e., diagnostic) lumbar puncture.
- To facilitate CNS delivery, the volume of CSF removed should equal the volume administered and patients should remain prone for 30 minutes.
- Intrathecal chemotherapy is dosed by age as follows:

Age (yr)	Methotrexate (mg)	Hydrocortisone (mg)	Cytarabine (mg)	Volume (mL)
<1	7.5	7.5	15	5
1	8	8	16	6
2	10	10	20	7
3–8	12	12	24	8
≥9	15	15	30	10

Induction Schedule
- CNS-1: Every 2 weeks × 2 doses
- CNS-2 or CNS-3: Weekly × at least 4 doses and until 2 successive CNS-1.

Consolidation Schedule
- Every 1–4 weeks

Maintenance Schedule
- Every 4–12 weeks for 1–2 years of treatment

CNS, central nervous sytem; CSF, cerebrospinal fluid.

CNS and testes. Importantly, patients with isolated extramedullary relapse also require systemic therapy.

NEW TREATMENT APPROACHES

A variety of targeted therapies with potential applications in ALL have recently become available. The bcr/abl tyrosine kinase inhibitor, imatinib mesylate (Gleevec), can induce

TABLE 12–8. *Radiation guidelines*

- CNS radiation should be avoided in children younger than 2 years of age.
- Radiation dose should be based on the specific indication and overall treatment regimen.

Site	Total dose (cGy)	Fractional dose (cGy)
Cranium	1,200–2,400	150–200
Spine	600–1,200	150–200
Testes	1,800–2,400	200–300

remission in some patients with Philadelphia chromosome positive ALL, but CR duration is inevitably short. Combination trials with this agent and chemotherapy are being conducted. Studies of anti-CD20 monoclonal antibody (rituximab) with chemotherapy for mature B-ALL are in progress.

MANAGEMENT OF RELAPSE

The likelihood of durable DFS decreases substantially after relapse. Reinduction of a second remission is critical and usually can be achieved with standard four- or five-drug regimens (Table 12-6A). The likelihood of prolonged DFS with standard regimens varies based on the duration of the initial complete remission and the intensity of the prior treatment. For those with CR1 durations of more than 12 to 18 months who received standard-risk therapy, approximately 20% to 30% will achieve prolonged DFS with high-risk disease regimens. With shorter CR1 durations, the likelihood of durable remission is extremely low. Curative salvage using standard chemotherapy and radiation is more likely in the setting of isolated extramedullary relapse.

Allogeneic Stem Cell Transplantation

For those with HLA-matched sibling donors, allogeneic SCT in second CR is considered standard. The risks of transplant-related morbidity and mortality are increased with alternative donors (unrelated and HLA-mismatched related). Consequently, alternative donor transplants are often reserved for those who have had short CR1 durations or subsequent relapses.

SUPPORTIVE CARE

Aggressive monitoring and supportive care are essential throughout all phases of treatment.

Antiemetics

Nausea and vomiting are common during induction, consolidation, intensification, and CNS-directed therapy. Routine antiemetic prophylaxis and treatment should be used.

Tumor Lysis Syndrome

Rapid blast lysis can result in life-threatening metabolic complications. Tumor lysis syndrome is usually seen within the first few hours to days of initiation of induction chemotherapy. Patients with WBC higher than 100,000 per microliter, elevated serum lactate dehydrogenase (LDH), and/or elevated uric acid are at increased risk and those with mature B-cell disease (i.e., L3 or Burkitt's) are at extreme risk. Tumor lysis precautions should be started as soon as possible after diagnosis and at least 12 hours prior to the start of induction. Prophylaxis and monitoring should continue until disease burden is reduced (e.g., peripheral blasts clear) and it is apparent that no tumor lysis has developed (usually for 3 to 7 days). The following is indicated for all patients around initial induction:

- Allopurinol: 100 mg/m^2 per dose orally, three times daily. Urate oxidase (Uricase) is a new alternative for management of extreme hyperuricemia.
- Hydration: Intravenous fluids at a rate of 2 or more times maintenance (120 mL/m^2 or more per hour) should be titrated to maintain urine specific gravity 1.010 or less and normal urine output. Because of the risk of hyperkalemia, potassium should be *avoided.*
- Alkalinization: To decrease the risk of uric acid nephropathy, urine may be alkalinized with sodium bicarbonate. Caution: It is recommended that the urine pH be maintained between 6.5 and 7.5 because a high pH is associated with hypoxanthine crystallization. In addition,

to decrease the risk of calcium/phosphate precipitation, alkalinization should be avoided or minimized if possible in the setting of hyperphosphatemia.
- Frequent serial laboratory monitoring is required during initiation of induction chemotherapy. Complete blood count (CBC), potassium, phosphorous, calcium, creatinine, blood–urea nitrogen (BUN), and uric acid should be assayed every 4 to 6 hours for the first 24 to 48 hours, then less frequently once stable.

Transfusions

Blood transfusion should be used to prevent complications related to severe cytopenias. To decrease the risk of transfusion-associated complications, specialized products should be used.

- Platelets: To prevent bleeding, platelet counts should routinely be maintained above 10,000 per microliter. Higher levels are recommended for management of bleeding, prior to invasive procedures such as lumbar puncture, and to reduce the risk of leukostasis-induced CNS hemorrhage in the setting of hyperleukocytosis. Single donor platelets are recommended whenever possible to decrease donor exposure and the risk of HLA-alloimmunization (20).
- Red blood cells (RBCs): Concomitant anemia partially offsets the hyperviscosity associated with severe hyperleukocytosis. Thus, RBC transfusion should be avoided if possible when the WBC is higher than 100,000 per microliter. If transfusion is necessary, the hemoglobin and hematocrit should be increased slowly using small aliquots of packed RBCs until the peripheral blast count is reduced.
- Irradiation: To reduce the risk of transfusion associated graft-versus-host disease, all cellular blood products should be irradiated.
- Leukodepletion: Platelets and red cells should be leuko-reduced to decrease the risk of febrile reactions, HLA-alloimmunization with subsequent platelet-refractoriness, and transmission of cytomegalovirus (CMV) infection.

Infection Prophylaxis

Aggressive surveillance, prophylaxis, and treatment for bacterial, fungal, viral, and opportunistic infections are essential to prevent morbidity and mortality.

- *Pneumocystis carinii* pneumonia (PCP): All patients should receive PCP prophylaxis. The standard regimen is trimethoprim/sulfamethoxazole (TMP/SMX) at a dose of 75 mg/m^2 dose of TMP (maximum 160 mg of TMP = 1 double-strength tablet) orally two to three three times per week. For patients who are allergic to these drugs or who develop myelosuppression with TMP/SMX, an alternative regimen should be substituted. PCP prophylaxis should continue until 6 months after chemotherapy is completed.
- Management of neutropenic fever: Patients with an absolute neutrophil count (ANC) less than 500 per microliter and temperature of 38.3°C or higher should be evaluated for possible infection and treated empirically with parenterally administered broad-spectrum antibiotics. Antifungal therapy should be initiated for neutropenic fever that persists for 5 to 7 days. Antibiotics should be continued until the ANC rises to more than 500 per microliter, fever resolves, cultures are negative, and any suspected infection is fully treated.
- Intravenous immunoglobulin (IVIG): Hypogammaglobulinemia is common during treatment for ALL. Immunoglobulin G (IgG) levels should be assayed for those with recurrent infections, and if low, IVIG supplementation is recommended at a dose of approximately 500 mg/kg every 4 weeks as needed to maintain an IgG level of 500 mg/dL or higher.
- Myeloid growth factors: Granulocyte colony-stimulating factor (G-CSF) during induction has been shown to improve outcome for adults, although no benefit was demonstrated in a pediatric study. Myeloid growth factor support should be employed during treatment of mature B-cell ALL (i.e., Burkitt's or L3) in both children and adults.

Chemotherapy Prophylaxis

Agent-specific prophylaxis should be utilized as clinically indicated. For example, gastritis prophylaxis is recommended during corticosteroid administration. To reduce the risk of conjunctivitis associated with high-dose Ara-C, corticosteroid ophthalmic solution should be administered during and for 24 to 48 hours after treatment. Mesna uroprophylaxis should be used in an attempt to prevent hemorrhagic cystitis caused by ifosfamide.

Nutritional Support

Nutritional status should be monitored and supplementation provided as indicated. Routine folic acid use should be avoided with methotrexate administration because it may counteract the therapeutic efficacy of folate antagonism. (In contrast, leucovorin rescue is indicated to prevent severe toxicity after high-dose methotrexate.)

Psychosocial Support

Multidisciplinary support for the patient and family is an important part of successful treatment.

EVALUATIONS

Serial evaluations to monitor for response, relapse, complications, and therapy-associated toxicity should be conducted throughout all treatment phases.

Evaluations During Treatment

- History, physical examination, and routine laboratory assessments including CBC and chemistry panel should be performed regularly throughout treatment.
- Bone marrow aspiration should be obtained at the following times:
  - Induction day 7 or 14 to assess early response.
  - Induction day 28 to assess remission status. If indeterminate, repeat weekly until recovery in order to confirm remission or induction failure.
  - At the end of therapy.
  - Bone marrow should also be performed at suspicion of relapse.
  - Flow cytometry, cytogenetics, and/or molecular genetic studies can be used to monitor minimal residual disease, which is prognostic.
- CSF cell count and cytospin should be performed at the time of all intrathecal chemotherapy administrations. Lumbar puncture should also be performed for suspicion of CNS relapse.

Evaluations After Treatment

- Follow-up evaluations to include history, physical examination, and routine laboratory studies (CBC, chemistry panel) should be conducted to monitor for toxicity and recurrent disease until at least 5 years posttreatment on the following schedule (or as clinically indicated):
  - Every 1 to 2 months during the first year.
  - Every 2 to 3 months during the second year.
  - Every 3 to 4 months during the third year.
  - Every 6 months during the fourth year.
  - Yearly thereafter.
- Late Effects: Life-long follow-up to monitor for a variety of possible late complications of treatment is recommended. The following are among the most frequent late effects:

- Cardiomyopathy: To decrease the risk of cardiotoxicity, cumulative anthracycline doses are usually limited to less than 400 mg/m^2. Echocardiograms for left ventricular function determination should be performed at baseline, at completion of treatment, every 1 to 2 years after treatment until serial studies remain normal, and as clinically indicated.
- Neurologic toxicity: Children are at especially high risk of neurotoxicity from chemotherapy and radiation. All patients should be monitored for neurologic toxicity including neurodevelopmental dysfunction.
- Endocrinologic dysfunction: Patients should be monitored for endocrinopathies including growth retardation, infertility, and hormonal dysfunction.
- Osteonecrosis: Corticosteroids, especially dexamethasone, are associated with a high incidence of osteonecrosis in survivors of ALL.
- Secondary malignancy: Patients should be monitored for secondary malignancies as these continue to develop even in the second decade after treatment (21).

REFERENCES

1. Smith M, Arthur D, Camitta B, et al. Uniform approach to risk classification and treatment assignment for children with acute lymphoblastic leukemia. *J Clin Oncol* 1996;14:18–24.
2. Mosquera-Caro M, Helman P, Veroff R, et al. Identification, validation, and cloning of a novel gene (OPAL1) and associated genes highly predictive of outcome in pediatric acute lymphoblastic leukemia using gene expression profiling. *Blood* 2003;102:4a (abst).
3. Pui C-H, Crist WM: Acute lymphoblastic leukemia. In: Pui C-H, ed. *Childhood Leukemias.* 1st ed. New York: Cambridge University Press, 1999:288–312.
4. Pui C-H, Rellins MV, Downing JR. Acute lymphoblastic leukemias. *N Engl J Med* 2004;350: 1535–1548.
5. Schrappe M, Reiter A, Ludwig W, et al. Improved outcome in childhood acute lymphoblastic leukemia despite reduced use of anthracyclines and cranial radiotherapy: results of trial ALL-BFM 90. *Blood* 2000;95:3310–3322.
6. Pui C-H, Boyett JM, Rivera GK, et al. Long-term results of Total Therapy studies 11, 12 and 13A for childhood acute lymphoblastic leukemia at St. Jude Children's Research Hospital. *Leukemia* 2000;14:2286–2294.
7. Silverman LB, Gelber RD, Dalton VK, et al. Improved outcome for children with acute lymphoblastic leukemia: results of Dana-Farber Consortium Protocol 91-01. *Blood* 2001;97:1211–1218.
8. Faderl S, Jeha S, Kantarjian HM: The biology and therapy of adult acute lymphoblastic leukemia. *Cancer* 2003;98:1337–1354.
9. Gökbuget N, Hoelzer D. Recent approaches in acute lymphoblastic leukemia in adults. *Rev Clin Exp Hematol* 2002;6:114–141.
10. Larson RA, Dodge RK, Burns CP, et al. A five-drug induction regimen with intensive consolidation for adults with acute lymphoblastic leukemia: Cancer and Leukemia Group B Study 8811. *Blood* 1995;84:2025–2037.
11. Annino L, Vegna ML, Camera A, et al. Treatment of adults with acute lymphoblastic leukemia (ALL): long-term follow-up of the GIMEMA ALL 0288 randomized study. *Blood* 2002;99:863–871.
12. Kantarjian HM, O'Brien S, Smith TL, et al. Results of treatment with hy per-CVAD, a dose-intensive regimen, in adult acute lymphocytic leukemia. *J Clin Oncol* 2000;18:547–561.
13. Nachman JB, Sather HN, Sensel MG, et al. Augmented post-induction therapy for children with high-risk acute lymphoblastic leukemia and a slow response to initial therapy. *N Engl J Med* 1998; 338:1663–1671.
14. Richards S, Burrett J, Hann I, et al. Improved survival with early intensification: combined results from the Medical Research Council childhood ALL randomised trials, UKALL X and UKALL XI. *Leukemia* 1998;12:1031–1036.
15. Durrant IJ, Prentice HG, Richards SM. Intensification of treatment for adults with acute lymphoblastic leukemia: results of U.K. Medical Research Council randomized trial UKALL XA. *Br J Haematol* 1997;99:84–92.
16. Barrett AJ, Horowitz MH, Pollock BH, et al. Bone marrow transplants from HLA-identical siblings as compared with chemotherapy for children with acute lymphoblastic leukemia in a second remission. *N Engl J Med* 1994;331:1253–1258.
17. Amylon MD, Shuster J, Pullen J, et al. Intensive high-dose asparaginase consolidation improves

survival for pediatric patients with T cell acute lymphoblastic leukemia and advanced stage lymphoblastic lymphoma: a Pediatric Oncology Group study. *Leukemia* 1999;13:335–342.

18. Thomas DA, Cortes J, O'Brien S, et al. Hyper-CVAD program in Burkitt's type adult acute lymphocytic leukemia. *J Clin Oncol* 1999;17:2461–2470.

19. Magrath I, Adde M, Shad A, et al. Adults and children with small non-cleaved-cell lymphoma have a similar excellent outcome when treated with the same chemotherapy regimen. *J Clin Oncol* 1996; 14:925–934.

20. Slichter SJ. Optimizing platelet transfusions in chronically thrombocytopenic patients. *Semin Hematol* 1998;35:269–278.

21. Pui C-H, Cheng C, Leung W, et al. Extended follow-up of long-term survivors of childhood acute lymphoblastic leukemia. *N Engl J Med* 2003;49:640–649.

13

Chronic Myelogenous Leukemia

A. John Barrett

Although chronic myelogenous leukemia (CML) is rare, it has achieved disproportionate prominence in the medical literature because its biologic basis has been elucidated in unprecedented detail, and also because CML has become a model for developing effective immune-based and molecularly targeted treatments for leukemia. The era of significant discoveries in CML began in 1960 when Nowell and Hungerford (1) first observed the occurrence of a unique unusually small G group chromosome in patients with CML. Following convention, they named it the Philadelphia (Ph) chromosome. This, the first association of a malignant disease with a chromosomal marker, focused attention on the Ph chromosome as a means to understand the molecular basis of CML. In the 1980s the fusion partners of the chromosomal translocation were identified as the c-*abl* oncogene on chromosome 9 and the breakpoint cluster region (BCR) on chromosome 22 (2,3). The BCR/ABL gene product was found to have tyrosine kinase activity (4,5), and the gene inserted into mouse stem cells induced leukemia in recipient mice (6). Two major advances have been made in CML treatment: (i) allogeneic stem cell transplantation (SCT); CML is readily cured by SCT because it is highly susceptible to a graft-versus-leukemia effect from transplanted donor lymphocytes (7) and (ii) imatinib mesylate (Gleevec), a drug engineered to block the BCR/ABL tyrosine kinase promises to achieve long-term disease control and possibly cure with minimal side effects (8). Despite progress in CML biology and treatment, fundamental questions about its origin remain unanswered. Evidence suggests that a predisposition to develop CML precedes the clonal expansion of BCR/ABL translocated stem cells, and the discovery of very low levels of BCR/ABL in the marrow of normal individuals who do not develop CML raises the possibility that the BCR/ABL translocation is not alone sufficient to cause leukemia (9).

EPIDEMIOLOGY

- Rare: incidence of 1 in 10,000.
- Represents 7% to 15% of all leukemias.
- Occurs at any age, most common in adults.
- Male predominance.
- Worldwide distribution: no sociogeographic preponderance.
- Ionizing radiation is the only known causative factor, leukemia occurs usually within 6 to 8 years of exposure.
- No known genetic factors determine susceptibility to CML.

PATHOPHYSIOLOGY

- Leukemic hematopoiesis originates in a myeloid stem cell: The Ph-positive chromosome is found in all cells of the myeloid lineage (red cell and granulocyte precursors and megakaryocytes) as well as in B cells but not in T cells. The BCR/ABL translocation is thus placed at the stage of an early myeloid/B cell progenitor. The most primitive pluripotent, nonproliferating (CD38 negative, HLA-DR negative) precursors in the CD34 stem cell compartment are BCR/ABL-negative. It is the unregulated proliferation of BCR/ABL translocated stem cells that is responsible for the massive expansion, primarily in granulocyte production, that leads to leucocytosis.

- Clonal dominance: The Ph-positive clone outcompetes normal hematopoiesis. At diagnosis it is common to find a mixed population of Ph-positive and Ph-negative cells in the bone marrow. With time, normal stem cells are progressively replaced by CML stem cells. An explanation for the clonal dominance of CML cells comes from a recent finding that neutrophil elastase enzymatically destroys granulocyte colony-stimulating factor (G-CSF) as well as other hematopoietic growth factors. Elastase production by neutrophils may regulate granulopoiesis by limiting growth factor availability when the neutrophil count (and thus elastase production) is high. In CML the production of elastase in large amounts by the expanded granulocyte compartment, together with the relative insensitivity of CML hematopoiesis to growth factors, allows CML cells to continue proliferating while growth of normal factor-dependent hematopoietic cells is prevented.
- Relationship of CML behavior to BCR/ABL translocation (10): The BCR/ABL fusion gene phosphorylates intermediate molecules in three important pathways, affecting proliferation through *ras* gene activation, maturation through statin activation, and cell adhesion via Crkl gene products. Alterations in these three pathways are sufficient to cause the leukemic phenotype.
- Clonal instability: CML is characterized by progression to a refractory acute leukemia. CML usually starts as a relatively benign disorder that changes into an accelerated phase where the leukemia is more difficult to control and additional chromosomal abnormalities appear, followed by a progressive increase in blast cells in blood and marrow, termed the blastic phase or blast crisis when the disease transforms to an acute myeloid or B lymphocytic leukemia. Clonal evolution, which is matched by increasing malignant behavior of the leukemia, has a variable pace but is inevitable.

PRESENTATION

- Classic presentation: insidious history of increasing fatigue, lassitude, weight loss, night sweats, massive splenomegaly and gout. Some patients have leucocyte counts greater than 300,000 per cubic millimeter and experience symptoms of leucostasis with headache, focal neurologic deficits, and priapism.
- Typical presentation in the developed world: overt symptoms and signs are rarely encountered because the diagnosis is made earlier. Commonly, patients present with symptoms of fatigue, with or without moderate weight loss, abdominal discomfort and early satiety from an enlarged spleen, or simply with the chance observation of an elevated leucocyte count. CML should be considered in the differential diagnosis of a patient at any age presenting with splenomegaly and with white blood cell count.
- Rare presentations: include chloroma, petechiae, and bruising. These features suggest progression of CML to an accelerated or blastic phase.
- Note: Unlike other leukemias, CML seldom if ever presents with bacterial or fungal infection because neutrophil function is preserved.

DIAGNOSIS

While blood and bone marrow examination share features with other myeloproliferative disorders, the typical presentation with high leucocyte count, hypercellular marrow and basophilia is diagnostic of CML. Chromosome and molecular analysis are used to confirm the presence of a BCR/ABL translocation.

- Blood count: the leucocyte count varies between being slightly elevated to over 200,000 per cubic millimeter. Leucocyte counts as high as 700,000 per cubic millimeter can occasionally be encountered. The platelet count is normal or elevated and there is often a mild normochromic normocytic anemia.

- Blood film: of great diagnostic value, because many of the typical features of CML are unique: there is a left shift with circulating myeloblasts, myelocytes, metamyelocytes, and band forms. The hallmark of CML is *basophilia* with basophil counts often exceeding 1,000 per cubic millimeter. Sustained basophilia is almost never encountered outside CML and some cases of mastocytosis. Eosinophilia and occasional nucleated red blood cells are also common findings. Platelet morphology is usually normal but giant forms can be seen.
- Bone marrow aspirate and biopsy: the aspirate shows cellular spicules and the biopsy is hypercellular with almost complete effacement of the fat spaces. There is granulocytic hyperplasia of the neutrophil eosinophil and basophil series. Megakaryocytes are normal or increased and may show reduced numbers of nuclei. Sea-blue histiocytes are commonly seen in CML marrow. Fibrosis of the marrow is a feature of accelerated phase CML, as is an increase in blasts over 15%. Patients presenting in blastic phase have more than 20% blasts.
- Chromosome analysis: the typical karyotype of CML shows the t(9:22) in the majority of metaphases. Variants include three-way translocations between chromosomes 9, 22 and 11, or 19. An additional chromosome abnormality or Ph chromosomes duplication indicates disease progression to an accelerated or blastic phase. The fluorescent in situ hybridization (FISH) technique is a rapid way of detecting the Ph chromosome directly in blood or marrow since it does not rely on dividing cells (Fig. 13-1).)
- Molecular diagnosis: more than 95% of patients presenting with the clinical and morpho-logic features of CML picture will have Ph chromosomes in the marrow. Of the 5% who are Ph-negative, half have a cryptic BCR/ABL transcript detected by Southern blot or by polymerase chain reaction (PCR) (Fig.13-2). Remaining patients are described as atypical Ph-negative CML. A few such patients are morphologically indistinguishable from Ph-positive CML but most have atypical features on careful examination and are considered to have a form of myelodysplastic syndrome or a neutrophilic leukemia. Molecular analysis provides further information of the precise transcript. Depending on the BCR breakpoint, four variants (b2a2, b3a2, e1a2, e1a3) and are possible. No

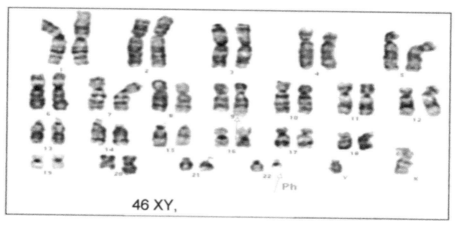

FIG. 13-1. The Philadelphia chromosome. G-banded metaphase preparation showing the diminutive Ph-positive chromosome and extra chromosomal material on the long arm of chromosome 9.

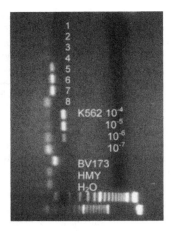

FIG. 13-2. Polymerase chain reaction for BCR/ABL. Patients 1, 2, 3, 4, and 8: negative for BCR/ABL at a sensitivity of less than 10^6 copies. Patients 5, 6, 7 BCR/ABL–positive (b2a2 transloca-tion) *Positive control* K562 cell line (b3a2) and BV173 cell line (b2a2). *Negative control* HMY cell line and H_2O.

prognostic or diagnostic significance is attached to having either the commoner b2a2 or the b3a2 variant. The e1a2 transcript occurs with Ph-positive acute lymphoblastic leukemia and the e1a3 form characterizes a rare relatively benign chronic neutrophilic leukemia.
• Other features: the neutrophil alkaline phosphatase (NAP) stain is typically low or absent in CML. This is believed to be a consequence of low levels of G-CSF. Serum elastase levels, lactic dehydrogenase, and vitamin B_{12} are elevated.

DIFFERENTIAL DIAGNOSIS

The diagnosis of CML is reached in three stages (Fig. 13-3):

• Persisting leucocytosis without any obvious infective cause suggests a myeloproliferative disease prompting further examination of the blood and bone marrow.
• Morphology and blood count will show either typical features of CML (basophilia being especially significant) or suggest other myeloproliferative disorders (high platelet counts, essential thrombocythemia; high red cell count, polycythemia vera; teardrop red cells, my-elofibrosis). The presence of dysplasia suggests a hyperproliferative myelodysplastic syn-drome.
• Definitive diagnosis requires chromosome analysis. This will identify the Ph-positive chro-mosome and the BCR/ABL translocation in all but a small percentage of patients with a morphological diagnosis of CML. Chromosome analysis is also useful in detecting the rare forms of Ph-positive leukemia with an e1a3 translocation and a morphologically atypical CML (11).

COURSE OF CHRONIC MYELOGENOUS LEUKEMIA

CML is a polyphasic disease which progresses from its chronic phase (CP) to an accelerated phase (AP) and then to a blastic phase (BP) (Fig. 3-4).

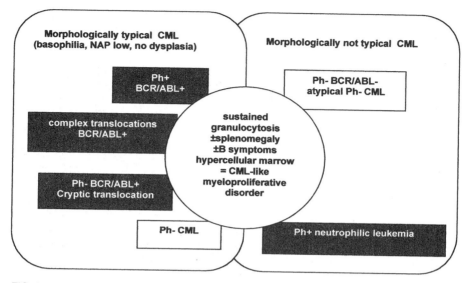

FIG. 13-3. Differential diagnosis of chronic myelogenous leukemia (CML) and related disorders.

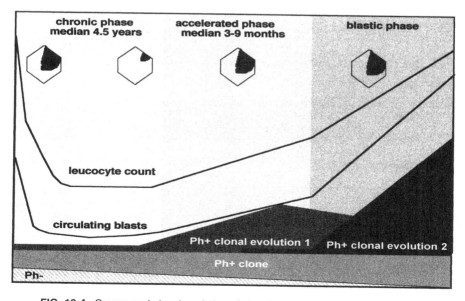

FIG. 13-4. Course and clonal evolution of chronic myelogenous leukemia (CML).

CHRONIC PHASE

- Untreated patients in CP show a gradual rise in the leucocyte count with emergence of splenomegaly and ultimately the full picture of a myeloproliferative disorder with B symptoms, weight loss, and hyperleucocytosis.
- Duration of the CP is highly variable: some patients can progress within months of diagnosis directly to AP and BP, while others remain for more than a decade in a stable CP. Sometimes patients present in AP or BP without any clear preceding CP. In the latter case it is important to distinguish CML presenting as acute leukemia from de novo (Ph-negative) acute leukemia since the treatment approaches are distinct.
- Median time to progression from CP to AP has been slowly increasing, in part because of better treatment and in part because the diagnosis of CML tends to be made earlier. Recent estimates of a median time to progression of 4 to 5 years do not reflect the likely further prolongation of time to progression in the imatinib era.

ACCELERATED PHASE

AP is characterized by one or more of the following (Table 13-1):

- Clonal evolution by a further mutation. Patients may acquire new chromosomal abnormalities such as a second Ph chromosome.
- Escape of the blood counts from treatment control.
- Organomegaly.
- Leucocytosis, basophilia, thrombocytosis, or thrombocytopenia in a patient previously well controlled with therapy.
- Myelofibrosis with teardrop cells in the blood smear and increased marrow reticulin.
- Chloromas in external soft tissues, the retroperitoneal spaces, paraspinal areas (leading to nerve root compression) and in intramedullary spaces.

BLASTIC PHASE

- Signs and symptoms of acute leukemia: bone pains, weight loss, and B symptoms, increasing numbers of blasts in the blood and marrow.
- Marrow failure: decreasing red cell count and platelets. (Neutrophil counts are better conserved.)
- Clonal evolution: further chromosomal abnormalities.

TABLE 13–1. *Characteristics distinguishing chronic myelogenous leukemia at different stages of evolution*

	CP	AP	BP
Blasts in blood	<15%	>15%–30%	>30%
Blasts in marrow	<20%	>20%–50%	>50%
Basophils	<20%	>20%	
Karyotype	Ph+	Second Ph+	7q-, t(15;17), other
NAP score	low	Low	normal
Marrow fibrosis		+	+
Escape from control		+	+
Cytopenias			+

CP, chronic phase; AP, acute phase; BP, blastic phase.

CHARACTERIZATION OF THE ACUTE LEUKEMIA IN BLASTIC PHASE

Approximately 60% of patients develop acute myeloid leukemia (AML); the remainder has acute lymphoblastic leukemia (ALL). In both phenotypes, blasts are poorly differentiated. Auer rods are not seen and the lymphoid or myeloid origin of the leukemia is only reliably determined by cytochemical stains and surface phenotype revealing either a pre-B ALL (PAS block-positive, TdT-positive, $CD10^+$, $CD19^+$, $CD33^\pm$, $CD34^\pm$) or an undifferentiated AML (peroxidase weak-positive, $CD33^+$, $CD34^+$, $CD13^\pm$). A peculiar feature of CML is the variability of its subsequent evolution. Patients achieving remission from AML can reenter a chronic phase only to relapse again with ALL or vice versa.

PROGNOSTIC FACTORS

Poor prognosis (tendency to rapid progression to BP):

- High leucocyte counts (>100,000 per cubic millimeter)
- Massive splenomegaly and constitutional symptoms
- Patients of African origin
- Patients with high basophil counts

Several predictive scores have been used to determine duration of CP (12). However, they were all validated in the era when patients received interferon treatment and may not be applicable for patients receiving imatinib.

TREATMENT OF CHRONIC MYELOGENOUS LEUKEMIA

Treatment of CML involves diverse approaches listed in Table 13-2. The drugs commonly used to treat CML are detailed in Box 1.

CML treatment is guided by disease monitoring using regular blood counts and bone marrow examination to document hematologic changes, chromosome analysis of marrow or FISH anaylsis of blood or marrow to detect response or progression at the karyotypic level and PCR for BCR/ABL monitoring of the blood to quantitate response at the molecular level. The degree of disease bulk reduction determines the appropriate monitoring approach. This approach is used to define the degree of response as hematological

TABLE 13–2. *Treatment modalities in chronic myelogenous leukemia*

Chemotherapy for cytoreduction in CP and AP
    Hydroxyurea
    Other agents: cytosine arabinoside, busulfan, anthracyclines
Chemotherapy to induce remission in BP
    Combination chemotherapy as used in *de novo* ALL or AML
Nonchemotherapy agents
    Interferon-α
    Imatinib mesylate (Gleevec, STI-571)
Bone marrow stem cell transplantation
    Standard myeloablative allogeneic
    Reduced intensity allogeneic
    Autologous

CP, chronic phase; AP, acute phase; BP, blastic phase; ALL, acute lymphoblastic leukemia; AML, acute myelogenous leukemia.

Box 13–1. *Agents Commonly Used to Treat Chronic Myelogenous Leukemia*

Hydroxyurea (Hydrea)

Action: Blocks cell proliferation in S phase. Used to control leukocyte count. Achieves rapid responses but is required daily to control counts.
Formulation: Tablets, 500 mg.
Dose: 500–2000 mg daily.
Cost: $
Side effects: Leukopenia, thrombocytopenia, anemia, occasionally nausea, rarely skin rash, fluid retention.

Busulfan (Myleran)

Action: Alkylating agent, kills noncycling and cycling hematopoietic stem cells. Used to control leukocyte counts. Responses less rapid but more sustained than hydroxyurea. Largely outmoded for chronic myelogenous leukemia (CML) treatment except as a conditioning agent for stem cell transplantation.
Formulation: Tablets/capsules: 2 mg, 50 mg; intravenous: 50-mg vials.
Dose: Oral, 2 mg daily until counts are controlled or single-dose intermittent treatment 50 to 100 mg every 4 to 8 weeks depending on response
For transplant conditioning: intravenous busulfan, twice daily in divided doses over 2 to 4 days to a total of 6.4 to 12.8 mg/kg.
Cost $
Side effects (dose and schedule-related): Prolonged cytopenia, pulmonary fibrosis, skin pigmentation, hair loss, infertility.

Cytosine arabinoside (Cytosar)

Action: Kills dividing cells in S phase. Has been used as an adjunct to interferon or imatinib or an alternative to hydroxyurea. Used in combination with anthracyclines to treat blastic phase (BP).
Formulation: Subcutaneous or intravenous use, 100 to 1000 mg.
Typical dose: 100 mg subcutaneously daily for 5 days.
Cost: $$
Side effects: Cytopenia, nausea, diarrhea, but uncommon with low doses used in CML.

Imatinib mesylate (Gleevec)

Action: Blocks ATP phosphorylation at the SH2 domain of the ABL gene. Inhibits downstream activation by BCR/ABL gene in CML. The agent of choice to achieve minimal residual disease (MRD) and prolongation of chronic phase (CP). Effective at all stages of CML but resistance develops with increasing rapidity and frequency the later into the disease the agent is introduced.
Formulation: Capsules, 100 mg, 400 mg
Dose: 300 to 800 mg daily
Cost: $$$$
Side effects: Dose-related fluid retention, limb pains, nausea, gastritis.

Interferon-a (Roferon)

Action: Antiproliferative, normalizes stem cell contact interactions. Used to achieve MRD state in CP CML. Largely outmoded by imatinib, which is more effective and better tolerated. Can be used in patients intolerant to imatinib, or in conjunction with other agents to control progressing disease.
Formulation: 1–5 million units vials for subcutaneous injection
Typical dose: 3–6 million units 2–5 × weekly depending on tolerance
Cost $$$$
Side effects: (often limiting) fevers, flu-like symptoms, mental slowing, depression, baldness, impotence, wasting, worse during first few weeks.

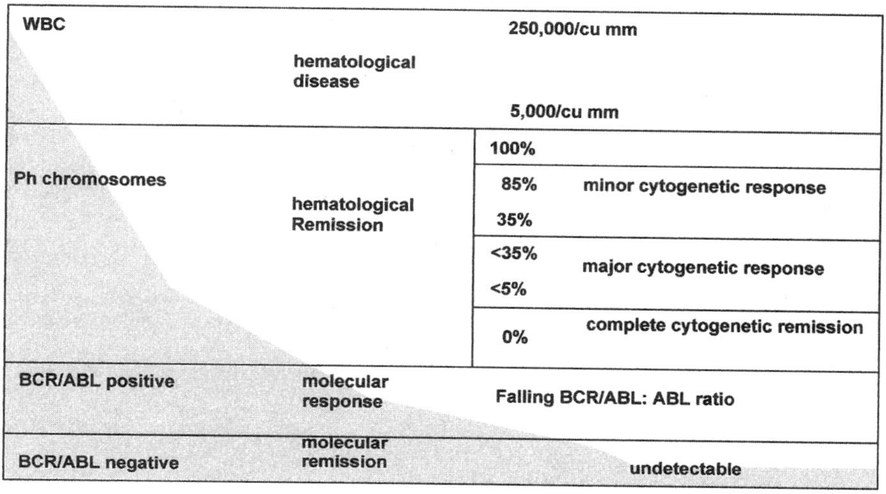

WBC		250,000/cu mm	
	hematological disease		
		5,000/cu mm	
Ph chromosomes		100%	
	hematological Remission	85%	minor cytogenetic response
		35%	
		<35%	major cytogenetic response
		<5%	
		0%	complete cytogenetic remission
BCR/ABL positive	molecular response	Falling BCR/ABL: ABL ratio	
BCR/ABL negative	molecular remission	undetectable	

FIG. 13-5. Disease monitoring in chronic myelogenous leukemia (CML)/

remission, minor karyotypic response, major karyotypic response and molecular response or molecular cure (Fig. 13-5) (13).

TREATING NEWLY DIAGNOSED CHRONIC MYELOGENOUS LEUKEMIA

Initial treatment is aimed at reducing disease bulk and obtaining hematological remission (i.e., a normalization of blood counts).

- Imatinib, 400 to 800 mg daily.
- Add hydroxyurea 1 to 2 g daily for patients with leucocyte counts over 100,000 per cubic millimeter or with massive splenomegaly.
- Allopurinol, 300 mg daily until blood counts normalize.

ACHIEVING MINIMAL RESIDUAL DISEASE

- Give imatinib, 800 mg daily or at the maximum tolerated dose.
- Continue for at least 2 years, possibly indefinitely.
- Stop if disease progresses on maximum dose treatment.

With this regimen, 95% of patients achieve a complete karyotypic response and 90% have a 3 log reduction in BCR/ABL. Because experience with imatinib is still recent, it is not yet known whether this minimal residual disease (MRD) status will translate into prolonged survival and ultimately a molecular cure of CML. However there is reasonable optimism that early treatment with higher doses of imatinib may arrest the clonal evolution that normally precedes disease progression, and permanently freeze the disease process in a MRD state. An unanswered question at present is how long to continue imatinib and at what dose.

INCOMPLETE RESPONSE OR LOSS OF RESPONSE TO IMATINIB TREATMENT

- A bone marrow at 6 and 12 months is required to assess karyotypic response. The degree of response has prognostic value. Only patients who have a complete or good partial response are likely to have a prolonged period without disease progression (see definitions in Fig. 13-5).

- Patients who respond but then progress may have developed resistance to imatinib and may still respond to higher doses of imatinib.
- Failure to achieve a hematologic remission with a combination of imatinib and hydroxyurea is uncommon unless the disease has already progressed to an accelerated phase.
- Where stable MRD is not achieved or disease progression not responding to higher doses of imatinib is encountered other treatment is indicated to prevent disease progression.
- Patients who have not achieved a good karyotypic response, or who have progressed after an initial response should be offered an allogeneic SCT from a human leukocyte antigen (HLA)-identical sibling or a well-matched unrelated donor.
- For patients unsuitable for SCT or without a matched donor, cytosine arabinoside (ARA-C) and interferon-α (IFN-α) have been used to improve the degree of response and trials combining imatinib with ARA-C or IFN-α demonstrate some benefit.
- Experimental approaches with autologous SCT, peptide vaccines and combinations of G-CSF with chemotherapy are being evaluated.

ALLOGENEIC STEM CELL TRANSPLANTATION: TREATMENT WITH CURATIVE INTENT

- SCT from an HLA-matched sibling in CP within a year of diagnosis, achieve long-term disease control and survival of 70% or more and approximately 60% for patients with CP who undergo transplantation more than a year from diagnosis (14). Age has a major impact on outcome, results being especially favorable for the minority pediatric CML population, while patients older than 40 years of age have a lower disease-free survival. Disease stage is the other major variable affecting transplantation success. Both transplant-related mortality (TRM) and relapse are higher in transplants for AP and BP (Fig. 13-6). However, patients who achieve a second CP have a better chance of disease-free survival (DFS). Most reported results analyze survival in the first 5 years. However, longer term follow-up indicates that late relapses and deaths from chronic graft-versus-host disease (GVHD) continue to

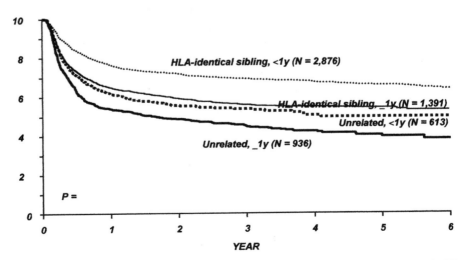

FIG. 13-6. A. Probability of survival for CML in CP by donor type and time from diagnosis (IBMTR data 1994–1999).

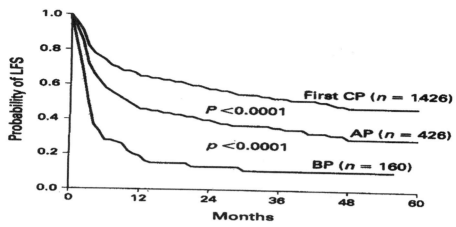

FIG. 13-6. B. Probability of leukemia-free survival showing the impact of disease state on transplant outcome for 2012 patients with chronic myelogenous leukemia (CML) receiving human leukocyte antigen (HLA)-identical sibling transplants reported to the IBMTR in the 1980s.

occasionally cause late mortality many years after transplant. In evaluating outcome after transplant for CML, measuring DFS underestimates the final cure rate because donor lymphocyte infusions can cure relapsed disease. With these provisos, it appears that in the long-term, allogeneic SCT from a matched sibling provides a cure in approximately 65% of individuals in CML CP.

- Unrelated donor transplants. There is now a large experience in transplants for CML using unrelated volunteer donors. Age, timing of transplant (early or late CP, more advanced disease) and degree of matching strongly affect success of the transplant. For low-risk patients (defined as patients younger than 40 years, in first CP, less than 1 year from diagnosis and with an HLA-matched unrelated donor) a DFS of approximately 60% can be achieved; poorer results can be anticipated from patients with less favorable presentations. However, reduced intensity transplants have improved the outlook for older patients. Thus, it is not inappropriate to offer lower intensity SCT to patients with CML up to the age of 70 if they have no significant comorbidities.
- Autologous SCT: It is possible to mobilize a high percentage of normal CD34 cells into the blood of patients with CML with a combination of chemotherapy and G-CSF. High-dose chemotherapy followed by autologous transplantation can produce prolonged periods of hematologic and cytogenetic remission but does not appear to be curative. Autologous transplantation is not generally used to treat CML and should be regarded as experimental treatment.
- Selecting patients for allogeneic transplantation: Gratwohl et al. (15) described a simple scoring system to predict the chance of a successful transplant outcome (Box 2). While it is possible to predict patients with CML who have a favorable outcome, the place of SCT as an elective procedure is constantly under review given the apparent success of imatinib. While imatinib treatment does not usually result in undetectable residual disease it is not known whether it is necessary to achieve the level of molecular cure seen after SCT to provide long-term survival without disease progression. It is argued that because SCT has a definite curative potential and a particularly low morbidity and mortality in young patients it is appropriate to consider elective transplantation in early chronic phase at least for patients under the age of 30 in whom long-term survival over many decades is only known to be

BOX 13–2. *Gratwohl score for predicting outcome after bone marrow transplantation*

Score	0	1	2	3	4	5	6
Survival at 5 years %	72	70	62	48	40	18	22
Transplant-related mortality%	20	23	31	46	51	71	73

Score	0	1	2
Donor type	HLA-identical sibling	matched unrelated	–
Disease stage	First CP	AP	BP, CP2+
Recipient age	<20 yr	20–40 yr,	>40 yr
Donor/recipient gender	M/M, F/F, M/F	F/M	–
Diagnosis-to-transplantation	<12 months	12 months	–

achieved with the transplant. For other patients it seems appropriate to use imatinib as first-line treatment and reserve SCT for patients who fail to respond, progress, or present with CML beyond CP.

- Treatment of accelerated phase: Patients with CML AP may still respond hematologically to increased doses of their current treatment with hydrea or imatinib. Alternatively interferon or chemotherapy with cytosine arabinoside can achieve disease control either as a substitution or as an addition to current therapy. The only chance of prolonged survival for CML AP is with an allogeneic SCT. Patients with an HLA-identical or nonidentical donor should be offered allogeneic SCT. Experimental treatment approaches include SCT from a mismatched-related donor and high-dose chemotherapy or radiation followed by autologous SCT.
- Treatment of blastic phase: The first step in managing CML BP is to determine whether the leukemia has developed into ALL or AML. Patients who have not already developed resistance to imatinib should be treated immediately with 800 mg daily. Many patients treated *de novo* with imatinib will have a complete or at least a partial response. Imatinib-refractory patients and those with rapidly progressing leukemia require induction chemotherapy with standard regimens: daunorubicin 45 mg/m^2 day 1 and 2, vincristine 2 mg/m^2 weekly, prednisolone 60 mg/m^2 daily for 3 weeks for ALL, and combinations of daunorubicin 50 mg/m^2 daily for 2 to 3 days with cytosine arabinoside 200 mg/m^2 daily for 5 to 7 days for patients with AML. Patients usually respond to initial chemotherapy but relapse rapidly. Another problem is sensitivity to remission induction therapy with prolonged cytopenia after successful eradication of blasts. For this reason moderate intensity remission induction chemotherapy is often used (e.g., "2 + 5" for AML, and avoidance of high-dose cytosine arabinoside regimens such as hyper-CVAD [cyclophosphamide, vincristine doxorubicin, dexamethasone] for patients with ALL). Patients achieving a remission may enter a second CP, or less commonly have a brief Ph-negative phase of normal hematopoiesis. Patients who are Ph-negative or in a second chronic phase have a relatively favorable outcome with an allogeneic stem cell transplant, which although considered salvage therapy, offers the only chance of cure. Patients who do not have a stem cell transplant relapse rapidly. Sometimes further remissions can be induced, especially when the relapse occurs in the alternate lineage.

SPECIAL PROBLEMS IN CHRONIC MYELOGENOUS LEUKEMIA MANAGEMENT

- Treatment of relapse after transplantation. Durable molecular remissions after donor lymphocyte infusion (DLI) are achieved between 3 and 12 months after DLI in up to 80% of patients relapsing in CP and more than 90% of molecular relapses. Predictably, the occurrence of GVHD results in a much higher probability of leukemic response and the antileukemic effect of DLI is greatest in the absence of immunosuppression. While DLI is often effective, it may cause bone marrow failure and lethal GVHD. Bone marrow failure is a greater risk in patients with no detectable residual donor marrow cells at relapse. Marrow aplasia in these patients can prevented or treated by infusing more donor stem cells. Despite concerns that DLI in the setting of unrelated donor transplants would result in excessive toxicity, results show response and durable remission rates similar to those seen after the use of matched sibling DLI. While GVHD remains a hazard it does not appear to be more frequent or more severe than that encountered after matched-sibling DLI.

- Leucostasis is an uncommon problem in CML and only occurs in a minority of patients with high leucocyte counts (over 300,000 per cubic millimeter). In patients with priapism or neurologic deficit emergency leukapheresis can be effective but may require several large-volume apheresis sessions to lower the leucocyte count significantly. At presentation such patients should receive high-dose hydroxyurea (up to 4 g daily) or cytosine arabinoside 1 g/m^2 daily for 2 to 3 days with allopurinol 300 mg daily, adequate hydration, and monitoring of blood chemistry. Imatinib may be started once control of the leucocyte count has been achieved.
- Splenic infarcts occur mostly when the disease in uncontrolled. Treatment is symptomatic, while attempts to lower the blood count are made. Splenectomy is not usually indicated.
- Myelofibrosis causing significant cytopenias can be treated by splenectomy but this maneuver is frequently followed by increasing symptomatic hepatomegaly. Myelofibrosis diminishes after successful allogeneic stem cell transplantation and is not a contraindication for SCT.
- Chloromas often respond poorly to chemotherapy and are best treated with local radiotherapy.
- Psychological responses of patients with CML to their disease. Patients presenting with CML are often asymptomatic and may have difficulty accepting that they have a potentially lethal disease. It is perhaps because of this that some CML patients explore alternative treatments and attempt psychosomatic techniques to control their leukemia. The complexity of disease evolution and the dilemmas of treatment in CML make it essential to educate patients about their leukemia, in order to provide them an informed basis for making treatment decisions.

REFERENCES

1. Nowell PC, Hungerford DA. Chromosome studies in human leukemia. II. Chronic granulocytic leukemia. *J Natl Cancer Inst* 1961;27:1013–1035.
2. Lindgren V, Rowley JD. Comparable complex rearrangements involving 8;21 and 9;22 translocations in leukaemia. *Nature* 1977;266:744–745.
3. Heisterkamp N, Stephenson JR, Groffen J, et al. Localization of the c-abl oncogene adjacent to a translocation break point in chronic myelocytic leukaemia. *Nature* 1983;306:239–242.
4. Konopka JB, Watanabe SM, Singer JW, et al. Cell lines and clinical isolates derived from Ph1-positive chronic myelogenous leukemia patients express c-abl proteins with a common structural alteration. *Proc Natl Acad Sci USA* 1985;82:1810–1814.
5. Stam K, Heisterkamp N, Grosveld G, et al. Evidence of a new chimeric bcr/c-abl mRNA in patients with chronic myelocytic leukemia and the Philadelphia chromosome. *N Engl J Med* 1985;313:1429–1433.
6. Daley GQ, Van Etten RA, Baltimore D. Induction of chronic myelogenous leukemia in mice by the P210bcr/abl gene of the Philadelphia chromosome. *Science* 1990;247:824–830.
7. Kolb HJ, Mittermuller J, Clemm C, et al. Donor leukocyte transfusions for treatment of recurrent chronic myelogenous leukemia in marrow transplant patients. *Blood* 1990;76:2462–2465.
8. Druker BJ, Talpaz M, Resta DJ, et al. Efficacy and safety of a specific inhibitor of the BCR-ABL tyrosine kinase in chronic myeloid leukemia. *N Engl J Med* 2001;344:1031–1037.

9. Biernaux C, Loos M, Sels A, et al. Detection of major bcr-abl gene expression at a very low level in blood cells of some healthy individuals. *Blood* 1995;86:3118–3122.
10. Deininger MWN, Goldman JM, Melo JV. The molecular biology of chronic myeloid leukemia. *Blood* 2000;96:3343–3356.
11. Al-Ali HK, Leiblein S, Kovacs I, et al. CML with an e1a3 BCR-ABL fusion: rare, benign, and a potential diagnostic pitfall. *Blood* 2002;100:1092–1093.
12. Hasford J, Pfirrmann M, Hehlmann R, et al. Prognosis and prognostic factors for patients with chronic myeloid leukemia: nontransplant therapy. *Semin Hematol* 2003;40:4–12.
13. Goldman JM, Melo JV. Chronic myeloid leukemia—advances in biology and new approaches to treatment. *N Engl J Med* 2003;349:1451–1464.
14. Barrett J. Allogeneic stem cell transplantation for chronic myeloid leukemia. *Semin Hematol* 2003; 40:59–71.
15. Gratwohl A, Hermans J, Goldman JM, et al. Risk assessment for patients with chronic myeloid leukaemia before allogeneic blood or marrow transplantation. Chronic Leukemia Working Party of the European Group for Blood and Marrow Transplantation. *Lancet* 1998;352:1087–1092.

14

Chronic Lymphocytic Leukemia

Salah Abbasi and Bruce D. Cheson

Chronic lymphocytic leukemia (CLL) is the most common leukemia in adults in the United States and most of Western Europe, where it accounts for approximately 25% of all leukemias.

The estimated number of new CLL cases expected in the United States in 2004 is 7,200, although the incidence of CLL has actually decreased in the recent years.

- Race: In the U.S. population, the incidence of CLL is similar in different races. However, the incidence is much lower in Asia, Latin America, and Africa than in the Western countries (1).
- Age: CLL is extremely rare among persons younger than age 30 but increases steeply beginning in the fifth decade. The median age at diagnosis is 65 to 70 years (1).
- Gender: The male to female ratio is 2:1. However, this trend decreases with age. The male: female ratio is 2.3:1 for patients younger than 50 years old, compared to 1.1:1 for those 75 years of age or older.

ETIOLOGY AND RISK FACTORS

CLL results from the clonal expansion of a subset of the normal B-lymphocyte compartment. This expansion is a consequence of prolonged cell survival, despite a relatively low rate of proliferation.

The etiology of CLL remains unknown. Recent evidence suggests a role for chronic antigenic stimulation. No consistent causal relationship has been found with exposure to radiation, chemicals, or alkylating agents. However, exposure to some chemicals used in agriculture may increase the risk of developing CLL (2); some reports suggest an association with exposure to the defoliant Agent Orange.

Familial Chronic Lymphocytic Leukemia

A family history of CLL or other lymphoproliferative disorders is one of the strongest risk factors for development of CLL, increasing the risk by twofold to sevenfold, with familial anticipation such that the disease tends to occur in younger individuals with subsequent generations. Numbers of CD5$^+$ monoclonal B cells can be identified in 0.5% to 0.8% of normal population, and in 18% of unaffected relatives of CLL patients (3).

Viral Infections

There is no conclusive evidence of a causal relationship exists between CLL and human T-cell leukemia virus (HTLV)-I, HTLV-II, Epstein-Barr virus (EBV), or other known viruses.

CHROMOSOMAL ABNORMALITIES

Acquired cytogenetic abnormalities can be detected in 50% to 80% of all patients with CLL, with a higher yield using fluorescence *in situ* hybridization (FISH). The most frequent abnormality is a deletion in 13q (55%), followed by normal genotype, trisomy 12q, a deletion in 11q, a deletion in 17p, and a deletion in 6q, in the same mentioned order (4).

Genomic aberrations in CLL are important independent predictors of disease progression and survival. Döhner et al. (4) noted that the longest median survival was for patients with an isolated 13q- (133 months) and shortest for patients with 17q- and 11q- (32 and 79 months, respectively).

Immunoglobulin variable heavy chain (IgVH) genes may be either mutated or unmutated and this finding has prognostic importance as discussed below (5).

ONCOGENESIS

In CLL, there is a progressive accumulation of leukemic lymphocytes that have defects in apoptosis and are arrested in the G_0 phase of the cell cycle. Although, no single gene has been implicated in the pathogenesis of CLL, most patients have increased expression of the *bcl-2* gene, which inhibits apoptosis.

DIAGNOSIS OF CHRONIC LYMPHOCYTIC LEUKEMIA

The National Cancer Institute-Working Group (NCI-WG) recommended the following three diagnostic requirements (6):

1. Absolute lymphocytosis in the peripheral blood, with a count of 5×10^6 per liter or more, and cells morphologically mature in appearance, unexplained by other causes.
2. At least 30% lymphocytes in a normocellular or hypercellular bone marrow.
3. A monoclonal B-cell population with lymphocytes that express low levels of surface immunoglobulins, simultaneously with CD5, CD23, CD19, and CD20 positivity.

CLINICAL MANIFESTATIONS

Symptoms

Most patients are asymptomatic at presentation. Disease-related symptoms most often include weakness, fatigue, fever, night sweats, and weight loss. Other findings include bacterial and viral infections and autoimmune anemia and thrombocytopenia. Some patients have symptoms related to enlarged lymph nodes or splenomegaly.

Physical Examination

The most frequent abnormal finding is lymphadenopathy; lymph nodes range from small to massively enlarged. Enlargement of the spleen and the liver when present may range from barely palpable to more than 20 cm below the costal margin.

LABORATORY EVALUATION

- Absolute lymphocytosis: increase in blood of mature appearing lymphocytes, with a lower limit of 5×10^6 per liter.
- Absolute neutrophil count is variable; may be low secondary to extensive bone marrow involvement, or related to autoimmune neutropenia.
- Thirty percent of patients with CLL may have some degree of anemia or thrombocytopenia at presentation, but only 15% have a hemoglobin less than 11 mg/dL or platelets less than 100×10^6 per liter.
- Autoimmune complications: 35% of patients with CLL have a positive Coomb's test; 10% to 25% of these patients have autoimmune hemolytic anemia during the course of the

disease. Immune thrombocytopenia occurs in 15% to 20% of CLL cases. Pure red cell aplasia is observed less frequently.

- Hypogammaglobulinemia is a common finding in CLL, especially in advanced disease. Patients with CLL tend to have defective specific antibody responses to infection and to immunization.
- Bone marrow can be hypercellular or normocellular, but the most characteristic feature is the presence of at least 30% mature lymphocytes.
- No characteristic abnormality of the blood chemistry profile. Lactate dehydrogenase (LDH), β_2-microglobulin, and uric acid may be elevated in advanced disease.

DIFFERENTIAL DIAGNOSIS

The differential diagnosis of CLL includes a spectrum of lymphoid malignancies. The immunophenotypic profile of lymphocytes is the most helpful tool for differentiation as summarized in Table 14-1 (7). B-CLL lymphocytes coexpress CD19 and/or CD20 with CD5. The expression of CD23 on CLL cells differentiates them from mantle cell lymphoma. Expression of surface immunoglobulins is usually weak.

STAGING

Patients with CLL are staged utilizing either the Rai or the Binet system as summarized in Table 14-2 (8). The Rai system is used mainly in North America, while the Binet system is often used in Europe.

Both of these systems discriminate CLL by the sites of disease and/or degree of cytopenias induced by leukemic marrow replacement. Both fail to consider prognostic factors such as age and recently identified genetic or molecular markers.

PROGNOSTIC FACTORS

The clinical course of CLL is variable. Some patients decline rapidly and die within months to a year after diagnosis, whereas others have a very benign indolent disease and live a normal lifespan without major problems from CLL.

Several prognostic features have been identified in patients with poor outcome.

TABLE 14–1. *Immunophenotype of B-cell chronic lymphocytic leukemia and lymphomas that resemble it*

Antigen	B-CLL	Mantle cell lymphoma	SLVL	Follicular lymphoma
sIg	Weak+	+ +	+ +	+ +
CD5	+ +	+ +	−	−
CD19	+ +	+ +	+ +	+ +
CD20	+	+ +	+ +	+ +
CD22	Weak or−	+ +	+ +	+ +
CD23	+ +	−	−	−
CD79b	Weak or−	+ +	+ +	+ +
CD10	−	−	−	+ +

B = CLL, B = cell chronic lymphocytic leukemia; sIg, surface immunoglobulin; SLVL, splenic lymphoma with villous lymphocytes.

TABLE 14–2. *Staging of chronic lymphocytic leukemia*

Rai	Lymphocytosis	Lymph node enlargement	Spleen/liver enlargement	Hemoglobin <11 g/dL	Platelet <100 × 10^9/L	Survival years
0	Yes	No	No	No	No	>13
I	Yes	Yes	No	No	No	8
II	Yes	±	Yes	No	No	6
III	Yes	±	±	Yes*	No	4
IV	Yes	±	±	±	Yes*	2

Binet	Lymphocytosis	Lymph node areas	Hemoglobin <11 g/dL	Platelet <100 × 10^9/L	Survival years
A	N/A	<3	No	No	12
B		≥3	No	No	5
C		±	Yes* (or low plt)	Yes* (or low Hb)	2

* Not autoimmune related.

CLINICAL RISK FACTORS

- Clinical staging. Median survival correlates inversely with the clinical stage: Rai stage 0, 13 + years; stage I, 8 years; stage II, 6 years; stage III, 2 to 6 years; and stage IV, 1.5 to 4 years (9).
- Pattern of bone marrow involvement. Some studies suggest a more rapid rate of disease progression in patients with a diffuse pattern than a nondiffuse pattern of bone marrow involvement. The pattern also correlates closely with the clinical stage.
- Lymphocyte doubling time. Rapid doubling time (less than 12 months) is associated with worse prognosis than a slower doubling time (12 months or longer).

MOLECULAR AND GENETIC RISK FACTORS

- Cytogenetics. Patients with single abnormality of 13q deletion, a normal karyotype, or trisomy 12 have a better prognosis than those with 11q deletion and 17p deletion (4,10).
- CD38 expression. CD38 is a signaling transmembrane glycoprotein expressed on the surface of leukemic cells in 40% to 50% of patients with CLL. CD38 expression identifies a subgroup of CLL with an aggressive clinical presentation and worse outcome.

Patients with unmutated IgVH and positive CD38 cells (more than 30%) respond poorly to chemotherapy (including fludarabine) and have shorter survival than do CD38-negative patients (11).

CD38 expression is associated with atypical morphology, a diffuse bone marrow involvement, Rai stage of 2 or higher, high LDH, high β_2-microglobulin and a higher lymphocyte count (12). CD38$^+$ patients require treatment earlier and more frequently and have higher CLL-related mortality.

- IgVH gene mutation status. The recombination of variable (V), diversity (D), and joining (J) immunoglobulin gene segments and the process of somatic hypermutation physiologically occurs in the germinal center. Somatically mutated variable region heavy chain genes (VH) are present in approximately half of all cases of CLL. Patients with unmutated IgVH genes experience a more aggressive clinical course and shorter survival than patients with mutated IgVH genes. Binet stage A patients without somatic mutations have a projected median survival of 8 years; those with somatic mutations have a projected median survival of 25 years (10,13). High-risk genomic aberrations such as 17p- and 11q- occur more often in the IgVH unmutated subgroup, whereas favorable aberrations such as 13q- are mainly seen in the IgVH-mutated subgroup (10).

• In some studies, high CD38 expression level correlated with the presence of unmutated IgVH genes and an unfavorable clinical outcome, but the relationship between CD38 expression and IgVH mutation status and survival remains unsettled.

• ZAP-70. Identifying IgVH mutation status is costly, time consuming, and unavailable in most laboratories. Investigations using DNA microarray have shown that CLL cells exhibit a characteristic gene expression profile in which a small subset of genes, including ZAP-70, correlates with the mutational status of IgVH genes. ZAP-70 is a member of the Syk/ZAP-70 protein kinase family and can be used as a surrogate marker for IgVH mutations in CLL. Most patients with ZAP-70–positive cells have unmutated IgVH, whereas IgVH mutations are found in most patients with ZAP-70–negative cells. Patients with Binet stage A CLL who had ZAP-70–positive cells (20% or more) had more rapid progression and poorer survival than those with ZAP-70–negative cells (14).

• Other poor prognostic features suggested in some studies include high LDH, high microglobulin level, increased serum-soluble CD25 receptors, and increased serum soluble CD23.

TREATMENT

Early-Stage Disease

Because most patients with early-stage CLL have a good long-term prognosis and prompt intervention with alkylating agents has not changed the outcome of the disease, these patients should not be treated unless specific indications exist (Table 14-3), or in the context of a clinical trial. A meta-analysis of 2,048 early-stage patients randomized between immediate or deferred treatment with chlorambucil demonstrated no benefit from early intervention (15). At present, watchful waiting is still the standard of care for patients with early stage CLL. Meanwhile, prospective clinical trials should evaluate whether any of the newer prognostic factors can be used successfully to guide early treatment of early-stage B-CLL that is destined to be progressive.

Indications for Treatment

The National Cancer Institute (NCI)-sponsored working group on CLL (6) established guidelines for initiation of treatment (Table 14-3).

TABLE 14–3. *Suggested indications for therapy for chronic lymphocytic leukemia*

Disease-related symptoms (e.g., fever, chills, night sweats, weight loss)
Bone marrow involvement with progressive anemia and thrombocytopenia
Progressive or massive splenomegaly
Progressive or bulky lymphadenopathy
Autoimmune hemolytic anemia or thrombocytopenia
Recurrent bacterial infections
Rapidly increasing lymphocytosis

CHOICES OF THERAPEUTIC MODALITIES

Nucleoside Analogues

Fludarabine and cladribine, which are purine analogues resistant to deamination by adenosine deaminase, and pentostatin, which is an adenosine deaminase inhibitor, are often used in CLL.

Three large phase III trials in symptomatic patients with untreated CLL have compared fludarabine (at a dose of 25 mg/m2 intravenously daily for 5 days, repeated every 28 days, for a maximum of 6 cycles) to chlorambucil or other combination therapies such as CAP (cyclophosphamide, doxorubicin, prednisone) or mini-CHOP (cyclophosphamide, doxorubicin, vincristine and prednisone). Fludarabine in general produced a higher response rate and prolongation of progression-free survival, but no significant difference in overall survival (16,17). The use of other purine analogues in the treatment of CLL has been more limited.

Fludarabine Combination Therapies

Multiple phase II trials have combined fludarabine at 30 mg/m^2 intravenously, days 1 to 3, and cyclophosphamide at 250 to 500 mg/m^2 intravenously, days 1 to 3 (FC), in patients with CLL. Cycles were repeated every 28 days. Patients receiving FC at relapse show response rates of 70% to 94%, with 11% to 34% complete remission rates. A phase III study comparing fludarabine with cyclophosphamide versus fludarabine alone in patients with previously untreated CLL showed similar response rates of 92% and 87% and complete response rates of 25% and 12%, respectively. There was also no significant difference in progression-free survival or overall survival. On the other hand, myelosuppression and infections were significantly more frequent in patients receiving combination therapy (18,19).

A small phase II study used a pentostatin and cyclophosphamide combination in patients with refractory or relapsed CLL and showed an overall response rate of 74% and a complete response rate of 17%.

Alkylators

Prior to the introduction of purine analogues, the initial treatment of symptomatic patients primarily involved chlorambucil, given as either 0.1 mg/kg per day, 0.4 to 1.0 mg/kg every 4 weeks, or 20 mg/m^2 every 2 weeks. While chlorambucil is effective in palliating symptoms in most patients, randomized studies in early stage patients indicated few complete responses and failed to demonstrate improved survival, compared to observation alone. Prednisone is often included with chlorambucil despite three randomized trials failing to demonstrate a survival advantage.

Alkylator-Based Combination Chemotherapy

Various chemotherapy combinations have been used in CLL. Randomized studies comparing regimens such as mini-CHOP, CAP, and COP (cyclophosphamide, vincristine, and prednisone) to chlorambucil-based or fludarabine-based regimens in previously untreated CLL did not show any survival superiority for one regimen over another (15).

Monoclonal Antibodies

Alemtuzumab (Campath-1H) is a humanized anti-CD52 antibody. CD52 is expressed on more than 95% of mature B and T lymphocytes. Phase II studies in fludarabine refractory patients showed an overall response rate of more than 30% (20,21). Alemtuzumab was given at a target dose of 30 mg intravenously, 3 times weekly, for a maximum of 12 to 18 weeks.

TABLE 14–4. *Selected clinical trials results with rituximab and fludarabine-based combinations in patients with previously untreated chronic lymphocytic leukemia*

Regimen	No. pts	CR	ORR	MS
Flu + Ritux versus	51	47	90	NR
Flu then Ritux (25)	53	28	77	NR
Flu + Cy + Ritux	60	66	95	NR

Flu, fludarabine; Ritux, rituximab; Cy, cyclophosphamide; CR, complete response; ORR, overall response rate; MS, median survival; NR, not reported.

Infection prophylaxis with bactrim, acyclovir, and fluconazole was initiated on day 8 and continued for a minimum of 2 months after treatment.

Common toxicities include self-limited cytokine release syndrome (fever, rigors, vomiting), immunosuppression with opportunistic infections, occasionally severe, and neutropenia.

Subcutaneously administered alemtuzumab monotherapy at a target dose of 30 mg, 3 times weekly for 18 weeks in patients with untreated CLL induced a 29% complete response and an 87% overall response rate with effective tumor elimination in nodal sites of involvement (22). Subcutaneous administration of alemtuzumab was not associated with infusion-related toxicity, but caused localized skin reactions.

Rituximab is a chimeric anti-CD20 antibody that has limited activity in relapsed or refractory CLL when administered at a dose of 375 mg/m^2 every week for 4 weeks. Response rates of 50% have been reported when used as initial therapy. In two studies, dose escalation or more frequent administration (375 mg/m^2, 3 times weekly for 4 weeks) increased only the partial response rate. Toxicity is minimal (23,24).

Two recent studies combining rituximab with fludarabine-based therapies in previously untreated CLL showed an overall response rate between 90% and 95% (Table 14-4) (25).

Bone Marrow Transplantation

Results of some phase II studies suggest that autologous stem cell transplantation may prolong progression-free survival in patients with CLL and low-risk features. Results may be better when patients undergo transplantation while in complete remission or with minimal residual disease. The role of allogeneic stem cell transplantation in CLL is less defined, except for young patients with high-risk features, because of the high treatment-related mortality. Nonmyeloablative transplant has produced encouraging results with less acute morbidity, but with substantial chronic GVHD. It should be considered in the setting of a clinical trial, particularly for older patients.

CURRENT RECOMMENDATIONS

- The standard first-line therapy for CLL has become a fludarabine-based regimen, either alone, or with rituximibarth or without cyclophosphamide. Fludarabine is administered at a dose of 25 mg/m^2 intravenously each day for 5 days, every 28 days, for a maximum of 6 cycles. Prophylactic use of sulfamethoxazole/trimethoprim during the course of therapy and 2 months after is highly recommended in some patients at risk of immunosuppression.
- Current studies compare the efficacy of fludarabine with or without other agents like cyclophosphamide, rituximab, alemtuzumab, or other new novel therapies. Chlorambucil or combinations such as CHOP or CAP are currently not used unless fludarabine is contraindicated or not feasible.

- Patients who relapse after a long disease-free period (longer than 1 year) may benefit from retreatment with the same regimen. Early relapse or refractory disease cases should be offered participation in a clinical trial, if available. Other options are alemtuzumab or a purine analogue-based combination. Hematopoietic stem cell transplants should not be used outside a research protocol as its role remains controversial.

COMPLICATIONS
Infections

Infections are the most important cause of morbidity and mortality in CLL. Advanced disease, hypogammaglobulinemia, neutropenia, defective complement activation, and immunosuppressive effects of chemotherapy are the main risk factors. The prophylactic use of antibiotics in untreated patients and in the absence of infection is not recommended because of the broad spectrum of infections and the risk of resistance. Replacement therapy with intravenous γ-globulin (250 to 500 mg/kg per month) may provide protection against moderate bacterial infections in high-risk patients (with hypogammaglobulinemia and prolonged immunosuppressive therapy, recurrent bacterial infections, or advanced disease).

Autoimmune Cytopenias

Autoimmune hemolytic anemia can often be treated successfully with prednisone. In cases refractory to prednisone, splenectomy and intravenous immunoglobulins may be beneficial. Recent studies showed rituximab to be effective in refractory cases (26), and the same approach may also serve for autoimmune thrombocytopenia. Pure red cell aplasia is a rare cause of anemia in CLL. Therapy with cyclosporine at a dose of 5 mg/kg per day may be effective.

Transformation
Richter's syndrome

Up to 15% of patients with CLL may transform into a large-cell lymphoma. Richter's syndrome usually presents with sudden onset of B symptoms, progressive lymphadenopathy, and a high serum LDH. The prognosis is poor, and therapy with combination chemotherapy or marrow transplantation generally ineffective.

Prolymphocytic Leukemia

More rarely, CLL may transform into prolymphocytic leukemia (PLL), characterized by an increase in prolymphocytes to higher than 55% on the peripheral blood smear, progression of splenomegaly, and worsening cytopenias. Therapy is generally unsatisfactory. The most active agents are alemtuzumab and nucleoside analogues.

Second Malignancies

Patients with CLL have a higher incidence of second malignancy related to the disease and its treatment. Most common are skin, gastrointestinal, and lung cancer.

REFERENCES

1. Ahmedin J, Taylor M, Alicia S, et al. Cancer Statistics, 2003. *CA Cancer J Clin* 2003;53:5–26.
2. Brown LM, Blair A, Gibson R, et al. Pesticide exposures and other agricultural risk factors for leukemia among men in Iowa and Minnesota. *Cancer Res* 1990;50:6585–6591.

3. Marti GE, Carter P, Abbasi F, et al. BCML and B-cell abnormalities in the setting of familial B-CLL. *Cytometry* 2003;52B:1–12.
4. Döhner H, Stilgenbauer S, Banner A, et al. Genomic aberrations and survival in chronic lymphocytic leukemia. *N Engl J Med* 2000;343:1910–1916.
5. Hamblin TJ, Davis Z, Gardiner A, et al. Unmutated 1gV(H) genes are associated with a more aggressive form of chronic lymphocytic leukemia [see comments]. *Blood* 1999;94:1848–1854.
6. Cheson BD, Bennett JM, Grever M et al. National Cancer Institute-sponsored working group guidelines for chronic lymphocytic leukemia: revised guidelines for diagnosis and treatment. *Blood* 1996; 87:4990–4997.
7. Harris NL, Jaffe ES, Diebold J, et al. World Health Organization classification of neoplastic diseases of the hematopoietic and lymphoid tissues: Report of the Clinical Advisory Committee Meeting—Airlie House, Virginia, November 1997. *J Clin Oncol* 1999;17:3835–3849.
8. Kay NE, Hamblin TJ, Jelinek DF, et al. Chronic lymphocytic leukemia. *Hematology (Am Soc Hematol Educ Program)* 2002;193-213.
9. Rai KR, Switsky A, Cronkite EP et al: Clinical staging of chronic lymphocytic leukemia. *Blood* 1975;46:219.
10. Kröber A, Seiler T, Benner A, et al. V_H mutation status, CD38 expression level, genomic aberrations, and survival in chronic lymphocytic leukemia. *Blood* 2002;100:1410–1416.
11. Damle RN, Wasil T, Fais F, et al. IgV gene mutation status and CD38 expression as novel prognostic indicators in chronic lymphocytic leukemia. *Blood* 1999;94:1840–1847.
12. Domingo-Domenech E, Domingo-Claros A, Gonzalez-Barca E, et al. CD38 expression in B-chronic lymphocytic leukemia: association with clinical presentation and outcome in 155 patients. *Haematologica* 2002;87:1021–1027.
13. Oscier DG, Gardiner AC, Mould SJ, et al. Multivariate analysis of prognostic factors in CLL: Clinical stage, V_H gene mutational status, and loss or mutation of the p53 gene are independent prognostic factors. *Blood* 2002;100:1177–1184.
14. Crespo M, Bosch F, Villamor N, et al. ZAP-70 expression as a surrogate for immunoglobulin-variable-region mutations in chronic lymphocytic leukemia. *N Engl J Med* 2003;348:1764–1775.
15. B-CLL Trialists Collaborative Group. Chemotherapeutic options in chronic lymphocytic leukemia: a meta-analysis of the randomized trials. *J Natl Cancer Inst* 1999;91:861–868.
16. Rai KR, Peterson BL, Appelbaum FR, et al. Fludarabine compared with chloramucil as primary therapy for chronic lymphocytic leukemia. *N Engl J Med* 2000;343:1750–1757.
17. Leporrier M, Chevret S, Cazin B, et al. Randomized comparison of fludarabine, CAP, and CHOP in 938 previously untreated stage B and C chronic lymphocytic leukemia patients. French cooperative Group on Chronic Lymphocytic Leukemia. *Blood* 2001;98:2319–2325.
18. O'Brien SM, Kantarjian HM, Cortes J, et al. Results of the fludarabine and cyclophosphamide combination regimen in chronic lymphocytic leukemia. *J Clin Oncol* 2001;19:1414–1420.
19. Eichhorst BF, Hopfinger G, Hallek M, et al. First-line therapy in patients with advanced CLL with Fludarabine vs fludarabine plus cyclophosphamide: interim analysis of the CLL4 protocol, a cooperative phase III study of the German CLL Study Group (GCLLSG). Poster Presentation, X international Workshop on CLL, Stresa, Italy. October 10–12, 2003.
20. Rai KR, Freter CE, Mercier RJ, et al. Alemtuzumab in previously treated chronic lymphocytic leukemia patients who also had received fludarabine. Long Island Jewish Medical Center. *J Clin Oncol* 2002;20:3891–3897.
21. Keating MJ, Flinn I, Jain V, et al. Therapeutic role of alemtuzumab (Campath-1H) in patients who have failed fludarabine: results of a large international study. *Blood* 2002;99:3554–3561.
22. Lundin J, Kimby E, Bjorkholm M, et al. Phase II trial of subcutaneous anti-CD52 monoclonal antibody Alemtuzumab (Campath-1H) as first-line treatment for patients with B-cell chronic lymphocytic leukemia (B-CLL). *Blood* 2002;100:768–773.
23. O'Brien SM, Kantarjian H, Thomas DA, et al. Rituximab dose-escalation trial in chronic lymphocytic leukemia. *J Clin Oncol* 2001;19:2165–2170.
24. Byrd JC, Murphy T, Howard R, et al. Rituximab using a thrice weekly dosing schedule in B-cell chronic lymphocytic leukemia and small lymphocytic lymphoma demonstrates clinical activity and acceptable toxicity. *J Clin Oncol* 2001;19:2153–2164.
25. Byrd JC, Peterson BL, Morrison VA, et al. Randomized phase 2 study of fludarabine with concurrent versus sequential treatment with Rituximab in symptomatic, untreated patients with B-cell chronic lymphocytic leukemia: results from Cancer and Leukemia Group B 9712 (CALGB 9712). *Blood* 2003;101:6–14.
26. Hegde UP, Wilson WH, White T, et al. Rituximab treatment of refractory fludarabine-associated immune thrombocytopenia in chronic lymphocytic leukemia. *Blood* 2002;100:2260–2262.

15

Hodgkin's Lymphoma

Jame Abraham, Wyndham H. Wilson, and Elaine S. Jaffe

Hodgkin's lymphoma (HL) is a neoplastic disorder of the lymphoid system characterized by the presence of binucleated giant cells, known as Reed-Sternberg (RS) cells. It is one of the few malignancies for which effective therapy has been developed, with more than 75% of patients cured with chemotherapy and/or radiation. The steady decline in mortality resulting from HL is primarily because of excellent results achieved with effective combination chemotherapy.

EPIDEMIOLOGY

HL is among the most common malignancies of young adults (1). It constitutes approximately 1% of all malignancies and 18% of all lymphomas. In 2003, approximately 7,600 patients were diagnosed with HL and 1,300 patients died of HL. In Europe and North America, there is a bimodal age distribution, with an increasing frequency between the second and third decades, and a second peak in the seventh decade.

PATHOLOGIC CLASSIFICATION

WHO/REAL Classifications

Table 15-1 lists the World Health Organization Revised European American Lymphoma classifications, in comparison with older historical schemes (2).

- Classic HL
  - Nodular sclerosis Hodgkin's lymphoma (NSHL)
  - Mixed-cellularity Hodgkin's lymphoma (MCHL).
  - Lymphocyte-depletion Hodgkin's lymphoma (LDHL)
  - Lymphocyte-rich classic Hodgkin's lymphoma (LRCHL)
- Nodular lymphocyte-predominant Hodgkin's lymphoma (NLPHL).

NLPHL is a clinicopathologic entity of B cell phenotype that is distinct from classic HL. The immunophenotypes for classic HL and NLPHL are described in Table 15-2. (3,4)

PATHOLOGY

HL is somewhat unique among the malignant lymphomas in that the RS cells and variants, the malignant cells, constitute the minority of cells present in the tumor mass (Fig. 15-1). The neoplastic cells in classic HL are associated with a rich inflammatory background containing lymphocytes, eosinophils, neutrophils, histiocytes, and plasma cells in varying proportions. While molecular studies in recent years have provided evidence for the B-cell origin of the neoplastic cell in both classic HL and NLPHL, in classic HL the neoplastic cells are "crippled B-cells" that fail to synthesize immunoglobulin (Ig) (5). The failure may be because of

TABLE. 15–1. *Historical evolution of the classification of Hodgkin's lymphomas*

Jackson-Parker	Lukes-Butler	Rye	REAL/WHO
Paragranuloma	L&H, nodular LP	LPHL ⟶	NLPHL
	L&H, diffuse	↘	LRCHL
Granuloma	NS	NS	NS
	MC*	MC*	MC
Sarcoma	LD, diff fibrosis	LD	LD
	LD, reticular		

* Defined as a category of exclusion, not with specific features. L&H, lymphocytic and histiocytic; LP, lymphocyte-predominant; LPHL, lymphocyte-predominant Hodgkin's lymphoma; NLPHL, nodular lymphocyte-predominant Hodgkin's lymphoma; LRCHL, lymphocyte-rich classic Hodgkin's lymphoma; NS, nodular-sclerosis; MC, mixed-cellularity; LD, lymphocyte depletion.

mutations in the Ig genes, or absence of the transcription machinery, manifested by absence of transcription factors OCT-2 and BOB.1 (6).

NSHL requires the presence of (i) a nodular growth pattern, (ii) broad bands of fibrosis, and (iii) a characteristic variant of the RS cell known as a lacunar cell. The lacunar cell has abundant clear cytoplasm with a sharply demarcated cell membrane. In formalin-fixed tissue a characteristic artifact often occurs; the cytoplasm of the cell retracts, leaving a clear space or lacunus. NSHL is graded according to the proportion of neoplastic cells and the presence of necrosis, as well as depletion of normal lymphocytes. Two grades of NSHL are identified in the World Health Organization (WHO) classification (2).

MCHL is characterized by classic RS cells in a rich inflammatory background, fine reticular fibrosis, and an absence of distinct fibrous bands. MCHL is more common in males than females. It is frequently associated with disseminated disease at presentation. B symptoms are also common. It is one of the variants of HL, along with lymphocyte depletion, that is seen in association with human immunodeficiency virus (HIV) infection. MCHL is the subtype most often positive for Epstein-Barr virus (EBV) sequences (2).

LDHL is the rarest form of HL, constituting no more than 5% of cases. Epidemiologically, it is seen in regions of the world of lower socioeconomic status, and is also increased in frequency in HIV-infected individuals. It may be thought of as representing a further evolution of MCHL, with more frequent malignant cells, a depletion of normal lymphocytes, and usually greater fibrosis, which is often diffuse and reticular in nature.

TABLE. 15–2. *Immunophenotypic criteria for the classification of Hodgkin's lymphoma*

Marker	NLPHL	Classic HL
CD30	−	+
CD15	−	+
CD20	+	−/+
EMA	+/−	−
LCA	+	−
BCL-6	+	−
Oct2, BOB.1	+	−(+)

NLPHL, nodular lymphocyte-predominant Hodgkin's lymphoma; HL, Hodgkin's lymphoma.

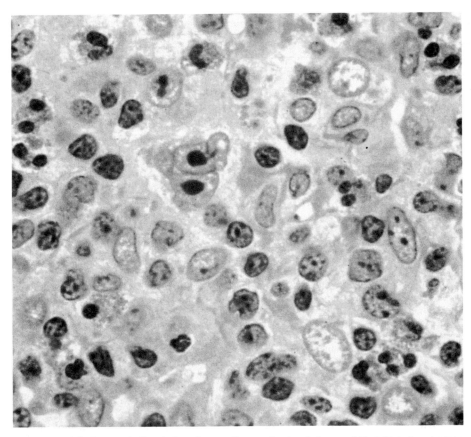

FIG. 15-1. **(A)** Diagnostic Reed–Sternberg cell, seen in classic types of Hodgkin's lymphomas (mixed cellularity, nodular sclerosis, lymphocyte depletion). **(B)** Neoplastic cells in nodular lymphocyte-predominant Hodgkin's lymphomas are termed popcorn cells or L and H cells (lymphocytic or histiocytic predominance). Reed–Sternberg cells of the classic type generally are not seen in a nodular lymphocyte-predominant Hodgkin's lymphoma.

LRCHL is characterized by a cellular milieu rich in normal lymphocytes, and a paucity of malignant cells that have the immunophenotype of classic RS cells. LRCHL may have a diffuse or nodular growth pattern, and especially in its nodular form may be mistaken for nodular lymphocyte predominant HL. It tends to present in older individuals, often with isolated peripheral lymphadenopathy (3,4).

NLPHL differs from classic HL in its immunophenotypic profile, histologic characteristics, and clinical behavior (3,4). Classic RS cells are not seen. The neoplastic cells are referred to as lymphocytic and histiocytic (L&H) cells or popcorn cells. They have a lobulated nuclear contour, dispersed chromatin, and inconspicuous nucleoli. They generally cluster within nodules associated with lymphocytes and histiocytes. Early on the background lymphocytes are predominantly of B-cell phenotype, but T cells may predominate in later stages. The neoplastic cells, the popcorn cells, stain for CD20 and are generally negative for CD15 and negative or weakly positive for CD30.

ETIOLOGY AND RISK FACTORS

EBV has been linked to many cases of classic HL, but is absent in NLPHL (1). EBV is most commonly found in MCHL and LDHL. Infectious mononucleosis appears to be a predisposing risk factor for subsequent EBV-positive HL but not EBV-negative HL (1). NSHL is most common in North America, and is more prevalent among individuals of higher socioeconomic status, whereas MCHL and LDHL are seen in underdeveloped regions of the world. The risk of EBV-positive classic HL is slightly increased in HIV-positive individuals. Familial cases of HL have been reported, and siblings of patients with HL are at slightly increased risk (7). There is a weak association with certain human leukocyte antigen (HLA) types.

CLINICAL FEATURES

- More than 80% of patients have cervical lymph node enlargement, and more than 50% will have mediastinal adenopathy.
- Lymph nodes are usually nontender, firm, and rubbery.
- Constitutional symptoms (B symptoms):
  - Unexplained fever (temperature, higher than 38°C).
  - Drenching night sweats.
  - Unexplained weight loss (more than 10% of body weight, over 6 months before the diagnosis).
- Other symptoms include fatigue, weakness, anorexia, alcohol-induced nodal pain, and pruritus.

Staging (Ann Arbor/AJCC and Cotswold) is outlined in Table 15-3 (8–10).

PRETREATMENT EVALUATION

1. Excisional biopsy of a prominent node is highly recommended to make a proper diagnosis.
2. Detailed history with attention to B symptoms, particularly fever and weight loss.
3. Complete physical examination, including the lymph node examination and evaluation for hepatosplenomegaly.
4. Laboratory tests include:

TABLE. 15–3. *Staging*

Stage I—Involvement of single lymph node region or lymphoid structure (spleen, thymus, Waldeyer's ring), or involvement of a single extralymphatic site (IE)

Stage II—Involvement of two or more lymph node regions on the same side of the diaphragm (II), which may be accompanied by localized contiguous involvement of an extralymphatic organ or site (IIE). The number of anatomic sites may be indicated by numeric subscript

Stage III—Involvement of lymph node regions on both sides of the diaphragm (III), which may also be accompanied by localized involvement of an associated extralymphatic organ or site (IIIE), by involvement of the spleen (IIIS), or both (IIIE+S)

Stage IV—Disseminated involvement of one or more extralymphatic organs, with or without associated lymph node involvement, or isolated extralymphatic organ involvement with distant (nonregional) nodal involvement

---

Each stage is divided into A and B categories: B for those with defined systemic symptoms, and A for those without.

X, A mass >10 cm or a mediastinal mass larger than one-third of the thoracic diameter; E, Involvement of a single extranodal site contiguous to a known nodal site; CS, Clinical staging; PS, Pathologic staging.

- Complete blood count (CBC), erythrocyte sedimentation rate (ESR).
- Biochemical tests of liver function, renal function, and serum uric acid.

   5. Radiologic studies:

- Chest radiograph and computed tomography (CT) scan of the chest, abdomen, and pelvis.
- Positron emission tomography (PET) scans have replaced gallium scans in many centers due to higher specificity and sensitivity. PET scans are optional pretreatment if systemic chemotherapy is used, but may be useful during and after treatment in some cases.
- Bone scan or radiographs if bone pain or tenderness is present.

   6. Bone marrow biopsy of the posterior iliac crest for those with abnormal CBC or clinical stage IIB, III, or IV.

- Staging laparotomy and splenectomy for patients with early-stage disease above the diaphragm is no longer performed to assess occult advanced stage disease because of more accurate radiologic staging and the equivalency of systemic treatment.

PROGNOSTIC FEATURES

Favorable prognostic features include:

1. Sedimentation rate less than 50.
2. Patient 50 years of age or younger.
3. Lymphocyte predominant or nodular sclerosing histology.
4. Absence of B symptoms (primarily fever and loss of weight).
5. Fewer than three sites of involvement.
6. No bulky adenopathy (e.g., involvement of more than one-third of the mediastinum).

The International Prognostic Factors Project on Advanced Hodgkin's lymphoma prognostic score:

1. Albumin level of less than 4.0 g/dL.
2. Hemoglobin level of less than 10.5 g/dL.
3. Male gender.
4. Age of 45 years or older.
5. Stage IV disease.
6. White cell count of at least 15,000 per cubic millimeter.
7. Absolute lymphocytic count of less than 600 per cubic millimeter or a lymphocyte count that was less than 8% of the total white cell count.

The 5-year progression free survival according to the international prognostic factor score are as follows: 0 or no factors, 84%; 1 factor, 77%; 2 factors, 67%; 3 factors, 60%; 4 factors, 51%; and 5 or higher, 42%.

MANAGEMENT OF NEWLY DIAGNOSED HODGKIN'S LYMPHOMA

The goal of therapy for HL is cure. Advances in the systemic treatment of HL have dramatically improved the response rate and survival. This is mainly because of careful staging, understanding of the pattern of spread, and advances in radiation and chemotherapy (10).

In general, the management of HL with radiation therapy consists of treating regions of known disease plus adjacent nodal groups. Radiation therapy is reserved for the early stages of HL without B symptoms (11). Chemotherapy with or without radiation is reserved for the advanced stages and is being used increasingly in patients with early-stage disease as well. Treatment selection is influenced by stage, prognostic factors, and short and longer toxicity.

Radiation Treatment

Because of the availability of effective chemotherapy regimens options, radiation as a single mode of treatment is becoming increasingly less common (10,11). In adult HLs, the appropriate dose of radiation is 2,500 cGy to 3,000 cGy to clinically uninvolved sites, and 3,500 cGy to 4,400 cGy to regions of initial nodal involvement. In advanced-stage adult patients, when combined with chemotherapy, these recommendations are modified with careful treatment technique; the risk of cardiac and pulmonary complications is small.

While considering radiation treatment, it is important to consider long-term complications such as breast cancer in young woman and risk of lung cancer in a patient with history of smoking.

Radiation therapy is delivered to three major fields, known as the mantle, para-aortic, and pelvic or inverted-Y fields. Extended field (EF) radiation refers to the inclusion of adjacent clinically negative nodal sites (Fig. 15-2).

Chemotherapy

Aggressive chemotherapy produces long-term disease-free remissions in advanced HL. The first curative regimen was mechlorethamine, oncovin, procarbazine, and prednisone (MOPP), which resulted in a 70% complete remission in stage III and stage IV patients. Subsequently many regimens have been developed, including MOPP variants, doxorubicin (adriamycin), bleomycin, vinblastine, and dacarbazine (ABVD) and its variants, and hybrids of MOPP and ABVD (12). Chemotherapy is usually administered for two cycles beyond complete response or stable disease, for a minimum of six cycles.

ABVD and MOPP contain different agents. Studies have shown that ABVD is less toxic and more effective than MOPP, with a higher freedom from progression and overall survival. At 10 years, the risk of developing treatment-related leukemia with the MOPP regimen is 2% to 3%, whereas with ABVD it is 0.7% (13).

Recently published data showed that increased-dose BEACOPP regimen for advanced HL (bleomycin, etoposide, doxorubicin, cyclophosphamide, vincristine, procarbazine and prednisone) had an overall 5-year survival of 91% and freedom from treatment failure of 87% (14).

Commonly used regimens are:

1. ABVD: doxorubicin + bleomycin + vinblastine + dacarbazine (15).
2. BEACOPP: bleomycin + etoposide + doxorubicin + cyclophosphamide + vincristine + procarbazine + prednisone.
3. COPP/ABVD: cyclophosphamide + vincristine + procarbazine + prednisone/doxorubicin + bleomycin + vinblastine + dacarbazine.
4. MOPP: mechlorethamine + vincristine + procarbazine + prednisone.
5. MOPP/ABV hybrid: mechlorethamine + vincristine + procarbazine + prednisone/ doxorubicin + bleomycin + vinblastine (16–19).
6. Stanford V: doxorubicin + vinblastine + mechlorethamine + etoposide + vincristine + bleomycin + prednisone. Radiation therapy is added to patients with bulky disease in addition to the Stanford regimen (20).

CHOOSING A REGIMEN

Historically, MOPP was considered the standard treatment for advanced HL. But ABVD is currently the standard treatment in North America. In a randomized study, the Cancer and Leukemia Group B (CALGB) compared leading regimens with an 8-year follow-up (Table 15-4). The results indicate that ABVD alone or MOPP/ABVD was superior to MOPP alone, in terms of remission, freedom from progression, and survival. A randomized study of ABVD versus MOPP-ABV showed equivalency but higher toxicity with MOPP-ABV.

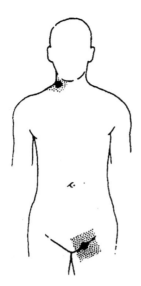

A Involved field irradiation

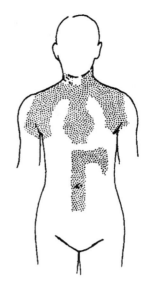

B Subtotal nodal irradiation
including mantle and spade fields

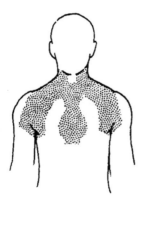

C Mantle field irradiation

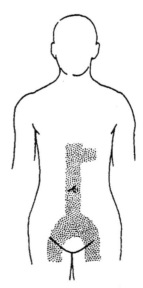

D Inverted-Y field irradiation

FIG. 15-2. Radiation therapy fields used in treating Hodgkin's disease. When the fields shown in (**C**) and (**D**) are combined, this is commonly called total nodal irradiation (TNI). From Haskell CM. *Cancer Treatment.* 4th ed. Philadelphia: WB Saunders, 1995:965.

TABLE. 15–4. *Response and Survival from different regimens (CALGB study and German Lymphoma Group study)*

Regimen	Complete response rate	Survival rate	Follow-up
MOPP	*67%*	*64%*	*8 years*
ABVD	*82%*	*72%*	*8 years*
MOPP/ABVD	*83%*	*73%*	*8 years*
BEACOPP (standard dose)	*88%*	*88%*	*5 years*
BEACOPP (increased dose)	*96%*	*91%*	*5 years*

MOPP, merchlorethamine, oncovin, procarbazine, and prednisone; ABVD, doxorubicin (adriamycin), bleomycin, vinblastin, and dacarbazine; BEACOPP, bleomycin, etoposide, doxorubicin, cyclophosphamide, vineristine, procarbazine; and prednisone.

The 12-week chemotherapy regimen, Stanford V, alone or in combination with irradiation to bulky disease was introduced with objectives maintaining or improving the rate of cure and minimizing the acute and longterm side effects. Stanford V is an abbreviated 12-week course of treatment in which myelosuppresive and nonmyelosuppressive treatments are alternated weekly. Clinical trials are ongoing to compare the efficacy of ABVD versus Stanford V.

A recent German study for patients with advanced-stage HL using COPP/ABVD, BEACOPP, or increased-dose BEACOPP, and consolidative radiation therapy to sites of initial bulky disease (5 cm or larger) showed a 5-year overall survival of 83% for COPP/ABVD, 88% for BEACOPP, and 91% for increased-dose BEACOPP. The actuarial rate of secondary acute leukemias 5 years after diagnosis of HL was 0.4% for COPP/ABVD, 0.6% for BEACOPP, and 2.5% for increased-dose BEACOPP ($p = 0.03$). Although this study suggests that dose intensity improves the survival of HL, this improvement must be balanced against the increased toxicity and risk of leukemia.

Treatment Options

For treatment selection, patients can be divided into two major risk groups:

1. Stages I and II without B symptoms or bulky disease are considered "favorable early stage" and at low risk for recurrence. Cure rate is greater than 90%.
2. Stage IIB and stage I-II B with bulk are variably considered "early" or "advanced" by different study groups. Most U.S. groups treat them as "unfavorable early disease." Cure rate is greater than 80%.
3. Stage III and IV are considered "advanced stage" and are at significant risk for recurrence. Cure rate is approximately 60% to 70%.

Treatment Recommendations

In addition to the information following, Table 15-5 details commonly used treatment regimens.

1. Favorable early disease (21).
   a. ABVD six cycles alone or ABVD two to four cycles with involved-field radiation.
   b. Extended-field radiation alone.

TABLE. 15–5. *Commonly used treatment regimens*

ABVD

Doxorubicin, 25 mg/m^2 per dose IV push for two doses, days 1 and 15 (total dose/cycle, 50 mg/m^2)
Bleomycin, 10 U/m^2 per dose IV push for two doses, days 1 and 15 (total dose/cycle, 20 U/m^2)
Vinblastine, 6 mg/m^2 per dose IV push for two doses, days 1 and 15 (total dose/cycle, 12 mg/m^2)
Dacarbazine, 375 mg/m^2 per dose IV infusion for two doses, days 1 and 15 (total dose/cycle, 750 mg/m^2)
Treatment cycle repeats every 28 days

MOPP

Mechlorethamine, 6 mg/m^2 per dose IV push for two doses, days 1 and 8 (total dose/cycle, 12 mg/m^2)
Vincristine, 1.4 mg/m^2 per dose IV push for two doses, days 1 and 8 (total dose/cycle, 2.8 mg/m^2)
Procarbazine, 100 mg/m^2 per day orally for 14 doses, days 1–14 (total dose/cycle, 1,400 mg/m^2)
Prednisone, 40 mg/m^2 per day orally for 14 doses, days 1–14 (cycles 1 and 14 only) (total dose/cycle, 560 mg/m^2)
Treatment cycle repeats every 28 days

Alternating MOPP/ABVD

Alternate MOPP and ABVD cycles by 28 days

MOPP/ABV hybrid

Mechlorethamine, 6 mg/m^2 IV push day 1 (total dose/cycle, 6 mg/m^2)
Vincristine, 1.4 mg/m^2 IV push day 1 (total dose/cycle, 1.4 mg/m^2; maximal dose, 2 mg)
Procarbazine, 100 mg/m^2 per day orally for 7 doses, days 1–7 (total dose/cycle, 700 mg/m^2)
Prednisone, 40 mg/m^2 per day orally for 14 doses, days 1–14 (total dose/cycle, 560 mg/m^2)
Doxorubicin, 25 mg/m^2 IV push day 8 (total dose/cycle, 25 mg/m^2)
Hydrocortisone, 100 mg IV day 8, before bleomycin (total dose/cycle, 100 mg)
Bleomycin, 10 U/m^2 IV push day 8 (total dose/cycle, 10 U/m^2)
Vinblastine, 6 mg/m^2 IV push day 8 (total dose/cycle, 6 mg/m^2)
Treatment cycle repeats every 28 days

BEACOPP standard dose

Bleomycin 10 mg/m^2 (day 8), etoposide 100 mg/m^2 (days 1–3), doxorubicin 25 mg/m^2 day 1, Cyclophosphamide 650 mg/m^2 (day 1), vincristine 1.4 mg/m^2 (day 8), procarbazine 100 mg/m^2 (day 1–7), and prednisone 40 mg/m^2 (day 1–14)
Regimen was repeated on day 22.
The maximum dose of vincristine is 2 mg

Increased dose BEACOPP

Bleomycin 10 mg/m^2 (day 8), etoposide 200 mg/m^2 (days 1–3), doxorubicin 35 mg/m^2 day 1, Cyclophosphamide 1,200 mg/m^2 (day 1), vincristine 1.4 mg/m^2 (day 8), procarbazine 100 mg/m^2 (day 1–7), and prednisone 40 mg/m^2 (day 1–14)
Regimen was repeated on day 22.
The maximum dose of vincristine is 2 mg

Stanford V

Mustard, 6 mg/m^2 IV week 1, 5, 9
Vincristine, 1.4 mg/m^2 IV week 2, 4, 6, 8, 10, 12 (maximal dose, 2 mg)
Prednisone, 40 mg/m^2 per day orally every other day week 1–9, taper
Doxorubicin, 25 mg/m^2 IV week, 1, 3, 5, 7, 9, 11
Bleomycin, 5 U/m^2 IV week 2, 4, 6, 8, 10, 12
Vinblastine, 6 mg/m^2 IV week, 1, 3, 5, 7, 9, 11
VP-16 60 mg/m^2 IV × 2 week 3, 7, 11
1. The maximum dose of vincristine is 2 mg
2. All drugs are administered on day 1, except for VP-16, which is given on days 1 and 2
3. Taper prednisone by 10 mg of the total dose qod (every other day) on weeks 10 and 11
4. Reduce the dose of vinblastine to 4 mg/m^2 if on weeks 9 and 11 for patients over the age of 50 years old
5. Reduce the dose of vincristine to 1 mg on weeks 10 and 12 for patients over the age of 50 years
6. If mustard is not available, a substitution with 650 mg/m^2 of cyclophosphamide can be made on weeks 1, 5, 9
7. Patients will receive total of 12 weeks of treatment.

IV, intravenous; ABVD, doxorubicin (adriamycin), bleomycin, vinblastin, and dacarbazine; MOPP, merchlorethamine, on-covin, procarbazine, and prednisone; BEACOPP, bleomycin, etoposide, cyclophosphamide, vincristine, procarbazine, and prednisone.

2. Unfavorable early disease
   a. ABVD six to eight cycles alone or ABVD four cycles with involved- or extended-field radiation. One European randomized trial showed no difference in freedom from treatment failure or overall survival when extended field radiation was replaced by involved field radiation (30 Gy to field, 10 Gy to bulk).
   b. Massive mediastinal disease (defined as a mediastinal mass width greater than one-third of the maximum chest diameter or 10 cm mass). Most patients with massive mediastinal disease will receive combined modality therapy. Chemotherapy regimens such as ABVD plus radiation therapy to a mantle or modified mantle field should be considered. Or patients can be considered for clinical trial evaluating ABVD with or without radiation therapy versus Stanford V with or without radiation therapy. Patients with an early and a complete radiographic and PET response may not require radiation consolidation.
3. Advanced disease
   a. ABVD for six to eight cycles is the current standard. Treatment is usually continued two2 cycles after resolution of disease by imaging studies. Increased-dose BEACOPP for patients with or without radiation treatment for poor prognosis disease should be considered in younger patients.
   b. Addition of involved field radiation is usually considered, particularly for bulky disease. Recent evidence from a randomized trial suggests there may be no need to add radiation, if a complete response can be achieved with combination chemo-therapy.
   c. Stanford V is an effective regimen with shorter treatment duration (3 months) and is currently undergoing randomized comparison with ABVD based treatment in inter-group trial E2496.

Lymphocyte Predominant Hodgkin's Lymphoma

This subtype has the propensity to cause multiple relapses even up to 15 years.

- Early stages of LPHL without risk factors are treated with radiation alone.
- Advanced stages are rare at diagnosis and have a poor prognosis. They are treated similar to classic HL. Because the tumor is of B-cell derivation, consideration of non-HL–type regimens may be reasonable. Phase 2 trials show single agent activity of rituximab for the usually CD-20–positive LPHL. It is possibly effective in the chemotherapy refractory setting, though the effect is of short duration (22). The use of rituximab has to be considered investigational and affected patients should be referred for trials because of the rarity of the disease.

COMPLICATIONS OF THERAPY

Radiation Therapy

Early Complications

- Mantle field radiation may cause mouth dryness, pharyngitis, cough, and dermatitis.
- Subdiaphragmatic radiation may cause anorexia and nausea.
- Radiation can cause myelosuppression or thrombocytopenia.

Late Complications

- Hypothyroidism.
- Pericarditis and pneumonitis.
- Lhermitte's sign: 15% of patients receiving mantle radiation may experience electric shock

sensation radiating down the back of the legs when the head is flexed, 6 to 12 weeks after the treatment. May be caused by transient demyelinization of the spinal cord; it usually resolves spontaneously.

- Coronary artery disease (CAD): increased risk in patients who received cardiac radiation. Patients should be monitored and evaluated for other risk factors for CAD.
- Secondary neoplasms (lung, breast, stomach, and thyroid).
- Lung cancer: twofold to eightfold increase in lung cancer is observed more than 5 years after the radiation treatment and persists through the second decade.
- The increase of lung cancer occurs mostly in smokers.
- Smokers should be encouraged stop smoking.
- Breast cancer is inversely proportional to the age at radiation treatment. The relative risk (RR) is 136 if the patient is younger than 15 years. RR is 19 for age group 15 to 24 years. RR is 7 for age group 24 to 29 years.
- The high risk is restricted to women irradiated before age 30 years.
- Average interval between radiation and diagnosis of breast cancer is 15 years.
- Breast examination should be part of follow-up for women at risk.
- Routine mammography should begin approximately 8 years after completion of the radiation.

Chemotherapy

Early Complications

- Nausea and vomiting
- Alopecia
- Myelosuppression
- Infection

Late Complications

- Sterility (primarily with MOPP-based regimens).
- Neuropathy (primarily with vincristine).
- Cardiomyopathy (doxorubicin).
- Pulmonary fibrosis (bleomycin).
- Secondary leukemia (MOPP with or without radiation).

TREATMENT OF HODGKIN'S LYMPHOMA IN RELAPSE

For successful management of patients with relapsed HL, one should have a clear understanding of:

1. Sites of relapse.
2. Time since the last treatment.
3. Details of previous treatment.

- If the relapse is because of inadequate initial treatment, retreatment with chemotherapy or radiation is considered.
- Relapse after primary radiation is best managed with chemotherapy.
- Generally relapse after primary combination chemotherapy should be consolidated with autologous stem cell transplant.

Salvage Chemotherapy Regimens

Nonanthracycline-Containing Regimens

1. ESHAP (etoposide, methylprednisolone, high-dose cytarabine, and cisplatin).
2. ICE (ifosfamide, carboplatin, and etoposide).
3. EIP (Etoposide, ifosfamide, and cisplatin).
4. DHAP (Dexamethasone, high dose cytarabine, and cisplatin).
5. MINE (mitoguazone, ifosfamide, vinorelbine, and etoposide).

Anthracycline-Containing Regimens

1. Dose-adjusted-EPOCH.
2. EVA (etoposide, vincristine and doxorubicin).
3. ASHAP (regimen doxorubicin, cisplatin, high dose cytarabine, and methylprednisolone).

POTENTIALLY CURATIVE TREATMENT APPROACH

1. High-dose chemotherapy with autologous stem cell transplantation.
2. Combination chemotherapy.
3. Extended-field radiation therapy.

PALLIATIVE TREATMENT

1. Investigational treatment.
2. Radiation treatment.
3. Sequential single-agent chemotherapy.

REFERENCES

1. Hjalgrim H, Askling J, Rostgaard K, et al. Characteristics of Hodgkin's lymphoma after infectious mononucleosis. *N Engl J Med* 2003;349:1324–1332.
2. Jaffe ES, Harris NL, Stein H, Vardiman J. *Pathology and Genetics of Tumours of Haematopoietic and Lymphoid Tissues.* World Health Organization Classification of Tumours. 2001, Lyon, France: IARC Press, pp 237–254.
3. Anagnostopoulos I, Hansmann ML, Franssila K, et al. European Task Force on Lymphoma project on lymphocyte predominance Hodgkin disease: histologic and immunohistologic analysis of submitted cases reveals 2 types of Hodgkin disease with a nodular growth pattern and abundant lymphocytes. *Blood* 2000;96:1889–1899.
4. Diehl V, Sextro M, Franklin J, et al. Clinical presentation, course, and prognostic factors in lymphocyte-predominant Hodgkin's disease and lymphocyte-rich classical Hodgkin's disease: report from the European Task Force on Lymphoma Project on Lymphocyte-Predominant Hodgkin's Disease. *J Clin Oncol* 1999;17:776–783.
5. Kuppers R, Klein U, Hansmann ML, et al. Cellular origin of human B-cell lymphomas. *N Engl J Med* 1999;341:1520–1509.
6. Stein H, Marafioti T, Foss HD, et al. Down-regulation of BOB.1/OBF.1 and Oct2 in classical Hodgkin disease but not in lymphocyte predominant Hodgkin disease correlates with immunoglobulin transcription. *Blood* 2001;97:496–501.
7. Harty LC, Lin AY, Goldstein AM, et al. HLA-DR, HLA-DQ, and TAP genes in familial Hodgkin disease. *Blood* 2002;99:690–693.
8. Lister TA, Crowther D, Suteliffe SB, et al. Report of a committee convened to discuss the evaluation and staging of patients with Hodgkin's disease: Cotswolds meeting. *J Clin Oncol* 1989;7:1630–1636.
9. Mauch P, Larson D, Osteen R, et al. Prognostic factors for positive surgical staging in patients with Hodgkin's disease. *J Clin Oncol* 1990;8:257–265.
10. Urba WJ, Longo DL. Hodgkin's disease. *N Engl J Med* 1992;326:678–687.

11. Sears JD, Greven KM, Ferree CR, et al. Definitive irradiation in the treatment of Hodgkin's disease: analysis of outcome, prognostic factors, and long term complications. *Cancer* 1997;79:145–151.
12. Canellos GP, Anderson JR, Propert KJ, et al. Chemotherapy of advanced Hodgkin's disease with MOPP, ABVD, or MOPP alternating with ABVD. *N Engl J Med* 1992;327:1478–1484.
13. Swerdlow AJ, Douglas AJ, Hudson GV, et al. Risk of second primary cancers after Hodgkin's disease by type of treatment: analysis of 2846 patients in the British National Lymphoma Investigation. *BMJ* 1992;304:1137–1143.
14. Diehl V, Franklin J, Pfreundschuh M, et al. The German Hodgkin's Lymphoma Study Group Standard and Increased-dose BEACOPP chemotherapy compared with COPP–ABVD for advanced Hodgkin's disease. *N Engl J Med* 2003;348:2386–2395.
15. Bonfante V, Santoro A, Viviani S, et al. ABVD in the treatment of Hodgkin's disease. *Semin Oncol* 1992;19(2 suppl 5):38–45.
16. Klimo P, Connors JM. MOPP/ABV hybrid program: combination chemotherapy based on early introduction of seven effective drugs for advanced Hodgkin's disease. *J Clin Oncol* 1985;3: 1174–1182.
17. Connors JM, Klimo P. MOPP/ABV hybrid chemotherapy for advanced Hodgkin's disease. *Semin Hematol* 1987;24:35–40.
18. Connors JM, Klimo P, Adams G, et al. Treatment of advanced Hodgkin's disease with chemotherapy: comparison of MOPP/ABV hybrid regimen with alternating courses of MOPP and ABVD. A report from the National Cancer Institute of Canada clinical trials group [published erratum appears in *J Clin Oncol* 1997;15:2762]. *J Clin Oncol* 1997;15:1638–1645.
19. Connors JM. An update on the Vancouver experience in the management of advanced Hodgkin's disease treated with the MOPP/ABV hybrid program. *Semin Hematol* 1988;25:34–40.
20. Horning SJ, Hoppe RT, Breslin S, Bartlett NL, Brown BW, Rosenberg SA. Stanford V and radiotherapy for locally extensive and advanced Hodgkin's disease: mature results of a prospective clinical trial. *J Clin Oncol* 2002 Feb 1;20(3):630–637.
21. Mauch PM. Controversies in the management of early stage Hodgkin's disease. *Blood* 1994;83: 318–329.
22. Ekstrand BC, Lucas JB, Horwitz SM, et Al. Rituximab in lymphocyte-predominant Hodgkin disease: results of a phase 2 trial. *Blood* 2003;101:4285–4289.

16

Non-Hodgkin's Lymphoma

Richard F. Little, Martin Gutierrez, and Wyndham H. Wilson

The non-Hodgkin's lymphomas (NHL) are a heterogeneous group of lymphoid tumors that have distinctive clinical and biologic behaviors. NHL is thus not a single disease, but a group of diseases.

- Accurate diagnosis of the specific NHL subtype is therefore critical to understanding management.
- Treatment approaches must take into account if the particular NHL is potentially curable.
- Even within a designated histopathologic classification, such as diffuse large B-cell lymphoma (DLBCL), there is considerable biological and clinical heterogeneity.
- Refinement in diagnostic resolution is an evolving science and is dependent on morphologic, immunophenotypic, and genetic features. Recent advances have led to resolution of clinically relevant molecular-based distinctions among lymphomas through the identification of a tumor's histogenetic origins and gene transcription programs.

EPIDEMIOLOGY

A steady increase in the age-adjusted incidence per 100,000 persons has been documented with 11.1 cases in 1976 and 19.0 in 2000.

- Approximately one-third of the increase may be attributed to a combination of iatrogenic immunosuppression and the AIDS epidemic. Other potential causes include increased exposures to environmental carcinogens.
- NHL occurs more commonly in males, and whites are affected more than blacks.
- In acquired immune deficiency syndrome (AIDS)-related lymphomas (ARL), certain chemokine receptor variants are associated with different risks of B-cell NHL subtypes. These chemokine variants appear to be racially distributed, paralleling differences in ethnic incidence.
- There are other differences in the epidemiology of lymphoma in human immunodeficiency virus (HIV)-infected and noninfected patients. For example, diffuse large B-cell lymphoma (DLBCL) comprises approximately 30% of lymphomas in HIV-noninfected and 70% to 80% of lymphomas in HIV-infected cases.
- The incidence of ARL has substantially decreased since the advent of highly active antiretroviral therapy (HAART) for HIV infection, but the risk remains substantially higher (100-fold) than in the HIV-noninfected population. Immunoblastic DLBCL subtypes mainly account for the decrease in incidence tumors, whereas the incidence of Burkitt's lymphoma has not been affected by HAART. The median survival of patients with ARL has increased from approximately 4 to 11 months pre-HAART to almost 24 months since the advent of HAART.

PATHOPHYSIOLOGY

A major known risk factor for NHL appears to be an abnormality of immune function (either immune deficiency or dysregulation) as in:

- HIV infection.
- Iatrogenic immune suppression.
- Autoimmune diseases.
- Congenital immune deficiencies.
  - Wiskott-Aldrich, X-linked lymphoproliferative disorder.

Infectious agents have been implicated:

- Gamma herpesviruses are linked to certain NHL subtypes, especially lymphomas associated with immune deficiency states.
- Epstein-Barr virus (EBV) is highly associated with African Burkitt's lymphoma and AIDS-related DLBCL.
- The Kaposi's sarcoma-associated herpes virus (KSHV) (also known as human herpes virus-8 or HHV-8) is etiologically linked to:
  - Primary effusion lymphomas that tend to occur specifically in AIDS.
  - Multicentric Castleman's disease, a rare lymphoproliferative disorder; affected persons have markedly increased risk developing aggressive NHL.
- Human retroviruses and RNA viruses.
  - HTLV-1 is causative of adult T-cell leukemia/lymphoma.
  - Hepatitis C virus is associated with splenic marginal zone lymphoma.
- Environmental and occupational exposures, especially organic compounds such as organo-phosphate insecticides.

CLASSIFICATION

Lymphoma classification has evolved since Hodgkin's lymphoma was first described, and new technology has made it possible to move from purely histopathologic typing to the current World Health Organization (WHO) classification that includes immunophenotypic, molecular, genetic, and clinical elements to distinguish NHL subtypes (Tables 16-1 to 16-4).

TABLE. 16–1. *Molecular characteristics of B-cell lymphomas*

			Immunoglobulin gene rearrangements	
Histology	Cytogenetics	Oncogene/protein	Heavy	κ λ
CLL/SLL[a]	t(14;19)	Bcl-3	+	
Lymphoplasmacytoid	Trisomy 12, 13q		+	+
Follicular center cell[b] Grade I, II, or III	t(14;18)	Bcl-2	+	+
Marginal zone[c]	Trisomy 3 t(11;18)		+	
Mantle cell lymphoma	t(11;14)	Bcl-1/Cyclin-D1	+	
Diffuse large B-cell[d]	t(3;22)(q27;q11)	Bcl-6 Bcl-2		+
Primary mediastinal (thymic) large B-cell		MAL gene	+	+
Lymphoblastic lymphoma/leukemia			+	+/−
Burkitt's lymphoma	t(8;14)(q24;q32) t(2;8)(11p;q24) t(8;22)(q24;q11)	c-*myc*	+	λ+ κ+

[a] Trisomy 12 is seen in 30% of cases and abnormalities in 13q are present in 25% of patients.
[b] t(14;18) is present in 75% to 95% of FCC-NHL.
[c] Cytogenetic abnormalities have been seen in extranodal marginal zone NHL.
[d] Bcl-2 rearrangements up to 30% and Bcl-6 up to 45% of cases of DLBCL, c-myc uncommon

TABLE. 16–2. *Molecular characteristics of T-cell lymphomas*

Histology	Cytogenetics	Oncoprotein	TCR gene rearrangements
T-CLL/T-PLL	Inv14(q11;q32), Trisomy 8q	Bcl-3	+
Mycosis fungoides			+
Peripheral T-cell lymphoma, unspecified			+/−
Extranodal NK/T-cell	EBV +		−
Angioimmunoblastic[a] T-cell lymphoma	Trisomy 3 or 5, EBV +		+
ATLL	HTLV 1 integration +		+
Enteropathy T cell	EBV-		β +
Hepatosplenic γ/δ T-cell lymphoma			$\delta\gamma$+
Systemic ALCL[b,c]	t(2;5)	Alk+	+
Precursor T-lymphoblastic lymphoma/leukemia	Variable t(7;9)	Tcl-4	Variable

[a] TCR gene rearrangement is present in 75% and IgH in 10%.
[b] TCR gene rearrangement in 60%+.
[c] Alk: Anaplastic lymphoma kinase gene.
NK, natural killer cells; EBV, Epstein-Barr virus; ATLL, agressive T-cell lymphoma; ALCL, anaplastic large cell lymphoma; HTLV-1, human T-cell leukemia virus 1.

TABLE. 16–3. *B-cell immunophenotype*

Histology	SIg	CIg	CD 5	10	11	15	20	23	30	34	43	45
CLL/SLL*	+/−	−/+	+	−	−/+		weak	+			+	
Lympho-plasmacytoid[a]	+	+	−	−	−/+		+	−			+/−	
Follicular center cell grade I–III[b,c]	+	−	−	+	−		+	−/+				
Marginal zone[a,c]	+	+	−	−	+/−		+	−			−/+	
Mantle cell lymphoma[a,d]	+	−	+	−	−/(+ few)		+	−			+	
Diffuse large B-cell[a]	+/−	−/+	−/+	−/+	−/+		+	−				+/−
Primary mediastinal large cell[a,e]	−	−	−/+	−/+		−	+	−	−/+			+/−
Precursor B lymphoblastic lymphoma/leukemia[a,f]	−	−/+		+/−			+			+/−		
Burkitt's lymphoma[a]	+		−	+			+	−				
Burkitt's like-lymphoma[a]	+/−	−/+	−	−/+			+					

[a] Positive B – Cell-associated antigens: CD19, CD20, CD22, and CD79.
[b] SIg$^+$: IgM$^{+/−}$, IgD >IgG>IgA.
[c] SIg M>G>A and IgD; CIg$^+$ in 40%.
[d] SIgM$^+$ usually IgD$^+$, $\kappa > \lambda$ and CD11c$^-$.
[e] M>G>A and IgD$^-$; CIg$^+$ in 40%.
[f] TdT$^+$, HLA – Dr$^+$ and CD20$^{-/+}$.

TABLE. 16–4. *T-cell immunophenotype*

Histology	CD									
	1a	2	3	4	5	7	8	25	56	TdT
T-CLL/T-PLL[a]		+	+	+	+	+	+	−		
Mycosis fungoides		+	+	+	+	−/+	−	−		
Peripheral T-cell lymphoma[b]		+/−	+/−	+	+/−	−/+	+/−			
Angioimmunoblastic T-cell lymphoma		+	+	+	+					
Extranodal NK/T		+	−	−	+/−	+/−	−		+	
Enteropathy T Cell[c]		+	−			+	+/−			
Adult T cell lymphoma/leukemia		+	+	+	+	−	−	+		
Systemic anaplastic large cell Lymphoma[d]		−/+						+/−		
Hepatosplenic γ/δ		+	−				−		+	
Precursor T lymphoblastic lymphoma/leukemia	+/−	+/−	+	+	+/−	+	+			+

[a] T-CLL: 60% are CD4[+] and 21% CD4[+] 8[+], rare cases are CD4[−] 8[+] and CD25[−].

[b] Peripheral T-cell are most commonly CD4 > CD8 and it can be CD4[−]8[−], CD45RA may be + and CD45RA[−].

[c] Intestinal T cell is CD103[+].

[d] ALCL are CD30[+], CD45[+/−], EMA[+] and CD15[+].

- NHLs are broadly classified as B-cell or T-cell lymphomas, depending on the lymphocyte lineage giving rise to the tumor.
  - B lymphocytes give rise to B-cell NHL, 88% of all NHL.
  - T lymphocytes give rise to T-cell NHL, 12% of NHL.
- Expression (or its lack thereof) of cell surface antigens and immunoglobulin proteins is dependent on the type of lymphocyte and its stage of differentiation. Analysis of these proteins in tumor cells is diagnostically useful as well as for determining tumor histogenesis.

There is an increasing appreciation of the relationship between tumor tissue origin and clinical behavior.

- DLBCL subtypes deriving from germinal center B-cells have a better prognosis than those DLBCL of postgerminal center B-cell histogenic origin.
- In chronic lymphocytic leukemia/lymphoma (CLL), cases can be grouped according to whether the variable region of the immunoglobulin genes (IgV_H) show sequence homology to germline IgV_H genes or evidence of somatic mutations. Prognosis is poorer in cases with unmutated IgV_H genes (pregerminal center histogenic origin) compared to cases with somatic mutations (postgerminal center B-cell histogenic origin).

WHO recognizes three major categories of lymphoid neoplasms:

1. B cell neoplasms.
2. T and natural killer (NK) cell neoplasm.
3. Hodgkin's lymphoma.

Both lymphomas and lymphoid leukemias are included in the WHO classification.

- Solid and leukemic phases are present in many lymphoid neoplasms.
- The WHO classification stratifies these neoplasms primarily by lineage.

- Within each category, distinct diseases are defined according to a combination of morphology, immunophenotype, genetic features, and clinical syndromes.
- A cell of origin is postulated for each neoplasm. For many, this cell of origin represents the state of differentiation of the tumor cells that are seen in the tissues, rather than the cell in which the initial transforming events occurs (not possible to know in many cases).

Further information regarding the WHO classification of tumors and to order the monograph for *Tumors of Haematopoietic and Lymphoid Tissues,* see http://www.iarc.fr/who-bluebooks/

STAGING

Staging evaluation for systemic NHL includes:

I. Diagnostic confirmation by tissue biopsy
   A. Sufficient material is critical in order to conduct the studies needed to insure accurate diagnosis
   B. Needle biopsies generally yield inadequate tissue for these studies and should be avoided for primary diagnosis
   C. Important studies for diagnostic confirmation often include:
      1. Assessment of clonality
      2. Immunophenotypic, cytogenetic, and molecular studies
      3. Markers of histogenesis (B- versus T-cell origin and germinal center versus nongerminal center histogenesis)
      4. Oncogene rearrangement can be diagnostically useful
         a. t(8;14) or MYC in Burkitt lymphoma
         b. t(14;18) or bcl-2 in follicular lymphoma
         c. t(2;5) or ALK in anaplastic large cell lymphoma
         d. t(11;14) or bcl-1 in mantle cell lymphoma
         e. Trisomy 3 or trisomy 18 (marginal zone lymphoma)
   D. Some tumors (e.g., T-cell–rich B-cell lymphoma or lymphomatoid granulomatosis) have excess reactive T cells that may obscure the minority of diagnostic malignant B cells if inadequate tissue is obtained
II. History and physical examination
III. Viral testing if indicated by risk or lymphoma subtype
   A. HIV serology in all aggressive NHL
   B. HTLV-1 serology
   C. Hepatitis B and C serology
IV. Clinical and laboratory assessment of organ function
   A. Include CD4 cell count if HIV-positive
   B. In addition to routine blood tests:
      1. Lactact dehydrogenase (LDH; indirect measure of tumor burden and prognosis)
      2. Serum β_2 microglobulin
      3. Serum α-fetoprotein or β-human chorionic gonadotropin young males with an isolated mediastinal mass where the differential diagnosis includes mediastinal germ cell tumor
VI. Chest x-ray, computed tomography scans of chest, abdomen, and pelvis
VII. Bone marrow biopsies
VIII. Lumbar puncture with cytology should be performed in patients at risk of central nervous system (CNS) disease:
   A. DLBCL with elevated LDH and more than 1 extranodal sites and/or lymphomatous involvement in the bone marrow
   B. All Burkitt's lymphoma and all ARL cases (regardless of bone marrow and extranodal sites)

TABLE. 16–5. *Ann Arbor staging system*

Stage	Description
I	Single lymph node region or single extralymphatic organ or site (IE)
II	Two or more lymph node regions on the same side of the diaphragm or single extranodal site with adjacent nodes (IIE)
III	Nodal regions on both sides of the diaphragm (III) or involving single extranodal site with adjacent nodes (IIIE), or spleen (IIIS), or both (IIISE)
IV	Diffuse or disseminated involvement of one or more extralymphatic organs; bone marrow, liver, brain involvement.

Absence of associated symptoms is designated A; presence of symptoms is designated B. B symptoms include unexplained fevers, unexplained weight loss of more than 10%, sweats.

IX. Positron emission tomography (PET) is useful for identifying sites of disease and for response assessment. Gallium scans are less sensitive and specific than PET, so of limited utility

X. The Ann Arbor Staging System, initially developed for patients with Hodgkin's lymphoma, also is used in NHL. This system does not apply to lymphoblastic leukemia/lymphoma or to mycosis fungoides (Table 16-5)

RESTAGING FOR RESPONSE EVALUATION

At completion of therapy, repeat all restaging studies. Generally restaging after four cycles is indicated in aggressive lymphomas (repeat all abnormal tests). In indolent lymphomas, response to therapy may be slower; restaging can be performed less frequently.

- The rate of response to treatment may have prognostic value.
- Disease progression or no response implies extremely poor prognosis
- Biopsy of residual masses after therapy may be required.
- PET scan may help to resolve whether a residual mass is malignant or not.
- Repeat staging procedures at regular intervals after treatment is completed.

PROGNOSTIC FEATURES

Prognostic features are related to disease and the individual patient.

- Disease-related
  - Tumor bulk, stage, number of extranodal sites
  - Histologic type and tumor histogenesis
  - Indolent lymphomas are rarely curable but may have prolonged natural history.
  - In DLBCL, better prognosis with gene expression patterns similar to germinal center B cells (GCB) compared to those with gene expression patterns similar to activated B-cells (postgerminal center histogenic derivation).
  - Tumor proliferation as measured by immunohistochemistry (such as MIB-1) or molecular profiling.
  - High proliferation associated with cyclophosphamide, doxorubicin, vincristine and prednisone (CHOP) failure may be overcome with infusional regimens such as dose-adjusted EPOCH (etoposide, prednisone, vincristine, cyclophosphamide, doxorubicin)
  - β_2-microglobulin
  - Bcl-2 expression is associated with CHOP failure, may be partially overcome with rituximab

TABLE. 16–6. *International Prognostic Index for diffuse large B-cell lymphomas*

Risk Category	Score	Patients in risk group (%)	Complete responses (%)	Five-Year disease-free survival (%)	Five-year survival (%)
Low	0 or 1	35	87	70	73
Low–intermediate	2	27	67	50	51
High–intermediate	3	22	55	49	43
High	4 or 5	16	44	40	26

- P53 mutation is associated with CHOP failure and may not be relevant in ARL
- Bcl-6 expression is an independent predictor of improved disease-free survival in aggressive lymphomas
- Patient-related
  - Age, performance status

Prognostic assessment and modeling have been developed to predict the outcome based on clinical presentation. Most commonly used model is International Prognostic Index (IPI) (Table 16-6). The IPI was initially developed for aggressive NHL, but is applicable to other NHL subtypes. In the IPI, 1 point is assigned for each of the following:

1. Older than 60 years of age
2. Eastern Cooperative Oncology Group (ECOG) performance status 2 or more
3. LDH above normal
4. Two or more extranodal sites
5. Stage III or IV disease

In age-adjusted international index for patients younger than 60 years of age, 1 point each is assigned for:

1. Performance status 2 or more
2. LDH above normal
3. Stage III or stage IV disease

In ARL, the primary prognostic determinant is the CD4 cell count. The IPI validity is not well established.

TREATMENT PRINCIPLES

Treatment of NHL is guided by clinical behavior. Approaches can been broadly classified by cell type and clinical behavior as indolent, aggressive, or highly aggressive. Conventional treatment has been chemotherapy, radiotherapy, or a combination of these modalities. Novel treatments, including monoclonal antibodies, are now in everyday practice. Ongoing clinical research will refine how newer treatments are used to augment or supplant current standards of care.

Indolent B-Cell and T-Cell Lymphomas

The natural history is one of a relatively slow-growing lymphoma with low potential for cure but with median survival measured in years to decades. Examples include:

- Grades I and II follicular lymphoma
- B-chronic lymphocytic leukemia/small lymphocytic lymphoma

- Marginal zone B-cell lymphoma
- Mycosis fungoides

Indolent lymphomas transform into high-grade malignancies in approximately 40% of patients and lead to death; treatment for transformed lymphoma is similar to that of aggressive lymphomas, but outcomes are not as favorable. Initial treatment depends on type of lymphoma, pace of the disease, and disease-associated morbidity. A slow-growing indolent lymphoma without associated symptoms may not require immediate treatment. Responses are not often durable and early treatment of asymptomatic patients does not improve survival. An alternative approach to watchful waiting is to offer participation in research protocols.

Newer treatments may change the natural history (as with CHOP-R). Research treatments may be curative (as with active immunotherapy with tumor-specific idiotype vaccine or nonmyeloablative stem-cell transplantation). In all cases, stratify by prognostic features so that treatment can be directed more effectively toward those with the worst prognosis.

Most cases are disseminated at diagnosis and standard chemotherapy is not curative. Regimens include (Table 16-7):

- Oral chlorambucil
- Cyclophosphamide, vincristine, and prednisone)(CVP)
- Fludarabine
- Rituximab (monoclonal anti-CD20 antibody):
  - As a single agent in previously untreated follicular lymphoma, yields up to 75% response rates. Maintenance rituximab may prolong remission (at 3 years of median follow-up, duration of remission was 23 months versus 12 months, favoring rituximab maintenance group receiving 375 mg/m² every 2 months for 4 doses postinduction
  - As a single agent in previously treated follicular lymphoma, rituximab can yield responses in 50% to 60% of cases, with a median response duration of 6 to 16 months
  - Rituximab with CHOP induces complete responses in up to 95% of previously untreated follicular lymphomas with a median response duration not reached at 50 months of follow-up
  - Rituximab combined with fludarabine yields results similar to CHOP plus rituximab
- Radioimmunotherapy for relapsed disease

TABLE. 16–7. *Indolent lymphoma treatment*

Combination chemotherapy	Treatment description	Reference
CVP	**Cyclophosphamide** 400 mg/m² PO daily for 5 days, days 1–5 (total dose/cycle = 2000 mg/m²) **Vincristine** 1.4 mg/m² IV on day 1 (maximum dose/cycle = 2 mg; total dose/cycle = 1.4 mg/m²) **Prednisone** 100 mg/m² PO daily for 5 days, days 1–5 (total dose/cycle = 500 mg/m²) · treatment is repeated every 21 days	[1]

Single Agents	Treatment Description	Reference
Fludarabine Rituximab	**Fludarabine** 25 mg/m² per day IV for 5 days, days 1–5 (total dose/cycle = 125 mg/m²) · treatment is repeated every 28 days	[2–4]
	Rituximab 375 mg/m² IV weekly (total dose/week = 375 mg/m²)	[5]

PO, orally; IV, intravenously.

- Yttrium 90-ibritumomab tiuxetan (Zevalan) is Food and Drug Administration (FDA)-approved and is well tolerated. In a randomized trial, Zevalan resulted in statistically and marginally clinically significant higher objective response rate (ORR) and complete response (CR) but not response duration compared with rituximab alone in relapsed or refractory low-grade, follicular, or transformed B-cell NHL
- Tositumomab and iodine-131 Tositumomab (Bexxar) are approved by the FDA for the treatment of patients with CD20-positive, follicular, NHL, with and without transformation, when disease is refractory to rituximab and has relapsed after chemotherapy.

Indolent B-positive T-cell lymphomas at stage I disease may be curable with 10-year disease-free survival of approximately 50% with radiation alone. Because of the long natural history, this is a difficult disease to study. For example, a large phase 2 trial of more than 100 patients was initiated in 1984 but was not complete and published until 2003. A 10-year disease-free survival of 76% was reported, suggesting that combined radiation and chemotherapy may be superior to radiotherapy alone in stage I and II disease. Based on these results, a randomized trial has been initiated. There is interest in newer treatments (including immunotherapy) as potentially more effective. Large retrospective databases indicate that the observational strategy does not compromise survival compared to early intervention. Thus, combined modality therapy cannot be recommended as standard of care.

Stage II to IV disease treatment options include:

- Watchful waiting
- Conventional chemotherapy plus rituximab
- Autologous transplantation associated with high risk of relapse
- Research approaches
  - Vaccine immunotherapy
  - Allogeneic transplantation

For chronic lymphocytic leukemia/small lymphocytic lymphoma treatment options include:

- Fludarabine and rituximab, given concurrently or sequentially increase response rates
- Alemtuzumab is approved for fludarabine-refractory disease, with response rates of approximately 30%
- Cladribine may also be used

For lymphoplasmacytoid lymphoma/Waldenström macroglobulinemia treatment options include:

- Initial therapy with rituximab has produced overall response rates of 30% to 60%
- Conventional therapies include alkylating agents (especially chlorambucil), with or without corticosteroids. CHOP is sometimes used
- Purine analogues such as fludarabine are also active. Response rate (RR) to first-line therapy range from 38% to 85%. RR to fludarabine in previously treated patients range from 30% to 50%

For marginal zone lymphoma:

- Associated with *Helicobacter pylori*, effective eradication of the infection can result in lymphoma regression and likely cure
- Associated with autoimmune disease (such as Sjögren syndrome or Hashimoto's thyroiditis), chemotherapy with or without rituximab may be useful

Local therapy such as surgery or regional irradiation may yield relatively long-term disease control. Splenectomy may be indicated for splenic marginal zone lymphoma. Cases associated with hepatitis C virus (HCV) infection may regress with effective HCV therapy.

Mycosis Fungoides

Mycosis fungoides is a cutaneous T-cell lymphoma that often has multiple skin plaques, nodules, and/or generalized erythroderma. Sezary syndrome is the late occurrence of nodal and leukemic disease. Prognosis depends on a number of features including disease extent. Median survival of approximately 10 years is seen in relatively indolent disease, but in those with poor prognostic features (older than 65 years of age, stage IVB), median survival may be only 1 year.

A variety of treatments have been reported for limited stage disease, but the extent to which outcomes are related to therapy or to the disease natural history is often not well documented.

Topical treatment should be used for local disease:

- Topical gel formulation combining methotrexate and laurocapram, and topical nitrogen mustard.
- Low-dose oral methotrexate.
- Topical bexarotene gel.
- Combined modality therapy including subcutaneous interferon-α and oral isotretinoin, followed by total-skin electron beam therapy, and long-term maintenance therapy with topical nitrogen mustard and interferon-α has been reported as useful. Some reports suggest that interferon alone is just as effective.
- Extracorporeal photopheresis with or without other modalities has been reported.
- Denileukin diftitox (recombinant diphtheria toxin and interleukin [IL]-2).
- Alemtuzumab.

Primary Cutaneous Anaplastic Large Cell Lymphoma/Lymphomatoid Papulosis (CD30$^+$)

These are chronic recurrent skin diseases usually of a benign course. Lymphomatoid papulosis is considered to be an atypical lymphoproliferation rather than a true lymphoma but may develop into a lymphoma. Low-dose methotrexate, and psoralen/UVA therapy can reduce the skin lesions, but chronic therapy is required. The anaplastic lymphoma kinase (ALK) protein has been shown to identify a subgroup of patients with systemic anaplastic large cell lymphoma (ALCL) with an excellent prognosis, whereas ALK-negative ALCLs are more heterogeneous. ALK positive cases are associated with younger age and more limited disease state, and better prognosis. ALK negative cases are associated with older age, advanced disease stage, and poor prognosis.

AGGRESSIVE B-CELL LYMPHOMAS

Mantle Cell Lymphoma

Most patients present with advanced-stage disease. The median age is in the seventh decade, and the male to female ratio is high. Splenomegaly and gastrointestinal involvement is common. Unlike other aggressive lymphomas, it is incurable and has a short median survival of 3 to 5 years. The blastic variant may be more aggressive with a propensity for central nervous system (CNS) involvement (25%) and shorter survival. There may be a survival advantage in younger patients with stage IA or IIA treated with radiation therapy.

Diffuse Large B-Cell Lymphoma

Morphologic variants of DLBCL include centroblastic, immunoblastic, T-cell histiocyte rich, anaplastic, and plasmablastic variants.

- A subtype of DLBCL, mediastinal (thymic) large B-cell lymphoma (Med-DLBCL), arises in the mediastinum and is of putative thymic B-cell origin. Med-DLBCL has distinctive

clinical, immunophenotypic, and genotypic characteristics. Presenting features include localized disease, and signs and symptoms related to a large anterior mediastinal mass. Dissemination to multiple organs can occur. CD19 and CD20 are present, CD10 and CD5 are absent. Gains in chromosome 9p and REL gene support the concept of a subtype distinct from DLBCL arising in other sites.
- Follicle center lymphoma grade III is an aggressive lymphoma with follicles present in the lymph node, but having more than 15 centroblasts per high-power field. This tumor is potentially curable with aggressive therapy. Thus, care must be taken to distinguish this tumor from mantle cell and from grades I and II follicle center cell lymphoma.

Primary Effusion Lymphoma (PEL)

All cases are associated with the KSHV, also known as human herpes virus-8 (HHV-8); more than 70% are coassociated with EBV. The tumor presents as effusions in the body cavities with an absence of nodal disease, giving rise to its alternative designation of body-cavity lymphoma. PEL occurs most often in the setting of HIV infection. There is no defined effective standard of care, and median survival is generally 4 to 6 months with therapy.

- Primary cutaneous large cell lymphoma often has an indolent course.
- Lymphomatoid granulomatosis has a variable clinical course depending on its grade. Interferon may be useful in low grade disease (grades I to II). Dose-adjusted EPOCH-R is useful in grade III disease.

TREATMENT PRINCIPLES

- Rituximab with cyclophosphamide, doxorubicin, vincristine, and prednisone (R-CHOP) is the standard of care for curative intent in DLBCL (Table 16-8). Probability of cure can be estimated using prognostic models, such as the IPI.

TABLE. 16–8. *Standard therapy for aggressive non-Hodgkin's lymphoma*

Combination chemotherapy	Treatment description	Reference
R-CHOP	**Rituximab** 375 mg/m^2 IV day 1 **Cyclophosphamide** 750 mg/m^2 IV day 1 (total dose/cycle = 750 mg/m^2) **Doxorubicin** 50 mg/m^2 IV day 1 (total dose/cycle = 50 mg/m^2) **Vincristine** 1.4 mg/m^2 IV day 1 (maximum dose/cycle = 2 mg; total dose/cycle = 1.4 mg/m^2) **Prednisone** 50 mg/m^2 per day PO for 5 days, days 1–5 (total dose/cycle = 250 mg/m^2) treatment is repeated every 21 days	[6,7]
Possible alternatives include: DA-EPOCH-R ACVBP CHOP every 14 days **CHOEP**	**(See Table 16–9)**	

IV, intravenously, PO, orally, DA-EPOCH-R, dose-adjusted EPOCH, ACVBP, doxorubicin, cyclophosphamide, vindesine, bleomycin, and prednisone; CHOP, cyclophosphamide, doxorubicin, vincristine, and prednisone; CHOEP, etoposide plus CHOP.

- For stage I to II disease, three cycles of CHOP plus involved-field radiotherapy results in 5-year progression-free survival (PFS) of 77% and overall survival (OS) of 82%, better than with 8 cycles of CHOP alone (64% and 72%, respectively). However, R-CHOP now is commonly used in early stage disease without radiation.
- In advanced-stage disease, the OS and PFS are approximately 50% and 32%, respectively, at 5 years with CHOP.
- Randomized trials show that addition of rituximab on day 1 of each CHOP cycle resulted in improved outcome in patients 60 to 80 years of age: complete response higher with rituximab (76% versus 63%), 2-year event-free survival with rituximab (57% versus 38%), 2-year overall survival with rituximab (70% versus 57%), and rituximab appears to confer greater benefit in tumors with bcl-2 overexpression.
- A preliminary report of an intergroup phase 3 trial of R-CHOP versus CHOP has raised questions regarding the best way to combine CHOP and rituximab: the report did not indicate an increased response rate with the addition of rituximab. The trial design includes a second randomization to maintenance rituximab or observation in patients 60 years of age and older. Time to treatment failure favored R-CHOP, but overall survival was not significantly different in the two groups. Maintenance rituximab appeared to increase time to treatment failure in those treated with CHOP alone.
- Possible alternatives to R-CHOP as front-line therapy, or as salvage therapy (Table 16-9):
  - Dose-adjusted-EPOCH-R
  - Biweekly R-CHOP
  - Doxorubicin, cyclophosphamide, vindesine, bleomycin, and prednisone (ACVBP)

HIGHLY AGGRESSIVE B-CELL LYMPHOMA

- Precursor B-lymphoblastic lymphoma/leukemia (PBLL). Most cases (80%) present as leukemia. In lymphoma cases, nodal, cutaneous, and osseous involvement is common. PBLL should be distinguished from Ewing's sarcoma (ES) or primitive neuroectodermal tumor (PNET). PBLL may be negative for CD45 (leukocyte common antigen, a widely used marker for lymphoma), and may express CD99 (a marker for ES or PNET). PBLL accounts for approximately 2.5% of childhood NHL. ALL therapy strategy can yield 73% EFS at 10 years, superior to short-pulse B-NHL therapy.
- Burkitt lymphoma/B-cell ALL. Immunophenotype, molecular, and cytogenetic analyses of the bone marrow or peripheral blood, or both, should be done. Surface immunoglobulin expression is characteristic. Cytogenetics shows t(8;14), t(2;8), or t(8;22).

Treatment may provoke tumor lysis syndrome and prophylaxis should be used: alkalinize the urine with D5W plus 100 mEq sodium acetate at 100 to 150 mL/hr, add allopurinol, 600 mg, orally daily for 2 days, then 300 mg per day orally until resolution of the tumor lysis syndrome. Aggressive chemotherapy:

- CODOX-M/IVAC risk-stratified regimen (Tables 16-10–16-13)
  - Three cycles of CODOX-M for low risk (all of the following: normal LDH, WHO performance status 0 or 1, Ann Arbor stage I to II, and no tumor mass 10 cm or larger)
  - Four cycles of alternating CODOX-M and IVAC for high risk (e.g., do not meet criteria for low risk above)
- Hyper-CVAD regimen (Tables 16-14 and 16-15).

TREATMENT OF RECURRENT AND REFRACTORY B-CELL LYMPHOMA

Many patients with NHL require additional therapy because of disease recurrence or refractoriness to therapy. Although grades I and II follicular lymphoma are not curable, high-dose chemotherapy followed by autologous transplant improves PFS. In aggressive NHL, approximately 40% to 50% of patients fail to achieve remission with conventional chemother-

TABLE. 16–9. *Alternative or salvage regimens for aggressive non-Hodgkin's lymphoma*

Combination chemotherapy	Treatment description	Reference
EPOCH (dose adjusted)[a]	**Etoposide** 50 mg/m^2 per day by continuous IV infusion for 4 days, days 1–4 (total dose/cycle = 250 mg/m^2)	
	Doxorubicin 10 mg/m^2 per day by continuous IV infusion for 4 days, days 1–4 (total dose/cycle = 40 mg/m^2)	
	Vincristine 0.4 mg/m^2 per day by continuous IV infusion for 4 days, days 1–4 (total dose/cycle = 1.6 mg/m^2 [no cap])	
	Prednisone 60 mg/m^2 per dose PO every 12 h for 5 days, days 1–5 (total dose/cycle = 600 mg/m^2)	[8, 9]
	Cyclophosphamide 750 mg/m^2 IV day 5 (total dose/cycle = 750 mg/m^2)	
	Filgrastim 5 μg/kg per day SC starting day 6; continues until ANC >5,000 cells/mm^3	
	• Treatment is dose-adjusted based on neutrophil nadirs and repeated every 21 days	
CHOEP	**CHOP with etoposide** 100 mg/m^2 IV days 1, 2, and 3	[10]
R-ICE	**Rituximab** 375 mg/m^2 IV 48 hours prior to cycle 1 and on day 1 of cycles 1–3	
	Etoposide 100 mg/m^2 IV days 3, 4, and 5	
	Carboplatin AUC 5: dose = 5 × [25 + creatinine clearance] capped at 800 mg IV on day 4	[11]
	Ifosfamide 5,000 mg/m^2 mixed with an equal amount of MESNA CIV for 24 hours on day 4	
DHAP	**Cisplatin** 100 mg/m^2 by CIV infusion for 24 hours on day 1 (total dose/cycle = 100 mg/m^2)	
	Cytarabine 2,000 mg/m^2 per dose IV over 3 hours every 12 hours for 2 doses on day 2 (total dose/cycle = 4000 mg/m^2)	
	Dexamethasone 40 mg per day PO or IV for 4 days, days 1–4 (total dose/cycle = 160 mg/m^2) treatment is repeated every 21–28 days	[12]
ESHAP	**Etoposide** 40 mg/m^2 per day over 1 hour IV for 4 days, days 1–4 (total dose/cycle = 160 mg/m^2)	
	Methylprednisolone 250–500 mg per day IV for 5 days, days 1–5 (total dose/cycle = 1,250–2,500 mg)	[13]
	Cytarabine 2,000 mg/m^2 IV over 2 hours on day 5 (total dose/cycle = 2,000 mg/m^2)	
	Cisplatin 25 mg/m^2 per day by C IV infusion for 4 days, days 1–4 (total dose/cycle = 100 mg/m^2)	
	• treatment is repeated every 21–28 days	
ACVBP	**Doxorubicin** 75 mg/m^2 IV day 1	
	Cyclophosphamide 1,200 mg/m^2 per dose IV day 1	[14]
	Vindesine 2 mg/m^2 IV days 1 and 5	
	Bleomycin 10 mg IV days 1 and 5	
	Prednisone 60 mg/m^2 per day PO days 1–5	

[a] Etoposide, cyclophosphamide, and doxorubicin dosages may be increased by 20% from the previous cycle's dosage if there was no evidence of absolute neutropenia (ANC <500/mm^3) or thrombocytopenia (platelet count <25,000/mm^3).

[b] Increments in the doses of cyclophosphamide by 50 mg/m^2 and etoposide by 15 mg/m^2 each cycle is allowed if patient could tolerated without significant neutropenia.

IV, intravenously; PO, orally; SC, subcutaneously; ANC, absolute neutrophil count; AUC, area under the curve; MESNA, 2-mercaptoethane sulfonate; CIV, continuous intravenous infusion.

TABLE. 16–10. *Outcome in adults and children with Burkitt's and Burkitt's-like lymphoma with CODOX-M/IVAC regimen*

Number	CR	EFS at 2 years
Children: 21	90%	85%
Adults: 20	100%	100%
Total: 41	95%	92%

From Magrath I, Adde M, Shaa A, et al. Adults and children with non-cleaved–cell lymphoma have a similar excellent outcome when treated with the same chemotherapy regimen. *J Clin Oncol* 1996;14:925–934, with permission. (ref 16)

apy. Among those who do achieve a CR, 30% to 40% will relapse. These patients may benefit from salvage therapy (Table 16-9).

Principles of Salvage Therapy

Conventional wisdom promotes the use of non–cross-resistant chemotherapy such as (cisplatin, cytarabine, and devamethasone), ESHAP (etoposide, methyl prednisolone, cytarabine, and cisplatin), and ICE (ifosfamide, carboplatin, etoposide). However, evolving understanding of cellular apoptotic response to chemotherapeutic stimuli suggests that true non–cross-resistance drugs may not exist—as mechanisms for tumor resistance may not be entirely drug-specific—because of the intrinsic high apoptosis thresholds in refractory tumors. Both *in vitro* and empiric clinical data provide evidence that tumor resistance can be overcome by using drugs already administered, but with different infusion schedules (e.g., by prolonged infusion regimens such as dose-adjusted EPOCH-R). In addition, other agents such as in ICE or ESHAP have also shown utility in the setting of relapsed and refractory NHL.

Rituximab added to conventional chemotherapy increases efficacy in CD20$^+$ tumors.

High-dose chemotherapy and autologous stem cell transplantation (ASCT) may confer curative advantage in some patients whose disease is responsive to salvage chemotherapy. ASCT achieves long-term survival in up to 50% of patients with chemotherapy-sensitive

TABLE. 16–11. *Estimate of one-year event-free survival for subgroups of high-risk patients treated with CODOX-M/IVAC regime for HIV-unrelated Burkitt lymphoma*

Variable	n	1-year EFS (%)	(95% CI)	Log-rank *p* value
International Prognostic Index score				
0–1	6	83.3	(53.5–99.0)	
2	19	63.2	(41.5–84.9)	
3	14	57.1	(31.2–83.1)	0.8852

EFS, event-free survival; HIV, human immunodeficiency virus. From Mead GM, Sydes MR, Walewski J, et al. An international evaluation of CODOX-M and CODOX-M alternating with IVAC in adult Burkitt's lymphoma: results of United Kingdom Lymphoma Group LY06 study. *Ann Oncol* 2002;13:1264–1274, with permission. (ref 17)

TABLE. 16–12. *CODOX-M regimen (17)*

Day	Drug	Dose	Route	Time
1	Cyclophosphamide	800 mg/m²	IV	
	Vincristine	1.5 mg/m² (max 2 mg)	IV	
	Doxorubicin	40 mg/m²	IV	
	Cytarabine	70 mg	IT	
2–5	Cyclophosphamide	200 mg/m²	IV	Daily
3	Cytarabine	70 mg	IT	
8	Vincristine	1.5 mg/m² (max 2 mg)	IV	
10	Methotrexate	1200 mg/m²	IV	Over 1 hour
		240 mg/m²	IV	Each hour over 23 hours
11	Leucovorin	192 mg/m²	IV	At hour 36
		12 mg/m²	IV	Every 6 hours until MTX level $<5 \times 10^{-8}$M
13	G-CSF	5 μg/kg	SC	Daily until AGC $>10^9$/L
15	Methotrexate	12 mg	IT	
16	Leucovorin	15 mg	PO	24 hours after IT methotrexate

Begin next cycle on the day that unsupported ANC is $>1.0 \times 10^9$/L, and unsupported platelet $>75 \times 10^9$/L.

IV, intravenously; IT, intrathecally; SC, subcutaneously; PO, orally; G-CSF, granulocyte colony-stimulating factor; AGC, absolute granulocyte count; ANC, absolute neutrophil count.

relapsed DLBCL, and some prospective randomized studies have documented the superiority of ASCT over salvage chemotherapy for relapsed DLBCL. Patients with low-risk IPI are most likely to benefit. Patients with well controlled HIV with relapsed NHL should not be routinely excluded from consideration for ASCT.

Allogeneic transplantation remains investigational. Nonmyeloablative or reduced intensity stem cell transplantation (RIST) attempts to exert immunologic effects against the tumor without the risk of high-dose chemotherapy. High-dose chemotherapy does not appear to overcome tumor resistance in the majority of cases. Graft engineering to enhance graft-versus

TABLE. 16–13. *IVAC regimen (17)*

Day	Drug	Dose	Method	Time
1–5	Etoposide	60 mg/m²	IV	Daily over 1 hour
	Ifosfamide	1500 mg/m²	IV	Daily over 1 hour
	MESNA	360 mg/m² (mixed with ifosfamide) then 360 mg/m²	IV	3 hourly (seven doses/ 24 hours period)
1 and 2	Cytarabine	2 g/m²	IV	Over 3 hours, 12 hourly (total of 4 doses)
5	Methotrexate	12 mg	IT	
6	Leucovorin	15 mg	PO	24 h after IT MTX
7	G-CSF	5 μ/kg	SC	Daily until ANC $>1.0 \times 10^9$/L

Begin next cycle (CODOX-M) on the day the unsupported ANC is $>1.0 \times 10^9$/L, and unsupported platelet $>75 \times 10^9$/L

MESNA, 2-mercaptoethane sulfonate; IV, intravenously; IT, intrathecally; PO, orally; SC, subcutaneously; MTX, methotrexate; ANC, absolute neutrophil count.

TABLE. 16–14. Treatment outcome with hyper-CVAD program by B-ALL Features: FAB, Immunophenotype, and Karyotype

Features	No.	%	% age>60 years	Outcome CR No.	CR %	Relapse No.	Relapse %	% 3-year survival
Total	26		46	21	81	9	43	49
L3, t(8;14), t(2;8), or t(8;22)	7	31	14	7	100	1	14	86
L3, CALLA, t(8;14), t(2;8), or t(8;22)	2	8	50	1	50	None		50
L3, other, sIg+	11	38	64	8	73	4	50	36
L3, CALLA, other, sIg+	3	12	33	3	100	2	67	33
L2, t(8;14), sIg+ >90%	1	4	All	1	100	All		None
L1/L2, other, sIg+ > 90%[b]	2	8	50	1	50	All		None

CALLA, common acute lymphocytic anemia antigen; CR, complete remission.
From Thomas DA, Cortes J, O'Brien S, et al. Hyper-CVAD program in Burkitt's-type adult acute lymphoblastic leukemia. J Clin Oncol 1999; 17: 2461–2470, with permission. (ref. 15)

TABLE. 16–15. *Hyper-CVAD alternating with high-dose methotrexate and Ara-C (15)*

Cycle	Day	Drug	Dose	Route	Time
Odd numbers 1, 3, 5, and 7	1–3	Cyclophos-phamide	300 mg/m^2 (total dose 1,800 mg/m^2)	IV	Each dose given over 2 hours every 12 hours for six doses
	1–3	MESNA	600 mg/m^2	CIV	Infused over 24 hours daily for 3 days. Start 1 hour before cyclophosphamide and continue for 12 hours after last dose
	4	Doxorubicin	50 mg/m^2	IV	Over 2 hours
	4 and 11	Vincristine	2 mg	IV	
	4–11 and 11–14	Dexametha-sone	40 mg/day	PO or IV	
		G-CSF	10 µg/kg	SC	Daily starting 24 hours after the last dose of doxorubicin, until granulocytes are >30,000/µL or until day 21 (whichever comes first).
Even 2, 4, 6, and 8	1	Methotrexate	1 g/m^2	CIV	Infused over 24 hours
		Leucovorin	50 mg IV or PO, is given	IV or PO	12 hours after the completion of methotrexate, followed by 15 mg IV or PO every 6 hours for 8 doses. At the end of the methotrexate infusion, 24 hours and 48 hours after completion, the methotrexate level is checked. If the level is >1 µM at 24 hours or >0.1 µM at 48 hours, the leucovorin dose is increased to 50 mg IV every 6 hours until the level is <0.1 µM
	2–3	Ara-C	3 g/m^2	IV	Given over 2 hours every 12 hours for 4 doses
		G-CSF	5 µg/kg,	SC	Begin after chemotherapy completion until the ANC is >30,000/µL or until day 21 (whichever comes first). Then it is held for 1 day and the next cycle is started

Central nervous system (CNS) prophylaxis: MTX 12 mg IT on day 2 and Ara-C 100 mg IT on day 8 of each cycle for 16 IT treatments in high-risk patients, four IT treatments in low-risk patients.

MESNA, 2-mercaptoethane sulfonate; G-CSF, granulocyte colony-stimulating factor; IV, intravenously PO, orally; SC, subcutaneously; MTX, methotrexate; IT, intrathecal; CIV, continuous intravenous.

lymphoma benefit and to decrease graft-versus-host complications remains an active area of investigation. Studies have not consistently shown strong graft-versus-lymphoma effects in the majority of patients.

ACQUIRED IMMUNE DEFICIENCY SYNDROME-RELATED LYMPHOMA (SYSTEMIC) TREATMENT CONSIDERATIONS

- Many experts recommend CNS prophylaxis for all systemic ARL (Table 16-16).
- Standard dose-chemotherapy has supplanted low-dose therapy in the HAART era.
- Some studies have suggested a role for dose-intense regimens for Burkitt lymphoma in AIDS (e.g., hyper-CVAD or CODOX-M), but toxicity is high and may not be acceptable for this patient population.
- Burkitt lymphoma in AIDS appears to respond to infusional chemotherapy (e.g., dose-adjusted EPOCH, Table 16-17).
- The use of concurrent HAART is unsettled. There are inadequate data to make evidence-based recommendations. A phase 2 trial of dose-adjusted EPOCH in ARL suggested that concurrent HAART is not necessary to achieve favorable results, provided effective antiretroviral therapy is initiated after treatment for lymphoma. Reasons to omit HAART during ARL therapy include: overlapping toxicity, pharmacokinetic interactions, HAART adherence problems related to chemotherapy, and because chemotherapy will deplete CD4 cells regardless of HAART.
- Rituximab in ARL cannot be recommended as standard care at the current time. In preliminary reporting of a large multicenter randomized trial of R-CHOP versus CHOP alone (both groups received HAART) conducted by the NCI-sponsored AIDS-Malignancy Consortium, rituximab did not increase the RR but there was a 15% occurrence of treatment-related death in the rituximab group compared to 2% in the CHOP only group. Rituximab with infusional cyclophosphamide, doxorubicin, and etoposide given with HAART has shown a high response rate in preliminary reports of a phase 2 trial.

TABLE. 16–16. *Selected regimens and outcomes for Acquired immune deficiency syndrome-associated non-Hodgkin's lymphoma*

Regimen	Evaluable patients	Median baseline CD4 cells/mm^3	Complete response rate (%)	Median overall/ disease-free survival (mo)	Reference
Low- or standard-dose m-BACOD[a]	175	100 (low) 107 (standard)	41 (low) 52 (standard)	8/8	(18)
Low- or standard-dose CHOP plus HAART	53	119	35 (low) 37 (standard)	Not available (limited follow-up)	(19)
Infusional CDE	48	70	46	8/15	(20)
Infusional CDE + rituximab + HAART	29	132	86	Not available (limited follow-up)	(21)
Dose-adjusted EPOCH (HAART deferment until chemotherapy completion)	39	198	74	Not yet reached (At 53 months, OS is 60% and DFS is 92%)	(22)

[a] Data from pre-HAART era. There is less emphasis on low-dose chemotherapy for ARL in the HAART era.

m-BACOD, bleomycin, doxorubicin, cyclophosphamide, vineristine, and dexamethasone; CHOP, cyclophosphamide, doxorubicin, vincristine, and prednisone; HAART, highly active antivetroviral therapy; CDE, cyclophosphamide, doxorubicin, and etoposide; OS, overall survival; DFS, disease-free survival; ARL, acquired immune deficiency syndrome-related lymphomas.

TABLE. 16–17. *Dose-adjusted EPOCH for ARL*

Etoposide Doxorubicin Vincristine)	50 mg/m^2 per day CIV days 1–4 (total dose/cycle = 250 mg/m^2) 10 mg/m^2 per day CIV days 1–4 (total dose/cycle = 40 mg/m^2) 0.4 mg/m^2 per day CIV days 1–4 (total dose/cycle = 1.6 mg/m^2 (no cap)
Prednisone	60 mg/m^2 PO daily, days 1–5
Cyclophosphamide	Cycle 1 dependent on CD4 cell count

CD4/mm^3	<100	187 mg/m^2 IV on day 5
	≥100	375 mg/m^2 IV on day 5

Cycles 2 and beyond dependent on ANC nadir

ANC nadir	<500	Decrease dose by 187 mg/m^2
	≥500	Increase dose by 187 mg/m^2 (maximum dose is 750 mg/m^2)

Filgrastim	300 μg per day SC starting day 6; continues until ANC >5,000 cells/mm^3 Treatment is repeated every 21 days

HAART suspended until completion of all EPOCH cycles.
PCP prophylaxis for all patients and continues until CD4 >200 cells/mm^3.
MAC prophylaxis for all patients with CD4 <100 cells/mm^3.
CIV, continuous intravenous; PO, oral; IV, intravenously; SC, subcutaneously; ANC, absolute neutrophil count; HAART, highly active antiretroviral therapy; PCP, *Pneumocystis carinii* pneumonia; MAC, *Mycobacterium avium* complex.
From Little RF, Pittaluga S, Grant N, et al. Highly effective treatment of acquired immunodeficiency syndrome-related lymphoma with dose-adjusted EPOCH: impact of antiretroviral therapy suspension and tumor biology. *Blood* 2003; 101 : 4653–4659.

ACQUIRED IMMUNE DEFICIENCY SYNDROME-RELATED PRIMARY BRAIN LYMPHOMA

For diagnosis, a major recent advance has been the ability to diagnose AIDS primary brain lymphoma (AIDS-PBL) more easily. Essentially 100% of AIDS-PBL are EBV associated. Combined EBV and PET or single photon emission computed tomography (SPECT) thallium can be used in a relatively noninvasive diagnostic approach, and brain biopsy can be avoided if the tests are concordant:

- If both EBV and PET/SPECT are positive, the positive predictive value for lymphoma is 100%.
- If both EBV and PET/SPECT are negative, the negative predictive value for lymphoma is 100%.

For treatment, the use of high-dose systemic methotrexate has not been adequately evaluated in HIV-infected patients. As AIDS-PBL virtually never occurs until CD4 cells are less than 50 per cubic millimeter, the importance of immune reconstitution with treatment should be considered a high priority in treatment, in order to help prevent disease recurrence. High-dose chemotherapy may retard immune recovery.

- Standard of care remains radiotherapy.
- HAART, especially among those naïve to antiretroviral therapy, may result in substantial immune recovery and tumor control, and thus should be initiated as soon as possible in patients with AIDS with focal brain lesions.

AGGRESSIVE T-CELL LYMPHOMA

Adult T-Cell Leukemia/Lymphoma

Rare in Western countries, this is the most common lymphoma in Asia and is caused by the human retrovirus, HTVL-1. Adult T-cell lymphoma (ATLL) may behave aggressively, but some clinical variants have a relatively indolent course. ATLL cannot be cured. Ameliorative treatments include interferon and doxorubicin-based combination chemotherapy.

Clinical variants include:

- Acute ATLL has a survival time ranging from a few weeks to more than 1 year. There is a leukemic phase with elevated white blood count, skin rash, generalized lymphadenopathy, organomegally, constitutional symptoms, and high LDH. Hypercalcemia is common. Opportunistic infections occur as a result of an associated T-cell immunodeficiency.
- For lymphomatous ATLL, survival also ranges from a few weeks to more than 1 year. The lymphoma is characterized by prominent lymphadenopathy without peripheral blood involvement. Hypercalcemia is less frequent than in the acute form, but generally patients have advanced stage disease.
- Chronic variant generally has a more protracted clinical course with longer survival, but it can transform into an acute phase with an aggressive course. There may be skin lesions, and absolute lymphocytosis but without numerous atypical lymphocytes in the peripheral blood. Hypercalcemia is absent.
- Smoldering ATLL is characterized by a more protracted clinical course and longer survival, but can acutely transform into an aggressive tumor. More generally, the ATLL is indolent with normal white blood count and less than 5% circulating neoplastic cells. Skin or pulmonary lesions are common, but hypercalcemia is absent. Progression from chronic and smoldering to acute variants occurs in 25% of cases, usually after a long duration.

Enteropathy-Type T-Cell Lymphoma

Adult patients usually have a history of gluten-sensitive enteropathy. The geographic distribution is that of intestinal enteropathies, and hence the disease is rare in Western countries. Patients may present with abdominal pain and small bowel perforation. The prognosis is usually poor.

Extranodal Natural Killer/T-Cell Lymphoma, Nasal-Type

This is most prevalent in Asia, Mexico, and Central and South America, occurs most often in adults (males more than females), and is almost always EBV-associated. The disease usually presents in the nasopharyngeal area with symptoms of obstruction, pain, or epistaxis. Tumors may cause extensive midfacial destructive lesions, termed lethal midline granuloma. Upper aerodigestive tract involvement may present with perforation. The skin is commonly involved. Treatment for localized disease is primarily radiation. Optimal outcome is dependent on careful planning of radiation fields and higher doses (50 to 60 Gy). The role of chemotherapy is unclear. At relapse (and less commonly at presentation), the disease may disseminate to extranodal sites such as the bone marrow and blood.

Angioimmunoblastic T-Cell Lymphoma

Angioimmunoblastic T-cell lymphoma or angioimmunoblastic lymphadenopathy with dysproteinemia (AILD) occurs most often in the middle aged and elderly with equal gender incidence, usually at an advanced stage with systemic symptoms. A pruritic skin rash is common. Laboratory findings include: polyclonal hypergammaglobulinaemia, circulating immune complexes, cold agglutinins with hemolytic anemia, positive rheumatoid factor, and anti-smooth muscle antibodies. The aggressive clinical course is responsive to steroids and chemotherapy, but most patients relapse and die from disease.

Peripheral T-Cell Lymphoma, Unspecified

Peripheral T-cell lymphoma (unspecified) accounts for nearly 50% of the peripheral T-cell lymphomas in Western countries, and most commonly occurs in adults with equal gender incidence. Nodal involvement is the most common presentation, but bone marrow, liver, spleen and extranodal involvement including skin is not uncommon. The clinical course is aggressive and the disease responds poorly to therapy. The median survival at 5 years is poor at 20% to 30%.

Anaplastic Large Cell Lymphoma: Systemic and Primary Cutaneous Forms

- Systemic form occurs in both children and adults, and has either a T-cell or null phenotype; true anaplastic large-cell lymphomas with a B-cell phenotype are rare. It may involve lymph nodes or extranodal sites, including the skin, and half of patients have B-symptoms and advanced states at presentation. It is highly responsive to chemotherapy and curable with OS and FFS of 75% and 60%, respectively, at 7 years.
- Primary cutaneous form occurs mostly in adults and presents with isolated skin nodules. The clinical course is indolent. Skin lesions may spontaneously regress. Systemic disease is uncommon and occurs late in the disease course. This form may be incurable. Some cases appear to be within the spectrum of lymphomatoid papulosis type A.

Hepatosplenic γ/δ

Hepatosplenic γ/δ is a rare tumor that comprises fewer than 5% of T-cell neoplasms. Its peak incidence is in adolescents and young adults, and males are more often affected than females. The aggressive clinical course is associated with a median survival less than 2 years.

TREATMENT PRINCIPLES

T-cell lymphomas tend to have a poorer PFS and OS than aggressive B-cell lymphomas. Systemic ALCL is an exception and is among the most curable subtypes with doxorubicin-based treatment. Some T-cell subtypes have no potential for cure and should be approached palliatively, as in ATL and primary cutaneous anaplastic lymphoma. Other T-cell subtypes, including angioimmunoblastic and PTL, have low curative potential with conventional dose treatment and should be considered for trials targeting high risk patients.

REFERENCES

1. Bagley CM Jr, Devita VT Jr, Berard CW, et al. Advanced lymphosarcoma: intensive cyclical combination chemotherapy with cyclophosphamide, vincristine, and prednisone. *Ann Intern Med* 1972;76: 227–234.
2. Hutton JJ, Von Hoff DD, Kuhn J, et al. Phase I clinical investigation of 9-beta-D-arabinofuranosyl-2-fluoroadenine 5'-monophosphate (NSC 312887), a new purine antimetabolite. *Cancer Res* 1984; 44:4183–4186.
3. Danhauser L, Plunkett W, Keating M, et al. 9-beta-D-arabinofuranosyl-2-fluoroadenine 5'-monophosphate pharmacokinetics in plasma and tumor cells of patients with relapsed leukemia and lymphoma. *Cancer Chemother Pharmacol* 1986;18:145–152.
4. Hersh MR, Kuhn JG, Phillips JL, et al. Pharmacokinetic study of fludarabine phosphate (NSC 312887). *Cancer Chemother Pharmacol* 1986;17:277–280.
5. McLaughlin P, Grillo-Lopez AJ, Link BK, et al. Rituximab chimeric anti-CD20 monoclonal antibody

therapy for relapsed indolent lymphoma: half of patients respond to a four-dose treatment program. *J Clin Oncol* 1998;16:2533–2833.

6. Coiffier B, Lepage E, Briere J, et al. CHOP chemotherapy plus rituximab compared with CHOP alone in elderly patients with diffuse large-B-cell lymphoma. *N Engl J Med* 2002;346:235–242.

7. Habermann TM, Weller EA, Morrison VA, et al. Phase III trial of rituximab-CHOP (R-CHOP) vs. CHOP with a second randomization to maintenance rituximab (MR) or observation in patients 60 years of age and older with diffuse large B-cell lymphoma (DLBCL). 45th Annual Meeting of the American Society of Hematology, San Diego, December 6–9, 2003.

8. Wilson WH, Bryant G, Bates S, et al. EPOCH chemotherapy: toxicity and efficacy in relapsed and refractory non-Hodgkin's lymphoma. *J Clin Oncol* 1993;11:1573–1582.

9. Wilson WH, Grossbard ML, Pittaluga S, et al. Dose-adjusted EPOCH chemotherapy for untreated large B-cell lymphomas: a pharmacodynamic approach with high efficacy. *Blood* 2002;99: 2685–2693.

10. Kaiser U, Uebelacker I, Abel U, et al. Randomized study to evaluate the use of high-dose therapy as part of primary treatment for "aggressive" lymphoma. *J Clin Oncol* 2002;20:4413–4419.

11. Kewalramani T, Zelenetz AD, Nimer SD, et al. Rituximab and ICE (RICE) as second-line therapy prior to autologous stem cell transplantation for relapsed or primary refractory diffuse large B-cell lymphoma. *Blood* 2004;103:3684–3688.

12. Velasquez WS, Cabanillas F, Salvador P, et al. Effective salvage therapy for lymphoma with cisplatin in combination with high-dose Ara-C and dexamethasone (DHAP). *Blood* 1988;71:117–122.

13. Velasquez WS, McLaughlin P, Tucker S, et al. ESHAP—an effective chemotherapy regimen in refractory and relapsing lymphoma: a 4-year follow-up study. *J Clin Oncol* 1994;12:1169–1176.

14. Tilly H, Lepage E, Coiffier B, et al. Intensive conventional chemotherapy (ACVBP regimen) compared with standard CHOP for poor-prognosis aggressive non-Hodgkin lymphoma. *Blood* 2003;102: 4284–4289.

15. Thomas DA, Cortes J, O'Brien S, et al. Hyper-CVAD program in Burkitt's-type adult acute lymphoblastic leukemia. *J Clin Oncol* 1999;17:2461–2470.

16. Magrath I, Adde M, Shad A, et al. Adults and children with small non-cleaved-cell lymphoma have a similar excellent outcome when treated with the same chemotherapy regimen. *J Clin Oncol* 1996; 14:925–934.

17. Mead GM, Sydes MR, Walewski J, et al. An international evaluation of CODOX-M and CODOX-M alternating with IVAC in adult Burkitt's lymphoma: results of United Kingdom Lymphoma Group LY06 study. *Ann Oncol* 2002;13:1264–1274.

18. Kaplan LD, Straus DJ, Testa MA, et al. Low-dose compared with standard-dose m-BACOD chemotherapy for non-Hodgkin's lymphoma associated with human immunodeficiency virus infection. National Institute of Allergy and Infectious Diseases AIDS Clinical Trials Group. *N Engl J Med* 1997;336:1641–1648.

19. Ratner L, Lee J, Tang S, et al. Chemotherapy for human immunodeficiency virus-associated non-Hodgkin's lymphoma in combination with highly active antiretroviral therapy. *J Clin Oncol* 2001; 19:2171–2178.

20. Sparano J, lee S, Chen M, et al. Phase II trial of infusional cyclophosphamide, doxorubicin, & etoposide (CDE) in HIV-associated non-Hodgkin's lymphoma (NHL): an Eastern Cooperative Oncology Group (ECOG) Trial (E1494). Third Annual AIDS Malignancy Conference, Bethesda, MD, May 26–27, 1999.

21. Tirelli U, Spina M, Jaeger U, et al. Infusional CDE with rituximab for the treatment of human immunodeficiency virus-associated non-Hodgkin's lymphoma: preliminary results of a phase I/II study. *Recent Results Cancer Res* 2002;159:149–153.

22. Little RF, Pittaluga S, Grant N, et al. Highly effective treatment of acquired immunodeficiency syndrome-related lymphoma with dose-adjusted EPOCH: impact of antiretroviral therapy suspension and tumor biology. *Blood* 2003;101:4653–4659.

17

Multiple Myeloma

Sandeep S. Dave and Cynthia E. Dunbar

The epidemiology and risk factors of multiple myeloma are (1–3):

- Annual incidence in the United States is approximately 4 per 100,000.
- There is a slight male predominance and the incidence in African Americans is almost twice that in Caucasians.
- Median age at diagnosis is 66 years.
- The role of genetic factors is uncertain. There have been a few reported cases of familial clustering, but the vast majority of cases are sporadic.
- Exposure to radiation may play a role. An increased incidence has been noted in atomic bomb survivors exposed to more than 50 Gy, as well in workers in nuclear power plants.
- There is little evidence to implicate other environmental causes.

PATHOPHYSIOLOGY

- Multiple myeloma is characterized by the proliferation and accumulation of clonal plasma cells. The presence of somatic mutations in the complementarity determining regions (the antigen binding portion) of the clonal immunoglobulin indicates the transforming event occurred in a postgerminal center B cell or a plasma cell itself (1).
- The commonest chromosomal abnormality involves the heavy chain locus on chromosome 14, but there is no single cytogenetic abnormality that is characteristic of the disease. Chromosome 13 abnormalities are also common and associated with poor prognosis.
- At the gene-expression level, monoclonal gammopathy of unknown significance (MGUS) cannot be distinguished from multiple myeloma. However, normal plasma cells can be clearly distinguished from plasma cells of both MGUS and myeloma (4).
- The clinical features of the disease result from bone marrow infiltration by the malignant clone, secretion of osteoclast-activating factors and cytokines, high levels of circulating immunoglobulin and/or free light chains, and depressed immunity.

DIAGNOSIS AND CLINICAL FEATURES
Clinical Features (2,5)

- The most common presenting symptom is bone pain, found in 60% of patients. Pain is most frequent in the back or chest.
- Weakness and fatigue are common and are often associated with a normochromic, normocytic anemia.
- Twenty-five percent of patients have renal insufficiency.
- Twenty percent of patients have hypercalcemia.
- Less than 5% of patients have clinically significant amyloidosis or hyperviscosity.

Diagnostic Criteria

The following minimal criteria have been established for diagnosis (6):

- Ten percent of plasma cells in the bone marrow or a plasmacytoma and one of the following:
- More than 3 g/dL of serum monoclonal protein (M-protein) or
- Urine M-protein or
- Lytic bone lesions

The distribution of monoclonal protein type in multiple myeloma patients is as follows:

- Immunoglobulin (Ig) G in 60% of patients
- Light chain only (Bence-Jones proteinuria) in 20% of patients
- IgA in 17% of patients
- IgD in 2% of patients
- Biclonal in 1% of patients

Bone marrow involvement can be quite patchy. Repeated bone marrow biopsies may be needed to make the diagnosis.

STAGING OF MULTIPLE MYELOMA

The Durie-Salmon Staging System (Table 17-1) is based on factors related to tumor burden. The system does not correlate well with prognosis because the majority of patients are stage III at diagnosis. Other prognostic factors have shown better predictive value, including β_2 microglobulin, lactate dehydrogenase (LDH), and the presence or absence of chromosome 13 abnormalities.

INITIAL EVALUATION

- Complete history and physical examination.
- Blood counts with differential and examination of the peripheral smear.
- Serum electrolytes, blood urea nitrogen (BUN), and creatinine.
- Calcium, magnesium, and phosphorus.
- Uric acid.
- β_2 microglobulin.
- Serum lactate dehydrogenase (LDH).
- Serum protein electrophoresis (SPEP) with immunofixation and quantitation of immunoglobulins.

TABLE. 17–1. *Durie-Salmon staging system*

Stage I (myeloma mass, $<0.6 \times 10^{12}$ cells/m²)	All of the following: Hgb, >10 g/dL; serum Ca, ≤12 mg/dL; ≤1 lesion on skeletal survey; IgG M-protein, <50 g/L; IgA M-protein, <30 g/L; urinary light chains, <4 g/24 hours
Stage II (myeloma mass, 0.6–1.2 × 10¹² cells/m²)	Results fit neither stage I nor stage III
Stage III (myeloma mass, >1.2 × 10¹² cells/m²)	Any of the following: Hgb, ≤8.5 g/dL; serum Ca, >12 mg/dL; >1 lesion on skeletal survey; IgG M-protein, >70 g/L; IgA M-protein, >50 g/L; urinary light chain excretion, >12 g/24 hours
Subclassification A	Serum creatinine, <2 mg/dL
Subclassification B	Serum creatinine, ≥2 mg/dL

Hgb, hemoglobin; Ca, calcium; IgG, immunoglobulin G; IgM, immunoglobulin M.

- Urine protein electrophoresis (UPEP) and quantitation of light chains.
- Radiographic skeletal survey.
- Bone marrow biopsy and aspirate, with standard cytogenetics, and if possible FISH (fluorescent in situ hybridization) analysis for chromosome 13 abnormalities. Standard cytogenetics are much less sensitive.
- Consider magnetic resonance imaging (MRI) of the spine, in particular if there are any symptoms of back pain or suggestive neurologic findings.

SPEP alone is inadequate because some forms of multiple myeloma only secrete light chains, which are rapidly cleared to the urine.

A nuclear medicine bone scan is of no value because the disease produces osteolytic and not osteoblastic bone lesions.

DIFFERENTIAL DIAGNOSIS

MGUS is characterized by:

- M-protein less than 3 g/dL.
- Less than 10% plasma cells in the bone marrow.
- Lack of symptoms.
- Normal blood counts and renal function.
- Absence of lytic lesions and evidence of end-organ involvement.

Approximately 1% of patients per year will experience progression to typical multiple myeloma.

Smoldering multiple myeloma (SMM) is characterized by:

- M-protein greater than 3 g/dL and/or greater than 10% plasma cells in the bone marrow.
- Lack of symptoms.
- Absence of lytic lesions and evidence of end-organ involvement.

Approximately 3% of patients per year will experience progression to typical multiple myeloma. Factors predicting progression include greater than 10% plasma cells in the bone marrow, detectable Bence-Jones proteinuria, and IgA subtype.

Primary Amyloidosis

This disease also is a clonal expansion of plasma cells resulting in the overproduction of monoclonal light chains. However, the clinical manifestations are different and result from specific characteristics of the light chains that lead to their deposition as amyloid fibrils and multi-organ involvement. The proportion of bone marrow plasma cells may exceed 10% but rarely is more than 20%. Lytic lesions are rare. The diagnosis is established by demonstrating the deposition of amyloid in a biopsy of affected tissue.

Metastatic Carcinoma

A number of malignant processes can produce lytic lesions and plasmacytosis. In the absence of significant M-protein in the blood or urine, the diagnosis of metastatic carcinoma must be excluded before the diagnosis of multiple myeloma is established.

TREATMENT

Not all patients who fulfill the minimal criteria for the diagnosis of multiple myeloma should be treated. SMM or asymptomatic stage I multiple myeloma often remains stable over many years, and has not been shown to prolong survival or to prevent progression in presymptomatic disease therapy.

The main options include conventional chemotherapy, high-dose corticosteroids, dose-intensive chemotherapy with autologous hematopoietic cell rescue, allogeneic stem cell transplantation, as well as newer therapies such as thalidomide or its analogs or the proteosome inhibitor bortezomib. Biphosphonate treatments can prevent or slow bone destruction and may also have antitumor activity.

No modality with the possible exception of allogeneic stem cell transplantation is curative in multiple myeloma. However, event-free survival and overall survival are improved by approximately a year after autologous hematopoietic stem cell transplantation (HSCT) compared to conventional chemotherapy, and newer agents such as thalidomide and bortezmib are effective in a significant percentage of patients with relapsed or refractory disease. The management of myeloma has become more complicated with this expanding set of alternatives, but the lack of overlapping toxicities means that many patients even with advanced disease can be managed effectively as outpatients with reasonable quality of life.

Treatment regimens are summarized in Table 17-2; a flow chart summarizing options for patients is shown in Figure 17-1 (6,7).

INITIAL THERAPY

All patients younger than 60 to 70 years of age should be considered for high-dose chemotherapy with autologous stem cell transplantation as consolidation after initial treatment. The most convincing data regarding survival advantage for transplantation is in patients younger than 55 to 60, with somewhat conflicting evidence in the 60 to 70 year age group. In symptomatic patients older than 70 and in younger patients who are not candidates for transplantation, chemotherapy with alkylating agents such as oral melphalan remains standard. More aggressive chemotherapy regimens such as VMBCP (vincristine, melphalan, bischloroethylnitrosourea (BCNU)/carmustine, cyclophosphamide, and prednisone), VMCP, VBAP (adriamycin), have failed to demonstrate consistent superiority over melphalan and prednisone (8–10).

Alkylating agents damage hematopoietic stem cells and autologous hematopoietic cells should be collected from the peripheral blood or bone marrow prior to any exposure to alkylators if autologous transplantation is a possible future treatment option. Stem cell-sparing options include high dose dexamethasone alone, or in combination with thalidomide or vincristine and adriamycin. High-dose decadron alone is also useful for patients requiring concurrent radiation therapy or in those with significant marrow involvement and cytopenias.

- Chemotherapy should be administered for at least three cycles and, in responders, continued until the disease reaches a plateau phase. However, more than five to six cycles is generally not necessary and in the case of alkylating agents, is associated with a higher risk of secondary myelodysplastic syndrome/acute myeloid leukemia (MDS/AML).
- The plateau phase is defined as a stable M-protein in the serum and the lack of evidence of disease progression. Partial remission is defined at more than 50% reduction in serum paraprotein or more than 90% reduction in urine light chains. Complete remission is defined as no detectable serum or urine paraprotein and marrow plasma cells less than 5%. Complete remission (CR) is extremely rare with conventional chemotherapy but can be reached in 20% to 50% of patients following a single or a double autograft.
- There is no evidence of additional efficacy of chemotherapy once patients enter a plateau phase. The value of continuation of maintenance thalidomide or pulse steroids is under investigation.
- Continued treatment may result in the development of resistance to therapy and increases the risk of myelodysplasia.
- Overall survival is significantly impacted by the ability to achieve an objective response, even if it is partial.

The combination of oral melphalan and prednisone produces a response in about 50% of patients, with rare CR. Median survival is roughly 3 years in responders (11). In patients

TABLE. 17–2. *Treatment regimens*

Regimen	Treatment description	Toxicities
Melphalan + prednisone (MP)	Melphalan, 10 mg/m^2 per day PO for 4 days (day 1–4; total dose/cycle, 40 mg/m^2) + Prednisone, 60 mg/m^2 per day PO for 4 days (day 1–4; total dose/cycle, 40 mg/m^2) Cycle duration, 4–6 weeks. Start at low doses and increase if tolerated. Decrease doses if myelosuppression is prolonged.	Myelosuppression. Therapy-related myelodysplastic syndrome.
Vincristine + adriamycin + dexamethasone (VAD)	Vincristine, 0.4 mg/day continuous IV infusion for 4 days (day 1–4; total dose/cycle, 1.6 mg) Doxorubicin, 9 mg/m^2 per day continuous IV infusion for 4 days (day 1–4; total dose/cycle, 36 mg/m^2) Dexamethasone, 40 mg per day PO for 4 days, repeated every 8 days (day 1–4, 9–12, and 17–20; total dose/cycle, 480 mg) Cycle repeats every 25 days	GI and myelotoxicity
High-dose chemotherapy and autologous stem cell transplantation	Conditioning regimen: Melphalan, 200 mg/m^2 IV as a single agent	Mucositis Up to 5% transplant-related mortality
Interferon-α	Interferon-α, 3 million units/m^2 SC, three doses/wk (total dose/wk, 9 million units/m^2)	CNS changes, cytopenias, fever and myalgias
Thalidomide	Dosing is not thoroughly established. Doses 400 mg/day needed for relapsed/refractory disease. Smaller doses (<400 mg/day) may be sufficient for untreated disease.	Peripheral neuropathy (dose-limiting toxicity). Somnolence, constipation, higher incidence of deep venous thrombosis when used in combination with adriamycin containing regimens. Consider placing such patients on prophylactic low molecular weight heparin.
Bortezomib	1.3 mg/m^2 as an IV bolus 2×/week for 2 weeks, on days 1, 4, 8, and 11 in a 21-day cycle.	Thrombocytopenia, GI symptoms, fatigue, and sensory neuropathy.
Pamidronate	Pamidronate, 90 mg IV infusion over 2–4 hours, monthly	Fever, nausea, hypokalemia, hypocalcemia
Zolendronic acid	Zolendronic acid 4 mg IV infusion over 15 minutes, monthly	Renal toxicity has been reported with higher doses and shorter infusions, Fatigue, fever, hypophosphatemia, hypokalemia

IV, intravenously; PO, orally; SC, subcutaneously; GI, gastrointestinal; CNS, central nervous system.

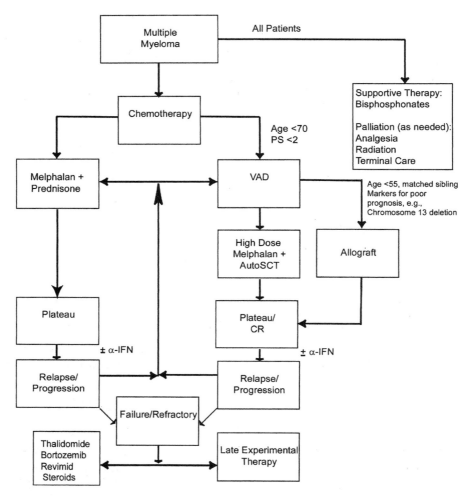

FIG. 17-1. Treatment Strategy (Adapted from UK Myeloma Forum. British Committee for Standards in Haematology. Diagnosis and management of multiple myeloma. *Br J Haematol* 2001; 99:3163–3168.)

with renal insufficiency (creatine clearance less than 50% of predicted), the melphalan dose should be reduced by 25% to prevent severe myelosuppression. The dose can be gradually escalated in the following courses if severe myelosuppression does not occur. At least three courses (or 3 months) of initial therapy should be administered before disease is deemed refractory.

Vincristine, adriamycin, and dexamethasone (VAD) has been used as initial therapy, often in the setting of preparation for autologous stem cell transplantation with response rates comparable to melphalan plus prednisone. Typically three to four cycles of VAD are administered prior to transplantation (12).

AUTOLOGOUS TRANSPLANTATION

- Several trials have shown a survival advantage of approximately a year for autologous transplantation over conventional chemotherapy (13).
- Data from a randomized trial show that there is no survival benefit to early transplantation versus late transplantation, although up-front autotransplantation resulted in a longer progression-free survival (14).
- There are conflicting data on whether tandem (two transplants back-to-back) autologous transplantation is better than conventional single autologous transplantation; a recent controlled trial showed benefit for tandem transplants (15).
- Melphalan, 200 mg/m^2 without radiation is considered the standard induction regimen (16).
- There in no proven benefit to purging the graft of tumor cells by either positive stem cell selection or antibody removal of tumor cells.
- In patients older than age 70 and in patients with renal failure, melphalan is frequently dose-reduced to 140 mg/m^2 or 100 mg/m^2 to decrease toxicity. Thus age and renal failure are not absolute contraindications to autologous transplantation approaches.
- Treatment-related mortality should be less than 5%. Younger patients can receive outpatient transplants.

ALLOGENEIC TRANSPLANTATION

- After being screened for the presence of a human leukocyte antigen (HLA)-matched sibling donor, and assessing cardiac, pulmonary and renal function, only approximately 10% of patients with multiple myeloma are candidates for standard myeloablative allogeneic transplantation.
- Although allogenic transplantation has the advantages of a tumor-free graft and the ability to effect a graft-versus-myeloma affect, the majority of patients who undergo allogeneic transplantation still relapse. In a series of 80 patients with newly diagnosed disease, as well as in relapse, treated with allogeneic transplantation, only 5 patients were in continuous remission at 4 to 7 years after transplantation (17).
- Patients with myeloma patients have increased treatment-related mortality from allogeneic transplantation, with high rates of serious infection presumed caused by poor underlying immune function secondary to their disease.
- Nonmyeloablative strategies as well approaches that decrease the likelihood of graft-versus-host disease, such as T-cell depletion, may improve outcomes in allogeneic transplantation. At some centers, initial autografts in high-risk patients may be immediately followed by a nonablative allograft.

Thalidomide

Thalidomide alone or in combination with dexamethasone has been studied primarily in refractory or relapsed disease. Inclusion of thalidomide in initial treatment regimens does not appear to diminish the success of later stem cell collection. In previously untreated patients, thalidomide and dexamethasone produced response rates of 36% (thalidomide alone) and 72% (both drugs), suggesting synergy between the two drugs (18).

MAINTENANCE THERAPY

Interferon-α

Data from the clinical trials are conflicting. Several have shown a benefit from interferon-α with increased freedom from progression for 6 to 12 months, other trials have shown no such benefit (19). A large number of patients are unable to tolerate the usual doses and a majority need to either reduce the dose or discontinue the drug altogether. At present, interferon maintenance is rarely utilized

Thalidomide

Thalidomide alone or in combination with corticosteroids is being investigated for use as maintenance in patients responding to autologous transplantation.

Corticosteroids

Prednisone as a maintenance therapy has only been studied in patients responsive to VAD. In this setting, both progression-free survival and overall survival were higher in patients receiving maintenance with prednisone 50 mg each day compared to 10 mg each day.

RELAPSED OR REFRACTORY DISEASE THERAPY

Patients who respond to their initial regimen will eventually relapse. If postchemotherapy relapse occurs more than 6 months after the plateau state has been achieved, the original regimen can be reinstated. Most patients will respond, but the response tends to be shorter in duration and more attenuated than initially. The highest rates of response in patients refractory to alkylating agents have been reported with VAD. At present, most relapsed patients are treated with thalidomide, with or without corticosteroids.

CHEMOTHERAPY

- VAD is most frequently used. Patients with relapsed or refractory disease had a response rate of 61% and median survival of 10 months.
- VMBCP and VBAP both produce response rates similar to those observed with VAD.

Thalidomide

- Thalidomide as a single agent produced a response in approximately 30% of patients with relapsed or refractory disease (20).
- In combination with dexamethasone, the response rate can be increased to 48% in this setting.
- Toxicities are frequent, including fatigue, constipation, and peripheral neuropathy.

Cortiscosteroids

Dexamethasone and intravenous pulsed methylprednisolone have produced response rates as high as 38% (21).

Bortezomid

- This proteosome inhibitor was shown to result in an overall response rate of 35% in a group of patients with at least two prior therapies (22).
- The dose-limiting toxicity is thrombocytopenia.

Revimid

This thalidomide analogue is undergoing phase 2/3 trials, and preliminary results indicate a response rate of approximately 30% in a group of heavily pretreated patients whose prior therapies included thalidomide (23).

SUPPORTIVE MEASURES

Bisphosphonates

- Bisphosophonates have been widely used for the treatment and prevention of osteoporosis and in the therapy of hypercalcemia.
- Bisphosophonates given at appropriate doses can prevent skeletal complications and improve quality of life in patients with advanced myeloma. There also is evidence for a survival benefit (24).
- Both intravenous pamidronate and zolendronic acid appear to be equally effective in preventing skeletal complication, with similar rates of renal toxicity.
- Oral bisphosophonates have failed to demonstrate similar efficacy in placebo-controlled trials.
- In the absence of significant toxicity or declining performance status, monthly treatment with intravenous bisphosophonates is recommended for all patients with multiple myeloma who have bone disease.
- Treatment should be continued even if a skeletal event develops during treatment.
- Bisphosphonates are frequently used in patients without bone disease, but prospective clinical trials documenting efficacy in this setting are lacking.
- Multiple in vitro and biologic studies indicate the potential for an antimyeloma effect, by stimulation of immune function or inhibition of interactions between myeloma cells and their microenvironment.

RADIATION

- Local radiation has a palliative role for symptomatic focal lesions. If pain is the sole symptom and there is no impending fracture or cord compression, responses to chemotherapy and in particular high-dose decadron can be equally rapid and effective.
- Radiation should be avoided to major bone-marrow regions in order to collect adequate hematopoietic stem cells as needed. Systemic therapy with dexamethasone and/or thalidomide can be undertaken while local irradiation is administered.

SURGICAL OPTIONS

Vertebroplasty and kyphoplasty are both frequently employed and effective in alleviating symptoms from vertebral collapse.

SPECIAL CONSIDERATIONS

Renal Failure

- Renal failure is usually multifactorial, secondary to light-chain nephrotoxicity, volume depletion, and hypercalcemia.
- Patients are treated with intravenous hydration, loop diuretics if hypercalcemia is present, chemotherapy (typically high-dose pulse dexamethasone because of more rapid onset of action as compared to melphalan and prednisone) to decrease light chain production.
- Dialysis is used as necessary.
- With the use of these modalities, at least partial recovery of renal function is possible in the majority of patients, with the exception of those with significant amyloid deposition.
- Plasmapheresis may be used to decrease serum light chains (if detected on SPEP) but can only temporize until systemic therapy decreases their production.

Hyperviscosity Syndrome

- Hyperviscosity syndrome should be suspected in patients with unexplained mental changes, worsening respiratory status, renal insufficiency, or bleeding.

- The syndrome is more common in the IgA and IgG3 subtypes.
- Diagnosis is made by measuring serum viscosity.
- Plasmapheresis is effective for symptomatic hyperviscosity and should be continued until the serum viscosity has normalized. Therapy with a regimen containing high dose dexamethasone results in the most rapid decrease in paraprotein production and should be used instead of melphalan and prednisone in patients with hyperviscosity.

Anemia

- Erythropoietin has been shown to significantly decrease the frequency of transfusions, and improve performance status and quality of life in anemic multiple myeloma patients.
- The greatest incremental improvement in quality of life occurs in patients with mild anemia (hemoglobin levels of 11 to 12 g/dL). Thus, all anemic patients who respond to erythropoietin should be treated until their hemoglobin levels exceed 13 g/dL.

Follow-Up of Monoclonal Gammopathy of Unknown Significance and Smoldering Multiple Myeloma

Because both MGUS and SMM have a small but significant risk of progression to multiple myeloma, it is important to periodically evaluate patients with these conditions. The frequency of monitoring is based on the concentration of M-protein.

- If the serum M-protein is less than 2 g/dL with no other evidence of multiple myeloma, then the M-protein should be rechecked in 6 months, then annually if stable.
- If the serum M-protein is more than 2 g/dL with no other evidence of multiple myeloma, the M-protein should be rechecked in 3 months, then annually if stable.

Solitary Plasmacytoma

- Plasmacytomas are tumors that are composed of plasma cells that are histologically identical to those seen in multiple myeloma.
- Overt multiple myeloma must be excluded in all patients.
- Patients with soft tissue plasmacytomas can be cured with local radiation.
- A majority of patients with solitary plasmacytomas of the bone develop systemic disease after receiving local radiation, suggesting that the presumed plasmacytoma is part of the systemic disease.

Plasma Cell Leukemia

- A rare disease variant of multiple myeloma, occurring in approximately 2% to 4% of all cases.
- Approximately 60% of the cases present as primary disease.
- The diagnosis is made when the circulating plasma cell count is greater than 2000 per microliter, in addition to fulfilling all the criteria for multiple myeloma.
- The prognosis is extremely poor, with median survival less than a year. Transplantation should be considered.

REFERENCES

1. Hallek M, Bergsagel PL, Anderson KC. Multiple myeloma: increasing evidence for a multistep transformation process. *Blood* 1998;91:3–21.
2. Riedel DA, Pottern LM. The epidemiology of multiple myeloma. *Hematol Oncol Clin North Am* 1992;6:225–247.

3. Lynch HT, Sanger WG, Pirruccello S, et al. Familial multiple myeloma: a family study and review of the literature. *J Natl Cancer Inst* 2001;93:1479–1483.

4. Zhan F, Hardin J, Kordsmeier B, et al. Global gene expression profiling of multiple myeloma, monoclonal gammopathy of undetermined significance, and normal bone marrow plasma cells. *Blood* 2002;99:745–757.

5. Kyle RA, Gertz MA, Witzig TE, et al. Review of 1027 patients with newly diagnosed multiple myeloma. *Mayo Clin Proc* 2003;78:21–33.

6. UK Myeloma Forum. British Committee for Standards in Haematology. Diagnosis and management of multiple myeloma. *Br J Haematol* 2001;115:522–540.

7. Barlogie B, Shaughnessy J, Tricot G, et al. Treatment of multiple myeloma. *Blood* 2004;103:20–32.

8. Case DC Jr, Lee DJ III, Clarkson BD. Improved survival times in multiple myeloma treated with melphalan, prednisone, cyclophosphamide, vincristine and BCNU: M-2 protocol. *Am J Med* 1977; 63:897–903.

9. Oken MM, Harrington DP, Abramson N, et al. Comparison of melphalan and prednisone with vincristine, carmustine, melphalan, cyclophosphamide, and prednisone in the treatment of multiple myeloma: results of Eastern Cooperative Oncology Group Study E2479. *Cancer* 1997;79:1561–1567.

10. Combination chemotherapy versus melphalan plus prednisone as treatment for multiple myeloma: an overview of 6,633 patients from 27 randomized trials. Myeloma Trialists' Collaborative Group. *J Clin Oncol* 1998;16:3832–3842.

11. Blade J, Lopez-Guillermo A, Bosch F, et al. Impact of response to treatment on survival in multiple myeloma: results in a series of 243 patients. *Br J Haematol* 1994;88:117–121.

12. Anderson, H, Scarffe JH, Ransom M, et al. VAD chemotherapy as remission induction for multiple myeloma. *Br J Cancer* 1995;71:326–330.

13. Child JA, Morgan GJ, Davies, FE, et al. High-dose chemotherapy with hematopoietic stem-cell rescue for multiple myeloma. *N Engl J Med* 2003;348:1875–1883.

14. Fermand JP, Ravaud P, Chevret S, et al. High-dose therapy and autologous peripheral blood stem cell transplantation in multiple myeloma: up-front or rescue treatment? Results of a multicenter sequential randomized clinical trial. *Blood* 1998;92:3131–3136.

15. Attal M, Harousseau JL, Facon T, et al. Single versus double autologous stem-cell transplantation for multiple myeloma. *N Engl J Med* 2003;349:2495–2502.

16. Moreau P, Facon T, Attal M, et al. Comparison of 200 mg/m(2) melphalan and 8 Gy total body irradiation plus 140 mg/m(2) melphalan as conditioning regimens for peripheral blood stem cell transplantation in patients with newly diagnosed multiple myeloma: final analysis of the Intergroupe Francophone du Myelome 9502 randomized trial. *Blood* 2002;99:731–735.

17. Bensinger WI, Maloney D, Storb R. Allogeneic hematopoietic cell transplantation for multiple myeloma. *Semin Hematol* 2001;38:243–249.

18. Weber D, Rankin K, Gavino M, et al. Thalidomide alone or with dexamethasone for previously untreated multiple myeloma. *J Clin Oncol* 2003;21:16–19.

19. Browman GP, Berggsagel D, Sicheri D, et al. Randomized trial of interferon maintenance in multiple myeloma: a study of the National Cancer Institute of Canada Clinical Trials Group. *J Clin Oncol* 1995;13:2354–2360.

20. Singhal S, Mehta J, Desikan R, et al. Antitumor activity of thalidomide in refractory multiple myeloma. *N Engl J Med* 1999;34:1565–1571.

21. Gertz MA, Garton JP, Greipp PR, et al. A phase II study of high-dose methylprednisolone in refractory or relapsed multiple myeloma. *Leukemia* 1995;9:2115–2118.

22. Richardson PG, Barlogie B, Berenson J, et al. A phase 2 study of bortezomib in relapsed, refractory myeloma. *N Engl J Med* 2003;348:2609–2617.

23. Richardson PG, Schlossman RL, Weller E, et al. Immunomodulatory drug CC-5013 overcomes drug resistance and is well tolerated in patients with relapsed multiple myeloma. *Blood* 2002;100: 3063–3067.

24. Kyle RA. The role of bisphosphonates in multiple myeloma. Ann Intern Med 2000;132:734–736.

18

Hematopoietic Stem Cell Transplantation

Richard Childs and Ramaprasad Srinivasan

AUTOLOGOUS HEMATOPOIETIC STEM CELL TRANSPLANTATION

Autologous hematopoietic stem cell transplantation (auto-HSCT) was conceived to overcome lethal hematopoietic toxicity associated with high-dose chemotherapy in the treatment of dose-responsive malignancies (1, 2). A role for auto-HSCT has been clearly established in the management of multiple myeloma and aggressive non-Hodgkin's lymphoma. Initial enthusiasm for this approach in solid tumors such as metastatic breast, ovarian and lung cancer has been tempered by the failure of prospective randomized trials to demonstrate benefit over conventional treatments. The role of auto-HSCT continues to be explored in neuroblastoma and Ewing's sarcoma.

General Considerations

- Most auto-HSCTs are performed using peripheral blood stem cells collected after mobilization with granulocyte colony-stimulating factor (G-CSF), with or without chemotherapy priming.
- Curative potential resides solely in the ability of high-dose chemotherapy to eradicate the underlying malignancy; no immune-mediated graft-versus tumor effects are generated.
- The high-dose chemotherapeutic regimen utilized is tailored to the malignancy based on its chemosensitivity profile; for instance, melphalan (200 mg/m^2) is the most widely used high-dose agent for multiple myeloma.
- Infections related to chemotherapy-induced neutropenia and immunosuppression and extramedullary toxicities from high-dose chemotherapeutic agents account for the majority of complications occurring after auto-HSCT.
- There is a low risk of treatment-related mortality, typically less than 5% in most series.
- Contamination of the stem cell product by malignant cells may limit the beneficial effects of high-dose chemotherapy.
- Efforts to purge tumor cells contaminating hematopoietic grafts by CD34$^+$ cell selection or by in vitro incubation of the stem cell graft with cytotoxic drugs remain investigational and have met with only moderate success.

Results of Autologous Hematopoietic Stem Cell Transplantation

Autologous Hematopoietic Cell Transplantation in Hematologic Malignancies

Multiple Myeloma

- Large phase II trials have demonstrated high response rates (complete response 30% to 50%) and impressive disease-free (DFS) and overall survival rates (OS) (median, more than 5 years).
- Randomized phase III trials in relatively young patients (less than 65 years of age) have shown superior response rates, DFS, and OS for auto-HSCT versus conventional chemotherapy (3).

- Consecutive or tandem auto-HSCTs are being evaluated, with at least one randomized study indicating a survival benefit for tandem as opposed to a single auto-HSCT.
- Auto-HSCT is currently considered standard for relatively young patients with myeloma. Mature data from several ongoing trials are needed to determine whether tandem transplants offer an advantage over a single auto-HSCT in these patients.

Non-Hodgkin's Lymphoma

- The benefit of auto-HSCT has been most clearly observed in intermediate- and high-grade non-Hodgkin's lymphoma (NHL).
- Auto-HSCT results in improved event-free and OS in patients with relapsed chemosensitive intermediate-/high-grade NHL, compared to conventional salvage therapy (4).
- Results from a recent randomized study suggest that initial treatment with auto-HSCT may benefit some patients with intermediate-/high-grade NHL, compared to standard treatment with cyclophosphamide, doxorubicin, vincristine, and prednisone (CHOP) chemotherapy.

Acute Myeloid Leukemia

- Auto-HCT has been used both as postremission therapy in acute myeloid leukemia (AML) in first complete remission (CR1) and as therapy after relapse.
- Phase III studies in patients in CR1 suggest an improvement in DFS but not OS, compared to conventional postremission therapy.
- The benefit derived from auto-HSCT appears to be restricted largely to AML with good-risk cytogenetics.

Autologous Hematopoietic Stem Cell Transplantation in Solid Tumors

The knowledge that some malignancies exhibited dose-dependent responses to chemotherapy led to the investigation of high-dose chemotherapy followed by auto-HCT in the treatment of solid tumors. Based on negative results from phase III trials, auto-HCT has been largely abandoned in the management of some malignancies (particularly metastatic breast cancer) but remains under investigation in several other solid tumor types.

Breast Cancer

- While promising results from phase II studies in patients with metastatic breast cancer paved the way for randomized phase III studies of auto-HSCT, larger studies unfortunately yielded negative results.
- At least seven large trials have compared auto-HSCT to standard chemotherapy in patients with metastatic breast cancer. Six demonstrated superior event-free survival with auto-HSCT, but none showed a survival advantage (5).
- Similar results were obtained in patients with high-risk breast cancer undergoing adjuvant auto-HSCT.
- Because of a lack of survival benefit and higher toxicity, there is little enthusiasm for further investigation of auto-HSCT in breast cancer.

Germ Cell Tumors

- Phase II trials of auto-HSCT in relapsed or refractory germ cell tumors have yielded response rates of 40% to 65% and long-term survival rates of 15% to 40%.
- Patients with progressive disease or human chorionic gonadotropin levels greater than 1000 IU/L at transplantation, mediastinal primaries, and refractoriness to cisplatin based therapy have a worse outcome and may not benefit from auto-HSCT.

- An interim report from a European Group for Blood and Marrow Transplantation study suggested no advantage for auto-HSCT over standard salvage chemotherapy in patients failing cisplatin-based chemotherapy.
- Randomized studies are currently in progress to evaluate the role of auto-HSCT as initial therapy in germ cell tumors at high-risk of relapse.

Other Tumors

- Although still under study, available data do not suggest a clear benefit for auto-HSCT in ovarian and lung cancers.
- When administered after an initial course of standard induction chemotherapy, auto-HSCT appears to improve short-term disease-free survival in neuroblastoma compared to conventional dose maintenance chemotherapy. However, a large randomized study was unable to demonstrate a survival advantage for patients undergoing auto-HSCT.
- Some patients with Ewing's sarcoma/primordial neurectodermal tumor (PNET) and other soft tissue sarcomas may benefit from high-dose chemotherapy. In the absence of evidence to support a survival benefit, patients should be treated with auto-HSCT only in the setting of a clinical trial.

ALLOGENEIC HEMATOPOIETIC STEM CELL TRANSPLANTATION

Allogeneic HSCT can cure patients with advanced chemotherapy-resistant hematologic malignancies (6–8). The first successful allogeneic HSCTs in humans were reported in 1968. These transplants were performed in children with congenital immune deficiencies, with donor stem cells from human leukocyte antigen (HLA)-compatible sibling donors. In the early years after the advent of allogeneic HSCT, immune deficiency syndromes and disorders of hematopoiesis constituted the major indications for the procedure; more recently, hematologic malignancies have become the usual reason for an allogeneic HSCT. Approximately 7,000 allogeneic HCTs are performed annually in North America for a wide array of both malignant and nonmalignant disorders.

Indications for Allogenetic Hematopoietic Stem Cell Transplantation

Allogeneic HCT has been used in both malignant and nonmalignant diseases (Table 18-1). The vast majority of patients undergoing allogeneic HSCT (approximately 75%) suffer an underlying hematologic malignancy (acute and chronic myelogenous leukemia, acute lymphocytic leukemia, and NHL being the most common). Nonmalignant conditions that are potentially curable by HSCT include disorders of hematopoiesis (e.g., aplastic anemia), immunodeficiency syndromes (e.g., Chediak-Higashi disease, severe combined immunodeficiency syndrome), congenital disorders of erythropoiesis (e.g., thalassemias), and inborn errors of metabolism (e.g., mucopolysaccharidoses). The advent of new treatment options for certain diseases (such as the tyrosine kinase inhibitor STI 571, which is effective in the treatment of chronic myelogenous leukemia) as well as improvements in the toxicity profile associated with HCT are likely to alter the indications for allogeneic transplantation.

Antileukemic Potential of Allogenetic Hematopoietic Stem Cell Transplantation: Underlying Principles

In the 1960s and 1970s, allogeneic HSCT was largely viewed as a means of ensuring immuno-hematopoietic reconstitution or replacement after administration of high doses of chemotherapy with or without radiation. This premise still applies to the treatment of nonmalignant conditions, where the major goal is to provide normal cellular components to replace or rectify an underlying deficiency. For hematologic malignancies, the dose-intensive prepara-

TABLE. 18–1. *Indications for hematopoietic stem cell transplantation*

Acute leukemias
Acute lymphoblastic leukemia (ALL)
Acute myelogenous leukemia (AML)

Chronic leukemias
Chronic myelogenous leukemia (CML)
Chronic lymphocytic leukemia (CLL)
Juvenile chronic myelogenous leukemia (JCML)
Juvenile myelomonocytic leukemia (JMML)

Myelodysplastic syndromes
Refractory anemia (RA)
Refractory anemia with ringed sideroblasts (RARS)
Refractory anemia with excess blasts (RAEB)
Refractory anemia with excess blasts
   in transformation (RAEB-T)

Chronic myelomonocytic leukemia (CMML)

Stem cell disorders
Aplastic anemia (severe)
Fanconi anemia
Paroxysmal nocturnal hemoglobinuria (PNH)
Pure red cell aplasia

Myeloproliferative disorders
Acute myelofibrosis
Agnogenic myeloid metaplasia (myelofibrosis)
Polycythemia vera
Essential thrombocythemia

Lymphoproliferative disorders
Non-Hodgkin's lymphoma
Hodgkin's disease

Phagocyte disorders
Chediak-Higashi syndrome
Chronic granulomatous disease
Neutrophil actin deficiency
Reticular dysgenesis

Inherited metabolic disorders
Mucopolysaccharidoses (MPS)
Hurler's syndrome (MPS-IH)
Scheie syndrome (MPS-IS)
Hunter's syndrome (MPS-II)
Sanfilippo syndrome (MPS-III)
Morquio syndrome (MPS-IV)
Maroteaux-Lamy syndrome (MPS-VI)
Sly Syndrome, β-C glucoronidase
   deficiency (MPS-VII)
Adrenoleukodystrophy
Mucolipidosis II (I-cell disease)
Krabbe disease
Gaucher's disease
Niemann-Pick disease
Wolman disease
Metachromatic leukodystrophy

Histiocytic disorders
Familial erythrophagocytic lymphohistiocytosis
Histiocytosis-X
Hemophagocytosis

Inherited erythrocyte abnormalities
β-Thalassemia major
Sickle cell disease

Inherited immune system disorders
Ataxia-telangiectasia
Kostmann syndrome
Leukocyte adhesion deficiency
DiGeorge syndrome

Bare lymphocyte syndrome

Omenn's syndrome
Severe combined immunodeficiency (SCID)
SCID with adenosine deaminase deficiency
Absence of T & B Cells SCID
Absence of T cells, normal B cell SCID
Common variable immunodeficiency
Wiskott-Aldrich syndrome
X-linked lymphoproliferative disorder

Other inherited disorders
Lesch-Nyhan syndrome
Cartilage-Hair hypoplasia
Glanzmann thrombasthenia
Osteopetrosis

Inherited platelet abnormalities
Amegakaryocytosis/congenital thrombocytopenia

Plasma cell disorders
Multiple myeloma
Plasma cell leukemia
Waldenstrom's macroglobulinemia

Other malignancies
Breast cancer
Ewing sarcoma
Neuroblastoma
Renal cell carcinoma

(Adapted from list of transplant indications provided by the National Marrow Donor Program [NMDP])

tive or conditioning regimen was considered to be critical for the eradication of the underlying malignancy, with HLA-matched donor stem cells used merely to reverse the accompanying fatal bone marrow ablation. However, over the last two decades, it has become increasingly evident that a donor immune mediated anti-malignancy effect, termed graft-versus-leukemia (GVL) or graft-versus-tumor (GVT), is central for the successful eradication of malignancies after allogeneic HCT. The following clinical observations have provided incontrovertible evidence for the existence of GVL and highlight the role of donor T lymphocytes in mediating this effect (6,7,9–11):

- Decreased risk of leukemia relapse in patients experiencing acute or chronic graft-versus-host-disease (GVHD).
- Increased risk of leukemia relapse in patients undergoing T-cell–depleted transplants.
- Increased risk of leukemia relapse in recipients of a syngeneic as opposed to nontwin sibling donor allografts.
- Ability of donor lymphocyte infusions (DLI) to induce sustained remission in patients with chronic myeloid leukemia (CML) who relapse after transplantation.

Recognition of GVL has led to the recent development of low intensity or nonmyeloablative conditioning regimens, in which efficacy is largely dependent on the generation of donor immune mediated anti-tumor responses.

Planning Allogenetic Hematopoietic Stem Cell Transplantation

Allogeneic HSCT is a complex procedure requiring careful planning and a multidisciplinary approach to patient management. Factors including patient age, performance status, underlying disease, and donor availability need to be considered before decisions regarding the type of transplantation to be performed (e.g., conventional myeloablative versus nonmyeloablative) and GVHD prophylaxis regimen are made.

Evaluation of Transplant Recipients

- The degree of donor-host HLA-compatibilty is one of the most important factors affecting outcome after HSCT. Evaluation of the transplant recipient begins with HLA testing and a search for an appropriate donor. The initial donor search focuses on identifying a sibling matched at the allele level for HLA-A, B and DR loci. If a suitable sibling donor is not available, a search for an HLA-compatible unrelated donor can be made through the National Marrow Donor Program (NMDP).
- Thorough history and physical examination, with emphasis on the underlying diagnosis and its treatment, concomitant medical problems, performance status, transfusion history, and any history of opportunistic (particularly fungal) infections.
- Assessment of major organ function including pulmonary function testing and full cardiac evaluation.
- Serologic testing to detect prior exposure to cytomegalovirus, herpesvirus, Epstein-Barr virus, hepatitis viruses, HIV, and varicella.
- Counseling to focus on the potential benefits and risks of transplantation, need for a dedicated caregiver, and, when appropriate, fertility prospects.

Identification of a Suitable Donor

- Matched related donor: approximately one-third of patients screened will have a suitable HLA-compatible sibling donor. While donors with a less than complete (6/6) HLA match can be used, greater HLA disparity increases the risk of both graft rejection and GVHD.
- Syngeneic donor: identical twin transplants are rarely performed because high degrees of histocompatibility (including for minor histocompatibility antigens) minimize clinically

meaningful GVL effects. Syngeneic donors are most desirable in the transplantation of nonmalignant diseases (such as severe aplastic anemia) where GVL is not required.

- Matched unrelated donor (MUD): the NMPD search identifies a suitable donor for two-thirds of Caucasians. Some minority groups are much harder to match. The process should be initiated as early as possible because the time to transplant once a search is initiated is typically 3 to 4 months. For a given degree of donor-host HLA-disparity, the risk of GVHD is higher with unrelated compared with related donors.
- Haplo-identical donor: most patients have a sibling, parent, or child with one matched HLA haplotype who could serve as donor. Transplants from haplo-identical donors are associated with a higher incidence of GVHD, necessitating T-cell depletion in most circumstances to prevent life-threatening GVHD.
- Umbilical cord cells: blood collected from the placenta at the time of childbirth can be used as a source of hematopoietic stem cells. While umbilical cord transplants are associated with a lower incidence of GVHD (even with HLA mismatching), their wide use is limited by an increased risk of graft failure owing to the small numbers of stem cells harvested. Umbilical cord transplants are usually limited to children and young adolescents.

Procurement of Hematopoietic Stem Cells

The majority of hematopoietic stem cells reside within the bone marrow, which traditionally served as the source of the allograft. However, the ability of G-CSF to mobilize hematopoietic stem cells into the circulation has led to the widespread use of peripheral blood stem cell allografts.

- Obtaining stem cells from the bone marrow involves multiple aspirations from the iliac crests, a relatively safe procedure performed under general anesthesia.
- Mobilized stem cells are typically collected from the peripheral blood by apheresis after administration of G-CSF (10 to 15 μg/kg per day) for 4 to 6 days.
- G-CSF mobilized peripheral blood stem cell (PBSC) grafts usually contain higher numbers of $CD34^+$ progenitor cells as well as T cells ($CD3^+$ cells) compared to bone marrow grafts.
- Compared to bone marrow stem cells, transplants using PBSCs are associated with faster neutrophil and platelet engraftment, a reduction in transfusion requirements, and a similar incidence of acute GVHD. In patients with an underlying hematologic malignancy, PBSC transplants also appear to result in a survival advantage compared to bone marrow transplants.
- Given the ease of stem cell collection from both the practitioner and the donor perspectives, the higher progenitor cell yield, earlier engraftment, and a possible survival advantage, the majority of allogeneic HCTs worldwide employ mobilized peripheral blood as a source of hematopoietic stem cells.

Conditioning Regimen

A variety of conditioning regimens have been used in allogeneic HCT. The choice of conditioning regimen for a given patient is dictated by the underlying disease, the age of the patient, the presence of medical comorbidity, and the donor characteristics (especially the degree of HLA-compatibility). Table 18-2 lists some commonly used conditioning regimens.

Conventional or Myeloablative Conditioning

- Myeloablative conditioning regimens serve a dual purpose:
  - High doses of chemotherapy with or without radiation provide cytoreduction of the neoplasm, usually accompanied by eradication or ablation of host hematopoietic function.

TABLE. 18–2. *Preparative regimens commonly used in allogeneic stem cell transplantation*

Myeloablative Regimens	
Cy/TBI	
Cyclophosphamide	120mg/kg IV
TBI	1,000–1,575 cGy
Bu/Cy	
Busulfan	16 mg/kg PO or 12.8 mg/kg IV
Cyclophosphamide	120–200 mg/kg IV
Nonmyeloablative Regimens	
Flu/Low-dose TBI	
Fludarabine	90 mg/m^2 IV
TBI	200 cGy
Flu/Mel	
Fludarabine	125 mg/m^2 IV
Melphalan	180 mg/m^2 IV
Flu/Bu/ATG	
Fludarabine	180 mg/m^2 IV
Busulfan	8 mg/kg PO or 6.4 mg/kg IV
ATG	40 mg/kg IV
Cy/Flu	
Cyclophosphamide	120 mg/kg IV
Fludarabine	125 mg/m^2 IV

Cy, cyclophosphamide; TBI, total body irradiation; Bu, busulfan; ATG, antithymocyte globulin; Flu, fludarabine; Mel, melphalan; IV, intravenously; PO, orally.

- Suppresses the host's immune system, a prerequisite for preventing rejection of the transplant.
- The burden of tumor eradication in conventional transplants rests on both the transient cytoreductive properties of the conditioning agents and on more durable GVL effects mediated by donor immune cells.
- The two most commonly used regimens are cyclophosphamide in combination with either total body irradiation (TBI) or busulfan.
- TBI-based regimens have a higher incidence of secondary malignancies, growth retardation, and cataracts, while non-TBI regimens, particularly those containing busulfan, are associated with more veno-occlusive disease (VOD) and mucositis.
- The underlying condition often dictates the optimal conditioning regimen. For example, patients with acute lymphoblastic leukemia (ALL) appear to have a lower risk of relapse with TBI-based regimens

Nonmyeloablative Conditioning

- Nonmyeloablative preparative regimens were devised in an effort to minimize conditioning-related morbidities associated with conventional transplants, while retaining the immunosuppressive effects necessary to ensure engraftment.
- The burden of tumor eradication in nonmyeloablative transplants mainly rests on the donor immune-mediated GVL effect.
- These regimens are associated with a decrease in the incidence of some conditioning-related toxicities (i.e., VOD, mucositis, prolonged neutropenia, etc.).
- Nonmyeloablative regimens are well tolerated by patients of advanced age (up to 70 years) or in patients with medical comorbidities.

- Several transplant centers are currently evaluating nonmyeloablative transplantation in patients with hematological malignancies, solid tumors and in nonmalignant hematologic disorders.

Results of Allogeneic Hematopoietic Stem Cell Transplantation

Allogeneic HSCT is the only curative option for many patients with hematologic malignancies (2,6). Approximately 85% to 90% of all allogeneic transplants in the United States are performed for an underlying hematologic malignancy.

Chronic Myeloid Leukemia (CML)

CML is a myeloproliferative disorder characterized by the presence of a characteristic t(9; 22) (q34;q11) translocation, the Philadelphia chromosome. The natural history consists of a relatively indolent chronic phase with progression to the more aggressive accelerated phase and blast crisis. Allogeneic HSCT is the only proven curative therapy for this condition.

- When transplantation is performed in chronic phase, 65% to 80% of patients are cured; transplantation is less effective in accelerated phase or blast crisis.
- Younger patients and patients who undergo transplantation within a year of diagnosis have the best outcomes.
- Chronic phase CML is sensitive to GVL effects and a single DLI can reinduce remission in 70% of patients who relapse after transplantation.
- Imatinib (Gleevec), a well-tolerated, orally administered tyrosine kinase inhibitor that induces complete cytogenetic remissions in more than 70% of chronic-phase CML patients, is likely to supplant allogeneic HSCT as initial therapy.

Acute Myeloid Leukemia (AML)

The indication and timing for transplantation in AML and outcome after allogeneic HSCT depend on the risk category.

- Patients with intermediate or poor prognosis AML as determined by cytogenetics are at high risk for relapse after chemotherapy and should be evaluated for allogeneic HSCT in first remission (CR1) when an HLA-matched sibling donor is available.
- Patients transplanted in CR1 have a 45% to 60% probability of long-term DFS.
- Patients transplanted in first relapse or after induction of second complete remission (CR2) have only a 22% to 40% chance of long-term DFS.
- Outcomes after transplantation in first relapse or CR2 are comparable.
- Allogeneic HSCT in good prognosis AML is usually reserved for CR2 or first relapse, because the risk of transplant-related mortality outweighs the benefits from early transplantation (CR1) in this group.
- Less than 20% of patients with primary induction failure or those beyond CR2 have durable leukemia remission after allogeneic HSCT.

Acute Lymphoblastic Leukemia

While a significant proportion of childhood ALL is curable with chemotherapy, the majority (60% to 70%) of adults with this disease relapse following initial chemotherapy. Patients older than 60 years of age, those with a leukocyte count higher than 30,000 per microliter, or with adverse cytogenetics [t(4;11), t(1;19), t(8;14) or t(9;22)] have a particularly poor prognosis. Allogeneic HSCT in CR1 is recommended for patients with poor prognostic features. Long-term DFS in this category approaches 40% to 60%. In patients without adverse factors, allogeneic transplantation is usually reserved for CR2. Patients undergoing transplantation in CR2 have long-term DFS of approximately 40%.

Myelodysplastic Syndrome (MDS)

Allogeneic HSCT offers a 30% to 40% probability of long-term DFS in patients with MDS. The two most important factors predicting outcome after transplantation are blast percentage and cytogenetic risk group. Accordingly, patients with few blasts (refractory anemia or refractory anemia with ringed sideroblasts) enjoy a 50% to 75% long-term DFS, while more advanced stages (e.g., refractory anemia with excess blasts) are associated with a 30% DFS. Similarly, patients with good-risk cytogenetics have an approximately 50% probability of DFS compared to 10% or less for those with poor-risk cytogenetics. Nonetheless, allogeneic HSCT remains the only curative therapy for MDS and should be considered as a potential definitive therapy.

Non-Hodgkin's Lymphoma

Low-Grade Non-Hodgkin's Lymphoma

Experience with allogeneic HSCT in low-grade lymphomas is largely restricted to patients undergoing the procedure late in the course of their disease after multiple chemotherapeutic options have been exhausted. Approximately 30% to 50% will achieve long-term DFS. The typically indolent disease course and profound susceptibility to GVL effects renders low-grade lymphomas amenable to management and cure using nonmyeloablative conditioning approaches.

Aggressive Non-Hodgkin's Lymphoma

The role of allogeneic HSCT in patients with intermediate- and high-grade lymphomas is unclear. Most studies have reported a high incidence of transplant-related mortality (TRM) with myeloablative transplantation in this group. As a consequence, allogeneic HSCT is generally reserved for whom potentially curative autologous HSCT has failed or for those unlikely to benefit from an autologous transplant (patients with chemotherapy-resistant disease).

Multiple Myeloma

TRM rates in the range of 50% have discouraged the use of conventional myeloablative transplantation for multiple myeloma. Nevertheless, there is evidence that donor immune-mediated graft-versus-myeloma effects can be curative. Recently, nonmyeloablative conditioning has been explored as a potentially safer transplant approach to treat multiple myeloma. Transplant-related mortality has been reported to be significantly lower (less than 25%) compared to historical myeloma cohorts undergoing myeloablative conditioning; importantly, graft-versus-myeloma effects resulting in durable disease remission can be induced after reduced-intensity transplants. Autologous transplantation as myeloma cytoreduction followed by nonmyeloablative allogeneic transplantation as immunotherapy to eradicate minimal residual disease appears promising, with DFS of more than 50% in some studies.

Aplastic Anemia (AA)

Allogeneic HSCT is a curative option for patients with severe AA (SAA). Early studies of allogeneic HSCT in patients with SAA were characterized by a high incidence of graft rejection (up to 35% in some early series) and GVHD. Sensitization to histocompatibility antigens as a result of multiple transfusions and the use of cyclophosphamide alone as pretransplant conditioning accounted for these high rejection rates. Subsequent approaches added antithymocyte globulin (ATG) to cyclophosphamide to minimize graft rejection while preventing severe and potentially lethal GVHD. Additionally, the routine use of leukocyte-depleted and irradiated blood products has decreased the risk of graft rejection to less than 5% in most studies. A combination of cyclosporin A (CSA) and methotrexate is generally used as GVHD prophylaxis with delayed and gradual withdrawal of immunosuppression to minimize the risk of GVHD. Patients under the age of 40 years receiving an allogeneic HSCT from an HLA-matched sibling have an excellent chance for cure, with long-term survival rates approaching 90% in children.

Complications of Allogenetic Hematopoietic Stem Cell Transplantation

Complications of allogeneic HSCT are most commonly related to preparative regimen toxicities, infections occurring as a consequence of immunosuppression, or acute or chronic GVHD.

Conditioning-Related Toxicities

Conditioning-related toxicities vary depending on the type and doses of agents used in the preparative regimen.

- Nausea, vomiting, and mucositis occur commonly with myeloablative preparative regimens. Busulfan tends to be associated with more severe mucositis.
- Hemorrhagic cystitis occurring early in the course of transplantation is usually associated with preparative regimens containing high dose cyclophosphamide. In contrast, hemorrhagic cystitis more than 72 hours after conditioning is typically viral (polyoma virus BK or adenovirus). Attention to hydration and the routine use of 2-mercaptoethan sulfonate (MESNA) has virtually eliminated cyclophosphamide-associated hemorrhagic cystitis.
- Opportunistic infections occur with conditioning-related neutropenia. Bacteria and fungi that are normally present in the skin, gastrointestinal tract or respiratory tract cause the majority of these infections.
  - Damage to gut mucosa and indwelling venous catheters serve as the portal of entry for most life-threatening gram negative or aerobic gram-positive organisms. The use of oral antibiotics such as quinolones for gut decontamination has decreased the incidence of gram-negative bacteremia.
  - Candida and aspergillus fungal infections occur commonly during conditioning-induced neutropenia. Prophylactic fluconazole appears to protect against sensitive candida. Trials comparing newer antifungal agents with improved safety profiles compared to amphotericin-B and with activity against aspergillus or resistant candida species are currently being conducted.
- VOD is characterized by the triad of jaundice, tender hepatomegaly, and ascites occurring early posttransplant. Risk factors include:
  - Advanced age.
  - Conditioning with busulfan or cyclophosphamide.
  - Preexisting liver disease.
  - Development of acute GVHD.
  - Transplants from matched unrelated and haplo-identical donors.

Prophylaxis with oral ursodiol may be protective. VOD can be severe and life-threatening in approximately 25% of patients developing this complication. Treatment remains largely supportive, although defibrotide and recombinant tissue plasminogen activator have each been used with some success in severe VOD.

Graft-versus-Host Disease

GVHD is one of the most common complications of allogeneic HSCT. GVHD is a consequence of allogeneic donor T cells damaging normal recipient tissues. Based on the time of onset, clinical features and pathophysiology, GVHD is classified as either acute or chronic (13).

Acute Graft-versus-Host Disease

- Typically commences during the first 100 days after transplantation.
- Of HLA-matched sibling donor transplant recipients, 20% to 50% experience acute GVHD; the incidence is higher in transplants utilizing unrelated donors. The extent of donor-host HLA-disparity, recipient age, T-cell content of the graft, intensity of the conditioning regimen, and the type of GVHD prophylaxis regimen utilized all influence the incidence and severity of GVHD.
- The skin, gastrointestinal tract, and liver are the most common targets of alloreactive donor T-cells. The following clinical and laboratory features should arouse suspicion of GVHD.
  - Skin: erythematous maculo-papular rash frequently involving the palms and soles. Severe cases can present with skin desquamation.
  - Gastrointestinal: crampy abdominal pain and large volume watery diarrhea characterize GVHD of the colon and distal small bowel. In severe cases, bloody diarrhea or ileus may occur.
  - Hepatic: elevated alkaline phosphatase and direct bilirubin accompanied by less pronounced increases in transaminases characterize acute GVHD of the liver.
- Definitive diagnosis can be difficult because a variety of other conditions (such as drug-induced skin rash, viral colitis) can present with similar features. Biopsy and histopathologic examination of involved tissue is considered the gold standard for diagnosing GVHD.
- GVHD is a major contributor to transplant-related mortality; strategies directed at preventing this complication are an important aspect of transplant planning. Pharmacologic prophylaxis and graft T-cell depletion are established methods that effectively reduce the incidence and severity of GVHD. Cyclosporin A or tacrolimus combined with methotrexate are commonly used for GVHD prophylaxis. Effective T-cell depletion of the allograft can be achieved *in vitro* by $CD34^+$ cell selection or in vivo pharmacologically (i.e., Campath-1H). However, T-depleted transplants are associated with a higher risk of graft failure, leukemia relapse, and opportunistic viral infections.
- Treatment of established GVHD depends on the type and severity of involved organ (for grading of acute GVHD, see Table 18-3). While mild (grade I) skin GVHD can be managed effectively with topical steroids, visceral GVHD and more severe forms of cutaneous GVHD require systemic immunosuppressive therapy. Glucocorticoids (methylprednisone, typically at doses of 1 to 3 mg/kg per day) are the mainstay of therapy and are given in conjunction with cyclosporine or tacrolimus, with doses titrated to maintain therapeutic serum levels. Unfortunately, only approximately 50% of patients demonstrate durable responses to this form of therapy (for treatment of established acute GVHD, see Table 18-4).
- Nonresponding or steroid-refractory patients have a poor outcome, with mortality rates of more than 80%. The majority developing steroid-refractory GVHD die from infectious complications or organ damage related to relentless immune attack. Comprehensive management of steroid-refractory GVHD patients with novel agents such as daclizumab or infliximab accompanied by targeted infectious prophylaxis against enteric bacteria and aspergillus appears to be a promising strategy that deserves further study (Table 18-4) (4).

Chronic Graft-versus-Host Disease

- Typically presents between 100 days and 2 years after transplantation
- Affects 20% to 50% of recipients of allogeneic bone marrow transplants and up to 80% receiving an allogeneic peripheral blood stem cell transplant. Risk is increased by:

TABLE. 18–3. *Grading of Acute GVHD*

	Organ involvement		
	Skin	Liver	GI
Stage			
1	Rash <25% of skin	Bilirubin 2–3 mg/dL	Diarrhea >500 mL/day *or* persistent nausea with histologic evidence of upper GI GVHD
2	Rash 25%–50% of skin	Bilirubin 3–6 mg/dL	Diarrhea >1000 mL/day
3	Rash >50% of skin	Bilirubin 6–15 mg/dL	Diarrhea >1500 mL/day
4	Generalized erythroderma with bullae	Bilirubin >15 mg/dL	Severe abdominal pain with or without ileus
Grade			
I	Stage 1–2	0	0
II	Stage 3 *or*	Stage 1 *or*	Stage 1
III	—	Stage 2–3 *or*	Stage 2–4
IV	Stage 4 *or*	Stage 4	—

GI, gastrointestinal; GVDH, graft-versus-host disease. From Przepiorka D, Weisdorf D, Martin P, et al. 1994 Consensus Conference on Acute GVHD Grading. *Bone Marrow Transplant* 1995; 15:825–828, with permission.

- · Prior history of acute GVHD.
- · Older patient age.
- · Use of HLA-mismatched or unrelated donors.
- · DLI administration.
- · Use of peripheral blood stem cell allografts.
- • Patients may present with a myriad of clinical features including lichenoid or sclerodermatous skin changes, elevated liver function tests, xerostomia, dry eyes, diarrhea, bronchiolitis obliterans and thrombocytopenia with or without pancytopenia.
- • Most clinicians use a two-stage staging system: limited GVHD representing localized skin involvement and extensive GVHD includes patients with more diffuse skin involvement or involvement of other target organs.
- • Therapy typically consists of cyclosporine or tacrolimus given in conjunction with low dose corticosteroids. Alternative agents include mycophenolate mofetil, thalidomide, photochemotherapy with oral methoxypsoralen therapy followed by ultraviolet-A photophoresis (PUVA), and monoclonal antibodies directed against T lymphocytes or cytokines implicated in pathogenesis.
- • A high risk of bacterial infections in patients with chronic GVHD warrants routine use antibiotic prophylaxis against encapsulated bacteria and opportunistic pathogens.

Pulmonary Complications

Pulmonary complications may occur both early and late after transplantation, and they may be infectious or noninfectious in etiology.

Pulmonary Complications Attributable to Infections

- • Fungi (aspergillus and other agents) as well as viruses (cytomegalovirus, respiratory syncitial virus, influenza, parainfluenza, etc.) can cause life-threatening pneumonia in the posttransplant setting. Early diagnosis, prophylactic or preemptive therapy (e.g., ganciclovir or foscar-

TABLE. 18–4. *Treatment of acute graft-versus-host disease: The NHLBI approach*

Initial management
Grade I GVHD (stage 1–2 skin)
Topical corticosteroid therapy
Grade II–IV GVHD
- High dose methylprednisolone 1–10 mg/kg per day up to a maximum of 500 mg/day IV 3–6 days
and
- IV cyclosporine or IV tacrolimus
- Steroids tapered once response is evident over 10–14 days
- All patients receiving ≥1mg/kg of methylprednisolone undergo routine surveillance blood cultures every 3 days
- All patients with ≥grade III GI GVHD receive prophylactic antibiotic therapy against enteric organisms (e.g., ampicillin-sulbactam)
Management of steroid-refractory GVHD
(GVHD not responsive to 6 or more days of continuous therapy with ≥1 mg/kg methylprednisolone)
A) Treatment
- Rapid taper of methylprednisolone to ≤1mg/kg
- Daclizumab (monoclonal antibody to interleukin-2 receptor-α) 1 mg/kg on days 1, 4, 8, 15, 22
- Infliximab (monoclonal antibody to tumor necrosis factor-α) 10 mg/kg on days 1, 8, 15, 22
B) Supportive care
- All patients with GI GVHD are maintained NPO
- All patients with ≥grade III GI GVHD receive prophylactic antibiotic therapy against enteric organisms (e.g., ampicillin-sulbactam)
- All patients with steroid-refractory GVHD and those patients who receive ≥1 mg/kg methylprednisolone for more than 6 days receive prophylaxis against aspergillus (e.g., liposomal amphotericin, 5 mg/kg per day)
- All patients receiving ≥1mg/kg of methylprednisolone undergo routine surveillance blood cultures every 3 days

NHLBI, National Heart, Lung, and Blood Institute; GVHD, graft-versus-host disease; IV, intravenously; GI, gastrointestinal; NPO, nothing by mouth.

net for cytomegalovirus [CMV] antigenemia) and prompt institution of definitive therapy when available are the major principles guiding management of these complications. The risk of *Pneumocystis carinii* pneumonia is greatest in the first 6 months after transplantation, particularly in patients receiving T-depleted grafts or those suffering from chronic GVHD; prophylaxis with sulfa/trimethoprim or inhaled pentamidine virtually eliminates this complication.

- Idiopathic interstitial pneumonitis usually occurs early after transplantation and is characterized by fever, hypoxia and diffuse pulmonary infiltrates. Total body irradiation or drugs with pulmonary toxicity (i.e., busulfan) in the preparative regimen increase the risk of this complication.
- Diffuse alveolar hemorrhage is a relatively infrequent but frequently fatal complication of allogeneic HSCT. It is characterized by the rapid onset of dyspnea, cough, and hypoxia with diffuse bilateral infiltrates on radiography. High dose corticosteroids appear to be of therapeutic benefit.

Infectious Complications

Recipients of allogeneic HSCT continue to be at risk for infections beyond the period of conditioning-related neutropenia, with viral and fungal pathogens and encapsulated bacteria posing the greatest hazard (15). Factors influencing infectious risk include the presence of acute or chronic GVHD, the extent of immunosuppressive pharmacotherapy in the post-transplant period, T-cell depletion of the graft, and the use of partially HLA-mismatched or unrelated donors.

Bacterial Infections

- Gram-negative bacteremia associated with gastrointestinal GVHD and venous catheter-related infections (predominantly gram positive pathogens) occur with greatest frequency during the first 3 to 4 months after transplantation.
- Recurrent sinus and pulmonary infections are associated with chronic GVHD. Antibiotic prophylaxis against encapsulated organisms, using penicillin or an appropriate alternative, reduces the risk of these infections.
- Patients with recurrent infections and low serum immunoglobulin levels may benefit from prophylactic intravenous immunoglobulin (IVIG) infusions.

Fungal Infections

- Fungal infections constitute a major cause of mortality after allogeneic HSCT: 60% to 70% of patients developing invasive fungal infections die despite antifungal therapy.
- Yeast (candida species) and molds (aspergillus) account for the majority of opportunistic fungal infections in the posttransplant period.
- Candida infections typically occur early in the course of transplantation, often near the end of the neutropenic phase. Candidal infections can manifest as mucocutanoeus candidiasis, candidemia, or with visceral involvement (the liver and spleen are most commonly involved). Routine prophylaxis with fluconazole offers protection against sensitive strains of candida.
- Invasive aspergillus infections typically involve the lungs, para-nasal sinuses and the central nervous system, although dissemination to other visceral organs has been described. Predisposing factors are:
  - Corticosteroids.
  - Severe GVHD.
  - The use of non-HLA identical and unrelated stem cell donors.
  - Transplantation in rooms lacking laminar air flow.
- Invasive fungal infections are difficult to eradicate. Fluconazole may be effective against sensitive candida strains (e.g., *Candida albicans*). Amphotericin B, lipid formulation amphotericin, and newer agents such as the echinocandins (caspofungin) and voriconazole have demonstrated efficacy against aspergillus and a wide spectrum of candida species.
- The diligent application of preventive measures such as avoiding the indiscriminate use of corticosteroids remains the most effective strategy for minimizing mortality related to invasive fungal infections.

Viral Infections

Cytomegalovirus

While advances in screening and preventive therapy have reduced CMV-related mortality, CMV infection continues to be a major contributor to post-transplant morbidity.

- CMV is a DNA virus belonging to the herpesvirus family.
- Posttransplant CMV infection is most often a consequence of viral reactivation in patients with prior exposure to CMV, and is observed in 50% to 70% of CMV seropositive recipients.
- Reactivation typically occurs in the first 100 days after transplantation.

- Primary infection in CMV-seronegative recipients can follow transplantation from a seropositive donor. Acquisition of primary infection from CMV-positive transfusion products has been all but eliminated with routine use of leukocyte-depleted or CMV-negative blood products.
- GVHD, the use of T-cell–depleted allografts, and corticosteroid/CSA/tacrolimus use increase the risk of CMV reactivation.
- Interstitial pneumonitis is the most common and serious manifestation of CMV disease, followed by enteritis/colitis. Other manifestations include febrile episodes and marrow suppression resulting in thrombocytopenia with or without neutropenia.
- Mortality rates with CMV pneumonitis range from 65% to 85%. Ganciclovir or foscarnet given in conjunction with IVIG improves outcome associated with CMV disease (Table 18-5).
- Early detection methods including polymerase chain reaction (PCR) for viral DNA and immunofluorescence for detecting viral antigen in leucocytes predict the subsequent development of CMV disease.
- Preemptive therapy with ganciclovir or foscarnet (Table 18-5) begun when CMV reactivation is first detected (either PCR or immunofluorescence assay) has dramatically reduced the incidence of CMV pneumonitis/enteritis and consequently CMV-related mortality.
- Newer approaches for treatment of or prophylaxis against CMV disease include adoptive transfer of ex vivo expanded CMV-specific cytotoxic T lymphocytes.

Epstein-Barr Virus-Associated Lymphoproliferative Disorder

- Epstein-Barr virus (EBV)-related lymphoproliferative disorder is a B-cell malignancy arising as a consequence of impaired T-cell immunity against EBV.

TABLE. 18–5. *Surveillance and management of Cytomegalovirus: – The NHLBI approach*

Surveillance
(CMV antigenemia or qualitative PCR)
  - Weekly posttransplant until day 100
  - Continue surveillance beyond day 100 in the event of late CMV reactivation, continued immunosuppressive therapy, or if clinically indicated

Management of CMV antigenemia[a]
Induction:
Ganciclovir 5 mg/kg IV q12h or foscarnet 90 mg/kg IV q12h or valganciclovir 900 mg PO twice daily × 7 days
  - If number of positive cells decrease or are negative in 1 week, decrease to maintenance dosing (below).
  - If number of positive cells are unchanged or increase, continue induction and consider other treatment options (e.g., switching from ganciclovir to foscarnet)
Maintenance:
Ganciclovir 5 mg/kg IV every day five times per week (M–F) or Foscarnet 90 mk/kg IV every day five times per week (M–F) or daily valganciclovir 900 mg PO every day
  - Continue treating until 2 CMV antigenemia results are negative, 1 week apart

Management of CMV Disease[a]
Induction: Ganciclovir or foscarnet IV (at induction doses) q12h × 14 days and IVIG 500 mg/kg IV QOD × 14–21 days
Maintenance: Ganciclovir 5 mg/kg IV every day × 30 days

---

[a] Foscarnet may be the drug of choice in patients who have cytopenias and CMV reactivation or CMV disease.
CMV, cytomegalovirus; PCR, polymerase chain reaction; IV, intravenously; PO, orally; IVIG, intravenous immunoglobulin.

- It is relatively rare complication, affecting approximately 1% of all allogeneic transplant recipients, although certain transplants (especially T-cell depleted) are associated with a significantly higher risk.
- The natural course of untreated EBV-lymphoproliferative disorder is rapid progression culminating in death.
- Allograft T-cell depletion, transplants from HLA-mismatched and unrelated donors, and the use of immunosuppressive agents predispose to the development of this malignancy.
- Treatment with a monoclonal antibody to CD20 (rituximab), donor lymphocyte infusions, or adoptive infusion of EBV-specific cytotoxic T cells are all effective in eradicating this disease, particularly when combined with withdrawal of immunosuppression.

Other Viral Infections

Patients undergoing allogeneic HSCT are at risk for infectious complications associated with the herpesviruses, varicella zoster, and various respiratory viruses (respiratory syncitial virus, influenza, parainfluenza). Adenoviruses or polyoma virus BK may appear clinically as hemorrhagic cystitis. Because cellular immunity is impaired in the posttransplant setting, otherwise self-limiting viral infections can have fatal sequelae.

Graft Failure

Graft failure is the inability to achieve (primary) or maintain (secondary) persistent donor hematopoiesis. Graft failure mediated by the recipient immune system is referred to as graft rejection.

- Graft failure is relatively uncommon in patients undergoing transplantation from an HLA-identical sibling donor (less than 2%).
- T-cell depletion, the use of HLA-mismatched or unrelated donor grafts, and alloimmunization caused by repeated transfusions are factors that increase the risk of graft rejection.
- In myeloablative HSCT, primary graft failure presents as persistent pancytopenia (more than 3 to 4 weeks) after conditioning and is associated with a high mortality rate. Secondary graft failure is characterized by initial recovery of blood counts followed by a later loss of donor hematopoiesis.
- Up to 50% of patients with graft rejection can be salvaged by repeat conditioning or immunosuppression (e.g., OKT3 plus corticosteroids) followed by reinfusion of a T-cell–replete allograft.
- Graft failure can also result from infections, drugs, or chronic GVHD. Patients can often be salvaged with hematopoietic growth factors (e.g., G-CSF) with or without additional stem cells.

Late Sequelae of Transplantation

Secondary Malignancies

- In addition to EBV-related lymphomas, leukemias and solid tumors can complicate allogeneic HSCT.
- The risk of solid tumors in transplant survivors at 10 years is increased eightfold compared to age-matched controls. Melanomas, tumors of the bone, liver, central nervous system (CNS), and thyroid are commonly encountered secondary malignancies.
- Younger patient age at transplantation and TBI-based conditioning regimens predispose to the development of secondary solid tumors.

Other Late Complications

Growth retardation, infertility, restrictive pulmonary disease, cataracts, endocrine dysfunction, avascular necrosis of bones, osteopenia and neurocognitive defects are other delayed sequelae of allogeneic HCT.

Nonmyeloablative Hematopoietic Stem Cell Transplantation

The high risk of transplant-related mortality with conventional transplants and the appreciation that GVL effects can cure some hematological malignancies provided the impetus for the development of nonmyeloablative conditioning regimens (16,17). The basic principles underlying these regimens include:

- Reduced-intensity conditioning to induce adequate host immunosuppression for donor allograft "take" while minimizing toxicities related to dose-intensive conditioning.
- Manipulation of posttransplant immunosuppression and administration of DLIs to promote rapid transition to complete donor immuno-hematopoiesis.
- Reliance on the GVL effect for eradication of the underlying malignancy.

A variety of different conditioning regimens have been used, and the cumulative experience from various transplant centers has led to the following observations:

- Several conditioning-related toxicities such as VOD and mucositis are absent or mild compared to myeloablative transplants.
- Transplant-related mortality is substantially lower (7% to 20%) than the 25% to 40% mortality associated with standard or myeloablative transplants.
- The improved toxicity profile has expanded the eligibility of allogeneic transplantation to older patients (up to 70 years of age) and patients with comorbid medical conditions.
- GVL effects against several hematologic malignancies including acute and chronic myelogenous leukemia, acute lymphocytic leukemia, chronic lymphocytic leukemia, NHL, and myeloma have been observed.
- Pilot trials of nonmyeloablative HCT in solid tumors have shown for the first time the ability of the GVT effect to induce disease regression in treatment-refractory metastatic solid tumors. Renal cell carcinoma provides the best example of a tumor that may be susceptible to GVT effects (18); GVT effects have also been described in other solid tumors including breast, pancreatic, colon, and ovarian carcinoma (19).

REFERENCES

1. Blume KG, Thomas ED. A review of autologous hematopoietic cell transplantation. *Biol Blood Marrow Transplant* 2000;6:1–12.
2. Thomas ED. Bone marrow transplantation: a review. *Semin Hematol* 1999;36(4 Suppl 7):95–103.
3. Attal M, Harousseau JL, Stoppa AM, et al. A prospective, randomized trial of autologous bone marrow transplantation and chemotherapy in multiple myeloma. Intergroupe Francais du Myelome. *N Engl J Med* 1996;335:91–97.
4. Philip T, Guglielmi C, Hagenbeek A, et al. Autologous bone marrow transplantation as compared with salvage chemotherapy in relapses of chemotherapy-sensitive non-Hodgkin's lymphoma. *N Engl J Med* 1995;333:1540–1545.
5. Antman KH. Randomized trials of high dose chemotherapy for breast cancer. *Biochim Biophys Acta* 2001;1471:M89–98.
6. Childs RW. Allogeneic hematopoietic cell transplantation. In: De Vita VT Jr, Hellman, S, Rosenberg SA, eds. *Principles and Practice of Oncology.* 7th ed., London: Lippincott Williams & Wilkins, 2004.
7. Storb R. Allogeneic hematopoietic stem cell transplantation—yesterday, today, and tomorrow. *Exp Hematol* 2003;31:1–10.
8. Mathe G, Amiel JL, Schwarzenberg L, et al. Adoptive immunotherapy of acute leukemia: experimental and clinical results. *Cancer Res* 1965;25:1525–1531.

9. Antin JH. Stem cell transplantation-harnessing of graft-versus-malignancy. *Curr Opin Hematol* 2003; 10:440–444.
10. Riddell SR, Berger C, Murata M, et al, The graft versus leukemia response after allogeneic hematopoietic stem cell transplantation. *Blood Rev* 2003;17:153–162.
11. Horowitz MM, Gale RP, Sondel PM, et al. Graft-versus-leukemia reactions after bone marrow transplantation. *Blood* 1990;75:555–562.
12. Bensinger WI, Martin PJ, Storer B, et al. Transplantation of bone marrow as compared with peripheral-blood cells from HLA-identical relatives in patients with hematologic cancers. *N Engl J Med* 2001;344:175–181.
13. Vogelsang GB, Lee L, Bensen-Kennedy, DM. Pathogenesis and treatment of graft-versus-host disease after bone marrow transplant. *Annu Rev Med* 2003;54:29–52.
14. Srinivasan R, Chakrabarti S, Walsh T, et al. Improved survival in steroid-refractory acute graft-versus-host disease after nonmyeloablative transplantation using a daclizumab-based strategy with comprehensive infection prophylaxis. *Br J Hematol* 2004;124:777–786.
15. Leather HL, Wingard JR. Infections following hematopoietic stem cell transplantation. *Infect Dis Clin North Am* 2001;15:483–520.
16. Storb RF, Champlin R, Riddell SR, et al. Non-myeloablative transplants for malignant disease. *Hematology (Am Soc Hematol Educ Program)* 2001:375–391.
17. Anagnostopoulos A, Giralt S. Critical review on non-myeloablative stem cell transplantation (NST). *Crit Rev Oncol Hematol* 2002;44:175–190.
18. Childs R, Chernoff A, Contentin N, et al. Regression of metastatic renal-cell carcinoma after nonmyeloablative allogeneic peripheral-blood stem-cell transplantation. *N Engl J Med* 2000;343:750–758.
19. Childs RW, Srinivasan R. Allogeneic hematopoietic cell transplantation for solid tumors. In: Blume KG, Forman SJ, Appelbaum FR, eds. *Thomas' Hematopoitic Cell Transplantation.* 3rd ed. Malden, MA: Blackwell Science, 2004;1177–1187.

19

Thrombocytopenia

Patrick F. Fogarty and Cynthia E. Dunbar

PLATELET BIOLOGY

- Platelets are anucleate blood cells that participate in *primary hemostasis,* the formation of a platelet plug at sites of vascular injury.
- Platelets are produced from *megakaryocytes,* multinucleate hematopoietic cells located in the bone marrow. Cytokines such as thrombopoietin are necessary for normal platelet maturation and release.
- The average life span of a platelet in the blood is 7 to 10 days. Platelets are removed from the circulation when they are activated and utilized at sites of vascular injury or as they become senescent.
- Up to one-third of the platelet mass is stored in the spleen, providing a reserve of platelets that may be released during periods of physiologic stress.
- The normal platelet concentration in the blood is 150,000 to 350,000/mL.

ETIOLOGY AND CLINICAL FEATURES OF THROMBOCYTOPENIA

Thrombocytopenia may occur as a result of:

- Decreased production of platelets, or
- Increased consumption of platelets, or
- Increased sequestration of platelets, or
- Any combination of these mechanisms (Table 19-1).

Regardless of the cause of thrombocytopenia, platelet-type bleeding is typically mucocutaneous and is characterized by petechiae, ecchymoses, epistaxis, and gingival and conjunctival hemorrhages. Less commonly, severe thrombocytopenia may lead to gastrointestinal, genitourinary, or central nervous system bleeding.

Spontaneous bleeding or bruising normally does not occur until the platelet count has fallen below 10,000 to 20,000/mL. The rate of decline of the platelet count also may influence the likelihood of unprovoked bleeding, presumably as a result of compensatory processes that may occur over time in the setting of persistent thrombocytopenia. Patients with dysfunctional platelets may bleed at higher platelet counts. Patients with thrombocytopenia and platelet counts greater than 20,000 to 30,000/mL without bleeding usually do not require immediate treatment to increase the platelet count. A platelet count of 80,000 to 100,000/mL is generally regarded as adequate for hemostasis during most invasive procedures, including surgery (Table 19-2).

DISORDERS CHARACTERIZED BY DECREASED PRODUCTION OF PLATELETS

Bone Marrow Failure

- Congenital disorders, such as *Fanconi's anemia* or *dyskeratosis congenita,* typically present early in life; these syndromes often cause depression of other blood cell lineages (white

TABLE. 19–1. *Causes of thrombocytopenia*

Disorders characterized by decreased production of platelets
Bone marrow failure syndromes
   Congenital (amegakaryocytic thrombocytopenia, Fanconi's anemia, dyskeratosis congenita, Schwachmann-Diamond syndrome, thrombocytopenia-absent radii syndrome, Wiskott-Aldrich Syndrome)
   Acquired (aplastic anemia, amegakaryocytic thrombocytopenia)
Myelodysplasia
Marrow infiltration (neoplastic, infectious)
Chemotherapy-induced
Irradiation-induced
Folate, B_{12}, or iron (advanced cases) deficiency
Alcoholism
Disorders characterized by increased clearance of platelets
Immune thrombocytopenic purpura
Heparin-induced thrombocytopenia
Thrombotic thrombocytopenic purpura/hemolytic-uremic syndrome
Disseminated intravascular coagulation (HELLP syndrome)
Posttransfusion purpura
Neonatal Alloimmune Thrombocytopenia
VonWillebrand disease, type IIB
Antiphospholipid antibody syndrome
Mechanical destruction (aortic valvular dysfunction; extracorporeal bypass)
Disorders characterized by increased sequestration of platelets
Hypersplenism (Table 19–5)
Other conditions/combined mechanisms
Artifactual (pseudothrombocytopenia)
Drug-induced (Table 19–6)
Gestational thrombocytopenia
Cyclic thrombocytopenia
Infection- and sepsis-related thrombocytopenia
   HIV-associated thrombocytopenia
Hemophagocytosis
Qualitative platelet disorder-related (Bernard Soulier disease, Grey platelet syndrome, May-Hegglin anomaly)

HIV, human immunodeficiency virus.

cells and red cells) in addition to the platelet count, but in a significant minority of cases isolated thrombocytopenia can be the presenting abnormality.

- *Congenital amegakaryocytic thrombocytopenia* and the *thrombocytopenia with absent radius (TAR) syndrome* are characterized by isolated thrombocytopenia.

- *Wiskott-Aldrich Syndrome (WAS)* is an X-linked recessive disorder that comprises a triad of thrombocytopenia, eczema, and immunodeficiency. Thrombocytopenia occurs as a result of decreased megakaryocytopoiesis along with increased destruction of abnormal platelets. Thrombocytopenia may improve with splenectomy, but allogeneic hematopoietic stem cell transplantation alone is potentially curative.

- Adults patients with *acquired amegakaryocytic thrombocytopenia* initially may appear to have immune thrombocytopenic purpura (discussion following), but the bone marrow reveals markedly reduced or absent megakaryocytes instead of normal or increased numbers. The disorder may progress to aplastic anemia, and patients with acquired aplastic anemia occasionally can present with isolated thrombocytopenia. Marked bone marrow hypocellularity with decreased megakaryocytes would suggest this diagnosis (for further discussion of the treatment of these entities see Chapter 6).

TABLE. 19–2. *Target platelet count values for commonly encountered clinical scenarios[a]*

Goal or intervention	Desired platelet count (/μL)
Prevention of spontaneous intracranial bleeding	>5,000–10,000
Prevention of spontaneous mucocutaneous bleeding	>10,000–30,000
Placement of central vascular catheters	
Compressible site	>20,000–30,000
Non-compressible site/tunneled catheter	>40,000–50,000
Use of anticoagulant medications in therapeutic doses	>40,000–50,000
Invasive procedures	
Endoscopy with biopsy	>60,000
Liver biopsy	>80,000
Major surgery	>80,000–100,000

[a] Values are approximate and reflect target ranges for patients with otherwise intact hemostasis. Patients with thrombocytopenia and bleeding may benefit from augmentation of the platelet count (e.g., by platelet transfusion) irrespective of the platelet value.

Myelodysplasia

- Thrombocytopenia is a common feature of myelodysplasia (MDS). Mild thrombocytopenia with macrocytosis, and with or without anemia or neutropenia in an older individual is usual. In contrast, an isolated very low platelet count (less than 20,000 per microliter) without any other blood count abnormalities is not typical for MDS.
- Examination of the bone marrow aspirate and blood smear may suggest MDS if megakaryocytic dysplasia (including small and mononuclear micromegakaryocyte forms) and maturation abnormalities of erythrocytic and granulocytic precursor cells are present. Cytogenetic abnormalities (especially deletion of chromosome 5q or monosomy 7), also indicate MDS as the underlying diagnosis (see Chapter 7).
- Treatment of thrombocytopenia caused by MDS can be difficult (see Chapter 7). Hematopoietic cytokines such as granulocyte colony-stimulating factor (G-CSF) or interleukin (IL)-11 are not effective.
- Transfusion of platelets may be required if thrombocytopenia is severe and accompanied by bleeding. Because the platelets produced by the bone marrow in patients with MDS mature abnormally, they may be defective and bleeding can occur at counts adequate for hemostasis with normal platelets; thus, a higher threshold for prophylactic transfusion may be necessary.

Marrow Infiltration

Infiltration of the bone marrow by malignant cells may cause thrombocytopenia, but usually only after massive replacement of the marrow space by tumor cells or immature hematologic precursor cells. However, thrombocytopenia is rarely the sole blood count abnormality. Examination of the bone marrow biopsy and aspirate is required to diagnose marrow infiltration-related thrombocytopenia.

- The *acute and chronic leukemias*, *myeloma*, and *lymphoma* are the most common tumors resulting in cytopenias caused by neoplastic marrow infiltration.
- Certain *infections* (such as tuberculosis and ehrlichiosis) can result in formation of granulomas in the bone marrow that supplant the normal architecture and lead to decreased production of blood cells, including platelets.

- Effective treatment of the underlying condition should restore a low platelet count to the normal range, but platelet transfusions may be required initially if bleeding is present or invasive procedures are planned (Table 19-2).

Irradiation and Chemotherapy

- *Irradiation* and/or *myelotoxic chemotherapy* induce thrombocytopenia by direct toxicity to megakaryocytes or more immature hematopoietic stem and progenitor cells. The degree and duration of thrombocytopenia depends on the intensity and the type of the myelotoxic regimen.
- Chemotherapy-induced thrombocytopenia typically resolves more slowly than neutropenia and/or anemia, especially following repetitive cycles of treatment.
- A recombinant IL-11–like cytokine (Neumega) has been approved for the prevention of chemotherapy-induced severe thrombocytopenia, but its use is limited by significant side effects such as allergic reactions, fluid retention, and cardiovascular toxicities.

Cyclic Thrombocytopenia

This rare disorder is characterized by episodes of thrombocytopenia that occur cyclically, typically every 3 to 6 weeks. The thrombocytopenia is frequently severe and may be associated with significant bleeding. Treatment with oral contraceptives (female patients), androgens, immunosuppressive agents (such as azathioprine), or thrombopoietic growth factor has led to responses in some cases.

Nutritional Deficiencies

Folate deficiency (commonly associated with alcoholism) and *vitamin B_{12} deficiency* may cause decreased megakaryocytopoiesis and thrombocytopenia in conjunction with anemia. In contrast, thrombocytosis is typical in significant iron deficiency; in very severe iron deficiency, however, thrombocytopenia may occur. Replacement of the deficient vitamin or mineral should correct the thrombocytopenia.

DISORDERS CHARACTERIZED BY INCREASED CLEARANCE OF PLATELETS

Immune Thrombocytopenic Purpura

Immune thrombocytopenic purpura (ITP) is an acquired autoimmune disorder in which antiplatelet antibodies result in platelet destruction, causing thrombocytopenia that may lead to bleeding. Patients typically present with markedly reduced platelet counts and mucocutaneous bleeding, or they may have only a mildly or moderately depressed platelet count that is discovered on a routine blood count. Because most of the available treatments have considerable toxicity, therapy should be offered only to symptomatic patients or to those at high risk for serious bleeding.

- *Epidemiology*: The annual incidence of ITP in adults has been estimated to be 32 cases per million persons (1).
- *Pathophysiology*: Pathogenic antiplatelet antibodies can be identified in approximately 75% of patients with ITP. These autoantibodies are commonly directed against the platelet glycoprotein complexes IIb/IIIa and/or Ib/IX but other platelet protein targets have been identified. The antibody-coated platelets are then cleared via reticuloendothelial macrophages in the liver and/or spleen, resulting in a reduced life span of platelets from about 7 days to less than 2 days. Adult-onset ITP is generally idiopathic and becomes chronic but may occur in association with disorders of lymphoproliferation (lymphoma or chronic lymphocytic

leukemia) or immune dysregulation (systemic lupus erythematosis, human immunodeficiency virus [HIV] infection). In contrast, ITP in children typically follows a viral infection and frequently resolves spontaneously without specific therapy (2).

- ***Presentation***: New-onset severe ITP (platelets, less than 30,000/mL) manifests with petechial bruising and bleeding from mucous membranes, including conjunctival hemorrhages, gingival bleeding, and epistaxis. Milder disease (platelet count greater than 50,000/mL) often presents as an asymptomatically low platelet count on a routine blood count.
- ***Diagnosis***: Because no single test or group of tests is diagnostic for ITP, the diagnosis is primarily one of exclusion.
  - New-onset isolated thrombocytopenia with no other readily apparent cause (including medication-related) in an otherwise asymptomatic adult generally may be regarded as sufficient grounds for the diagnosis of ITP and subsequent initiation of medical therapies (if appropriate based on the degree of thrombocytopenia).
  - The presence of other cytopenias, age greater than 60 years, or failure of primary therapy (corticosteroids for a trial of 1 week) should prompt bone marrow examination before consideration of other therapies. Abnormal or decreased numbers of megakaryocytes or abnormal marrow cellularity redirect the evaluation away from ITP as a cause of the thrombocytopenia.
  - All patients should be screened for HIV infection (discussion following).
- ***Treatment***: Individuals with mild or moderate thrombocytopenia (greater than 20,000 to 30,000/mL) who do not require a higher count (for surgery or active bleeding) should not receive treatment; they may be observed at regular intervals for disease progression. Adults with platelet counts of less than 20,000 to 30,000/mL or those with significant bleeding generally should be treated (2,3).
- *Initial management* generally consists of a short course of *corticosteroids* (prednisone 1 mg/kg per day). A significant increase in the platelet count should be seen within 3 to 7 days; treatment with full-dose prednisone for longer than 7 to 10 days is rarely indicated. In the event of a platelet response, prednisone should be tapered rapidly until 20 mg per day is reached: thereafter, tapering should proceed slowly (dose decrements of no more than 5 mg per adjustment, occurring no more frequently than once every 3 weeks).
  - For patients with serious active bleeding and/or very severe thrombocytopenia (less than 5,000 to 10,000 per microliter), *intravenous immune globulin* (IVIG; 1 g/kg per day for 2 days) can be administered in addition to prednisone in order to decrease clearance of antibody-coated platelets. Responses are generally seen within 1 to 2 days of IVIG administration.
  - *Platelet transfusions* are indicated if the presentation is complicated by serious (for example intracranial) bleeding. Allogeneic platelets will be cleared very rapidly in the presence of antiplatelet antibodies but may provide at least temporary hemostasis. If platelet transfusion is given, documentation of a 1-hour and then a 1-day posttransfusion platelet count is important. If transfused platelets persist at a significant level for more than 24 hours, the diagnosis of ITP is unlikely.
- *Long-term treatment*: Unfortunately, despite a high initial response rate of 60% to 75%, the majority of adults with ITP do not sustain good platelet levels once prednisone is discontinued. Side effects of long-term corticosteroid therapy must be balanced against the risk of bleeding and the availability of other therapies for a chronic disease.
  - *Splenectomy* traditionally has been performed if the platelet count has failed to respond durably to prednisone. There is a lack of consensus regarding timing of and indications for splenectomy in adult patients. Laparoscopic splenectomy, at centers experienced with the procedure, results in decreased morbidity and shorter hospitalizations than with open splenectomy. All patients must receive the polyvalent pneumococcal vaccine (Pneumovax) several weeks prior to splenectomy if possible. A 65% to 75% response rate immediately postprocedure is typical; one recent survey reported a 66% durable response rate at 5 to 7 years (4).

- *IVIG* and *anti-D* (WinRho; 50 to 75 µg/kg per dose) may be used to decrease clearance of antibody-coated platelets by reticuloendothelial cells. Anti-D should be considered in Rh-positive patients only. Both IVIG and anti-D produce rapid increase the platelet count in a majority of patients; however, the effect is transient and the agents must be readministered every 2 to 3 weeks in most instances. They can be particularly useful for patients that require intermittent elevation of the platelet count for surgical procedures or other periods of increased bleeding risk.
- The monoclonal anti-B–cell antibody *rituximab* (anti-CD20) induces a response in some patients with chronic ITP (5).
- *Combination chemotherapy* or *high-dose chemotherapy with autologous stem cell support* (6) has resulted in durable complete remissions in a subset of patients with severe, refractory ITP, but these experimental approaches are best studied in a clinical trial.
- Other treatments for steroid and/or splenectomy-refractory ITP include *very high-dose pulse dexamethasone, single-agent vincristine, cyclosporine, danazol, mycophenolate mofetil, dapsone, Helicobacter pylori* treatment, *azathioprine, vitamin C, interferon, plasma exchange*, and *immunoadsoption over staphylococcal protein A columns* (2). Most of these therapies have response rates of 30% or less and can cause significant side effects.
- **Pregnancy-associated ITP**: Pregnant women with platelet counts less than 30,000/mL during the second or third trimester, or with platelet counts less than 10,000/mL or bleeding in any trimester, should be treated. Intermittent infusions of IVIG are standard. Splenectomy during the first or second trimester may be considered for women whose ITP has failed treatment with IVIG and steroids and who have platelet counts less than 10,000/mL with associated bleeding. Platelets may be administered prophylactically prior to cesarean section in women who have platelet counts less than 10,000/mL or mucocutaneous bleeding near the time of delivery. A platelet count of higher than 50,000 generally is regarded as adequate prior to cesarean section or vaginal delivery.

Heparin-Induced Thrombocytopenia

Heparin-induced thrombocytopenia (HIT) is an antibody-mediated disorder that results in platelet activation and clearance. Despite the thrombocytopenia, patients with HIT paradoxically are at high risk for thrombosis. If HIT is suspected, heparin should be discontinued immediately, and, if appropriate, alternative anticoagulation administered.

- **Epidemiology**: HIT occurs in approximately 3% of patients who are treated with unfractionated heparin (7); as many as half of these individuals will develop thrombosis.
- **Pathophysiology**: The pathogenesis of HIT begins with binding of the heparin molecule to platelet factor 4 (PF4), a platelet α granule protein that becomes antigenic when bound to heparin. The heparin-PF4 complex stimulates formation of an immunoglobulin G (IgG) antibody (HIT antibody) that binds both to the heparin-PF4 complex (via its Fab portion) and to platelet Fc receptors (via its Fc portion). Binding of the HIT antibody to platelets activates them, resulting in release of procoagulant microparticles, platelet clearance, and subsequent thrombocytopenia. PF4 also binds to polysaccharides (e.g., heparan sulfate) on the endothelial surface; recognition of these PF4-polysaccharide complexes by HIT antibodies may lead to endothelial damage, expression of tissue factor, and further hypercoagulability.
- **Presentation**: Typically in HIT, a hospitalized patient develops thrombocytopenia within 5 to 10 days of receiving heparin. Other presentations, however, are possible.
  - The presenting platelet count may be in the normal range, but a decline of 50% or more from the baseline value in a heparin-treated patient may signify HIT. Platelet counts generally do not decrease below 30,000/mL.

- Spontaneous bleeding (including petechiae) is not typical, even in patients who have markedly decreased platelet counts. Bleeding, elevated coagulation tests, or severe thrombocytopenia point the investigation away from HIT.
- Venous (upper or lower limb, dural sinus) or arterial (lower limb, CVA (cardiovascular accident), myocardial infarction, other locations) thromboses frequently occur in patients with HIT. The risk of HIT-related thrombosis persists for at least 30 days after discontinuation of heparin (8).
- In a minority of patients with HIT, thrombosis is the presenting clinical sign; in these cases, an unrecognized decline in the platelet count almost always has preceded the thrombosis.
- ***Delayed onset HIT*** describes new thrombocytopenia and venous or arterial thrombosis that occurs up to 14 days after uneventful completion of a course of heparin therapy. Thrombocytopenia and thrombosis typically worsen if heparin is readministered.
- ***Rapid onset HIT*** may occur within 1 to 4 days of reexposure to heparin in patients who have received heparin within the prior 100 days, because of prior formation and persistence of HIT antibodies. Sometimes, there is an acute systemic reaction, characterized by fever, chills, hypotension, and/or cardiovascular compromise immediately after exposure to heparin. An abrupt fall in the platelet count is then observed.
- ***Diagnosis***: The diagnosis of HIT requires both an appropriate clinical context and confirmatory laboratory testing (demonstration of HIT antibodies). Because of the limited availability of HIT-specific laboratory assays, however, any patient in whom clinical suspicion for the disorder is high should be managed as HIT, even if the results of diagnostic tests are pending or unavailable.
  - *Clinical factors*: Thrombocytopenia (or greater than 50% decline from the baseline platelet count) or thrombosis in a patient who has recently been exposed to heparin may indicate HIT. The timing of the decline in platelet count or appearance of thrombosis should be compared to the onset of exposure to heparin. An appropriate increase in the platelet count after discontinuation of heparin plus the absence of another plausible explanation for thrombocytopenia may be regarded as diagnostic for HIT in the absence of confirmatory laboratory testing. A careful review of the hospital chart (including nursing notes) may be necessary to document administration of heparin, especially if its use was transient (heparin flushes) or its form covert (heparin-impregnated catheters).
  - *Laboratory diagnosis* is achieved by one or both of two types of assays. Both tests have a sensitivity of approximately 90%. The *enzyme-linked immunosorbent assay (ELISA) for PF4-heparin–associated IgG* measures binding of HIT antibodies in the patient's serum to a PF4-heparin complex that has been used to coat wells of a microtiter plate; an anti-IgG antibody with a label is applied and the binding quantified. *Platelet activation assays* (less commonly available) measure activation of donor platelets in the presence of the patient's serum and a high and low concentration of heparin; increased release of adenosine triphosphate (ATP; chemiluminescence method) or ^{14}C-serotonin (9) in the presence of therapeutic concentrations of heparin (0.05–0.3 U/mL) indicates HIT. Some heparin-treated patients who have not demonstrated a decline in the platelet count (and thus do not have HIT) nonetheless show HIT antibodies by ELISA; in these cases, platelet activation assays (which have a higher specificity than ELISA) are likely to be negative.
- ***Treatment***.
  - *All forms of heparin must be discontinued immediately*. (In patients in whom laboratory testing for HIT eventually proves negative or in whom an alternative explanation for thrombocytopenia has been found, heparin may be subsequently restarted.)
  - Doppler ultrasound of the lower extremities should be performed to exclude subclinical deep vein thrombosis.

- Because patients with HIT rarely bleed and transfused platelets may worsen the already increased thrombotic risk by providing substrate for HIT antibodies, platelet transfusions are rarely indicated.
- *Warfarin is contraindicated as initial treatment* of clinically proven or suspected HIT, because of its propensity to exacerbate hypercoagulability by reduction of plasma levels of proteins C and S (see Chapter 23).
- An alternative anticoagulant (Table 19-3 and see Chapter 23) should be administered to a patient with HIT and any of the following features:

  1. Concomitant thrombosis.
  2. High risk for thrombosis (e.g., immobilized or postsurgical patients).
  3. Requirement for anticoagulation (e.g., after interventional cardiac procedures).

Note that some investigators recommend that all patients with HIT receive an alternative anticoagulant, at least initially.

- The alternative anticoagulant should be continued at least until significant recovery of the platelet count has occurred or, in patients with thrombosis, until the platelet count has recovered substantially and adequate anticoagulation with warfarin has been achieved (see below). If an alternative anticoagulant is not used, the patient should be closely observed until the platelet count has recovered for signs or symptoms of thrombosis.
- *Longer-term anticoagulation*: Patients with HIT who develop thrombosis should receive anticoagulation with warfarin for a total duration of 3 to 6 months at an international normalized ratin (INR) of 2.0 to 3.0. Warfarin should not be initiated, however, until therapeutic anticoagulation with an alternative anticoagulant has been achieved and the platelet count has recovered substantially. (Note: concomitant warfarin and argatroban use requires a special approach to interpretation of the INR; see Chapter 23.)
- *Thrombolysis/thromboembolectomy*: Low-dose or very low-dose thrombolytic agents may be indicated in acute limb ischemia or life-threatening pulmonary embolism caused by HIT-associated thrombi. Surgical removal of large-vessel, arterial thrombi may be needed if the limb is threatened and other treatments have failed. These patients require concomitant use of an alternative anticoagulant, regardless of the degree of thrombocytopenia.
- *IVIG, plasma exchange*, and *aspirin* are not used unless thrombocytopenia and/or life-threatening thromboses are worsening or persistent despite initiation of an alternative anticoagulant.
- *Retreatment with heparin*: HIT antibodies probably do not persist beyond 100 days from the initial episode of HIT (10), in which case very transient use of heparin subsequent to this time period may be safe. If possible, however, heparin should be avoided in all patients with a prior history of HIT, and an alternative anticoagulant used. If heparin is essential (as in cardiopulmonary bypass), it should not be given until absence of HIT antibodies has been confirmed by ELISA or platelet activation methods, and its use should be limited to the procedure.
- *Low molecular weight heparins*: The prevalence of HIT among patients treated with low molecular weight heparins (LMWHs) is much lower than that observed with unfractionated heparin (UFH). The smaller molecular size of the LMWHs decreases their binding to PF4 and their immunogenicity. The small but reproducible rate of cross-reactivity of HIT antibodies with LMWHs contraindicates their use in the treatment of acute HIT.
- ***Nonimmune HIT*** describes a small decrease in the platelet count observed after the initiation of heparin; this phenomenon is not immune-mediated and presumably is caused by heparin induced, PF4-independent platelet aggregation. The decrease in platelets (from baseline) generally is less than 10,000 to 30,000/mL and not significant enough to result in thrombocytopenia. Heparin does not need to be discontinued in this setting.

TABLE. 19-3. *Alternative anticoagulants in the treatment of heparin-induced thrombocytopenia*

Agent	Description	Indication	Dosing	Comment
Argatroban	Synthetic direct thrombin inhibitor	Prophylaxis or treatment of HIT, including postpercutaneous coronary intervention	Obtain baseline PTT. Start continuous infusion at 2 μg/kg/min. Titrate to achieve PTT of 1.5 to 3 times the baseline value. Do not allow PTT to exceed 100 seconds, nor the infusion rate to exceed 10 μg/kg/min.	• Patients with hepatic insufficiency: initial infusion rate = 0.5 μg/kg/min. • Increases the INR in warfarin-treated patients; interpret INR accordingly.
Lepirudin (*Refludan*)	Recombinant hirudin; direct thrombin inhibitor	Treatment of HIT with associated thrombosis	Obtain baseline PTT. Give slow bolus of 0.4 mg/kg then continuous infusion of 0.15 mg/kg/hr. Titrate to achieve PTT of 1.5–2.5 times baseline value. PTTs should be obtained 4 hours after starting the infusion and at least daily during treatment.	• Patients with renal insufficiency: initial bolus = 0.2 mg/kg. • 50% of patients develop antidrug antibodies that increase half-life; may necessitate a decrease in dose
Bivalirudin (*Angiomax*)	Semisynthetic derivative of hirudin; direct thrombin inhibitor	Unstable angina in patients undergoing percutaneous coronary angioplasty	—	• Renal insufficiency: may require dose reduction
Danaparoid sodium (*Orgaran*)[a]	Mixture of negatively charged glycosaminoglycans (heparin sulfate, dermatan sulfate, chondroitin sulfate)	—	—	• Monitoring difficult (requires anti-Xa levels and danaparoid calibration curve) • 10% cross-reactivity with HIT antibodies

[a] Not available in the United States. HIT, heparin-induced thrombocytopenia; PTT, partial thromboplastin time; INR, international normalized ratio.

Thrombotic Thrombocytopenic Purpura

Thrombotic thrombocytopenic purpura (TTP) and the related disorder, the hemolytic-uremic syndrome (HUS), are characterized by microangiopathic hemolytic anemia (MAHA) and the formation of platelet-rich thrombi in the arterial and capillary microvasculature; they also are known as thrombotic microangiopathies (TMA). As platelets are consumed, thrombocytopenia develops; anemia results from hemolysis and bleeding. Early aggressive intervention with plasma exchange is crucial in most cases because of the extremely high mortality rate.

- *Epidemiology*: The incidence of sporadic TTP is approximately 3 to 4 cases per 100,000 persons (11); there is a slight female predominance. Most cases of endemic HUS occur in children, are related to infection with enteropathogenic bacteria, and are more prevalent in summer or warm climates. TMA occurs at an increased rate during pregnancy and in the peripartum period.
- *Pathophysiology*: TMAs are thought to arise from factors that directly or indirectly cause platelet aggregation and/or endothelial cell damage, leading to the formation of microvascular thrombi and ischemia in involved organs. These factors include toxins, cytokines, drugs, or deficiencies in the function of the *von Willebrand factor cleaving protease* (VWFCP or ADAMTS-13). Red cells are sheared as they negotiate thrombotic obstructions and fibrin strands in the microvasculature, leading to hemolytic anemia. Consumption of platelets results in thrombocytopenia and bleeding.
  - Patients with *congenital TTP* have decreased activity of the VWFCP (12), a metalloproteinase which normally functions to cleave newly synthesized, ultra-large VWF (ULVWF) multimers released in the plasma into multimers of smaller size. ULVWF multimers bind to platelets more avidly than do smaller VWF molecules; thus, ULVWF in the plasma may incite platelet aggregation.
  - In *sporadic TTP*, an acquired deficiency of VWFCP results from production of an autoantibody against the VWFCP (13), leading to an accumulation of ULVWF in the plasma and excessive platelet aggregation.
  - *Pregnancy-associated TTP-HUS* may be due to decreased levels of the VWFCP that naturally occur in the second and third trimesters; in some cases an antibody to VWFCP is present (14).
  - In *endemic HUS*, Shiga toxin from *Escherichia coli* (especially type 0157:H7) promotes platelet aggregation by damaging endothelial cells or by other mechanisms.
  - *Drugs* such as cyclosporine, quinine, ticlopidine, clopidogrel, mitomycin C, and bleomycin may cause TMA by endothelial cell injury and/or proaggregatory effects on platelets. Antibodies inhibiting the VWFCP have been described in patients who received some of these medications (15,16).
  - TMA in the setting of *cancer, hematopoietic stem cell transplantation*, or *HIV infection* has not been linked to abnormalities of VWFCP.
- *Presentation*: All patients with TMA have MAHA. Varying degrees of bleeding and neurologic impairment (more typical of TTP) or symptoms related to renal failure (predominant in HUS) may also be present (Table 19-4). Microangiopathic hemolytic anemia, thrombocytopenia, fever, renal insufficiency and neurologic system abnormalities (the classic pentad) occur in less than half of patients with TTP (17). Most patients with HUS have a recent or current diarrheal illness.
  - Children with diarrhea-associated TMA usually are said to have HUS (hemolytic uremic syndrome) because of the degree of renal impairment. In adults, TTP and HUS are often difficult to distinguish because of overlapping symptoms, but if kidney dysfunction predominates, the syndrome usually is classified as HUS.
  - Manifestations of renal insufficiency include elevated creatinine, azotemia, proteinura, hematuria, and/or oliguria.
  - Neurologic impairment (from microthrombi in the cerebral vasculature) occurs in approx-

TABLE. 19–4. Features of thrombotic microangiopathes

Parameter	TTP	HUS	Pregnancy-related TTP-HUS	Therapy-related TTP-HUS
Patient-specific factors	Most cases in adults. Preceding upper respiratory illness in some patients. Minority of cases familial.	Most cases in children. Episode(s) of bloody diarrhea within prior 2 weeks in 90%.	Current or recent pregnancy	Recent (<200 days) HSCT, or use of TMA-associated drugs (especially cyclosporine)
MAHA	All patients	All patients	All patients; may resemble HELLP	All patients
Bleeding	Most patients	Less common	Most patients	Variable
Thrombocytopenia	Most patients; typically moderate-severe	Most patients, but mild or absent in 30%	Most patients; may resemble HELLP	Most patients; overlap with thrombocytopenia of graft-versus-host disease
Fever	Present in 75%	Typically absent	Variable	Variable
Renal insufficiency	May be mild	All patients	Most patients	Most patients; may be difficult to distinguish from CSA ATN or renal allograft rejection in KT patients
Neurologic impairment	Most patients	<50% of patients.	Most patients	Most patients
Corroborative specialized laboratory findings	Decreased activity of VWFCP (by collagen binding assay or other methods)	Positive stool culture for E. coli 0157:H7; positive (antibody to) Shiga(-like) toxin; VWFCP activity usually normal	In some cases, decreased activity of VWFCP	In some cases, decreased activity of VWFCP
Treatment	Immediate plasma exchange; supportive care. Few patients require dialysis. Usually, platelet transfusions contraindicated.	Most require (temporary) dialysis; supportive care. Adults may benefit from plasma exchange.	Immediate plasma exchange; supportive care. Usually, platelet transfusions contraindicated. Uterine evacuation probably unhelpful.	Discontinue offending drug(s). Plasma exchange less helpful in HSCT-associated TMA. Supportive care. Usually, platelet transfusions contraindicated.

MAHA, microangiopathic hemolytic anemia; HELLP, hemolysis, elevated liver enzymes, low platelets syndrome; HSCT, hematopoietic stem cell transplantation; KT, kidney transplantation; CSA, cyclosporine; ATN, acute tubular necrosis; VWFCP, von Willebrand factor cleaving protease; HUS, hemolytic-uremic syndrome; TTP, thrombotic thrombocytopenic purpura; TMA, thrombotic microangiopathy.

imately 75% and 30% of patients with TTP and HUS, respectively, and includes headache, somnolence, confusion, seizures, and (less commonly) paresis and coma.

- **Diagnosis**: TMA is a clinical diagnosis; the presence of new-onset MAHA and thrombocytopenia (and/or renal failure) in the absence of any other plausible explanation suffice for the diagnosis.
  - MAHA is essential to the diagnosis of TTP-HUS and is defined by anemia with positive markers of intravascular hemolysis (elevated lactate dehydrogenase [LDH], elevated indirect bilirubin, decreased haptoglobin, and reticulocytosis) and negative direct antiglobulin (Coombs) test (DAT). The blood smear shows more than three schistocytes per high-power microscopic field.
  - Clinical features such as an antecedent bloody diarrheal illness and/or renal insufficiency (more typically associated with HUS), or neurologic abnormalities with or without fever (more typically associated with TTP), or recent or current pregnancy, or treatment with associated drugs, or cancer, or recent hematopoietic stem cell transplantation are diagnostically corroborative.
  - Stool culture for *E. coli* 0157:H7 or assays for antibody against Shiga or Shiga-like toxins, or against specific bacterial lipopolysaccharide, may be positive in patients with endemic HUS.
  - Assays for the VWFCP may be abnormal in congenital or sporadic (acquired) TTP; these specialized tests are not available widely and most require substantial processing time, so treatment decisions must be made on clinical grounds.
  - The prothrombin time (PT), activated partial thromboplastin time (aPTT), and fibrinogen are typically within the normal range in TMA.
- **Treatment**: Without plasma exchange, the mortality rate of sporadic TTP exceeds 90% (11). For this reason, the diagnosis of TMA should be made promptly and treatment with plasma exchange instituted expeditiously. An important exception is children or adults with endemic (*E.coli* diarrhea-associated) HUS, who generally recover with supportive care within 3 weeks, without plasma exchange.
  - *Plasma exchange* should be initiated as soon as appropriate vascular access has been obtained. Exchange should be performed once daily until the LDH and platelet count are normal for 2 to 3 days—up to 3 weeks of treatment may be required. Failure to respond to once-daily therapy requires twice-daily treatments; once the LDH and platelet count indicate response, once-daily treatments can be resumed until these parameters have normalized for 2 to 3 days, and then the treatments can be continued every other day, then weekly, for a short period of time, before being discontinued.
  - *Platelet transfusions generally are contraindicated* in TMAs because of possible propagation or new formation of platelet-rich microthrombi (18). If computed tomography (CT)- or magnetic resonance imaging (MRI)-documented intracranial bleeding or other life-threatening bleeding is present, platelet transfusions may be necessary; transfuse platelets slowly and after plasma exchange is underway (19).
  - *Packed red cells* may be transfused commensurate with the pace of the MAHA and degree of bleeding.
  - Should plasma exchange be delayed, infusion of fresh-frozen plasma (FFP) may be helpful as a temporizing measure. Plasma infusion as sole treatment of TMA, however, is substandard because of (i) the possible role of plasma exchange in removing offending drugs, cytokines, bacterial proteins, ULVWF multimers, or antibodies to the VWFCP and (ii) the volume overload frequently incurred when the required large volumes of FFP are infused. An exception is familial relapsing TMA, as the congenital deficiency in the VWFCP can be corrected merely by infusion of smaller volumes of plasma.
- **Refractory and relapsing TMA**: If remission is not achieved with aggressive plasma exchange, second-line treatments can be considered: the addition of *steroids* or *IVIG* to plasma exchange, *vincristine*, *cyclophosphamide*, *cyclosporine* (in select cases of sporadic TTP) and *splenectomy*. The monoclonal antibody *rituximab* also has achieved responses in a limited number of refractory cases (20). Up to one-third of patients with sporadic TMA

relapse after discontinuation of plasma exchange. In these cases, plasma exchange should be reinitiated according to the guidelines above, and, if ineffective, immunosuppressive treatments should be considered.

- **Hemodialysis**: More than half of all patients with HUS (and a minority with TTP) require hemodialysis. Approximately half of these patients will attain durable restoration of renal function but 25% develop chronic renal failure. The remainder experience variable degrees of permanent renal insufficiency.

DISSEMINATED INTRAVASCULAR COAGULATION

Thrombocytopenia in disseminated intravascular coagulation (DIC) occurs as a result of uncontrolled activation of coagulation in the circulation. Platelets participate in these reactions, leading to their consumption. If bleeding is present, platelet transfusions may be administered to reach a platelet count target of 20,000 to 30,000 per microliter (most cases) or more than 50,000 per microliter (intracranial or life-threatening hemorrhage). Thrombocytopenia and the other clinical and laboratory manifestations of DIC are expected to resolve with effective treatment of the underlying, inciting disorder. (For a full discussion of DIC, see Chapter 21.)

Posttransfusion Purpura

Posttransfusion purpura (PTP) is characterized by the unexplained, sudden appearance of thrombocytopenia in an otherwise asymptomatic individual who recently has received a blood transfusion (red cells, platelets or plasma), usually within 1 week prior to development of thrombocytopenia. The precipitating events are unknown, but more than 90% of individuals with PTP display antibodies against the human platelet antigen Pl^{A1} (21).

- Most patients with PTP are postmenopausal females who are either multiparous or who have received prior transfusions; they commonly present with severe thrombocytopenia and bleeding.
- If untreated, thrombocytopenia typically persists for up to 2 to 3 weeks, concurrent with a mortality rate of 10% from bleeding; therefore, *IVIG* (1 gm/kg per day for 2 days) should be administered as soon as the diagnosis is suspected. Most patients will respond, but in the case of relapse, IVIG may be administered in a second course. Plasma exchange, adjunctive corticosteroids, and splenectomy are alternative treatments for refractory cases. Because transfused platelets are probably as susceptible to binding by antigen–antibody complexes as are the patient's own platelets, platelet transfusion is generally not performed unless severe bleeding is present; in this case, human leukocyte antigen (HLA)-matched platelets are preferred. Future transfusions should be administered judiciously, with washed or Pl^{A1}-negative blood products.

Neonatal Alloimmune Thrombocytopenia

- Neonatal aloimmune thrombocytopenia (NAIT) is a cause of severe thrombocytopenia in neonates. Fetal platelet antigens cross the placenta and trigger formation of maternal alloantibodies that can then enter the fetal circulation, bind platelets, and induce thrombocytopenia. Antibodies commonly have specificity for human platelet antigen [HPA]-1a, also known as Pl^{A1}. The presence of certain maternal platelet phenotypes (such as the homozygous HPA-1b state) influences the risk of the disorder, especially if the fetus inherits a different, paternal platelet phenotype.

- The thrombocytopenia is severe and there is a high prevalence of intracranial hemorrhage (ICH) during or after delivery, resulting in neonatal death in 5% of cases. Thrombocytopenia typically resolves by 2 to 3 weeks of age (22).
- *IVIG*, with or without *corticosteroids*, is recommended for any neonate with platelet counts less than 20,000 to 25,000/mL. Random donor or (ideally) irradiated maternally antigen-matched platelets are often administered in cases of ICH. Subsequent pregnancies are as high risk for recurrent NAIT.

Von Willebrand disease, Type IIb

This type of von Willebrand disease (vWD) is characterized by an abnormal von Willebrand factor (vWF) that has increased affinity for its platelet receptor, glycoprotein Ib. As a result of the bridging action of vWF, platelets aggregate in vivo and are cleared, typically resulting in a mild thrombocytopenia. vWD is discussed in detail in Chapter 21.

Extracorporeal Circulation-Related Thrombocytopenia

The passage of the blood for prolonged periods outside the body in an artificial circuit (as during cardiac bypass surgery) results in platelet activation and clearance. Thrombocytopenia generally is not severe. Other common concomitant causes of thrombocytopenia in the post-surgical patient (such as HIT, DIC, and sepsis-related and drug-induced thrombocytopenia) must be considered.

DISORDERS CHARACTERIZED BY INCREASED SEQUESTRATION OF PLATELETS

- Hypersplenism results in sequestration of blood cells (including platelets) in an enlarged or abnormal spleen. Mild to moderate thrombocytopenia is most commonly observed, but when the bulk of the platelet mass is contained within a massively enlarged spleen, thrombo-cytopenia can be severe.
- Splenomegaly with hypersplenism is almost always an acquired condition, resulting from many different underlying disorders (Table 19-5).

TABLE. 19–5. *Selected causes of splenomegaly*

Lymphoproliferation	**Congestion**
Lymphoma	Cirrhosis
Chronic lymphocytic leukemia	Heart failure
Collagen vascular disease	
(Felty syndrome, systemic lupus)	
Autoimmune lymphoproliferative disorder	**Hemolysis**
	Hereditary spherocytosis
Myeloproliferation	Paroxysmal nocturnal hemoglobinuria
Myeloid leukemia	Thalassemia
Polycythema vera	
Essential thrombocythemia	**Infection**
	Viral (CMV, EBV, hepatitis)
Inborn Errors of Metabolism	Parasitic (malaria, babesiosis)
Gaucher disease	
Niemann-Pick disease	**Immunodeficiency**
	Common variable immunodeficiency

CMV, cytomegalovirus; EBV, Epstein-Barr virus.

- If adequate production of platelets can be documented and significant splenomegaly with thrombocytopenia is present, splenectomy may be considered. Splenic embolization and splenic irradiation are alternatives but generally do not result in maximal platelet responses. They may be considered for significant hypersplenism in disorders such as chronic leukemia/ lymphoma (CLL) or lymphoma for patients unable to tolerate surgery.

OTHER MISCELLANEOUS CAUSES OF THROMBOCYTOPENIA

Pseudothrombocytopenia

For unclear reasons, calcium chelation induced by the anticoagulant ethylenediaminetetra-acetic acid (EDTA; present in blood-collecting tubes) causes changes on the platelet membranes of certain patients that expose cryptic antigens to which preformed, otherwise nonpathogenic agglutinating antibodies may bind, causing platelet clumping. Automated cell counters (such as those that are present in most hospital laboratories) will report a falsely low platelet count; examination of the blood smear reveals platelet clumps. Normalization of the platelet count upon automated determination from a blood specimen collected in citrate anticoagulant and/or disappearance of platelet clumps on a blood smear obtained from a fingerstick source yield a correct assessment of platelet number and confirms the presence of this harmless phenomenon.

Drug-Induced Thrombocytopenia

- By definition, drug-induced thrombocytopenia develops after initiation of a given drug, resolves when the offending medication is discontinued and may recur if the agent is reintroduced (23). The mechanisms by which many drugs may lead to a low platelet count have not been elucidated.
- *Chemotherapeutic agents* cause decreased platelet production by direct cytotoxicity.
- *Quinine purpura* is a type of drug-induced immune thrombocytopenia (DITP), in which antibody-mediated destruction of platelets occurs after exposure to a given drug. Quinine induces a conformational change in the platelet membrane, allowing exposure of an otherwise cryptic antigen; circulating antibodies then bind the antigen, but only in the presence of the drug. DITP presents with severe thrombocytopenia (less than 20,000/mL) and mucocutaneous bleeding, including purpura and ecchymoses. Thrombocytopenia should resolve within days to weeks of discontinuing the agent. In cases of severe bleeding, IVIG and platelet transfusions appear to be more effective than corticosteroids in inducing responses.
- Other medications frequently associated with thrombocytopenia are listed in Table 19-6.

Gestational Thrombocytopenia

The blood volume increases by as much as 40% to 45% over baseline during pregnancy, causing progressive hemodilution. Cytopenias result, but production of blood cells is normal or increased. Approximately 10% and fewer than 1% of pregnant women experience platelet counts less than 100,000/mL and less than 50,000/mL by the third trimester, respectively; the incidence of ITP is thought to be even lower. Severe thrombocytopenia in pregnancy (less than 50,000/mL) should prompt investigation to exclude a preexisting condition, preeclampsia, or a pregnancy-related thrombotic microangiopathy; if negative, the etiology may be presumed to be ITP and treated accordingly (see the Immune Thrombocyopenic Purpura section earlier).

Human Immunodeficiency Virus-Related Thrombocytopenia

Thrombocytopenia in HIV infection results both from immune-mediated phenomena leading to increased clearance of platelets and ineffective platelet production, possibly as a result

TABLE. 19–6. *Drugs associated with thrombocytopenia*

Antimicrobials	**Cardiovascular agents**
Amphotericin	Amiodarone
Ampicillin	Captopril
Isoniazid	Digoxin
Rifampin	Hydrochlorothiazide
Methcillin	Procainamide
Piperacillin	Quinidine
Sulfasoxazole	
Trimethoprim-sulfamethoxazole	**Neuropsychiatric agents**
	Carbemazepine
Antiplatelet agents	Chlorpromazine
Anagrelide	Diazepam
Abciximab	Haldoperidol
Eptifibatide	Lithium
Ticlopidine	Methyldopa
Tirofiban	Phenytoin
Analgesics/anti-inflammatory	**Other**
agents	Gold
Acetominophen	Heparin
Diclofenac	Mycophenolate mofetil

From DeLoughery T. Hemorrhagic and thrombotic disorders in the intensive care setting. In: Kitchens C, Alving BM, Kessler C, eds Consultative Hemostasis and Thrombosis. Philadelphia: W.B. Saunders Company, 2002:493–513.

of direct infection of megakaryocytes with HIV. Improvement or resolution of thrombocytopenia after initiation of antiretroviral therapy in newly diagnosed patients is commonly observed; if possible, *zidovudine* (AZT) (24) should be included in the antiretroviral regimen since data on the efficacy of other antiretroviral agents in the correction of thrombocytopenia are limited. If the thrombocytopenia proves refractory, therapies commonly used in the treatment of ITP (IVIG, anti-D, steroids, splenectomy, others) are used, but the potentially immunosuppressive effects of some of these approaches need to be considered.

Infection- and Sepsis-Related Thrombocytopenia

- Thrombocytopenia in the setting of infection or sepsis is common. DIC is often implicated in critically ill patients, but other causes, such as megakaryocyte-specific effects or increased clearance caused by fever or splenic enlargement, may be responsible.
- Transient thrombocytopenia is commonly observed with many viral infections. Certain bacterial infections, such as *ehrlichiosis, rickettsial disease*, and *dengue* characteristically produce thrombocytopenia. A corroborative travel history and directed microbiologic testing are usually necessary to make a diagnosis.
- If the platelet count does not return to baseline with effective antimicrobial treatment or after resolution of the infection, an alternative etiology should be sought.

Hemophagocytosis

- In hemophagocytosis, bone marrow macrophages (histiocytes) engulf cellular components of the marrow. Occasional phasocytosins histiocytis are nonspecific if they occur sporadically within an aspirate smear, but abundant histiocytes with intracytoplasmic white cells, red cells or platelets indicate pathology.

- In adults, *sepsis* (25) or *Epstein-Barr virus-related infection or malignancy* (26) can drive T cells to produce cytokines that mediate hemophagocytosis, leading to thrombocytopenia. In these cases, the treatment is principally immunosuppressive, but the disorder often is aggressive and unresponsive to treatment.
- *Familial hemophagocytic lymphohistiocytosis* (27) is an autosomal recessively-inherited disorder featuring hemophagocytosis, fever, organomegaly and hypertriglyceridemia or hypofibrinogenemia; it presents at a young age. The only curative treatment is allogeneic hematopoietic stem cell transplantation.

Qualitative Disorders

Several heritable platelet anomalies of structure or function (including the *May-Hegglin anomaly* and the *Bernard-Soulier syndrome*) are typically associated with a mild thrombocytopenia. These are discussed in more detail in Chapter 21.

REFERENCES

1. Frederiksen H, Schmidt K. The incidence of idiopathic thrombocytopenia in adults increases with age. *Blood* 1999;94:909–913.
2. Cines DB, Blanchette VS. Immune thrombocytopenic purpura. *N Engl J Med* 2002;346:995–1008.
3. George JN, Woolf SH, Raskob GE, et al. Idiopathic thrombocytiopenic purpura: A practice guideline developed by explicit methods for The American Society of Hematology. *Blood* 1996;88:3–40.
4. Schwartz J, Leber MD, Gillis S, et al. Long term follow-up after splenectomy performed for immune thrombocytopenic purpura (ITP). *Am J Hematol* 2003;72:94–98.
5. Stasi R, Pagano A, Stipa E, et al. Rituximab chimeric anti-CD20 monoclonal antibody treatment for adults with chronic idiopathic thrombocytopenic purpura. *Blood* 2002;99:3872–3873.
6. Huhn RD, Fogarty PF, Nakamura R, et al. High-dose cyclophosphamide with autologous lymphocyte-depleted peripheral blood stem cell (PBSC) support for treatment of refractory chronic autoimmune thrombocytopenia. *Blood* 2003;101:71–77.
7. Warkentin TE, Levine MN, Hirsh J, et al. Heparin-induced thrombocytopenia in patients treated with low-molecular-weight heparin or unfractionated heparin. *N Engl J Med* 1995;332:1330–1335.
8. Warkentin TE, Kelton JG. A 14-year study of heparin-induced thrombocytopenia. *Am J Med* 1996; 101:502–507.
9. Sheridan D, Carter C, Kelton JG. A diagnostic test for heparin-induced thrombocytopenia. *Blood* 1986;67:27–30.
10. Warkentin TE, Kelton JG. Temporal aspects of heparin-induced thrombocytopenia. *N Eng J Med* 2001;344:1286–1292.
11. Torok TJ, Holman RC, Chorba TL. Increasing mortality from thrombotic thrombocytopenic purpura in the United States—analysis of national mortality data, 1968–1991. *Am J Hematol* 1995;50:84.
12. Furlan M, Robles R, Galbusera M, et al. von Willebrand factor-cleaving protease in thrombotic thrombocytopenic purpura and the hemolytic-uremic syndrome. *N Engl J Med* 1998;339:1578–1584.
13. Tsai HM, Lian EC. Antibodies to von Willebrand factor-cleaving protease in acute thrombotic thrombocytopenic purpura. *N Engl J Med* 1998;339:1585–1594.
14. Lattuada A, Rossi E, Calzarossa C, et al. Mild to moderate reduction of a von Willebrand factor cleaving protease (ADAMTS-13) in pregnant women with HELLP microangiopathic syndrome. *Haematologica* 2003;88:1029–1034.
15. Moake JL. Thrombotic thrombocytopenic purpura and the hemolytic uremic syndrome. *Arch Pathol Lab Med* 2002;126:1430–1433.
16. Tsai HM, Rice L, Sarode R, et al. Antibody inhibitors to von Willebrand factor metalloproteinase and increased binding of von Willebrand factor to platelets in ticlopidine-associated thrombotic thrombocytopenic purpura. *Ann Intern Med* 2000;132:794–805.
17. Ridolfi RL, Bell WR. Thrombotic thrombocytopenic purpura: report of 25 cases and a review of the literature. *Medicine* 1981;60:413.
18. Bell WR, Braine HG, Ness PM, et al. Improved survival in thrombotic thrombocuytopenic purpura-hemolytic-uremic syndrome. *N Eng J Med* 1991;325:398–403.
19. De la Rubia J, Plume G, Arriaga F, et al. Platelet transfusion and thrombotic thrombocytopenic purpura. *Transfusion* 2002;42:1384–1385.

20. Chemnitz J, Draube A, Scheid C, et al. Successful treatment of severe thrombotic thrombocytopenic purpura with the monoclonal antibody rituximab. *Am J Hematol* 2002;71:105–108.
21. Shulman NR, Aster RH, Leitner A, et al. Immunoreactions involving platelets. V. Posttransfusion purpura due to a complement-fixing antibody against a genetically controlled platelet antigen. A proposed mechanism for thrombocytopenia and its relevance to "autoimmunity". *J Clin Invest* 1961; 40:1597.
22. Mueller-Eckhardt C, Grubert A, Weisheit M et al. 348 cases of suspected neonatal allo-immune thrombocytopenia. *Lancet* 1989;1:363.
23. George JN, Raskob GE, Shah SR, et al. Drug-induced thrombocytopenia: a systematic review of published case reports. *Ann Intern Med* 1998;129:886.
24. Hymes KB, Greene JB, Karpatkin S. The effect of azidothymidine on HIV-related thrombocytopenia. *N Engl J Med* 1988;318:516.
25. Stephan F, Thioliere B, Verdy E, et al. Role of hemophagocytic histiocytosis in the etiology of thrombocytopenia in patients with sepsis syndrome or septic shock. *Clin Infect Dis* 1997;25: 1159–1164.
26. Watson HG, Goulden NJ, Manson LM, et al. Virus-associated hemophagocytic syndrome: further evidence for a T-cell mediated disorder. *Br J Haematol* 1994;86:213.
27. Arico M, Janka G, Fischer A, et al. Hemophagocytic lymphohistiocytosis. Report of 122 children from the International Registry. *Leukemia* 1996;10:197.

20

Disorders of Hemostasis I: Coagulation

Patrick F. Fogarty and Margaret E. Rick

Abnormalities of the activity of coagulation proteins and related molecules, decreased platelet function, or disruption of the vasculature (by surgery or trauma) can lead to bleeding. Careful assessment of the clinical history and laboratory testing are necessary to establish the reason for bleeding.

Screening studies in a patient with new-onset or recent bleeding include a platelet count, activated partial thromboplastin time (aPTT), prothrombin time (PT), and fibrinogen. If the bleeding is moderate to severe, a hemoglobin level and specimen for red cell cross-matching should be sent.

- The *character, timing, and location* of the bleeding should be considered. Is the bleeding spontaneous or is it associated only with invasive procedures or trauma? If periprocedural, is the bleeding immediate or delayed? Mucocutaneous bleeding (epistaxis, gingival hemorrhage, petechiae/ecchymoses, gastrointestinal and urinary tract bleeding) is more characteristic of a defect in platelet activity, whereas soft-tissue bleeding or hemarthrosis suggests a deficiency in the activity of coagulation factors.
- The *clinical context* is important. Hemorrhage in a patient who has been receiving heparin or warfarin may indicate excess anticoagulation or presence of a previously undetected lesion. Bleeding after allogeneic transplantation or treatment with certain drugs occurs as a result of thrombotic microangiopathy (TMA). Bleeding in the setting of septic shock may point to disseminated intravascular coagulation (DIC). New-onset diffuse bleeding in a patient who is pregnant or postpartum may signify the HELLP (hemolysis, elevated liver enzymes, low platelets) syndrome or other entities. Postsurgical bleeding may stem from a number of causes, but an initial consideration should be deficient hemostasis caused by a traumatized bleeding vessel, as well as a coagulation factor defect or deficits.
- A positive *family history* raises the clinical suspicion for heritable disorders such as hemophilia A or B (X-linked recessive inheritance) or von Willebrand disease (autosomal dominant inheritance).
- Importantly, bleeding does not necessarily indicate an intrinsic abnormality of hemostasis. Individuals with perfectly normal coagulation and platelet function will bleed upon encountering a sufficient hemostatic challenge (trauma, surgery, invasive malignancy, etc.).

THE COAGULATION SYSTEM

Coagulation Factors: Background

- Most coagulation factors (clotting factors) are synthesized in the liver.
- Clotting factors II, VII, IX, X, XI, and XII are *serine proteases* that are inactive as synthesized and acquire enzymatic capability when cleaved (activated) by other proteins. Tissue factor and factors V and VIII are not enzymes, but serve as *cofactors* for coagulation reactions. A post-synthetic step in the production of factors II, VII, IX, and X and the

natural anticoagulant proteins C and S requires the activity of a *vitamin K-dependent carbox-ylase* that modifies the amino terminus of each factor, enabling it to function.

- The activity of all clotting factors culminates in a principal event: the generation of thrombin. Thrombin activates platelets and cleaves fibrinogen to form fibrin; therefore, it assists in both primary hemostasis (formation of an occlusive platelet plug) and secondary hemostasis (clot formation) at sites of blood vessel compromise.
- The normal *laboratory range* of factor activity levels is approximately 50% to 150% and is derived from plasma activity as observed in a reference pool of normal donors. The *hemostatic level* of a given clotting factor (the level of factor necessary to maintain normal hemostasis) typically is much lower. For instance, 5% activity of factor VIII is well below the laboratory reference range but usually is sufficient to prevent spontaneous bleeding.

The Coagulation Cascade

The *coagulation cascade* comprises the *extrinsic, intrinsic* and *common pathways of coagulation* (Fig. 20-1). *In vivo,* these pathways interact at multiple points and function in concert with the activation and aggregation of platelets to achieve hemostasis.

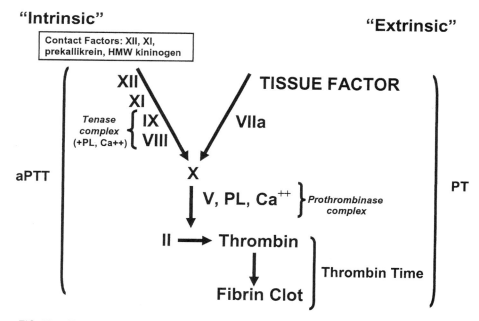

FIG. 20-1. The coagulation cascade. The extrinsic pathway of coagulation begins with the binding of activated factor VII (VIIa) to tissue factor (TF), which is provided by cell membranes. VIIa converts X to Xa. The *prothrombinase complex,* formed by the binding of Xa to Va in the presence of phospholipid (PL) and Ca^{2+}, converts II (prothrombin) to IIa (thrombin). The intrinsic pathway of coagulation begins with the activation of factor XII to XIIa by kallikrein. XIIa cleaves XI to XIa; XIa cleaves IX to IXa. IXa forms a complex with VIIIa in the presence of phospholipid and Ca^{2+} (*tenase complex*), and converts X to Xa. Xa, in the presence of Va, PL and Ca^{2+}, then cleaves II (prothrombin) to IIa (thrombin). The common pathway involves the cleavage of II by prothrombinase to yield thrombin, and thrombin cleavage of fibrinogen to form fibrin, which is then cross-linked via the action of XIIIa. Activation of coagulation usually begins with the extrinsic system, which provides feedback to the intrinsic system by IIa activation of factor XI. There are additional points of interaction between the pathways (not indicated).

- *Extrinsic pathway:* The extrinsic pathway of coagulation begins with the binding of activated factor VII (VIIa) to tissue factor (TF). The TF-VIIa complex mediates the conversion of X to Xa. The *prothrombinase complex,* formed by the binding of Xa to Va on a phospholipid (PL) surface (usually platelet membranes) in the presence of Ca^{2+}, converts II (prothrombin) to IIa (thrombin).
- *Intrinsic pathway:* Activation of contact factors at the site of vascular injury leads to the conversion of factor XII to XIIa, and the sequential conversion of XI to XIa and IX to IXa. IXa complexes with VIIIa, PL, and Ca^{2+}, forming the *tenase complex,* which converts X to Xa. Xa, in a complex with Va, PL and Ca^{2+} then cleaves II (prothrombin) to IIa (thrombin). The TF-VIIa complex can also activate IX leading to the subsequent formation of the tenase complex.
- *Common pathway:* Both the intrinsic and extrinsic pathways culminate in the common pathway, in which X is converted to Xa, and prothrombin (II) is cleaved to yield thrombin. Thrombin cleaves fibrinogen to form fibrin, which is then cross-linked via the action of XIII.

Common Coagulation Tests

An understanding of the basic laboratory tests for coagulation assists in the evaluation of bleeding disorders.

- The *PT* is performed by adding thromboplastin, composed of crude or recombinant TF plus Ca^{2+}, to plasma that has been anticoagulated with citrate, and the time to formation of a fibrin clot is measured. Because the PT comprises reactions of coagulation that occur in the extrinsic and final common pathways of coagulation, deficiencies in the activity of II, V, VII, X, or fibrinogen may prolong the PT.
  - The international normalized ratio (INR) was developed to standardize the reporting of PT values in warfarin-anticoagulated patients. Standardization is necessary because commercially available thromboplastin reagents have varying potencies that directly impact the PT; one thromboplastin may yield a different PT result than another when the same sample is tested. The potency of a given thromboplastin is expressed in terms of the international sensitivity index (ISI).
  - Because the INR was developed to report factors measured by the PT that are decreased by warfarin impairment of vitamin K-mediated synthesis (i.e., it is not standardized for abnormalities of factor V and fibrinogen), the INR should be used only to describe anticoagulation in patients who are receiving warfarin. In all other patients (e.g., patients with liver disease), the PT should be referenced.
  - The formula for the INR is: $(PT_{patient}/PT_{mean\ normal})^{ISI}$
- The *aPTT* begins with the addition of a contact activating agent to citrate-anticoagulated plasma. PL and Ca^{2+} are added, and the time to formation of a fibrin clot is measured. Because the aPTT reflects reactions of coagulation that occur in the intrinsic and final common pathways of coagulation, deficiencies in the activity of factors II, V, VIII, IX, X, XI, or XII may prolong the aPTT. Deficiency of other contact factors, prekallikrein and high molecular weight kininogen (HMWK), may also prolong the aPTT. Abnormalities of fibrinogen rarely impact the aPTT.
  - The *long-incubation aPTT* is performed by incubating the patient sample with activating agents for 10 minutes prior to the addition of PL and Ca^{2+}. If the contact factor prekallikrein is deficient, this extra incubation time allows activation of factor XII and correction of the aPTT.
- *Mixing studies* are performed using a mixture of 50% patient plasma and 50% normal control plasma; the PT or aPTT is then performed as usual. Correction of a prolonged PT or aPTT with mixing generally implies a qualitative or quantitative abnormality of one or more clotting factors in the patient plasma. In contrast, failure of the PT or aPTT to correct

completely upon mixing suggests the presence of an inhibitor in the patient plasma that neutralizes a component of the patient _and_ normal plasma. Both lupus anticoagulants and inhibitors to specific clotting factors can result in a prolonged aPTT or PT that does not correct upon mixing.

- When evaluating a prolonged aPTT, an aPTT is performed on the mixture, then the mixture is allowed to incubate for 1 hour and the aPTT is repeated; some inhibitors of factor VIII are maximally effective at 1 hour or more postmix. For instance, the aPTT on a 1:1 mixture of normal and patient plasma containing a factor VIII inhibitor may show correction initially but demonstrate prolongation at 1 hour.
- Occasionally, a weak lupus anticoagulant (LA) may produce a prolonged aPTT or PT that corrects on mixing (1).

- The _bleeding time_ involves making a controlled incision in soft tissue (usually at a site on the forearm) and measuring the time to cessation of bleeding. Anemia and abnormalities of coagulation factors, platelets, or the vasculature may prolong the bleeding time. The bleeding time does not correlate with risk of surgical bleeding in most patients (2). The PFA-100 (3) has been used in place of the bleeding time as a global assessment of platelet function (see Chapter 21).
- The _thrombin time (TT)_ involves the addition of exogenous thrombin to patient plasma, inducing cleavage of fibrinogen to fibrin and the formation of a fibrin clot.
  - The most common cause of a prolonged TT is the presence of heparin in the sample, which can be confirmed by documentation of a normalization of the TT when the test is repeated using a heparin-binding agent such as protamine or Heparsorb.
  - Abnormalities of fibrinogen and circulating heparin-like anticoagulants also cause a prolonged TT.
  - The _reptilase time_ is also used to assess abnormalities of fibrinogen (reptilase cleaves fibrinogen to fibrin). Unlike thrombin, however, reptilase is not inhibited by the presence of heparin. Thus, a prolonged TT in conjunction with a normal reptilase time usually indicates heparin contamination, whereas prolongation of both tests indicates a qualitative abnormality of fibrinogen.
- The _functional fibrinogen assay_ assesses fibrinogen concentration by addition of an excess of thrombin to a sample of diluted plasma.

Specialized Coagulation Tests

- The _anti-Xa assay_ provides information about the degree of anticoagulation that has occurred in the patient plasma as a result of the effect of heparin (unfractionated or low molecular weight) on factor Xa in the sample. By convention, samples should be drawn 4 to 6 hours after LMWH administration to estimate the degree of anticoagulation.
- Two common tests for lupus anticoagulants include the _dilute Russell's viper venom time_ (DRVVT) and the _Staclot assay._ These tests are used to identify an LA and distinguish an inhibitor of a clotting factor from a LA as the cause of a prolongation in the aPTT that does not correct with mixing. Other systems for the diagnosis of lupus anticoagulants are available (1).
  - _Russell's viper venom_ in the DRVVT directly activates X in the patient sample, ultimately leading to the conversion of fibrinogen to fibrin. Lupus anticoagulants inhibit the DRVVT, leading to a prolonged reaction time. If the DRVVT is prolonged, the presence of an LA is confirmed by repeating the test in a system that contains excess phospholipid (DRVVConfirm), which neutralizes the LA and prevents it from interfering in the reaction, resulting in normalization the DRVVT.
  - The _Staclot assay_ involves performance of an aPTT with or without hexagonal phase phospholipids (HPE). If an LA is present, the aPTT will be shorter in the HPE-containing sample because of neutralization of the LA by HPE.

- The *Bethesda assay* is a special type of mixing study that involves incubation of dilutions of patient plasma with normal (control) plasma to assess the potency of an inhibitor (generally, to factor VIII) in the patient plasma. After a 2-hour incubation phase, a factor VIII assay (or other appropriate factor assay, as indicated) is performed on each dilution (and on samples used to create a control curve); as the proportion of patient plasma in the mixture decreases, the effect of the inhibitor decreases, and the factor assay clotting time shortens.
  - The potency of the inhibitor is expressed in *Bethesda units (BU)*. The reciprocal of the dilution of the mixture of patient and normal control plasma that contains approximately 50% of normal factor VIII activity is the inhibitor titer in BU. For instance, if 50% inhibition of normal FVIII activity occurred at a 1:40 dilution, the inhibitor titer would be said to be 40 BU.
  - The Nijmegen modification to the Bethesda assay includes slightly different buffers to stabilize the proteins during the incubation period (4).
- *Assays for specific clotting factors:* Factor activity levels can be assessed by clot-based reactions (that use modifications of the aPTT or PT), and (some factors) by chromogenic systems.
  - Factor activity levels are generally reported as percentages (of normal activity) or in units per milliliter (U/mL), with 1 U/mL corresponding to 100% of the factor found in 1 mL of normal plasma.
  - Usually, levels of 25% to 40% are necessary to prolong the PT or aPTT. Mild or moderate deficiencies of a given clotting factor may lead to an elevated PT or aPTT, but still be adequate for hemostasis.
- The *euglobulin clot lysis time (ECLT)* measures time to dissolution of a fibrin clot; a shortened ECLT indicates activation of the fibrinolytic system. The most common cause of a shortened ECLT is DIC, in which fibrinolysis is activated in response to an activation of coagulation. Deficiencies in the activity of plasminogen activator inhibitor or α-2-antiplasmin also shorten the ECLT (discussion following).

DIFFERENTIAL DIAGNOSIS OF ABNORMAL COAGULATION TESTS

Conditions that predispose to bleeding or produce abnormal coagulation test results can be divided into those entities that prolong the aPTT, PT, or both (Table 20-1 and Figs. 20-2, 20-3, and 20-4).

Conditions Associated with a Prolonged Activated Partial Thromboplastin Time

- *Lupus anticoagulants:* LAs are a very common cause of a prolongation in the aPTT that does not correct completely on mixing.
  - LAs were so named because of their frequent presence in patients with systemic lupus erythematosis and tendency to prolong coagulation tests by interacting with phospholipid in the test sample. In contradistinction to their name, however, lupus anticoagulants are *not* physiologic anticoagulants; additionally, over one-half of patients with LAs do not have connective tissue disease (see Chapter 22).
  - LAs are diagnosed using the methods described above.
- *Hemophilia A and B:* More frequently than with any other factor essential to the aPTT reaction, a deficiency of factor VIII causes a prolongation in the aPTT that corrects completely on mixing. Congenital factor VIII deficiency is referred to as hemophilia A. (Factor VIII is also decreased in moderate and severe von Willebrand disease; see below.) Congenital deficiency of factor IX is referred to as hemophilia B.
  - *Hemophilia A* occurs in 1 in 5,000 to 10,000 live male births; *hemophilia B* is about one-fifth as common. The disorders are inherited in an X-linked recessive fashion: males are

TABLE. 20–1. *Common causes of abnormal coagulation studies*

Prolonged aPTT	Prolonged PT	Prolonged aPTT and PT	Prolonged BT
Lupus anticoagulant Heparin in sample (at clinically relevant concentrations) Deficiency of, or inhibitor to, factors VIII, IX, XI, XII Deficiency of, or inhibitor to, prekallikrein or HMWK Hypofibrinogenemia or dysfibrinogenemia Traumatic venipuncture	Lupus anticoagulant Liver disease Warfarin use Vitamin K deficiency Deficiency of, or inhibitor to, factors II, VII, X Hypofibrinogenemia or dysfibrinogenemia Heparin in sample (at high concentration only)	Lupus anticoagulant Liver disease Warfarin use Vitamin K deficiency Deficiency of, or inhibitor to, factors II, V, or X DIC Hypofibrinogenemia or dysfibrinogenemia Heparin in sample (PT prolonged at high concentration only)	Thrombocytopenia Disorders of platelet function Von Willebrand disease Disorders of vasculature (e.g., Ehlers-Danlos) Anemia

aPTT, activated partial thromboplastin time; PT, prothrombin time; HMWK, high molecular weight kininogen; DIC, disseminated intravascular coagulation; BT, bleeding time.

affected, whereas females are carriers and are generally not affected unless significant lyonization has occurred favoring the X chromosome bearing the abnormal copy of the FVIII gene. There is no race predilection (5).

- The presentation of the disease relates to the level of residual factor activity in the plasma. Severe hemophilia (less than 1% factor activity) typically presents in infancy with bleeding at circumcision, or in early childhood with spontaneous bleeding into soft tissues (muscles) or joints, and intracranial, gastrointestinal, or urinary bleeding. Moderate hemophilia (1% to 5% factor activity) is typified by less severe bleeding than that observed in severe disease, whereas individuals with mild hemophilia (greater than 5% activity) usually do not experience spontaneous bleeding (but hemorrhage can occur and become significant hemostatic challenges such as trauma or surgery).
- *Factor concentrates* are the mainstay of treatment. For acute bleeding, doses of 25 to 40 U/kg are administered every 8 to 12 hours (or by continuous infusion) for 1 to 14 days, depending on the anatomic location and severity of the bleeding. Prophylactic therapy (twice or thrice weekly infusions of factor) is used to prevent morbidity incurred from recurrent joint bleeding; generally, the practice is begun by the age of 4 years (6). Patients with mild hemophilia A may respond to infusion of DDAVP. The antifibrinolytic agent *aminocaproic acid* (Amicar) may be useful in cases of oral bleeding or bleeding associated with dental procedures. *Gene therapy* (delivery of normal factor VIII or IX genes to patients with hemophilia) is in initial phases of clinical investigation (5).
- *Inhibitors:* Hemophiliacs (usually with severe disease) who have received factor concentrates as treatment for bleeding are at risk for inhibitor formation. Approximately 25% of patients with hemophilia A and less than 5% of patients with hemophilia B will develop inhibitors to factor VIII or IX, respectively. The potency of the inhibitor is expressed in BU. Low-titer inhibitors (less than 5 BU) often may be overwhelmed by increasing the amount of factor concentrate infused. It is usually not possible to overcome high-titer inhibitors (greater than 5 BU) with excess human factor concentrates; rather, porcine

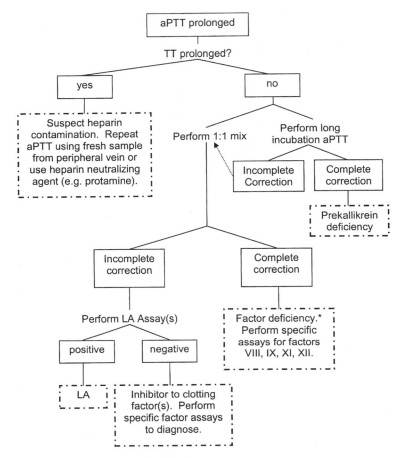

FIG. 20-2. Laboratory diagnostic algorithm for a prolonged aPTT and normal PT. *Occasionally, weak lupus anticoagulants can cause a prolongation in the aPTT that corrects completely on mixing. In this scenario, factor assays may be indicated in addition to LA testing, especially if demonstration of hemostatic factor levels is regarded as important (e.g., in a preoperative patient). aPTT, activated partial thromboplastin time; LA, lupus anticoagulant.

factor VIII (for hemophilia A), prothrombin complex concentrates or recombinant factor VIIa are used.

- *Von Willebrand disease (VWD):* The lack of adequate VWF to bind and protect circulating factor VIII from clearance can lead to low VIII levels and a prolongation in the aPTT, which corrects on mixing.
- *Factor XI deficiency* typically results in a prolonged aPTT that also corrects on mixing. It is inherited in an autosomal recessive manner and is most prevalent among Ashkenazi Jews, in whom the frequency of heterozygotes is approximately 12% (7). Factor XI deficiency causes a mild bleeding tendency that is worsened by trauma or surgery. Levels of factor XI do not correlate well with bleeding symptoms. Fresh-frozen plasma (FFP) may be used prophylactically or for treatment of bleeding.

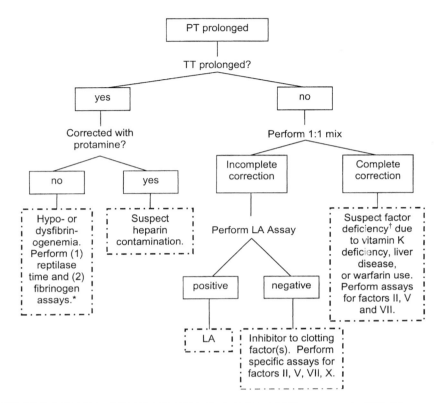

FIG. 20-3. Laboratory diagnostic algorithm for a prolonged PT and normal aPTT. *Decreased functional fibrinogen in conjunction with a normal immunologic fibrinogen indicates an abnormal fibrinogen (dysfibrinogenemia), whereas decreased functional and immunologic assays are typical of hypofibrinogenemia. †Occasionally, lupus anticoagulants can cause a prolongation in the PT that corrects on mixing. aPPT, activated partial tromboplastin time; PT, prothrombin time; TT, thrombin time; LA, lupus anticoagulant.

- *Factor XII deficiency and deficiencies of prekallikrein and HMWK:* Although they may lead to a prolonged aPTT, these conditions do not cause bleeding.
- *Acquired inhibitors to coagulation proteins:* Patients with hemophilia are not the only individuals to develop inhibitors to coagulation proteins. Occasionally, adults without a prior history of hemophilia develop high-titer inhibitors to factor VIII; a concomitant lymphoproliferative or immune disorder is often present. Immunosuppressive treatment with steroids or chemotherapy usually is effective (8).
- *Heparin contamination:* Presence of heparin in the sample used for the aPTT determination may be verified by documenting normalization of the aPTT after the test is repeated using a heparin-binding agent.
- *Warfarin* may mildly prolong the aPTT as a result of depletion of factors II, IX, or X.
- Occasionally, *traumatic venipuncture* causes the aPTT to be prolonged because of the direct activation of coagulation at the site of venipuncture, leading to depletion of crucial coagulation proteins in the collected specimen. The blood should be redrawn with careful technique during phlebotomy and the aPTT repeated to document normalization. (Traumatic

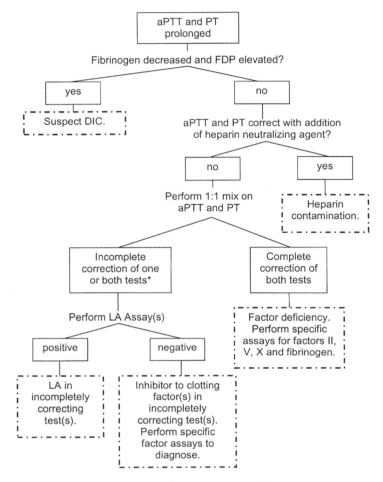

FIG. 20-4. Laboratory diagnostic algorithm for a prolonged aPTT and PT. *Coexisting conditions, such as vitamin K deficiency (leading to a prolonged PT) and a LA (leading to an elevated aPTT), are possible. aPTT, activated partial thromboplastin time; PT, prothrombin time; FDP, fibrin degradation products; DIC, disseminated intravascular coagulation; LA, lupus anticoagulant.

venipuncture may also lead to a *shortening* of the aPTT because of small amounts of thrombin generation.)

Conditions Associated with a Prolonged Prothrombin Time

- *Vitamin K deficiency* can cause an elevated PT that typically corrects completely on mixing. The vitamin-K–dependent factors that are measured by the PT are II, VII, and X. Malabsorption or deficient dietary intake of vitamin K (from green leafy vegetables such as cabbage, cauliflower, and spinach; cereals; soybeans; and other foods) or decreased production by intestinal bacteria (which may be destroyed by antibiotics) may lead to vitamin K deficiency.

- For treatment, *vitamin K* (phytonadione) is administered via parenteral, oral, or subcutane-ous routes (9). Intravenous administration (1 mg per day) results in faster normalization of a prolonged PT than subcutaneous dosing, but occasionally has been associated with anaphylaxis; therefore, intravenous doses should be administered slowly (over 30 minutes) while the patient is monitored. At least partial correction of the PT is expected within 24 hours after parenteral administration of phytonadione if vitamin K deficiency is the only reason for the prolongation in the PT.
- *Coagulopathy of liver disease:* Hepatic insufficiency leads to decreased synthesis of clotting factors, such as the vitamin-K–dependent factors and, with more severe disease, factors V, VIII, XI, XII, and fibrinogen, resulting in a prolonged PT (and with severe disease, aPTT) that correct(s) on mixing.
  - In contrast to coagulopathy caused by isolated vitamin K deficiency in liver disease, there may be reduced factor V in addition to decreased levels of factors II, VII, IX, and X.
- *Warfarin ingestion:* Warfarin inhibits the vitamin-K–dependent carboxylase that is impor-tant for the synthesis of factors II, VII, IX, and X. Decreased functional levels of factors II, VII and X prolong the PT and produce an elevated INR.
  - Supratherapeutic INRs that are not associated with bleeding generally are managed by temporarily withholding warfarin to allow the INR to descend into the desired range, and then restarting the warfarin at a lower dose.
  - Critically elevated INRs (greater than 9) may be addressed with temporary discontinuation of warfarin, plus administration of vitamin K or FFP if the patient is considered to be at very high risk of bleeding.
  - For treatment of warfarin-associated bleeding, warfarin should be discontinued and FFP should be administered along with parenteral or oral vitamin K. Recombinant human factor VIIa (rhVIIa) has been used in some cases to temporarily reverse over anticoagula-tion caused by warfarin (10).
- *LAs* can cause a mild prolongation in the PT (discussed previously).
- *Hypofibrinogenemia/dysfibrinogenemia:* Quantitative or qualitative abnormalities of fibrin-ogen typically produce a long TT and reptilase time (see above), but the PT also may be prolonged (Fig. 20-3). The PT is much more sensitive to hypo/dysfibrinogenemia than is the aPTT.
  - Acquired defects in the function of fibrinogen (occurring in liver disease) are more com-mon than congenital abnormalities of fibrinogen function. DIC produces an acquired hypofibrinogenemia.
  - Replacement of fibrinogen in a bleeding patient with hypofibrinogenemia/dysfibrinogene-mia is best accomplished by administration of *cryoprecipitate,* using a target plasma fibrinogen level of 80 to 100 mg/dL.
- *Deficiencies of individual clotting factors:* Congenital deficiencies of isolated coagulation factors (for example, factor VII) leading to a prolonged PT are extremely rare and typically are inherited in an autosomal recessive pattern.
- *Antibodies to bovine factor V:* Topical bovine thrombin (used in orthopedic, neurologic, and vascular surgery) contains bovine factor V, which is antigenic in some individuals. The resulting anti-bovine factor V antibody cross reacts with human factor V, resulting in an acquired factor V deficiency and prolongation of the PT. Bleeding has been reported in some of these patients (11). Patients also may develop antibodies to bovine thrombin that can prolong the TT if bovine thrombin is used in the assay. The TT normalizes when a human thrombin is used instead, because the bovine and human antibodies usually do not cross-react.

Conditions Associated with a Prolonged Activated Partial Thromboplastin Time and Prothrombin Time

- *Coagulopathy of liver disease:* If hepatic insufficiency is extreme, multiple factor deficien-cies can result in a prolonged PT and aPTT.

- *Deficiencies of individual clotting factors:* Isolated deficiencies of factors II, V, or X are rare but may prolong both the PT and aPTT.
- *DIC:* Depletion of coagulation factors by diffuse activation of coagulation may cause prolongation in both the PT and aPTT (see Chapter 21).
- *LAs* can prolong both the aPTT and PT (discussed previously).

Conditions Associated with Bleeding and Normal Coagulation Tests

- *Factor XIII deficiency:* Activated factor XIII cross-links fibrin strands, stabilizing the fibrin clot. Individuals with a deficiency of factor XIII develop delayed bleeding several hours to days after surgery or trauma. Traumatic soft tissue and joint bleeds, recurrent pregnancy loss, and spontaneous intracranial hemorrhages also have been described (12).
  - Clot lysis or enzymatic assays and sequencing of either of the two genes that encode the molecule may be diagnostic.
  - Treatment of bleeding consists of infusion of *cryoprecipitate* or *FFP.*
- *α-2-antiplasmin deficiency:* α-2-antiplasmin normally inhibits plasmin, thus limiting fibrinolysis. Patients with α-2-antiplasmin deficiency experience accelerated digestion of fibrinogen and fibrin clots and increased bleeding.
  - Heterozygous individuals have a mild bleeding tendency, often with trauma or invasive procedures, whereas homozygotes may experience severe and spontaneous bleeding (13).
  - Bleeding is treated with *FFP* (to replace antiplasmin); FFP also should be infused prior to surgery if a history of perisurgical bleeding is present. (Note: SDP [solvent-detergent treated] plasma does not contain antiplasmin.) *Aminocaproic acid (Amicar)* decreases unmitigated fibrinolysis, making it useful for chronic prophylaxis, oral bleeding, dental work, or minor surgical procedures.
- *Plasminogen activator inhibitor* (PAI)-*1 deficiency:* This extremely rare disorder causes a mild to moderate bleeding tendency due to an accelerated rate of lysis of fibrin clots (14).
- *Congenital and acquired abnormalities of the vasculature and integument* can cause increased fragility of blood vessels and bruising or bleeding, despite normal coagulation, fibrinolysis and platelet function. Such conditions include hereditary hemorrhagic telangiectasia (Osler-Weber-Rendu disease), heritable defects of collagen (Ehlers-Danlos syndrome, osteogenesis imperfecta), acquired collagen-associated conditions (scurvy, prolonged glucocorticoid administration, the normal aging skin) and other anomalies (Marfan syndrome, amyloidosis, vasculitis). There is no effective treatment for bruising associated with the congenital disorders; preventative measures to reduce the risk of trauma should be followed. Repletion of vitamin C (scurvy) and reduction of corticosteroids (glucocorticoid excess) ameliorate bruising associated with the acquired processes (15).

REFERENCES

1. Brandt JT, Tripplett DA, Alving B, et al. Criteria for the diagnosis of lupus anticoagulants: an update. *Thromb Haemost* 1995;74:1185–1190.
2. Lind SE. The bleeding time does not predict surgical bleeding. *Blood* 1991;77:2547.
3. Carcao MD, Blanchette VS, Dean JA, et al. The platelet function analyzer (PFA-100): a novel invitro system for evaluation of primary hemostasis in children. *Br J Haemotol* 1998;101:70.
4. Verbruggen B, Novakova I, Wessels H, et al. The Nijmegen modification of the Bethesda assay for factor VIII:C inhibitors. Improved specificity and reliability. *Thromb Haemost* 1995;73:247.
5. Bolton-Maggs PH, Pasi J. Haemophilias A and B. *Lancet* 2003;361:1801–1809.
6. Schramm W. Experience with prophylaxis in Germany. *Semin Hematol* 1993;30[Suppl 2]:12–15.
7. Seligsohn U. High gene frequency of factor XI (PTA) deficiency in Ashkenazi Jews. *Blood* 1978; 51:1223.
8. Ludlam CA, Morrison AE, Kessler C. Treatment of acquired hemophilia. *Semin Hematol* 1994;31: 16.
9. Raj G, Kumar R, McKinney WP. Time course of reversal of anticoagulant effect of warfarin by intravenous and subcutaneous phytonadione. *Arch Intern Med* 1999;159:2721–2724.

10. Deveras RA, Kessler CM. Reversal of warfarin-induced excessive anticoagulation with recombinant human VIIa concentrate. *Ann Intern Med* 2002;137:884–888.
11. Ortel TL, Charles LA, Keller FG, et al. Topical thrombin and acquired coagulation factor inhibitors: clinical spectrum and laboratory diagnosis. *Am J Hematol* 1994;45:128–135.
12. Mikkola H, Palotie A. Gene defects in congenital factor XIII deficiency. *Thromb Hemost* 1996;22: 393–398.
13. Saito H. Alpha 2-plasmin inhibitor and its deficiency states. *J Lab Clin Med* 1988;112:671–678.
14. Lee MH, Vosburgh E, Anderson K, et al. Deficiency of plasma plasminogen activator inhibitor 1 results in hyperfibrinolytic bleeding. *Blood* 1993;81:2357–2362.
15. Goodnight S. Primary vascular disorders. In: Colman R, Hirsch J, Marder VJ, et al., eds. *Hemostasis and Thrombosis: Basic Principles and Practice.* 4th ed. Philadelphia: Lippincott Williams and Wilkins, 2001:945–953.

21

Disorders of Hemostasis II

Patrick F. Fogarty and Margaret E. Rick

Thrombocytopenia (see Chapter 19) and primary deficiencies in the activity of coagulation proteins (see Chapter 20) are not the only causes of disordered hemostasis. Abnormalities in platelets themselves or inappropriate activation of normal coagulation (leading to a consumptive coagulopathy) can result in bleeding. Von Willebrand disease, which affects platelet function and the coagulation cascade, is also discussed here.

DISSEMINATED INTRAVASCULAR COAGULATION

Although it frequently manifests as bleeding, disseminated intravascular coagulation (DIC) begins as a result of an uncontrolled local or systemic *activation* of coagulation caused by an underlying disorder. DIC may be acute or chronic, limited or diffuse, and accompanied by thrombosis or hemorrhage. Disorders that are associated with DIC are listed in Table 21-1.

- *Pathophysiology.* The normal mechanisms that regulate clot formation and dissolution are imbalanced in DIC, allowing intravascular coagulation to proceed preferentially (1). The inciting events are numerous but generally involve either overwhelming release of tissue factor (see Chapter 20) by cellular, vascular, or hypoxemic injury, or the presence of endogenously or exogenously derived procoagulant molecules (such as bacterial lipopolysaccharide, proteins produced by neoplastic cells, or snake venom). As the acute primary process continues to drive coagulation, clotting factors and platelets are consumed, leading to bleeding commensurate with the degree of consumption. If activation of coagulation is chronic and low-grade, however, clotting factors and platelets may be replenished sufficiently so as to avert bleeding; in these patients, hypercoagulability predominates, manifest as thrombosis (as in Trousseau syndrome).
- *Presentation.* The appearance of DIC always indicates a serious underlying condition. A typical presentation of DIC involves a patient who has been hospitalized due to another disorder (Table 21-1) when unexplained bleeding and/or abnormalities in routine coagulation are observed.
  - The hemorrhage of DIC is typically diffuse and may involve bleeding at sites of surgical incisions or vascular access catheters, as well as urinary, gastrointestinal, pulmonary, central nervous system, or cutaneous hemorrhage. Acral cyanosis and petechial and ecchymotic lesions may also occur. Widespread DIC-associated truncal and extremity bruising (*purpura fulminans*) usually is limited to children or follows a viral infection.
  - Any degree of thrombocytopenia, hypofibrinogenemia, and prolongation of the activated partial thromboplastin time (aPTT) and prothrombin time (PT) is possible, but DIC rarely produces a platelet count less than 20,000 per microliter. Occasionally DIC will be manifest by only moderately abnormal laboratory tests, without clinically significant thrombosis or bleeding. Patients with thrombosis and chronic DIC resulting from malignancy may have a normal or even elevated platelet counts.

TABLE. 21–1. *Conditions associated with disseminated intravascular coagulation*

Condition	Example
Tissue damage	Trauma, burns
Sepsis	Gram-negative or -positive bacterial infection; rickettsial or viral infection
Shock	Cardiogenic, septic
Pregnancy-related	Toxemia, placental abnormalities (abruption or previa), amniotic fluid embolism, retained uterine placental or fetal tissue; HELLP syndrome
Vascular stasis	Cavernous hemangiomas (Kasabach-Merritt syndrome), abdominal aortic aneurysm
Fat embolism	Fracture of long bones, sickle cell crisis
Malignancy	Acute promyelocytic leukemia, adenocarcinoma (Trousseau syndrome)
Injection of toxic procoagulant molecules	Snake bites

- Severe systemic DIC may lead to widespread tissue hypoxia and multiorgan dysfunction; hepatic, neurologic, cardiac, and renal impairment can occur. Multiorgan failure is associated with a high mortality rate.
- *Diagnosis.* Typically, acute DIC is suspected when a patient with a predisposing condition (Table 21-1) develops bleeding or thrombosis and/or a perturbation in laboratory tests indicative of DIC. DIC is a dynamic condition, especially in the acutely ill patient; considerable variation in laboratory markers over time may make analysis of trends rather than isolated values more relevant to management. Laboratory testing may show:
  - Increased (prolonged) aPTT, PT, or thrombin time (TT) resulting from consumption of clotting factors and/or fibrinogen (most patients).
  - Decreased fibrinogen (compared to baseline) resulting from consumption of fibrinogen.
  - Increased products of fibrinogen and fibrin degradation (FDPs; D-dimer assay) resulting from plasmin-mediated cleavage of fibrinogen and fibrin. The D-dimer assay measures fibrin products that have been cross-linked by activated factor XIII.
  - Decreased platelet count (compared to baseline) from intravascular clearance due to activation and aggregation at the sites of local prothrombotic reactions (most patients). Especially in early DIC, the platelet count and fibrinogen may be reduced from the baseline value but still remain within the normal laboratory reference range.
  - Fragmented red cells (schistocytes) on peripheral blood smear resulting from microvascular hemolysis (10% to 20% of patients with DIC).
- *Treatment.* The clinical and laboratory manifestations of DIC should resolve with correction of the inciting disorder, such as by effective administration of antimicrobials in sepsis, treatment of malignancy, surgery to repair an aneurysmal dilatation, or removal of conceptus and placenta. If DIC is severe enough to cause multiorgan dysfunction, management in an intensive care unit is usually required.
  - *Blood products* should not be administered to patients with acute DIC unless clinically significant bleeding is present or if the risk of bleeding is felt to be high (e.g., thrombocytopenia in patient who has sustained major trauma); there is, however, no reason to withhold blood products for fear of "fueling the fire." If bleeding is present, *platelet transfusions* may be administered: a target platelet count of 20,000 to 30,000/mL (most cases) or more than 50,000 per microliter (intracranial or life-threatening hemorrhage) is reasonable. Higher thresholds may be desired for patients who are to undergo invasive

procedures such as major surgery, but the consumptive process may make achieving the goal difficult.

- *Cryoprecipitate* may be administered for bleeding in the setting of fibrinogen levels that are consistently less than 80 to 100 mg/dL. *Fresh-frozen plasma (FFP)* should be given only for significant bleeding and a prolonged PT and aPTT.
- Because of its potential to exacerbate hemorrhage, *heparin* should be considered only in cases of ongoing bleeding due to DIC, despite appropriate treatment. Heparin should not be administered unless the platelet count can be supported to 50,000 or more per microliter and there is no central nervous system or diffuse gastrointestinal bleeding. A low-dose infusion (6 to 10 U/kg per hour) with no bolus is recommended. An improving platelet count and fibrinogen concentration signifies that the treatment is effective. Heparin is contraindicated in patients with placental abruption or other obstetrical conditions that will require surgical management, because the anticoagulation is likely to complicate the curative treatment.
- The use of *fibrinolysis inhibitors* and *antithrombin concentrates* in acute DIC is controversial. Fibrinolysis inhibitors may have a role in patients with profuse bleeding who have failed to respond to other management, in whom FDPs are felt to be inhibiting platelets.
- Laboratory parameters (PT, PTT, fibrinogen and platelet count) should be monitored at least every 6 hours in the acutely ill patient with DIC, and clinical bleeding should be followed to assess efficacy of therapeutic measures.

- HELLP syndrome (*h*emolysis, *e*levated *l*iver enzymes, and *l*ow *p*latelets) is a severe form of DIC affecting women in the peripartum period. HELLP produces clinically significant hemolytic anemia and hepatocellular injury, and may be difficult initially to distinguish from thrombotic thrombocytopenic purpura (TTP; see Chapter 19) (hepatic dysfunction, or elevated transaminases, indicates HELLP syndrome). Introduction of placental proteins into the maternal circulation may be etiologic. Gross hemoglobinuria with renal dysfunction and hypotension are common; the mortality rate is high. As with other forms of DIC, management is principally supportive, but in HELLP it also must include evacuation of the uterus, either by delivery of a term or near-term infant or by dilatation and curettage to remove retained placental or fetal fragments.
- Acute promyelocytic leukemia (APL) is frequently associated with DIC, potentially as a result of procoagulant molecules (tissue factor and others) contained within circulating promyelocytes. Bleeding in a patient with APL who presents with laboratory parameters consistent with DIC should be treated emergently; in addition to the appropriate use of platelets and cryoprecipitate, initiation of chemotherapy within 24 hours of diagnosis is advised (see Chapter 11).
- Trousseau syndrome is a form of chronic DIC in which recurrent episodes of venous thromboembolism (VTE) complicate an underlying malignancy, especially adenocarcinomas. Anticoagulation with warfarin in not effective in preventing further VTE; instead, subcutaneous low molecular weight heparin in therapeutic doses is usually necessary to prevent recurrence of thromboembolism (see Chapter 23).

VON WILLEBRAND DISEASE

- *Epidemiology.* Von Willebrand disease (vWD) is the most common inherited bleeding disorder. Up to 1% of the population has levels of von Willebrand factor (vWF) below the laboratory reference range (not all of these individuals, however, will experience bleeding) (2).
- *Pathophysiology and classification.* vWF is an unusual, extremely large multimeric glycoprotein that is synthesized in endothelial cells and megakaryocytes. Binding of vWF to its receptor, platelet glycoprotein Ib (GPIb), tethers platelets to one another and to the subendothelial collagen matrix, localizing them to the site of injury. This interaction is especially important in vessels such as arterioles, where a high-shear state is present. vWF also binds to factor VIII (FVIII) in the circulation, protecting it from clearance. Types 1

and 3 vWD involve quantitative decreases in vWF, while type 2 disease is characterized by qualitative (functional) abnormalities in the vWF molecule.

- *Type 1* includes approximately 75% to 80% of patients, the majority of whom do not have an identified causal mutation in the vWF gene on chromosome 12. Patients usually have mild or moderate bleeding.

- *Type 2* includes four subtypes; patients usually have moderate to severe bleeding symptoms and present before adulthood. *Type 2A* (10% to 15% of vWD) involves mutations in vWF that cause either a defect in intracellular transport (2A, type 1) or make the molecule more susceptible to proteolysis (2A, type 2). Laboratory testing (Table 21-2) typically shows a more marked decrease in vWF activity assays compared to antigen. *Type 2B* (5% of vWD) mutations result in an abnormal structure in the binding site for platelet GPIb and are responsible for a gain-of-function defect that allows spontaneous binding of the abnormal vWF to circulating platelets. Patients typically have thrombocytopenia as a result of removal of vWF-bound platelet aggregates. The ristocetin-induced platelet aggregation (RIPA; Table 21-2) shows an increase in platelet aggregation to low concentrations of ristocetin. *Pseudo* or *platelet type vWD* is caused by a defect in the platelet GPIb molecule, allowing it to bind to the patient's normal vWF with increased avidity and producing a type 2B clinical phenotype. Mixing studies using a modified RIPA (patient's platelets and control plasma) distinguish it from type 2B vWD. *Type 2N* (uncommon) features mutations in vWF that decrease its ability to bind and protect FVIII from clearance, resulting in decreased FVIII levels in the plasma and a phenotype similar to hemophilia A. Soft tissue and joint bleeding are common. The presence of affected females in the family is an important clue to this diagnosis. Laboratory studies show decreased FVIII (2% to 10%) and normal vWF function and antigen. *Type 2M* (very uncommon) results from mutations affecting the A1 domain in a different area than mutations in type 2B. The result is decreased binding of platelets to vWF.

- *Type 3* vWD (rare) is caused by a variety of mutations of the vWF molecule, including larger deletions; patients may be homozygous for a given mutation or double heterozy-

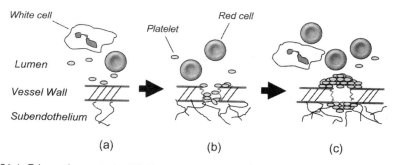

FIG. 21-1. Primary hemostasis. **(A)** Normal conditions. Under physiologic conditions, platelets do not interact with the endothelium. **(B)** Adhesion. On disruption of the blood vessel wall, subendothelial collagen and fibronectin are exposed, leading to platelet adhesion. In the arterial/arteriolar circulation, subendothelial von Willebrand factor (vWF) assists in the adherence of platelets to the site of injury via binding to the platelet glycoprotein (GP) Ib receptor. **(C)** Aggregation. Tissue factor interacts with factor VIIa, present locally, to catalyze the formation of thrombin. Thrombin, collagen, and other molecules bind to receptors on the platelet membrane, leading to platelet activation. Fibrinogen cross-links platelets via their GP IIb/IIIa receptors, promoting formation of an occlusive plug that prevents additional blood loss through the break in the vessel wall. vWF also bridges between platelets, via their GP Ib or GP IIb/IIIa receptors.

TABLE. 21–2. *Laboratory Evaluation of von Willebrand disease*

Laboratory test	Method or premise	Indication
vWF antigen (ELISA)	Binding to an anti-vWF antibody quantitatively measures vWF in plasma	Initial work-up
vWF activity (ristocetin cofactor assay)	Ristocetin promotes binding of patient plasma vWF to normal platelets (via GPIb); decreased platelet aggregation indicates abnormal or reduced vWF in patient's plasma	Initial work-up
Factor VIII activity level	FVIII levels are reduced in moderate or severe vWD	Initial work-up
Ristocetin-induced platelet aggregation (RIPA)	Type 2B mutation results in increased aggregation of patient PRP with low concentrations of ristocetin	Diagnosis of vWD type 2B
vWF multimer assay	Assess distribution of vWF multimers by electrophoresis	Diagnosis of vWD type 2
Platelet-associated vWF activity or antigen	Patient's platelets are lysed to assess amount and activity of intra-platelet (i.e., α-granule) vWF	Rarely indicated, but might be helpful if bleeding diathesis is present and other testing is negative

vWD, von WIllebrand disease; GPIb, platelet membrane receptor glycoprotein Ib; PRP, platelet-rich plasma; vWF, von Willebrand factor; ELISA, enzyme-linked immunosorbent assay; FVIII, factor VIII.

gotes. Severe bleeding manifests in childhood. FVIII is usually approximately 5%, and vWF levels usually are too low to detect.
- *Presentation.* Symptoms usually involve mucous membranes. Epistaxis, oral bleeding, menorrhagia, and gastrointestinal bleeding are common. Individuals with marked abnormalities of vWF usually present earlier in life with bleeding at the time of mucous membrane-related procedures (tooth extractions, tonsillectomy), or at menarche.
- *Diagnosis.* The diagnosis of vWD is based on a typical history of bleeding (usually mucous membrane-related) and confirmatory laboratory testing. Because many individuals with laboratory values of vWF that are below the reference range do not have bleeding, low vWF levels in a patient with bleeding may not necessarily be indicative of vWD. Other causes, such as structural anomalies in nasal vessels in an individual with epistaxis, should be sought concomitantly.
  - *Personal and family history* of bleeding must be carefully documented.
  - Initial testing for vWD (Table 21-2). A *vWF antigen level* (by enzyme-linked immunosorbent assay [ELISA]) and a *vWF activity* (by ristocetin cofactor assay) should be performed. The latter involves addition of ristocetin at 1.2 mg/mL to a mixture of patient plasma (the vWF source) and washed normal platelets. Ristocetin binds to vWF, allowing it, in turn, to bind GPIb on the platelet membrane, causing platelet aggregation. The *factor VIII activity* may be abnormal. A *vWF multimer study* detecting the distribution of multimers and a *RIPA* is performed once a diagnosis of vWD has been made, to assess for types 2A or 2B vWD.
  - Testing of family members, when possible, aids in the diagnosis of patients with borderline results.
- *Treatment.* The patient's previous response to bleeding challenges, current medications, and general medical condition should be considered (Table 21-3) (2).

TABLE. 21–3. *Treatment of von Willebrand disease*

Type	Treatment	Comment
1	DDAVP; vWF replacement concentrates	DDAVP effective in most patients
2A	DDAVP; vWF replacement concentrates	Response may not be as marked to DDAVP as in type I
2B	Possibly DDAVP; vWF replacement concentrates	DDAVP may worsen thrombocytopenia; perform therapeutic trial with measurement of post-DDAVP platelet count
2N	DDAVP; vWF replacement concentrates	FVIII half-life may be shortened due to lack of binding by abnormal vWF
2M	DDAVP; vWF replacement concentrates	
3	vWF replacement concentrates; platelet transfusions if inadequate response to vWF replacement	Increase initial dose of vWF replacement concentrate to 50 IU/kg

Desmopressin acetate (DDAVP) dose is 0.3 μg/kg intravenously in 50 mL of saline over 20 minutes, or nasal spray 300 μg for weight less than 50 kg or 150 μg for less than 50 kg, every 8 to 12 hours, maximum of 3 doses in a 48-hour period; monitor for hyponatremia. Nasal spray may be particularly helpful for home use in women with excessive menstrual bleeding due to von Willebrand disease (vWD). Replacement vWF concentrates are indicated for major bleeding or severe vWD; dose is 20 to 30 IU/kg every 12 hours (give for 3 to 10 days for major bleeding or after surgery). Intermediate purity plasma-derived factor VIII concentrates contain von Willebrand factor (vWF); recombinant or monoclonally purified factor VIII concentrates do not. Monitor clinical status and vWF antigen or activity to determine efficacy and need for dose modifications; patients may require an increase in dose despite an adequate vWF level. Antifibrinolytic agents (such as ε-aminocaproic acid, 50 mg/kg 4 times daily for 3 to 5 days; maximum 20 g/d) are often used in conjunction with other therapies; they are especially useful for mucosal bleeding (e.g., dental procedures).

- Desmopressin acetate (DDAVP) indirectly causes release of vWF and factor VIII from storage sites; after intravenous administration, levels of both factors are increased two- to fivefold for approximately 6 hours. Patients should undergo a therapeutic trial to document responsiveness to the medication (as assessed by increased vWF levels and lack of worsening thrombocytopenia, as may occur in patients with type 2B) prior to use in clinically significant bleeding or as prophylaxis for invasive procedures. Only two to three doses should be administered during a course of treatment. Tachyphylaxis and serious hyponatremia can occur after repeated dosing; nonsteroidal anti-inflammatory agents may aggravate this latter effect (3).
- vWF concentrates are used when bleeding is not controlled with DDAVP or as prophylaxis, when a therapeutic trial has indicated a poor response to DDAVP (most type 3 and some type 2B patients). Humate-P is an intermediate-purity antihemophilic factor that contains vWF and is labeled with vWF ristocetin cofactor units. Cryoprecipitate generally is not recommended because of its lack of viral inactivation.
- Antifibrinolytic agents such as epsilon aminocaproic acid (Amicar) and topical agents (including topical thrombin, gelfoam, and fibrin sealant) are used adjunctively; epsilon aminocaproic acid may be particularly helpful for dental procedures.
- Pregnancy and vWD. vWF levels increase two- to threefold during the last two trimesters of pregnancy; patients with type 1 vWD whose vWF levels have reached the normal range during the third trimester may not require treatment during delivery. In more severely affected patients, DDAVP can be administered prophylactically, beginning usually after the onset of labor. (Patients with type 2B vWD who have experienced worsening thrombocytopenia during pregnancy should receive vWF replacement therapy and platelets, not

DDAVP.) Because vWF levels decrease rapidly within 24 hours after delivery, DDAVP may be helpful for patients with vWD who have peripartum bleeding, and if ineffective, replacement vWF by concentrates undertaken (2).

QUALITATIVE PLATELET DISORDERS

Most disorders of platelet function are acquired; heritable qualitative platelet disorders are rare. When critical pathways of platelet biochemistry are perturbed, bleeding typically occurs, but because of redundancy of biochemical and receptor pathways that mediate the function of platelets, other defects may be detectable only on laboratory testing and do not produce clinically significant bleeding. In most cases, transfusion of platelets or other therapies will (temporarily) augment hemostasis in a patient with a congenital or acquired qualitative platelet disorder who has bleeding or who is to undergo an invasive procedure.

Platelet Biochemistry

Primary hemostasis describes the formation of a platelet plug at the site of vascular injury (Fig. 21-1). In a variety of reactions that are not entirely sequence-specific, individual circulating platelets must adhere to the denuded endothelial surface, undergo activation through receptor-ligand interactions, release the contents of their granules (the process of platelet secretion), and aggregate to form a physical barrier to continued blood loss. Additionally, phospholipid in the platelet membrane participates in localizing and promoting the activity of coagulation factors.

- *Adhesion.* Subendothelial molecules such as vWF, collagen, and fibronectin mediate adhesion of platelets to the exposed subendothelial matrix at sites of vessel wall compromise. In high-shear conditions as in arterioles, vWF is especially important, because it tethers the platelet to the endothelial surface via interaction with its receptor, platelet GPIb.
- *Activation.* Subendothelial collagen activates platelets; thrombin, which has been generated locally in reactions following the interaction of factor VIIa and tissue factor (provided by the membranes of cells) also activates platelets by binding to receptors on the platelet surface and initiating a series of signal transduction events.
- *Secretion.* Agonists such as collagen, thrombin, adensosine diphosphate (ADP), and epinephrine bind to their receptors on the platelet membrane and induce a series of biochemical events that cause platelets to release the contents of their granules (Table 21-4), which act to promote further activation and aggregation.
- *Aggregation.* Binding of agonists also promotes a conformational change in the platelet GP IIb/IIIa receptor, exposing its binding sites for fibrinogen and vWF; these molecules can then bridge between individual platelets at the site of vascular injury, promoting the formation and stability of the platelet plug.

TABLE. 21–4. *Characteristics of platelet granules*

	α-Granules	δ-(dense) Granules
Number per platelet	30–50	3–7
Visualization	Light microscopy (Wright's stain), electron microscopy	Electron microscopy
Contents	vWF, PDGF, PF4, TSP, FV, FXI, protein S, fibronectin; fibrinogen, IgG, P-selectin	ADP, ATP, serotonin, calcium

PDGF, platelet-derived growth factor; PF4, platelet factor 4; vWF, von Willebrand factor; FV, factor V; FIX, factor IX; IgG, immunoglobulin G.

• *Participation in coagulation reactions.* The platelet membrane is rich in phospholipid, a required component for reactions involving clotting factor complexes.

Platelet Function Testing

• *Platelet aggregation studies (platelet-rich plasma system).* The premise of platelet aggregation testing is that the cellular component (platelets) in a suspension of platelet-rich plasma (PRP) impedes transmission of light through the suspension. When any of a variety of agonists (collagen, thrombin, ADP, epinephrine) is added, aggregation occurs, consolidating the cellular component to the bottom of the reaction tube and allowing the passage of light through the plasma component. The increase in light transmission as aggregation occurs is plotted as a function of time. Ideally, the waveform shows two physiologic processes: a *primary wave* represents initial aggregation as platelet receptors are activated and become available to bind pro-aggregatory molecules such as fibrinogen, and a *secondary wave* indicates further aggregation that is stimulated by the release of platelet granule contents. Routinely, secretion of platelet granule contents (Table 21-4) is assessed in tandem with platelet aggregation; after stimulation of platelets with an agonist, release of adenosine triphosphate (ATP) into solution is measured through a chemiluminesence procedure, and plotted as a function of time.

• *Platelet function analyzer (PFA-100).* This device assesses the formation of a platelet plug. Citrated whole blood is aspirated through a capillary leading to an aperture in a collagen-impregnated membrane; either ADP or collagen is added as an agonist. Platelets are activated and aggregate, progressively occluding the aperture. The time to complete occlusion is measured and compared with a normal range. Although less sensitive, an advantage of the PFA is that it is less time-consuming and laborious than standard platelet aggregation studies (4).

• *Measurement of granule contents (rarely indicated).* Centrifugation of PRP produces a platelet pellet; the platelet membranes are then disrupted, liberating intracellular/intragranular proteins into the lysate. The molecule of interest is then assessed (vWF, by ristocetin cofactor assay, for intragranular vWF).

Acquired Disorders

• *Drugs.* The most common acquired qualitative platelet disorders are caused by the use of medications that directly or indirectly impair platelet function; of these, aspirin and the non-steroidal anti-inflammatory drugs (NSAIDs) are most frequently responsible (Table 21-5). Patients who present with bruising or platelet-type bleeding and whose platelet function testing shows abnormal aggregation or secretion should be questioned regarding current medications, especially recently initiated drugs and over-the-counter, naturopathic, and herbal agents. Treatment of clinically significant drug-induced platelet dysfunction first involves discontinuation of the offending agent, but may require additional measures (Table 21-6).
  • *Aspirin* irreversibly inhibits the platelet cyclooxygenase enzyme, which is responsible for the conversion of membrane-associated arachidonic acid to thromboxane A_2 (TxA_2); the inhibition is constant for the entire life span of the platelet (approximately 10 days). Once liberated from the platelet, TxA_2 binds to receptors on adjacent platelets, initiating secretion of platelet granule contents and further promoting aggregation. Platelet aggregation studies (Fig. 21-2) show decreased reactivity to most agonists, including low concentration of thrombin and collagen, but normal aggregation with high concentrations of thrombin and collagen. Using the PFA-100 system, aspirin-induced platelet dysfunction is evident in an increased time to aperture occlusion with the epinephrine/collagen reagent, while that of the ADP/collagen reagent is unaffected.
  • *NSAIDs* reversibly inhibit platelet cyclooxygenase; their inhibitory effect persists only as long as the drug is present in the circulation. *Selective inhibitors of cyclooxygenase-2* (COX-2) do not bind or impair platelet cyclooxygenase (COX-1).

TABLE. 21–5. *Substances associated with platelet dysfunction[a]*

Platelet-directed agents
  Aspirin
  NSAIDS (except COX-2 inhibitors)
  Dipyridamole (Aggrenox)
  Clopidigrel (Plavix)
  Ticlopidine (Ticlid)
  Abciximab (ReoPro)
Eptifibatide (Integrilin)
  Tirofiban (Aggrastat)
 	
Anesthetics
  Dibucaine
  Procaine
  Halothane
 	
Antibiotics
  Penicillins (penicillin G, ticarcillin, nafcillin,
  piperacillin, methcillin, ampicillin)
 	
Cephalosporins (cefazolin, cefotaxime)
  Nitrofurantoin
	Chemotherapeutic drugs
	  BCNU
	  Daunorubicin
	  Mithramycin
	
	Psychiatric medications
	  Selective serotonin reuptake inhibitors
	  (e.g., fluoxetine, paroxetine, sertraline)
	  Tricyclic antidepressants (e.g., imipramine,
	  amytriptyline, nortriptyline)
	
	Other agents
	  Nitrates
	  Antihistamines (diphenhydramine,
	  chlorpheniramine)
	  Ethanol
	  ω-3 fatty acids (eicosapentaenoic acid)
	  "Wood ear" mushrooms
	  Radiographic contrast dye

[a] Most of these agents have been reported to cause abnormalities in platelet aggregation or the bleeding time rather than bleeding.
NSAIDS, nonsteroidal anti-inflammatory drugs; COX-2, cyclooxygenase 2; BCNU, carmustine.
Adapted from George JN, Shattil SJ. Acquired disorders of platelet function. In: Hoffman R, Benz EJ, Shattil SJ, et al., eds. *Hematology: Basic Principles and Practice*. 3rd ed. New York: Churchill Livingstone, 2000:2174.

- *Platelet glycoprotein IIb/IIIa inhibitors* are used in the management of patients with acute coronary syndromes or before or following percutaneous coronary intervention, frequently in conjunction with heparin. *Eptifibatide* is a small molecule that binds the GP IIb/IIIa receptor, inhibiting the binding of its ligands, fibrinogen, vWF, and others, hindering platelet aggregation. The usual dose in patients with normal renal function is a bolus of 180 μg/kg, followed by continuous infusion of 2.0 μg/kg per minute. *Abciximab* is a monoclonal antibody against GP IIb/IIIa that also inhibits binding of these proaggregatory ligands; the usual dose is a 0.25 mg/kg intravenous bolus followed by a 12- to 24-hour intravenous infusion of 10 μg/min. Abciximab-bound platelets can be cleared at an accelerated rate due to interaction between the Fc portion of the antibody and Fc receptors on reticuloendothelial macrophages in the liver and spleen, producing thrombocytopenia that in some cases (less than 1.0%) is severe.
- *Ticlopidine* and *clopidogrel* irreversibly inhibit the binding of ADP to its receptor on the platelet membrane, impairing the ADP-dependent binding of fibrinogen to GPIIb/IIa, decreasing platelet aggregation. Neutropenia and aplastic anemia have been associated with ticlopidine (5); TTP has been described with use of ticlopidine and less frequently with clopidogrel (6,7).
- *Dipyridamole* is used to prevent recurrent stroke or transient ischemic attack, usually in conjunction with aspirin. Dipyridamole inhibits ADP- and collagen-induced platelet aggregation through an effect on intracellular cyclic adenosine monophosphate (cAMP).
- *Other substances. Serotonin reuptake inhibitors (SSRIs)* may impair the function of platelets by reducing the serotonin content of platelet dense granules. *Omega-3 fatty acids* can

TABLE. 21–6. *Treatment of qualitative platelet disorders*

Nature of defect in platelet function	Prophylaxis prior to invasive procedures	Treatment of bleeding
Acquired		
Drug-induced	If possible, discontinue drug at least 7 days prior to procedure (ASA, ticlopidine, clopidogrel), or at least 6–12 hours (eptifibitide) or 24–48 hours (abciximab) prior to procedure	Discontinue drug; platelet transfusion until drug has been cleared and/or hemostasis is achieved.
MDS/MPD	Platelet transfusion only if significant thrombocytopenia or prior history of bleeding	Platelet transfusion
Renal failure	DDAVP,[a] platelets; hemodialysis prior to procedure	Platelets, DDAVP, cryo, high-dose estrogens (see text); possibly, hemodialysis. Keep Hct >30%
Cardiac bypass-related	Not applicable	Platelet transfusions if clinically significant bleeding
Congenital		
Bernard-Soulier syndrome	Platelets, possibly DDAVP[a]	Platelets, possibly DDAVP. Menses suppression may be required, rhVIIa
Glanzmann's thrombasthenia	DDAVP,[a] platelets. Pregnancy: platelets at delivery and 3–7 days postpartum	Platelets, DDAVP, Amicar, rhVIIa
Storage pool disease (α-granule, δ-granule, or combined deficiency)	Platelets, DDAVP[a]	Platelets, DDAVP; possibly rhVIIa
Disorders of signal transduction	Platelets; possibly DDAVP[a]	Platelets, possibly DDAVP

[a]If DDAVP is to be used as prophylaxis prior to invasive procedures, a therapeutic trial confirming correction of a prolonged bleeding time after administration of DDAVP is recommended.
Amicar, aminocaproic acid; ASA, aspirin; DDAVP, desmopressin acetate; MDS/MPD, myelodysplasia/myeloproliferative disorders; cryo, cryoprecipitate; rhVIIa, recombinant human factor VIIa; Hct, hematocrit.

disrupt the phospholipid membrane of the platelet and interfere with reactions of coagulation that normally take place on the platelet surface.
- *Myelodysplasia (MDS)/myeloproliferation.* The platelets that are produced in MDS and the myeloproliferative disorders (chronic myeloid leukemia, essential thrombocythemia, polycythemia vera, and idiopathic myelofibrosis) often show abnormal receptor-ligand interactions, ineffective signal transduction, or decreased secretion of platelet granule contents; in a minority of patients these abnormalities lead to bleeding (8).
- *Renal failure/uremia.* Platelets from individuals with impaired kidney function frequently show abnormalities on aggregation testing. Although plasma urea itself may not be causative,

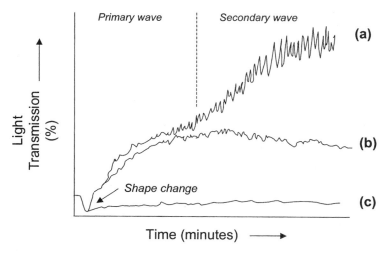

FIG. 21-2. Platelet aggregation studies. Platelet aggregation studies involve the addition of ago-nists (collagen, thrombin, adenosine diphosphate [ADP], arachidonic acid, or epinephrine) to a suspension of platelet-rich plasma (PRP); the agonist induces aggregation of platelets and allows transmission of light through the plasma component of the PRP. **(A)** In the normal scenario, the binding of an agonist to its platelet receptor initiates a *shape change* that temporarily decreases light transmission; subsequently, a *primary wave of platelet aggregation* is recorded (as increased light transmission) as fibrinogen binds its receptor, glycoprotein (GP) IIb/IIIa, and begins to cross-link platelets. Unlike the other agonists, collagen does not induce a primary wave. A *secondary wave* occurs as signal transduction events (resulting from platelet activation) eventuate in aug-mented binding of GP IIb/IIIa by fibrinogen and release of platelet granules, whose contents are able to induce further aggregation. **(B)** In storage pool disease (SPD), platelet aggregation to ADP and other agonists typically shows an initial wave of aggregation, but the aggregates subse-quently dissociate because of reduced or absent release of platelet granule contents. Because release of granules is largely dependent on thromboxane, the aspirin effect produces a similar platelet aggregation profile to that of SPD when ADP or epinephrine is used, but stronger agonists such as thrombin and collagen can circumvent the thromboxane pathway and produce a normal aggregation curve. **(C)** Because of lack of GP IIb/IIIa expression on the platelet surface, platelets from patients with Glanzmann's thrombasthenia show absent aggregation to all agonists except ristocetin.

other factors, such as increased levels of nitric oxide (9) or other products can cause de-creased binding of fibrinogen to platelet GP IIb/IIIa or impaired release of platelet granules. Some patients experience clinically important bleeding, especially gastrointestinal (9). DDAVP (standard doses) (3), cryoprecipitate, and high-dose estrogens (premarin, 50 mg single dose, [10]) have been suggested to be beneficial in uremia-related bleeding. Because the presence of adequate numbers of intravascular red cells may facilitate interaction of platelets with the vessel wall, red cell transfusions are recommended in patients with anemia related to renal failure who are bleeding, to maintain the hematocrit higher than 30% (11). Platelet transfusion may be beneficial temporarily if other measures fail and bleeding per-sists. If a dialyzable substance in uremic plasma is responsible for the defect in platelet function, hemodialysis also may be beneficial, albeit temporarily.

- *Cardiac bypass* causes defects in both platelet number and function. Platelets passing through the extracorporeal oxygenating circuit contact the artificial surfaces of the system and are activated; they also are fragmented by distortional trauma. Both mechanisms lead to their accelerated clearance. After bypass, a decrease in the platelet count, abnormalities in platelet morphology on the blood smear, and impaired *in vitro* platelet aggregation are observed in most patients (12), but these effects typically persist for only 24 to 72 hours. Platelet transfusion may be given for serious bleeding.

Congenital Disorders

Inherited disorders of platelet function are rare and produce varying degrees of bleeding, usually beginning within the first decade of life; they may also remain clinically silent until unmasked by a significant hemostatic challenge. Prophylaxis prior to invasive procedures and treatment of significant hemorrhage may require transfusion of normal platelets, or use of DDAVP (3), antifibrinolytic agents, or (refractory bleeding) recombinant human factor VIIa (3,13,14) (Table 21-6).

- *Bernard-Soulier syndrome* comprises a triad of large platelets, moderate thrombocytopenia, and a prolonged bleeding time; there is reduced or abnormal expression of platelet GPIb/IX (the receptor for vWF) on the surface of the platelets. Bernard-Soulier syndrome is autosomal recessively inherited. Platelet aggregation studies are normal with all agonists except ristocetin. Bernard-Soulier syndrome is distinguished from vWD in that the reduced RIPA in Bernard-Soulier syndrome is corrected by the addition of normal platelets, whereas in vWD it is corrected by the addition of normal plasma (which contains adequate vWF). The diagnosis can be confirmed by platelet flow cytometry.
- *Glanzmann's thrombasthenia* is a recessively-inherited qualitative or quantitative abnormality in GP IIb/IIIa expression on the platelet surface. Without adequate functional IIb/IIIa to bind fibrinogen and vWF (both of which cross-link platelets), platelet aggregation is markedly impaired (Fig. 21-2). Patients may present with mucocutaneous bleeding in infancy. The severity of clinical bleeding does not correlate well with the degree of deficiency of IIb/IIIa (15). Allogeneic hematopoietic stem cell transplantation (HSCT) has been used in the management of severe cases (16).
- *Storage pool disease* is characterized by abnormalities in number or content of platelet granules. Defects in α-granules, dense granules, or both (Table 21-4) may be present. Platelet aggregation to ADP (Fig. 21-2) typically shows an initial wave of aggregation, but the aggregates subsequently dissociate because of reduced or absent release of granule contents, which normally reinforce the aggregatory response. Most patients have a prolonged bleeding time. A variable bleeding diathesis results. More commonly, patients may have *release defects* wherein granules are present, but signaling necessary for release of granule contents is defective.
  - *Albinism-associated storage pool disease* appears in the context of disorders characterized by oculocutaneous albinism, such as the Hermansky-Pudlak and Chediak-Higashi syndromes. Impaired biogenesis of dense granules, lysosomes, and melanosomes may be responsible for the reduced number of dense granules in these patients (17).
  - *Nonalbinism-associated storage pool disease* occurs in a variety of other conditions (thrombocytopenia absent radii syndrome, Ehlers-Danlos syndrome, Wiskott-Aldrich syndrome, osteogenesis imperfecta). Defects in dense granules may relate more to granular content rather than number (18) and may be associated with α-granule abnormalities (α/δ- storage pool disease [SPD]). Decreased or empty dense granules can be visualized on electron microscopy.
  - The *gray platelet syndrome* (19) is a rare, inherited disorder characterized by abnormalities of platelet α-granules, thrombocytopenia, and fibrosis in the bone marrow. Consanguinity is common, and a lifelong history of mild to moderate mucocutaneous bleeding usually is present. Review of the blood smear shows agranular platelets that appear gray on Wright's staining because of a lack of azurophilic granules. In contrast to dense-granule deficiency, platelet aggregation to epinephrine, ADP, and arachidonic acid is often normal, while thrombin and collagen produce variable results. The diagnosis is confirmed by electron microscopy.

• The *Quebec platelet disorder* (20), extremely rare, is characterized by abnormal platelet factor V, mild thrombocytopenia, and prolonged bleeding time, leading to a moderate bleeding diathesis. Bleeding is unresponsive to platelet transfusion.
• *Scott syndrome* (21) is an extremely rare disorder characterized by spontaneous bleeding caused by a platelet membrane defect that does not support the binding of coagulation factors. Patients have a normal bleeding time and platelet aggregation studies.
• *Congenital disorders of signal transduction* include defects in receptor-agonist interactions, G-protein activation, platelet enzymatic activity and phosphorylation of signaling proteins (22).
• *Isolated laboratory-specific defects.* Individuals with phenotypically normal hemostasis occasionally demonstrate reduced or, less frequently, absent aggregation to one or more agonists on platelet aggregation testing. These abnormalities, which may be genetically determined, probably reflect interindividual differences in the reactivity of platelets to certain ligands and do not necessarily indicate an increased risk for spontaneous or trauma-induced hemorrhage, unless a tendency to bleed has been previously demonstrated.

Other Conditions

The *May-Hegglin anomaly* features mild to moderate thrombocytopenia, large platelets, and characteristic leukocyte azurophilic inclusions (Dohle bodies). While the large size of the platelets implies a qualitative abnormality, patients generally do not bleed excessively and aggregation studies are normal. An autosomal dominantly-inherited disorder, it is a manifestation of mutated nonmuscle myosin heavy chain IIA, which has been implicated in the related disorders Sebastian syndrome, Fechtner syndrome, and Epstein syndrome; these feature varying degrees of sensorineural hearing loss, nephritis, cataracts, and leukocyte inclusions (23).

REFERENCES

1. Bick RL. Disseminated intravascular coagulation current concepts of etiology, pathophysiology, diagnosis, and treatment. *Hematol Oncol Clin North Am* 2003;17:149–176.
2. Rick ME. Treatment of von Willebrand disease. In: Rose BD, ed. *UpToDate.* Wellesley, MA: UpToDate, 2003.
3. Mannucci PM. Desmopressin (DDAVP) in the treatment of bleeding disorders: the first twenty years. *Blood* 1997;90:2515.
4. Carcao MD, Blanchette VS, Dean JA, et al. The platelet function analyzer (PFA-100): a novel in-vitro system for evaluation of primary hemostasis in children. *Br J Haematol* 1998;101:70.
5. Symeonidis A, Kouraklis-Symeonidis A, Seimeni, U et al. Ticlopidine-induced aplastic anemia: two new case reports, review, and meta-analysis of 55 additional cases. *Am J Hematol* 2002;71:24–32.
6. Moake JL. Thrombotic thrombocytopenic purpura and the hemolytic uremic syndrome. *Arch Pathol Lab Med* 2002;126:1430–1433.
7. Bennett CL, Connors JM, Carwile JM. Thrombotic thrombocytopenic purpura associated with clopidogrel. *N Engl J Med* 2000;342:1773–1777.
8. Landolfi R, Marchioli R, Patrono C. Mechanisms of bleeding and thrombosis in myeloproliferative disorders. *Thromb Haemost* 1997;78:617.
9. Zuckerman GR, Cornette GL, Clouse RE, et al. Upper gastrointestinal bleeding in patients with chronic renal failure. *Ann Intern Med* 1985;102:588.
10. Boyd GL, Diethelm AG, Gelman S, et al. Correcting prolonged bleeding during renal transplantation with estrogen or plasma. *Arch Surg* 1996;131:160.
11. Turrito VT, Weiss HJ. Red blood cells: their dual role in thrombus formation. *Science* 1980;207:541.
12. Kestin AG, Valeri CR, Khuri SF, et al. The platelet function defect of cardiopulmonary bypass. *Blood* 1990;76:1680.
13. Bellucci S, Caen J. Molecular basis of Glanzmann's thrombasthenia and current strategies in treatment. *Blood Rev* 2002;16:193–202.
14. Buchanan GR. Quantitative and qualitative platelet disorders. *Clin Lab Med* 1999;19:71–86.

15. George JN, Caen JP, Nurden AT. Glanzmann's thrombasthenia: the spectrum of clinical disease. *Blood* 1990;75:1383.
16. Bellucci S, Devergie A, Gluckman E, et al. Complete correction of Glanzmann's thrombasthenia by allogeneic bone-marrow transplantation. *Br J Haematol* 1985;59:635–641.
17. Shalev A, Michaud G, Israels SJ, et al. Quantification of a novel dense granule protein (granulophysin) in platelets of pateitns with dense granule storage pool deficiency. *Blood* 1992;80:1231.
18. Weiss HJ, Lages B, Vicic W, et al. Heterogenous abnormalities of platelet dense granule ultrastructure in 20 patients with congenital storage pool deficiency. *Br J Haematol* 1993;83:282.
19. Raccuglia G. Gray platelet syndrome: a variety of qualitative platelet disorder. *Am J Med* 1971;51:818.
20. Hayward CPM, Rivard GE, Kane WH. An autosomal dominant, qualitative platelet disorder associated with multimerin deficiency, abnormalities in platelet factor V, thrombospondin, von Willebrand factor, and fibrinogen, and an epinephrine aggregation defect. *Blood* 1996;87:4967.
21. Sims PJ, Wiedmer T, Esmon CT, et al. Assembly of the platelet prothrombinase complex is linked to vessiculation of the platelet plasma membrane: studies in Scott syndrome, an isolated defect in platelet procoagulant activity. *J Biol Chem* 1989;264:17049.
22. Rao K, Gabbeta J. Congenital disorders of platelet signal transduction. *Arterioscler Thromb Vasc Biol* 2000;20:285–289.
23. Seri M, Pecci A, Di Bari F, et al. MYH9-related disease: May-Hegglin anomaly, Sebastian syndrome, Fechtner syndrome, and Epstein syndrome are not distinct entities but represent a variable expression of a single illness. *Medicine* 2003;82:203–215.

22

Venous Thromboembolism

Steven J. Lemery and Craig M. Kessler

As clinicians, we must maintain a high index of suspicion for the diagnosis of venous thrombo-embolism (VTE) because of its potential for significant morbidity and mortality. VTE is responsible for up to five times more deaths annually in the United States than is breast cancer. Deep venous thrombosis (DVT) is estimated to occur in 43.7 to 145 individuals per 100,000 population. Pulmonary embolism (PE), which is the cause of death in up to 200,000 patients per year in the United States, occurs with an incidence of 20.8 to 65.8 cases per 100,000 population. Approximately 12% of all in-hospital fatalities are attributed to VTE—a likely underestimate because autopsy studies indicate that there was no antemortem clinical suspicion in more than 50% of hospital deaths involving PE. Thus, PE may be one of the leading preventable causes of death in hospitalized patients. VTE most commonly affects the lower extremities, but virtually any venous vascular bed can be involved. We still recognize Virchow's triad of vascular stasis, endothelial injury, and hypercoagulability as factors leading to thrombosis. With modern laboratory techniques, many of the biochemical and heritable variables that lead to a hypercoagulable state can be detected and explained.

DEEP VENOUS THROMBOSIS AND PULMONARY EMBOLISM

Thrombosis of the deep veins of an extremity often is the initial manifestation of the more devastating entity of PE. The incidence of symptoms or signs that may alert a clinician to the diagnosis of DVT includes (1):

- Calf or leg swelling (88%)
- Pain (56%)
- Tenderness (55%)
- Warmth (42%)
- Erythema (34%)
- Homan's sign (13%)
- Palpable cord (6%)

Alternatively, a DVT may remain asymptomatic and be diagnosed only when a patient experiences symptoms of a PE. A patient who is experiencing a pulmonary embolus may experience (1):

- Dyspnea (77%)
- Chest pain (55%)
- Hemoptysis (13%)
- Syncope (10%)
- Sudden death

The signs that accompany PE are (1):

- Tachypnea (70%)
- Tachycardia (43%)
- Hypoxia/cyanosis (18%)
- Hypotension (10%)

DVT may also cause significant long-term morbidity related to chronic leg pain, cyanosis, venous dilatation and congestion, swelling, cutaneous ulceration, and decreased mobility. Within 6 years after initial treatment of DVT with heparin alone, postthrombotic syndrome develops in up to 80% of involved extremities; approximately 20% of contralateral extremities may also become symptomatic with postthrombotic manifestations (2).

A distinction is made between distal DVT in the distal calf veins and those designated as proximal DVT, which involve the popliteal and more proximal venous system. Calf vein DVT are considered low risk for PE in contrast to the high risk of PE associated with proximal DVT. Approximately 25% of distal DVT will propagate proximally within 1 to 2 weeks if left untreated, increasing the risks of subsequent PE and development of postthrombotic syndrome.

RADIOGRAPHIC DIAGNOSIS OF DEEP VENOUS THROMBOSIS

Because of its general availability, noninvasive nature, and sensitivity and specificity, ultrasound of the involved extremity is usually the first diagnostic test performed when the physician suspects DVT. The gold standard, against which all other tests are compared, is contrast venography. Detection of an intraluminal-filling defect on contrast venography is diagnostic of DVT. Although considered the most sensitive and specific of the diagnostic tests for VTE, contrast venography has the disadvantage of requiring the use of iodine-based contrast dye and its attendant allergenicity. Venography is also invasive, and can be uncomfortable or painful. Ultrasonography is considerably more sensitive for the detection of proximal DVT than for distal DVT. Venography often detects asymptomatic DVT, usually located distally in the venous vasculature of the lower extremities. The clinical relevance of distal DVT is questionable because they rarely embolize; however, if they propagate proximally, significant PE may develop. Impedance plethysmography is another method to evaluate for the presence of DVT and is often combined with ultrasonography. This test detects differences in the velocity of blood outflow through the venous circulation with electrodes; decreased blood flow is characteristic of an occlusive or partially occlusive thrombus. To ensure ultimate accuracy, the technique requires strict conditions regarding leg positioning, because conditions other than DVT may affect flow and decrease the test's specificity; examples include morbid obesity or a pelvic mass. As with ultrasonography, the sensitivity of impedance plethysmography to detect a distal calf vein DVT is reduced because of collateral venous flow in the calf.

Compression ultrasound with venous imaging combines features of the above techniques and is currently the most commonly used test for the diagnosis of DVT. The diagnostic criteria for DVT include the inability to compress a vein, direct visualization of an occlusive or partially occlusive thrombus, and/or lack of blood flow seen with Doppler. Sensitivity ranges from 89% to 100% and specificity ranges from 86% to 100% (3). Unfortunately, sensitivity may be lower in patients with asymptomatic DVT (3). Serial evaluations with ultrasound may improve sensitivity, as an undiagnosed distal DVT may be discovered when it propagates proximally. An additional advantage of ultrasound is that it can accurately diagnose a Baker's cyst, which occasionally may mimic DVT. One potential limitation of ultrasound is the challenge of differentiating between a new recurrent DVT in the ipsilateral extremity of a patient who has previously carried the diagnosis, especially true if the previous DVT has not resolved.

Magnetic resonance venography (MRV) is currently undergoing clinical evaluation to detect DVT. MRV has the advantages of direct visualization of either distal or proximal thrombi in a noninvasive manner, and it can image proximal veins in the pelvis. Major disadvantages are cost and availability.

ELECTROCARDIOGRAPHIC AND RADIOGRAPHIC DIAGNOSIS OF PULMONARY EMBOLISM

PE is a potentially fatal condition that usually results from the embolization of a thrombus from the distal extremities. PE also may complicate up to one-third of upper extremity DVT and occur as a consequence of removing an indwelling central venous access device. Less commonly, PE may arise from the inferior vena cava or the heart via a patent foramen ovale or mural thrombus in the right ventricle. The diagnosis of PE may be confounded when it is accompanied by concurrent arterial thromboembolic features such as a cerebrovascular accident, where there is paradoxical embolization of DVT through a patent foramen ovale.

Less specific methods for diagnosing PE include electrocardiography, echocardiography, and chest radiography. Electrocardiogram (ECG) findings of new right atrial or ventricular enlargement, a right bundle branch block, or the classic S1Q3T3 pattern increase suspicion for PE. A transthoracic echocardiogram is sensitive in the presence of a major PE. Right ventricular dilatation, often with myocardial hypokinesis, occurs on transthoracic echocardiograms in 50% to 90% of central/proximal PE. Pulmonary artery dilatation, right ventricular mural thrombi, tricuspid regurgitation, and loss of inspiratory collapse of the inferior vena cava are observed less commonly with PE. Transthoracic echocardiogram confirmation of right ventricular hypertension may assist in the decision regarding thrombolysis with right heart failure. The sensitivity of transesophageal echocardiography approaches 80% to 97% with 84% to 100% specificity, which is comparable to spiral computed tomography (CT). Both echocardiography and spiral CT have a low sensitivity for PE located in peripheral pulmonary vessels. Chest x-ray findings that may suggest a pulmonary embolus include a Hampton's hump or a focal paucity of blood vessel perfusion.

The gold standard for the diagnosis of PE remains pulmonary angiography. Angiography allows direct visualization of the pulmonary vascular tree; an intraluminal-filling defect is consistent with an embolus. Angiography is not the initial test used to diagnose PE because it requires an invasive procedure and is associated with risks of stroke, renal failure caused by contrast dye osmotic load, hematoma at the venous access site, anaphylaxis caused by iodine contrast dye, and even death, usually secondary to induced arrhythmias. Nevertheless, potential risks are usually outweighed by benefits of accurate diagnosis and facilitating the implementation of thrombolytic therapy or anticoagulation. Initiating extended oral or parenteral anticoagulation without a firm diagnosis of PE confers a considerable and potentially unwarranted risk of hemorrhagic complications.

The two most commonly ordered tests to diagnose PE are the ventilation/perfusion lung scan (V/Q) and a helical or spiral CT scan of the chest. CT is widely available and can diagnose other potential pathological causes of dyspnea. The advantages of V/Q scanning over CT include lack of need for contrast dye and ability to diagnose distal vascular PE, which the spiral CT frequently cannot detect.

Table 22-1 compares the advantages and disadvantages of different diagnostic modalities used for DVT and PE.

The V/Q scan evaluates mismatches in pulmonary perfusion compared to that of ventilation. The test was prospectively evaluated as part of the PIOPED study in 1990 (4). The clinical pretest probability of PE was combined with V/Q scan results to determine posttest probability for PE in 755 patients who underwent both pulmonary angiography and a V/Q scan. Only 41% of patients with a PE had a high-probability V/Q scan, but the specificity of a high-probability V/Q scan was high, at 97%. Conversely, 4% of patients with a normal or near-normal V/Q scan had a PE documented by pulmonary angiography. The PIOPED study investigators defined a high

TABLE. 22–1. *Radiologic methods used to diagnose DVT and PE*

	Advantages	Disadvantages
1. Compression ultrasound	Available, noninvasive, good sensitivity/specificity, and can diagnose Baker's cyst	Not sensitive for distal- or high-iliac DVT. Operator-dependent. Less sensitive for asymptomatic DVT
2. Contrast venography	Gold standard	Requires use of contrast dye and is invasive and painful
3. Impedance plethysmography	Often combined with ultrasound to increase sensitivity	Operator-dependent, requires strict positioning, and is less sensitive in conditions that affect distal blood flow (pelvic mass, morbid obesity).
4. Magnetic resonance venography	Can directly visualize both distal and proximal thrombi	Cost and availability.
5. Ventilation/Perfusion Scan	Extensively studied, noninvasive	Often nondiagnostic.
6. Helical CT scan	Availability, noninvasive, rapid, may suggest an alternative diagnosis	Not sensitive for distal PE, requires contrast dye, not as extensively studied
7. Pulmonary angiography	Gold standard	Invasive, requires contrast dye, arrhythmias (can be fatal). Also, risk of stroke

DVT, deep venous thrombosis; PE, pulmonary embolism; CT, computed tomography.

pretest clinical probability as conveying an 80% to 100% chance of having a PE while a low pretest clinical probability was associated with a 0% to 19% chance of having a PE. Forty percent of patients with a low-probability V/Q scan but a high pretest clinical probability of PE actually had a PE, thus underscoring the need for further testing in this subgroup. Likewise, 56% of patients with a high-probability V/Q scan but a low pretest clinical probability of PE had a PE (thus, 44% of patients with a high-probability V/Q scan would likely have been treated with long-term anticoagulation if a pulmonary angiogram had not been performed. Thus the V/Q scan is often a useful initial test, but many patients will require further testing, including pulmonary angiography in patients who are at high risk despite a low- or intermediate-probability V/Q scan. Serial Doppler examinations of the lower extremities are another option for patients at lower risk, such as a patient with an intermediate pretest probability for PE and a low- or intermediate-probability V/Q scan (16% and 28% chances of having a PE respectively). Figure 22-1 is an algorithm for the diagnosis of patients suspected of having a PE.

Helical or spiral CT scanning of the chest also is commonly used to evaluate patients for PE. Sensitivity in various trials has varied from 53% to 100% (3); large studies now being conducted may change the diagnostic approach to PE. Expert radiologists trained to evaluate for PE may not always be available in the community setting. To date, it appears from at least five published clinical trials that a negative spiral CT justifies withholding anticoagulation: negative spiral CT scans were associated with 0% to 1.8% incidence of nonfatal PE and 0% to 0.9% fatal PE.

Low Clinical Suspicion (<20% Chance of PE)

D-Dimer: (if sensitive ELISA assay is available)
If negative, PE unlikely, but if positive
↓

V/Q scan or Helical CT Angiogram

Normal V/Q Scan	Negative CT Scan or Low Probability V/Q Scan	Intermediate/High Probability V/Q Scan or Positive CT Scan
↓	↓	↓
Explore Alternative Diagnosis.	Explore Alternative Diagnosis. If none Exists, Consider Serial Ultrasound of Lower Extremities.	Consider Pulmonary Angiogram; or Consider Treatment with Positive CT, but Explore Embolic Source.

↓   ↓

Positive: Treat   Negative:
Explore Alternative
Diagnosis

Intermediate Clinical Suspicion

V/Q Scan or Helical CT Angiogram

High Probability V/Q Scan or Positive CT Scan	Intermediate Probability V/Q	Low Probability V/Q Scan
↓	↓	↓
Treat: Try to Find Embolic Source	Consider Pulmonary Angiogram	Serial Ultrasound of Lower Extremities, and Consider Other Diagnoses if Negative

High Clinical Suspicion (>80% Chance of PE)

V/Q Scan or Helical CT Angiogram

High Probability V/Q Scan or Positive CT Scan	Negative CT Scan or Low/Intermediate Probability V/Q Scan
↓	↓
Treat	Pulmonary Angiogram

Positive   Negative
↓   ↓
Treat   Explore Alternative Diagnosis

FIG. 22-1. Diagnosis of pulmonary embolus. ELISA, enzyme-linked immunosorbent assay; CT, computed tomography; PE, pulmonary embolism; V/Q, ventilation/perfusion lung scan.

LABORATORY DIAGNOSIS OF VENOUS THROMBOEMBOLISM

The D-dimer assay has been used as an adjunct to exclude DVT and PE. The D-dimer is a breakdown product of the end result of the coagulation cascade. When the cross-linked fibrin clot is degraded by plasmin, D-dimers are formed. Enzyme-linked immunosorbent assay (ELISA) and latex agglutination assays for D-dimers vary in their usefulness in the diagnostic algorithm for PE. A sensitive ELISA test, if negative, essentially excludes the likelihood of VTE, but its low specificity usually results in the need for further diagnostic testing. The latex agglutination test is less sensitive for the diagnosis of VTE. Elevated levels of D-dimers are produced by many other diseases, many of which are hypercoagulable states complicated by VTE: cancer, pregnancy, sepsis, sickle cell crisis, and surgery. A persistent elevation of D-dimers despite adequate anticoagulation is predictive for recurrent VTE.

Recently, elevated levels of troponin I and troponin T have been associated with right ventricular dysfunction (63%), an increased number of V/Q segmental defects (troponin I), and with massive or moderate PE (troponin T). These parameters may be additional tools in the laboratory to diagnose PE (5,6).

DEEP VENOUS THROMBOSIS IN SITES OTHER THAN THE DISTAL VEINS OF THE LOWER EXTREMITIES

DVT can have devastating consequences when it occurs in unusual sites. Increasing use of indwelling venous access devices means DVT of the subclavian and axillary veins is much more common. More worrisome are DVT that involve the hepatic, retinal, and renal veins, or the cerebral venous structures. DVT of the hepatic vein, also called the Budd-Chiari syndrome, results in abdominal pain caused by an engorged liver, ascites, and portal hypertension. Budd-Chiari is usually an acute phenomenon associated with acquired hypercoagulable states, including pregnancy and the myeloproliferative disorders, as well as hereditary hypercoagulable states, including deficiencies of proteins C and S. Paroxysmal nocturnal hemoglobinuria also causes thrombosis of the hepatic vein. Treatment options include thrombolysis, anticoagulation, and consideration for orthotopic liver transplantation in a patient with liver failure.

Retinal vein occlusion (RVO) is often observed in patients with diabetes or glaucoma, but RVO is also associated with hypercoagulable states, especially the antiphospholipid syndrome (7). Patients with RVO may note an acute decrease in visual acuity, with engorged veins and hemorrhage seen on fundoscopic evaluation. RVO may require anticoagulation in consultation with an ophthalmologist (7).

Cerebral venous thrombosis may be discovered in a patient with a new headache or central neurologic symptoms; papilledema is often but not always seen. Mortality is significantly higher when anticoagulation is withheld, despite the risk of bleeding (7).

Thrombosis of the renal vein often presents as acute or chronic renal failure; there may be hematuria and pain related to a swollen kidney. An antecedent nephrotic syndrome may lead to a hypercoagulable state and thus renal vein thrombosis. The benefit of anticoagulation is unknown, because many patients have chronic renal failure that will worsen without anticoagulation. Anticoagulation to resolve thrombosis may delay time to renal failure (7).

ACQUIRED THROMBOPHILIC STATES

Heparin-Induced Thrombocytopenia

Heparin-induced thrombocytopenia (HIT) is a thrombogenic state caused by antibodies formed after exposure predominantly to unfractionated heparin. These antibodies bind to the heparin-platelet factor 4 (PF4) complex and secondarily promote thrombosis in vivo in both venous and arterial sites by aggregating platelets. In general, platelet counts begin to decrease

5 to 9 days after heparin administration is initiated. Thrombocytopenia may occur earlier in patients who had previously received heparin in the past 100 days. HIT can be diagnosed in the coagulation laboratory by direct measurement by ELISA assays of PF4-heparin antibodies or by platelet aggregation assays, which detect spontaneous aggregation of platelets induced by the addition of heparin to platelet-rich plasma. Sensitivity of platelet aggregation assays can be increased when platelets are "loaded" with radioactive serotonin; serotonin release from platelets is detected as a marker of platelet activation in vitro, after the addition of heparin. The most sensitive test is the serotonin-loaded platelet aggregation assay, however false-positive platelet aggregation assays and ELISA for PF4-heparin antibodies are not uncommon (8). HIT may be precipitated by even small exposures to unfractionated heparin, such as used for flushes of intravenous lines. Low molecular weight heparins (LMWH) rarely precipitate HIT but can exacerbate HIT once it occurs in association with unfractionated heparin. Occasionally, HIT is complicated by the development of significant arterial and/or venous thromboembolic phenomena and is designated as heparin-induced thrombocytopenia with thrombosis syndrome (HITTS). This syndrome occurs most often in the presence of another hypercoagulable trigger, such as acquired protein C or S deficiency.

Multiple agents are available for the treatment of HIT or HITTS when anticoagulation is undertaken in the presence of thrombocytopenia. Traditional low molecular weight heparin preparations such as enoxaparin, dalteparin, and tinzaparin can cross-react with the PF4-heparin antibodies produced by unfractionated heparin and are not recommended for anticoagulation in HIT/HITTS. The synthetic pentasaccharide fondaparinux does not appear to cross-react and may prove to be an effective anticoagulation option for HIT/HITTS. Danaparoid sodium, a mixture of heparan sulfate, dermatan sulfate, and chondroitin sulfate, is an indirect thrombin inhibitor by its anti-Xa and IIa effects (anti-Xa/anti-IIa >22:1). Danaparoid has been used almost exclusively for anticoagulation during HIT, although it cross-reacts with anti-PF4-heparin antibodies in 25% of cases. Danaparoid is no longer marketed in the United States now that argatroban and the other direct thrombin inhibitors have proved successful and safe for the treatment of HIT/HITTS. Lepirudin (a recombinant form of hirudin), bivalirudin (a small synthetic molecule (molecular weight [MW] = 2,180 D) with homology to the two amino acids of hirudin), and argatroban (a small, synthetically derived compound [MW = 527] that binds to thrombin in a reversible manner) are direct thrombin inhibitors that have proven effective and safe for anticoagulation during the thrombocytopenia of HIT and for treatment of thrombosis in HITTS. Lepirudin is antigenic, and antibody formation results in excessive anticoagulation. Lepirudin is contraindicated in the presence of renal insufficiency. Bivalirudin and argatroban are both hepatic-excreted, nonantigenic, and short-acting and should be used with caution in patients with liver disease. None of these agents have specific antidotes if excessive bleeding occurs in association with their use.

Nephrotic Syndrome

Patients with nephrotic syndrome are at high risk of thromboembolic complications: renal vein thrombosis in 30% to 50% and concurrent PE in 20% to 30%. Predisposition toward hypercoagulability is due to reductions of modulators of coagulation, particularly antithrombin III and protein S, both of which are lost in the urine. In addition, the nephrotic syndrome is accompanied by elevations of C4b binding protein as an acute phase reactant, resulting in the inactivation of circulating protein S through complex formation. Increased levels of procoagulant factors, including factors V and VIII, and fibrinogen also occur (9). While anticoagulation is indicated in nephrotic patients who sustain an acute thrombosis, thrombolytic therapy may be of benefit for bilateral acute renal vein thrombi with renal failure. Nephrotic syndrome, caused by membranous glomerulonephritis or the antiphospholipid syndrome, poses an especially high thrombogenic risk: prophylactic anticoagulation should be considered with extreme albuminuria, which parallels urinary loss of antithrombin III and protein S (9). Low molecular weight heparin anticoagulation is contraindicated in renal insufficiency.

Antiphospholipid Syndrome

Different mechanisms have been proposed to explain how antiphospholipid antibodies (APA) mediate the development of thrombosis: binding of APA to β_2-glycoprotein I (β_2-GPI) complexed to phospholipid exposed on the surface of injured or activated endothelial cells, oxidant based injury to endothelin, and interference with regulatory proteins such as annexin V and protein C (10). Antiphospholipid antibodies can be related to an infection such as syphilis, but these APA are less thrombogenic and often transient.

Testing for APA is accomplished directly by using specific assays to quantitate levels by ELISA or indirectly through the detection of antiβ_2-GPI antibodies. The functional expression of APA is designated as the lupus anticoagulant (LAC), which prolongs phosphoplipid-dependent clotting assays. Assays include the dilute Russell viper-venom time, the dilute prothrombin or tissue thromboplastin inhibition test, and the kaolin clotting time. Because the APA is directed against phospholipid, a useful confirmatory test for the LAC is the platelet neutralization assay, in which the prolonged activated partial thromboplastin test, characteristic of the LAC, is shortened or normalized after incubating patient plasma with normal platelets; these platelets will provide enough phospholipid to adsorb the LAC and allow the coagulation test to proceed normally.

Two positive tests for APA, obtained at least 6 weeks apart, are required to fulfill the laboratory criteria for the APA syndrome. Clinical criteria for the diagnosis of the APA syndrome include detection of venous and/or arterial thrombotic events, autoimmune thrombocytopenic purpura, marantic endocarditis, or multiple fetal loss. Thrombosis can occur in virtually any vascular bed, and patients may present with a catastrophic syndrome with thrombosis in multiple vascular sites, including cerebrovascular accidents and DVT.

Treatment strategies should focus on modification and elimination of risk factors, such as smoking and oral estrogen contraceptives. The prophylactic use of aspirin, 81 mg daily, has been advocated to reduce the platelet activation component of the APA syndrome. For a thrombotic complication, systemic anticoagulation should be initiated with heparin or warfarin. A recent prospective study showed that dosing warfarin to an international normalized ratio (INR) of 2.0 to 3.0 was equally effective as higher intensity warfarin regimens to achieve an INR of 2.5 to 3.5, formerly recommended to prevent recurrent thromboses (11). In general, anticoagulation after a thrombotic event should be long term; future studies may delineate if certain subgroups may safely discontinue anticoagulation (10).

HYPERCOAGULABILITY OF MALIGNANCY

VTE is a frequent complication of malignancy and can result in significant morbidity and mortality. The estimated prevalence of venous thromboembolism in patients with cancer is 10% to 15% and as high as 28% in pancreatic cancer (12). Cancer may stimulate thrombosis through a variety of mechanisms: release of tissue factor, activation of factor X by a cancer procoagulant, endothelial-tumor cell interactions, and platelet activation. Hypercoagulability associated with malignancies is designated as the Trousseau syndrome and can manifest as disseminated intravascular coagulation, nonbacterial thrombotic endocarditis, PE, DVT, and arterial thromboses. Recurrent migratory thrombophlebitis and DVT in atypical sites, such as in the upper extremities and splanchnic vessels, also are characteristic. Occasionally, chemotherapy agents may promote thrombosis, possibly through direct injury to the vascular endothelium. Central venous indwelling catheters often complicate cancer care because of thrombus formation in the catheter itself and the vessel into which it has been inserted (13).

Treatment of the hypercoagulability of cancer can be challenging, with rethrombosis occurring despite adequate treatment with warfarin. Warfarin resistance has been observed in up to 30% of patients with cancer. In a recent study, a low molecular LMWH regimen (dalteparin) was more effective than oral anticoagulation in preventing recurrent thromboembolism in patients with cancer (Kaplan-Meier estimate of VTE recurrence at 6 months was 9% for low molecular weight heparin versus 17% with warfarin) (14).

PAROXYSMAL NOCTURNAL HEMOGLOBINURIA

Paroxysmal nocturnal hemoglobinuria is a rare clonal hematopoietic cell disorder, in which a mutation of the PIG-A gene results in the lack of glycosylphosphatidylinositol-linked membrane proteins. Diagnosis can be made rapidly by flow cytometric detection of deficient CD55 and CD59 on peripheral blood erythrocytes and neutrophils. Patients with large clones (greater than 50%) carry a high risk of thrombotic events, which include unusual sites such as the hepatic or mesenteric veins. Hypercoagulability is the most common cause of death in this disease. The etiology of the thrombogenicity has not been elucidated and treatment of thrombosis with anticoagulation can be difficult. One recent nonrandomized study showed significantly decreased risks of thrombosis in patients who were prophylaxed with warfarin (15).

SURGERY AS AN ACQUIRED RISK FOR THROMBOSIS

Surgery imparts a significant predisposing risk for thrombosis. Surgery and trauma may induce a hypercoagulable state through multiple mechanisms: direct endothelial injury, activation of the coagulation cascade (through the release of tissue factor), and platelet activation. Risk varies with the indications for surgery, anesthesia time, patient age, and the presence of underlying heritable or acquired hypercoagulable states. VTEs most frequently occur with hip or knee arthroplasty, hip fracture surgery, spinal cord injury, major trauma, and any surgery performed in the context of malignancy. Patients undergoing these procedures should receive prophylaxis against the formation of thrombosis; options include graduated pneumatic compression stockings plus LMWH, adjusted dose heparin, and oral anticoagulation with warfarin to achieve an INR goal of 2 to 3 (16). DVT prophylaxis should be individualized depending on bleeding risk, history of previous thrombosis, history of heparin-induced thrombocytopenia, and type of surgery. Outpatient surgical procedures performed in patients younger than 40 who can be made readily ambulatory do not require prophylactic anticoagulation. Prolonged prophylactic anticoagulation postsurgery may be indicated for patients undergoing total hip replacement (at least until the patient is mobile) and for those in whom a malignancy persists. Options include warfarin to an INR of 2 to 3 or LMWH (16).

OTHER ACQUIRED RISK FACTORS FOR THROMBOSIS

Microangiopathic hemolytic anemias are commonly associated with thrombosis. Thrombotic thrombocytopenic purpura (TTP) is the paradigm. TTP is characterized by:

• Thrombocytopenia
• Microangiopathy
• Renal insufficiency
• Fever
• Central nervous system abnormalities

TTP should be suspected when thrombocytopenia and microangiopathic hemolysis coexist. Thrombogenicity may be related to *in vivo* platelet activation mediated by the effects of the high molecular weight multimers of von Willebrand factor (vWF) protein. Thrombosis causes the secondary manifestations of renal insufficiency and central nervous system alterations. TTP may be precipitated by an acquired quantitative or qualitative deficiency of VWF protease, resulting in abnormally large, unprocessed circulating VWF multimers that have potent platelet-activating properties. Initial treatment for TTP involves immediate administration of corticosteroids combined with aggressive plasmapheresis and exchange of the patient's total plasma volume with normal plasma. Plasma exchange provides a source of normal vWF protein and vWF protease, and simultaneously removes neutralizing autoantibodies directed against host vWF protease activity. TTP is a readily treatable disease but has a mortality rate of approximately 20% (compared to almost 100% mortality untreated).

Disseminated intravascular coagulation (DIC) is characterized by systemic thrombosis, mediated by pathologic overproduction of thrombin. DIC is the consequence of other concurrent disease processes, especially evident in patients with active malignancy, obstetrical catastrophes, or trauma. Treatment for DIC is challenging, with primary therapy targeted toward eradicating the underlying precipitant and secondary therapy intended to ameliorate the bleeding and/or thrombotic consequences of the consumptive coagulopathy. Heparin anticoagulation should be used sparingly since it may exacerbate bleeding complications rather than prevent thrombin generation. When heparin is used in DIC, it is usually administered in lower doses (2,500- to 3,000-unit bolus followed by continuous infusion of 350 to 500 U/hr, titrated according to the recovery of fibrinogen concentrations and platelet counts). If bleeding ensues, supportive care in the form of cryoprecipitate and platelet transfusions may be useful. Even acute promyelocytic leukemia, traditionally treated initially with heparin to downregulate life-threatening DIC, is better approached with all-*trans*-retinoic acid for the underlying leukemia.

Myeloproliferative disorders (MPD) have been associated with thrombosis, especially true of polycythemia rubra vera and essential thrombocythemia (see Chapter 8). MPDs, paradoxically, are also associated with an increased risk of hemorrhage, but thrombotic complications are the most common cause of death in MPD. The thrombotic risk of polycythemia is often exacerbated by the hyperviscosity produced by a markedly increased red cell mass. Treatments for polycythemia vera include repeated phlebotomy to decrease red cell volume/hyperviscosity and cytotoxic agents, such as hydroxyurea, to reduce erythrocyte and platelet production, with the ultimate goal to minimize the risk of thrombosis.

Other acquired risk factors for thrombosis include increased age, immobility, prior VTE, myocardial infarction, pregnancy, and hormone therapy (17). Another recently discovered risk factor is thalidomide. In a study of patients with multiple myeloma who received combination chemotherapy with or without thalidomide, the thalidomide-treated patients had a much higher incidence of VTE (28% versus 4%), particularly if they had previously received therapy with adriamycin (18).

Table 22-2 lists acquired and heritable hypercoagulable states.

HERITABLE HYPERCOAGULABLE STATES

There is increasing appreciation that individuals who experience recurrent spontaneous VTE may have an underlying, inherited hypercoagulable state. Known congenital hypercoagulable states include:

- Activated protein C resistance (factor V Leiden gene polymorphism)
- Prothrombin gene mutation
- Deficiencies of protein C, protein S, and antithrombin III
- Hyperhomocysteinemia

There may also be heritable hypercoagulable states precipitated by persistent elevations of coagulation factors VIII, IX, and XI. Screening for a hypercoagulable state should be performed for a young patient with a positive family history of thrombosis, unprovoked thrombosis, or recurrent thrombosis. Appropriate genetic counseling should be performed before these tests are administered, and testing should be timed appropriately. For example, protein C, protein S, and antithrombin III levels may be reduced during an active thrombosis, which can create a false-positive test result. Warfarin will reduce the activities of the vitamin K-dependent modulators of clotting factors, protein C and protein S. Heparin and warfarin may affect test results for the lupus anticoagulant, and this diagnosis is best established after anticoagulation is discontinued.

TABLE. 22–2. *Hypercoagulable states*

Acquired hypercoagulable states
  Heparin-induced thrombocytopenia
  Nephrotic syndrome
  Antiphospholipid antibody syndrome
  Malignancy
  Paroxysmal nocturnal hemoglobinuria
  Surgery
  Microangiopathic hemolytic anemia (TTP/HUS/DIC)
  Myeloproliferative disorders
  Increased age
  Immobility
  Trauma
  Prior venous thromboembolism
  Myocardial infarction
  Pregnancy
  Hormone therapy
  Presence of a venous access device
Heritable hypercoagulable states
  Activated protein C resistance
  Prothrombin gene mutation (G20210A)
  Protein C deficiency
  Protein S deficiency
  Antithrombin III deficiency
  Hyperhomocyteinemia

TTP, thrombotic thrombocytopenic purpura; HUS, hemolytic-uremic syndrome; DIC, disseminated intravascular coagulation.

Testing may be useful for first-degree family members if they are in high-risk situations, including abdominopelvic surgery or orthopedic casting of the lower extremities, where more aggressive prophylactic anticoagulation would be recommended. In addition, oral estrogen contraceptive use is not recommended for these hypercoagulable females. Some hypercoagulable states, such as the antiphospholipid antibody syndrome, may require prolonged periods of anticoagulation, particularly during pregnancy. An elevated homocysteine level may prompt treatment with appropriate supplementation of vitamin B_6, B_{12}, and folate.

ACTIVATED PROTEIN C RESISTANCE (FACTOR V LEIDEN)

A mutation in coagulation factor V (Arg506Gln; factor V Leiden gene polymorphism) results in a protein that is no longer susceptible to inactivation by activated protein C proteolysis. Factor V Leiden is the most common known inheritable risk factor for VTE but has little effect on arterial thrombotic potential. Laboratory testing includes direct detection of an abnormal but characteristic gene mutation in factor V, accomplished by polymerase chain reaction (PCR), and indirectly, by evaluating the effects of factor V Leiden in an *in vitro* laboratory test for activated protein C resistance (this latter assay should not be performed while the patient is receiving warfarin). Factor V Leiden is common in the general population (5% incidence in a white cohort), but most people with the mutation do not develop a thrombosis. Approximately 20% of individuals with VTE do have evidence of factor V Leiden. Additive risk factors, however, including estrogen use and the coexistence of the prothrombin mutation, greatly increase the risk of VTE.

PROTHROMBIN MUTATION (G20210A)

The second most common gene mutation responsible for congenital hypercoagulability is the prothrombin G20210A polymorphism. As with factor V Leiden, VTE predominates in patients with the prothrombin gene mutation, with arterial thrombosis being unusual. This mutation is associated with elevated prothrombin levels, mainly in whites, and was found to have a crude 2.8 odds ratio for the development of thrombosis (19). G20210A can be indirectly assayed by measuring a prothrombin level, but direct genetic testing with PCR is more frequently performed.

DEFICIENCIES OF PROTEINS S, C, AND ANTITHROMBIN III

These three proteins are synthesized in the liver and have a modulatory function in homeostasis of the coagulation cascade. Protein S is a cofactor of activated protein C that serves to inactivate factors Va and VIIIa. Antithrombin III inhibits factors II, Xa, XIa, IXa, and XIIa (20). Heparin complexes to antithrombin III, greatly potentiating the serine protease inhibitory activity of antithrombin III. These enzymes can be quantitatively or qualitatively abnormal in hypercoagulable individuals. Severe deficiencies of these enzymes may result in VTE at a young age, in newborns as purpura fulminans. Arterial thrombotic complications are unusual. These deficiencies are uncommonly detected in the general population, but they are responsible for 5% to 15% of idiopathic VTE.

HYPERHOMOCYSTEINEMIA

Homocysteine can be metabolized to either methionine or cystathione by two pathways: remethylation of homocysteine to methionine and transsulfuration of homocysteine to cysteine. Different polymorphisms of enzymes of these pathways can result in hyperhomocysteinemia. The most common polymorphism, the heat labile variant of N5,N10-methylenetetrahydrofolate reductase, is present as a homozygous variant in up to 20% of whites and causes mildly elevated homocysteine levels. This polymorphism is not a primary cause of hypercoagulability but is probably an important secondary factor for thrombophilia in conjunction with other risks like factor V Leiden gene mutation. Other inborn errors of metabolism, involving homozygous cystathionine β-synthase deficiency, cause more marked hyperhomocysteinemia and are associated with early atherosclerosis and thrombosis. Proposed mechanisms to explain the development of thrombosis in hyperhomocysteinemia include direct endothelial injury with induction of tissue factor activity, downregulation of the vasodilatory effects of nitric oxide, inhibition of tissue plasminogen activator activity, suppression of heparan sulfate expression of endothelial cells, and upregulation of factor V (21). In a patient with hyperhomocysteinemia-associated thrombosis, treatment by dietary supplementation of vitamin B_{12}, folate, and vitamin B6, in addition to anticoagulation, is warranted.

TREATMENT FOR VENOUS THROMBOEMBOLISM

Anticoagulation is the main prophylaxis and first therapy for thrombosis and for prevention of recurrent VTE. In certain situations, treatment may include additional modalities, such as fibrinolytic therapy or insertion of an inferior vena cava filter.

DVT or PE should be treated initially with systemic anticoagulation in the form of unfractionated heparin (UFH) or LMWH. The goal is to prevent propagation of a clot while the endogenous fibrinolytic system dissolves the clot locally. Oral anticoagulation with warfarin should not be used as a single agent for the initial treatment of thrombosis. Warfarin, which inhibits the postribosomal modification of vitamin K-dependent proteins synthesized in the liver, will produce a rapid and early decrease in protein C activity, within hours after administration of the anticoagulant, and later will depress protein S activity. Warfarin-mediated decreases in the activity of these modulators of coagulation exacerbate the already depressed levels of proteins C and S, which are consumed during formation of VTE. These precipitous drops in protein C, particularly, have been associated with the development of severe skin necrosis, a manifestation of the unfavorable predisposition toward hypercoagulability that characterizes the first few days of warfarin therapy. Thus, the initial administration of warfarin as a single, unopposed anticoagulant for acute VTE may be detrimental unless it is part of a heparin-based regimen.

The choice of UFH versus LMWH as initial treatment for VTE depends on several factors. LMWH produces an earlier and more consistent antithrombotic state than does UFH, because LMWH does not complex with acute phase reactant proteins, such as fibrinogen and vWF protein, which are increased in response to the inflammatory effects of acute VTE. Second, LMWH is effective as a weight-based medication, and in contrast to UFH does not require dose adjustment or laboratory monitoring except in special situations, such as renal failure, pregnancy, and at both extremes of body mass index. LMWH is less likely than UFH to cause HIT. Cost may be an additional factor, because LMWH is more expensive than UFH; however, overall hospitalization and laboratory monitoring expenses are less with LMWH. UFH administration is dosed according to routine algorithms, based on aPTT results. LMWH should be followed with anti-factor Xa levels whenever laboratory monitoring is required. LMWH is contraindicated in renal failure and should be used with caution in patients with mild renal insufficiency, as the kidneys excrete LMWH. UFH may be preferred in a patient at risk for bleeding, because its half-life is shorter and its action can be reversed with protamine. In contrast, there is no specific antidote for LMWH if untoward hemorrhage occurs. Protamine sulfate's ability to reverse LMWH is unpredictable. In vitro studies suggest that recombinant factor VIIa may be a useful adjunct.

When a patient is receiving appropriate anticoagulation with UFH or LMWH for acute VTE, warfarin therapy can be initiated concurrently. Heparin overlap therapy as bridging for long-term anticoagulation with warfarin should continue for a minimum of 5 days and not be terminated until a therapeutic INR of 2 to 3 is reached. Standard practice is to start at 5 mg of warfarin per day because of possible overanticoagulation at higher doses. A recent double-blinded randomized study, however, showed that warfarin at 10 mg for 2 days was safe practice; the dose could then be adjusted by a nomogram (22). No increased bleeding risk was evident with the higher initial dose of warfarin in this trial. In patients with potential vitamin K deficiency, this strategy might increase the risk of overanticoagulation; vitamin K-deficient patients may have a mildly elevated prothrombin time prior to warfarin treatment. Common examples of patients who are at increased risk for vitamin K deficiency includes those who are malnourished, postsurgical, or on antibiotics.

Warfarin is currently the favored standard treatment for long-term anticoagulation because of the ease of oral administration. LMWH-based regimens for long-term anticoagulation are being used more often. Subcutaneously administered LMWHs do not require laboratory monitoring to assess safety or efficacy. Long-term LMWH use rarely, if ever, triggers heparin-induced thrombocytopenia, but the risk of osteopenia is real, if less than for UFH. Supplemental calcium should be provided during long term anticoagulation with UFH or LMWHs.

The ideal intensity of the INR for warfarin anticoagulation to prevent recurrent idiopathic VTE has been studied in two large prospective, randomized trials, which have yielded conflicting results. In the placebo controlled PREVENT trial, low-intensity anticoagulation with the target INR of 1.5–2.0 reduced the recurrent VTE rate by two-thirds (23). In a randomized, two-arm study of standard warfarin anticoagulation to achieve an INR between 2 and 3 versus a low-intensity INR arm with target INR between 1.5 and 2.0, the standard dosing regimen was over 60% more effective ($p = 0.03$) than low-intensity warfarin anticoagulation in reducing the cumulative probability of recurrent thromboembolism (24). There was no difference in bleeding complications between the two dosing intensities.

Different clinical situations determine the duration of time that anticoagulation is required. In general, for an unprovoked idiopathic DVT, at least 6 months of anticoagulation are recommended. In general, a massive life-threatening PE requires lifelong anticoagulation, similar to the recommendations for recurrent idiopathic VTE. The PREVENT trial corroborated that patients with idiopathic VTE have a high incidence of recurrent VTE and benefit from long-term anticoagulation (23). As previously discussed, the antiphospholipid antibody syndrome requires prolonged warfarin therapy. Individuals with cancer may be hypercoagulable and anticoagulation should probably be continued as long as the malignancy is present.

NEW CLASSES OF ANTICOAGULANTS

Numerous new classes of anticoagulants are being developed that may be more effective, safe, and convenient than currently available agents. Fondaparinux, a synthetic pentasaccharide LMWH derivative, is a specific inhibitor of factor Xa through its interaction with antithrombin (25). It has the convenience of once-daily weight-based dosing and is administered subcutaneously. Fondaparinux has been compared to adjusted dose UFH (followed by warfarin in both groups) in a randomized open label trial with 2,213 patients with acute PE: mortality, recurrent VTE, and bleeding were similar in both groups (26). Fondaparinux has also been compared to enoxaparin (30 mg twice daily) in clinical trials for the prevention of VTE in patients undergoing hip replacement surgery: the PENTATHALON study reported a nonstatistically significant trend toward decreased VTE in patients undergoing hip replacement surgery treated with fondaparinux (27).

A second new promising agent now in clinical evaluation for the treatment and prevention of VTE is ximelagatran. Unlike fondaparinux, ximelagatran acts independently of antithrombin and is a direct thrombin inhibitor (25). It has the clinical benefit of oral dosing without the need for laboratory monitoring (25). The THRIVE III trial evaluated patients treated for their VTE with 6 months of conventional anticoagulation and randomized them to placebo versus 24 mg of ximelagatran twice daily for 18 months: 12 of 612 patients in the ximelagatran group had a recurrent VTE versus 71 of 611 patients in the placebo group (28). Bleeding was higher in the ximelagatran group; however, the incidence of major hemorrhage was low (28). Transient transaminitis was higher in the ximelagatran group, and monitoring of hepatic enzymes may be necessary. Transaminitis was readily reversible upon discontinuation of the medication. Larger studies comparing ximelagatran and warfarin will be required to assess the efficacy and safety of this agent, especially given its greater cost and the longer track record of warfarin (25).

INFERIOR VENA CAVA FILTERS IN THE TREATMENT OF DEEP VENOUS THROMBOSIS OR PULMONARY EMBOLUS

Inferior vena cava (IVC) filters are inserted to prevent thrombi originating in the venous vasculature of the lower extremities from embolizing to the pulmonary circulation. The IVC filter is placed by an interventional radiologist. Major reasons for the placement of an IVC filter include strong contraindications to the use of anticoagulants, intolerance to or noncompliance with anticoagulants, and recurrent PE despite adequate systemic anticoagulation. A randomized study revealed that, in the short term, an IVC filter can decrease the incidence of pulmonary embolus, but at 2 years the difference was not statistically significant (29). In addition, there were more DVT in the IVC filter group, with the potential of greater morbidity from postphlebitic syndrome (29). Individuals with permanent IVC filters probably benefit from life-long anticoagulation. Temporary filters have been approved by the Food and Drug Administration; they may be used as bridge protection against VTE until patients can be anticoagulated effectively. Removal may prevent long-term risks associated with IVC filters.

FIBRINOLYTIC THERAPY

Fibrinolytic therapy has been used for patients with massive PE with hemodynamic compromise. Nevertheless, no clinical study has confirmed a survival advantage when using thrombolytic agents. Some practitioners also consider thrombolytic therapy for patients with new right heart failure or moderate to severe pulmonary hypertension in the setting of PE. Fibrinolysis is also used in selected patients with massive ileofemoral DVT to decrease development of postthrombotic complications. For DVT, thrombolytic therapy is often catheter directed, while catheter-directed lysis for PE has no advantage over systemic administration of the thrombolytic agent. Careful patient selection is critical to avoidance of the morbidity and mortality associated with thrombolysis: elderly individuals with systemic hypertension are at greatest risk. Major bleeding is common at the venotomy site if the venipuncture is not performed flawlessly. Because of an intracerebral bleed rate approaching 0.6%, and approximately 2% major bleeds elsewhere, thorough discussion with a patient regarding potential risks and benefits is important. Surgical thrombectomy is indicated for the small number of patients with massive PE who are not candidates for fibrinolytic therapy.

REFERENCES

1. Anderson FA, Wheeler HB, Goldberg RJ, et al. A population-based perspective of the hospital incidence and case-fatality rates of deep vein thrombosis and pulmonary embolism. the Worchester DVT Study. *Arch Intern Med* 1991;151:933–938.
2. Elliot MS, Immelman EJ, Jeffery P, et al. A comparative randomized trial of heparin versus streptokinase in the treatment of acute proximal venous thrombosis: an interim report of a prospective trial. *Br J Surg* 1979;66:838–843.
3. Tapson VF, Carroll BA, Davidson BL, et al. The diagnostic approach to acute venous thromboembolism. Clinical practice guideline. American Thoracic Society. *Am J Resp Crit Care Med* 1999;160: 1043–1066.
4. Saltzman HA, Alavi A, Greenspan RH, et al. Value of the ventilation/perfusion in acute pulmonary embolism: results of the Prospective Investigation of Pulmonary Embolism Diagnosis (PIOPED). *JAMA* 1990;263:2753–2759.
5. Meyer T, Binder L, Hruska N, et al. Cardiac troponin I elevation in acute pulmonary embolism is associated with right ventricular dysfunction. *J Am Coll Cardiol* 2000;36:1632–1636.
6. Giannitsis E, Muller-Bardoff M, Kurowski V, et al. Independent prognostic value of cardiac troponin T in patients with confirmed pulmonary embolism. *Circulation* 2000;102:211–217.
7. Kitchens CS. Venous thromboses at unusual sites. In: Kitchens CS, Alving BM, Kessler CM, eds. *Consultative Thrombosis and Hemostasis.* Philadelphia: W.B. Saunders Company, 2002:181–196.
8. Warkentin TE. Heparin-induced thrombocytopenia: pathogenesis and management. Br J Haematol 2003;121:535–555.
9. Orth SR, Ritz E. The nephrotic syndrome. *N Engl J Med* 1998;38:1202–1211.
10. Levine JS, Branch DW, Rauch J. The antiphospholipid syndrome. *N Engl J Med* 2002;346:752–763.
11. Crowther MA, Ginsberg JS, Julian J, et al. A comparison of two intensities of warfarin for the prevention of recurrent thrombosis in patients with the antiphospholipid antibody syndrome. *N Engl J Med* 2003;349:1133–1138.
12. Caine GJ, Stonelake PS, Lip GYH, et al. The hypercoagulable state of malignancy: pathogenesis and current debate. *Neoplasia* 2002;4:465–473.
13. Bick RL. Cancer-associated thrombosis. *N Engl J Med* 2003;349:109–111.
14. Lee AY, Levine MN, Baker RI, et al. Low-molecular-weight heparin versus a coumarin for the prevention of recurrent venous thromboembolism in patients with cancer. *N Engl J Med* 2003;349: 146–153.
15. Hall C, Richards S, Hillmen P. Primary prophylaxis with warfarin prevents thrombosis in paroxysmal nocturnal hemoglobinuria (PNH). *Blood* 2003;102:3587–3591.
16. Geerts WH, Heit JA, Clagett P, et al. Prevention of venous thromboembolism. *Chest* 2002;119: 132S–175S.
17. Anderson FA, Spencer FA. Risk factors for venous thromboembolism. *Circulation* 2003;107 (23 Suppl 1):I9–I16.

18. Zangari M, Anaissie E, Barlogie B, et al. Increased risk of deep-vein thrombosis in patients with multiple myeloma receiving thalidomide and chemotherapy. *Blood* 2001;98:1614–1615.
19. Poort SR, Rosendaal FR, Reitsma PH, et al. A common genetic variation in the 3N-untranslated region of the prothrombin gene is associated with elevated plasma prothrombin levels and an increase in venous thrombosis. *Blood* 1996;88:3698–3703.
20. Zwicker J, Bauer KA. Thrombophilia. In: Kitchens CS, Alving BM, Kessler CM, eds. *Consultative Thrombosis and Hemostasis.* Philadelphia: W.B. Saunders Company. 2002:181–196.
21. Lee R, Frenkel EP. Hyperhomocysteinemia and thrombosis. *Hematol Oncol Clin North Am* 2003;17:85–102
22. Kovacs MJ, Roger M, Anderson DR, et al. Comparison of 10-mg and 5-mg warfarin initiation nomograms together with low-molecular-weight-heparin for outpatient treatment of acute venous thromboembolism. A randomized, double-blind, controlled trial. *Ann Intern Med* 2003;138:714–719.
23. Ridker PM, Goldhaber SZ, Danielson E, et al. Long-term, low intensity warfarin for the prevention of recurrent venous thromboembolism. *N Engl J Med* 2003;348:1425–1434.
24. Kearon C, Ginsberg JS, Kovacs MJ, et al. Comparison of low-intensity warfarin therapy with conventional-intensity warfarin therapy for long-term prevention of recurrent venous thromboembolism. *N Engl J Med* 2003;349:631–639.
25. Shapiro SS. Treating thrombosis in the 21st century. *N Engl J Med* 2003;349:1762–1764.
26. Buller HR, Davidson BL, Decousus H, et al. Subcutaneous fondaparinux versus intravenous unfractionated heparin in the initial treatment of pulmonary embolism. *N Engl J Med* 2003;349:1695–1702.
27. Turpie AG, Bauer KA, Eriksson BI, et al. Postoperative fondaparinux versus postoperative enoxaparin for the prevention of venous thromboembolism after elective hip-replacement surgery. A randomized double-blind study. *Lancet* 2002;359:1721–1726.
28. Schulman S, Wahlander K, Lundstrom T, et al. Secondary prevention of venous thromboembolism with the oral direct thrombin inhibitor ximelagatran. *N Engl J Med* 2003;349:1713–1721.
29. Decousus H, Leizorovicz A, Parent F, et al. A clinical trial of vena caval filters in the prevention of pulmonary embolism in patients with proximal deep-vein thrombosis. *N Engl J Med* 1998;338:409–415.

23

Consultations in Anticoagulation

Pallavi P. Kumar and Barbara Alving

This chapter provides guidelines for the treatment of venous thromboembolism (VTE) in patients who require special consideration, such as those who have underlying cancer, are pregnant, have undergone surgery, or who have catheter–related thrombosis. The last section of the chapter addresses the treatment of postphlebitic syndrome and the recognition and management of peripheral vascular disease.

ANTICOAGULATION AND MALIGNANCY

Patients with malignancy frequently have an underlying hypercoaguable state, which includes induction of tissue factor (TF) by cytokines. The risk of thrombosis is further increased because of prolonged immobilization; obstruction of vascular flow caused by obstruction by the tumor; vascular damage induced by chemotherapy; and the presence of central venous access devices.

PROPHYLAXIS AND TREATMENT OF VENOUS THROMBOEMBOLISM IN THE PATIENT WITH MALIGNANCY IN SPECIFIC CLINICAL SETTINGS

As long as the cancer is active, patients remain at high risk for venous thromboembolism (VTE). In general, unfractionated heparin (UFH), low molecular weight heparin (LMWH), and oral anticoagulants have been the mainstay of therapy. An oral anticoagulant that may be available in the future is ximelagatran, a thrombin inhibitor that does not require laboratory monitoring. This drug, which is currently under review by the Food and Drug Admnistration (FDA), has not been tested specifically in patients with cancer.

This section discusses the clinical settings in which the patient with malignancy may require anticoagulation. The recommendations are based primarily on clinical trial data or small studies in which patients with malignancy were only a minor subset (fewer than 20% of participants).

- Primary prophylaxis in surgery.
- Primary prophylaxis during chemotherapy.
- Primary prophylaxis when hospitalized/immobilized.
- Primary prophylaxis and treatment of patients who have brain metastases or primary brain tumors.
- Treatment of patients with Trousseau's syndrome.
- General approach in treating an acute VTE.
- General approach in treating recurrent VTE.
- Indications for inferior vena caval filters.

Primary Prophylaxis in Patients with Cancer Undergoing Surgical Intervention

Once-daily LMWH appears to be as safe and effective as several daily injections of UFH for prophylaxis. In addition, the once-per-day injection provides convenience and a better quality of life (1,2). In the Clinical Center at the National Institutes of Health, enoxaparin is the LMWH utilized. However, other LMWH, such as nadroparin calcium, dalteparin, ardeparin, tinzaparin, and reviparin may be considered (Table 23-1).

Primary Prophylaxis in Patients with Cancer Receiving Chemotherapy

A double-blind randomized trial of very low dose warfarin (1 mg daily) in women with stage IV breast cancer showed an 85% relative risk reduction in the rate of VTE (p = 0.031) without an increase in risk for bleeding (11). However, in practice, most oncologists do not prophylactically anticoagulate patients with advanced cancer who are receiving chemotherapy. Candidates for prophylaxis include patients who have a history of VTE, have a large mass compressing a major vessel, or those who are receiving tamoxifen or an antiangiogenic agent, such as thalidomide. Treatment in these patients should be individualized; if prophylaxis is chosen, the following could be considered:

- Warfarin, 1 mg daily.
- Anticoagulation to continue 1 week after completing all cycles of chemotherapy.
- Monitoring not usually performed, except for patients who are at increased risk for bleeding (an appropriate international normalized ratio [INR] range for these patients is 1.3 to 1.9 (1,7,12).

Primary Prophylaxis in Patients with Cancer who are Immobilized/Hospitalized

Subcutaneous prophylactic doses of LMWH appear to be safe and efficacious for patients with cancer who are hospitalized for medical illnesses. This recommendation is based in part on the MEDENOX trial, a double-blind randomized study of 1102 patients with acute medical illnesses who received prophylaxis against VTE (14.9% of these patients had cancer or a history of cancer) (Table 23-2). Patients were assigned to one of three groups that would receive 40 mg of enoxaparin, 20 mg of enoxaparin, or placebo, respectively, subcutaneously once daily for 6 to 14 days. The primary outcome was lower extremity deep venous thrombosis (DVT) or pulmonary embolism (PE) with a follow-up duration of 3 months. The outcome favored prophylactic treatment with subcutaneous enoxaparin at a dose of 40 mg daily. Adverse events, which included hemorrhage, local reaction, thrombocytopenia, and death from any cause, were not different between the groups receiving enoxaparin and placebo.

Primary Prophylaxis in Patients with Cancer with Brain Metastases and Primary Brain Tumors

The causes of VTE in these patients appear to be multifactorial and include release of procoagulants, venous stasis, bulky tumor, and treatments that may induce a low-grade disseminated intravascular coagulation (DIC). The challenge in using anticoagulation is balancing the risk of thrombosis with the risk of hemorrhage. Studies have shown both increased risk as well as benefit with the use of LMWH (14). One protocol began treatment with LMWH before surgery but was terminated early because of the increased incidence of intracranial hemorrhage (15). In comparison, initiating LMWH within 24 hours after surgery appears to have minimal risks, and this is the recommended prophylaxis in patients with brain tumors (Table 23-3) (8,10).

TABLE. 23–1. *Primary prophylaxis in patients with cancer undergoing surgical intervention*

Surgical intervention	Drug of choice	Dose	Initiation of dose	Other	Duration of treatment
Abdominal/Pelvis (3–5)	Enoxaparin (LMWH)	40 mg SQ daily	10–14 hours preoperatively	Recommend use of compression stockings with anticoagulant	28 days
Orthopedic (6,7)	Enoxaparin	30 mg SQ q12hr **or** 40 mg SQ daily	12–24 hours postoperatively 10–12 hours preoperatively	Recommend use of compression stockings or intermittent pneumatic compression with LMWH	Under debate: 30–35 days showed significant reduction of VTE
Neurosurgery (8–10)	Enoxaparin	40 mg SQ daily	12–24 hours postoperatively	Use compression stockings and/or intermittent pneumatic compression with LMWH	Until hospital discharge

LMWH, low molecular weight heparin; SQ, subcutaneously; VTE, venous thromboembolism

TABLE. 23–2. *Primary prophylaxis in patients with cancer hospitalized for acute medical illnesses: the MEDENOX trials*

Recommended prophylaxis for VTE	Dose	Duration of treatment	Incidence of VTE	Other
Enoxaparin versus placebo	40 mg SQ daily	6–14 days (days of hospitalization or as long as patient is immobilized)	5.5% versus 14.9% p <0.001	Significant reduction in VTE with enoxaparin was maintained at three months.

[13]
VTE, venous thromboembolism; SQ, subcutaneously.

Treatment of Venous Thromboembolism in Patients with Primary Brain Tumors or Brain Metastases

Anticoagulation for VTE in patients with brain tumors or brain metastases is often perceived to lead to intracranial hemorrhage, but standard anticoagulation can be safely administered if closely monitored (14). The risk of hemorrhagic complications may be increased in patients with metastatic tumors that are very vascular or that have a high propensity for bleeding (such as melanoma). Other options include the placement of an inferior vena cava filter, although risks need to be carefully considered. Table 23-4 provides recommendations that have not been developed specifically for patients with brain tumors or with brain metastases and should be considered as a general guide.

At our institution, enoxaparin is the LMWH of choice, although direct comparisons of different LMWH in the treatment of VTE have not been made in clinical trials. Verification of the appropriate degree of anticoagulation by measuring anti-Xa activity is recommended in patients who have impaired renal function. For example, the elderly may have normal serum creatinine values despite underlying renal dysfunction; thus, calculating creatinine clearance is indicated prior to initiating therapy. In addition, careful monitoring of the anticoagulant effect must be considered in obesity (body mass index greater than 30 kg/m2), particularly if the patient has concurrent moderate to severe renal insufficiency (creatinine clearance less than 60 mL/min). Antifactor Xa levels should be monitored initially in severely obese patients receiving therapeutic LMWH (16).

TABLE. 23–3. *Evidence for favorable benefit/risk ratio with anticoagulation after neurosurgery*

Patient group	Recommended treatment	Duration of treatment	Outcome
Patients with brain tumors	40 mg enoxaparin subcutaneously daily with compressive stockings or compressive stockings alone	Begin within 24 hours after neurosurgery and continue for more than 7 days	Rate of VTE: 17% with LMWH + stockings versus 32% with stockings alone. P=0.004 3% in each group had major bleeding.

[8]
VTE, venous thromboembolism; LMWH, low molecular weight heparin.

TABLE. 23–4. *Treatment of venous thromboembolism in patients with primary brain tumors or brain metastases*

Treatment for VTE	Recommended dose	Duration of treatment	Other comments
LMWH (enoxaparin) + warfarin	Enoxaparin 1 mg/kg every 12 hours + warfarin daily (dose adjust to maintain INR goal 2.0–3.0)	LMWH for at least 5 days and concurrently INR goal maintained for 2 days before stopping LMWH	
UFH + warfarin	Initial bolus 5,000 units IV followed by 1,280 U/hr + warfarin daily (dose adjust to maintain INR goal 2.0–3.0)	UFH for at least 5 days and concurrently INR goal maintained for 2 days before stopping UFH.	UFH adjusted to maintain aPTT 60–85 seconds (a targeted aPTT should be equivalent to antifactor Xa activity level of 0.3–0.7 U/mL). Warfarin continued for at least 3 months
IVC filter			High rate of complications in patients with cancer reducing quality of life. Retrievable filter may be considered.

[17]
VTE, venous thromboembolism; LMWH, low molecular weight heparin; INR, international normalized ratio; IV, intravenously; UFH, unfractionated heparin; aPTT, activated partial thromboplastin time; IVC, inferior vena cava.

Treatment of Patients with Trousseau's Syndrome

Trousseau's syndrome is a spectrum of thromboembolic disorders of the venous and arterial systems associated with a malignancy. Patients with this syndrome, even if adequately anticoagulated with warfarin, according to the INR, may have recurrent thrombi. UFH and LMWH are efficacious, but each clinical situation may warrant variable dosing. For example, an acute DVT may necessitate enoxaparin at therapeutic doses, whereas DIC may be controlled with lower doses. Administration of LMWH reduces the rate of recurrent thrombi without increasing bleeding and may also improve quality of life (Table 23-5).

General Approach in Treating Venous Thromboembolism in Patients with Cancer

In general, treatment of PE or DVT in patients with cancer consists of LMWH or UFH followed by warfarin. However, for patients who may be bedridden and critically ill, continued long-term treatment with LMWH may be preferable to warfarin. Most institutions have a nomogram which guides the dosing and monitoring of UFH. General guidelines are provided in Table 23-6.

General Approach in Preventing or Treating Recurrent Venous Thromboembolism in Patients with Cancer

For patients without cancer, warfarin therapy is generally administered for at least 3 months after a first episode of proximal DVT or PE. However, patients with malignancy may be at continued risk of VTE even after 3 to 6 months of treatment with warfarin.

Anticoagulation Options

• For patients with recurrent VTE despite adequate anticoagulation with warfarin (INR 2 to 3), consider initiation of LMWH and discontinuation of warfarin. These patients may have underlying Trousseau's syndrome.

TABLE. 23–5. *Treatment of patients with Trousseau's syndrome*

Clinical manifestations	Recommended treatment	Dose	Length of treatment	Other comment
Spontaneous recurrent or migratory venous thrombosis Arterial thrombosis Microangiopathy Marantic endocarditis Acute/chronic DIC-thrombotic versus bleeding state (characterized predominantly by thrombosis with no clinically significant bleeding)	Enoxaparin	Dose is variable depending on clinical condition.	Requires treatment as long as tumor persists	Further studies are needed to compare efficacy, safety, and costs of LMWH with other anticoagulants

[1, 11, 18]
DIC, disseminated intravascular coagulation; LMWH, low molecular weight heparin.

TABLE. 23-6. General approaches in treating patients with cancer who develop venous thromboembolism

Treatment for VTE	Recommended dose	Duration of treatment	Other comments
LMWH (enoxaparin) + warfarin	1 mg/kg every 12 hours + warfarin daily (dose adjust to maintain INR goal of 2.0–3.0)	LMWH for at least 5 days, start warfarin on the 2nd day. Concurrently INR goal maintained for 2 days before stopping LMWH	Continue for at least 3 months
UFH + warfarin	Initial bolus 5,000 units IV followed by approximately 1,280 U/hr + warfarin daily (dose adjust to maintain INR goal of 2.0–3.0)	UFH for at least 5 days, start warfarin on the 2nd day. Concurrently INR goal maintained for 2 days before stopping UFH.	UFH adjusted to maintain an aPTT of 60–85 seconds (the targeted aPTT should be equivalent to antifactor Xa activity level of 0.3 to 0.7 U/mL) Warfarin continued for as long as the malignancy is present and for at least 3 months (assuming the bleeding risk is acceptable)

[7, 17, 19]
VTE, venous thromboembolism; LMWH, low molecular weight heparin; INR, international normalized ratio; IV, intravenously; UFH, unfractionated heparin; aPTT, activated partial thromboplastin time.

- For patients with a first event, consider long-term anticoagulation after the first 3 to 6 months using low-intensity warfarin. In a recent study, patients with idiopathic VTE who had received a median of 6.5 months of warfarin (INR 2 to 3) were randomly assigned to placebo or low-intensity warfarin (target INR 1.5 to 2.0); they were followed for up to 4.3 years. The trial was terminated early for benefit, because patients receiving warfarin had a risk reduction of 65% for recurrent VTE compared to the patients receiving placebo ($p < 0.001$) (7,20).

Indications for Inferior Vena Cava Filters in a Patient with Malignancy

Although inferior vena cava (IVC) filters are effective initially in preventing PE, their long-term complications include recurrent DVT, IVC thrombosis, and thrombosis at the insertion site. The use of IVC filters should be based on the contraindications to anticoagulation and failure of adequate anticoagulation. Filters that can be retrieved are now available and can help reduce morbidity associated with permanent IVC filters.

Examples of Newer Inferior Vena Cava Filters

- TrapEase filter. This filter has the advantages of being small and symmetrical. Delivery can be through an antecubital, jugular, or femoral vein approach with the potential of easy manipulation. This type of filter is not retrievable.
- Gunther Tulip Retrievable Vena Cava Filter. This retrievable filter, approved by the FDA, is ideal for a patient who has an acute VTE or who is at high risk for VTE and is actively bleeding. It can be inserted and removed within 7 to 10 days, as required.
- Bard Removable Vena Cava Filter. This retrievable filter, also approved by the FDA, is unique in that it does not have an indicated time limit for removal, but provides flexibility in extraction timing based on patient risk (1,21).

ANTICOAGULATION AND CATHETERS

One complication of long-term central venous catheters is thrombosis, which can involve the tip of the catheter alone, the length of the catheter forming a fibrin sheath, or the veins of the upper extremities, neck, and mediastinum (7). This section discusses prophylaxis against thrombosis, as well as the treatment of patients with catheter-related central venous thrombosis.

Prophylaxis

Studies on the use of anticoagulation in preventing thrombosis associated with chronic indwelling central venous catheters have had differing outcomes. One trial reported 82 patients at risk for thrombosis who were prospectively randomized to receive 1 mg warfarin daily or no anticoagulants. The occurrence of venographically proven thrombosis in the group receiving warfarin compared to the group not receiving warfarin was 10% versus 38% ($p = 0.001$) (22). In contrast, other studies have shown no benefit in routine prophylactic use of low-dose warfarin (23). At the present time, low-dose warfarin as prophylaxis is not routinely used in clinical practice.

Treatment

The goals of treating catheter-induced thrombosis are to prevent extension of the thrombus and to restore catheter patency, thus avoiding the need for catheter removal. Some clinicians advocate immediate catheter removal and full-dose heparin once a venous thrombus has been diagnosed; below is a guide to other options (Table 23-7).

TABLE. 23–7. *Treatment of patients with catheter-induced venous thromboembolism*

Event	Treatment for VTE	Recommended dose	Duration of treatment	Other comments
Thrombus at the tip of the catheter (ball-valve clot) or fibrin sheath	tPA or urokinase	2 mg (5,000 to 10,000 U)	Instill for 30–120 minutes into the catheter.	Success defined by withdrawing 3 mL of blood and infusion of 5 mL of saline through the catheter—successful 70%–90% of the time, repeat once if not successful.
Thrombus occlusion despite tPA (2 doses)	tPA	1 mg/hr	Infusion for 6 hours into the catheter	Prime IV tubing with 10–15 mL of a 1 mg/mL solution, then bolus 1–2 mL to fill lumen of catheter, then start infusion.[a]
	Urokinase	40,000 U/hr	Infusion for 6–12 hours into the catheter	
Venous thrombosis confirmed	Urokinase	500 to 2,000 U/kg per hr	Infusion into the catheter for 24–96 hours, then continue with heparin and warfarin to prevent rethrombosis	Use when indwelling catheter is essential and if catheter is close to the thrombus

[24–26]
[a] Horne M. *Personal Communication*, 2004.
VTE, venous thromboembolism; tPA, tissue plasminogen activator; IV, intravenously.

ANTICOAGULATION AND PREGNANCY

Although maternal mortality is rare in pregnant women who live in developed countries, pregnancy-associated PE remains one of the most frequent causes of death. The evaluation and management of VTE in pregnancy are complicated by difficulty in interpreting symptoms, concern about performing imaging that may be hazardous to the fetus, and the need to consider possible complications of anticoagulation in both the mother and the fetus. This section will summarize the following topics:

- Diagnosis of VTE during pregnancy.
- Management of pregnant patients at increased risk of VTE.
- Treatment of VTE during pregnancy.

Diagnosis of Venous Thromboembolism During Pregnancy

In pregnant women, symptoms of lower extremity edema, back pain, and/or chest pain are often attributed to pregnancy rather than to a possible VTE. D-dimer assays are not helpful in establishing a diagnosis of VTE in late pregnancy because of the high rate of false-positive test results. Radiologic studies have to be assessed carefully in terms of potential risks of ionizing radiation on the fetus. Compression ultrasonography of the proximal veins is recommended as the initial test for suspected DVT. If results are equivocal or an iliac vein thrombosis is possible, then magnetic resonance venography should be considered since it does not carry radiation risks and is reliable. Finally, evaluation of pregnant women for PE would include a ventilation/perfusion (V/Q) lung scan. If the V/Q scan is indeterminate and the patient has no lower extremity thrombosis, angiography with a brachial approach can be performed because the procedure carries less radiation exposure to the fetus than spiral computed tomography (CT) (27).

Management of Pregnant Women at Increased Risk For Venous Thromboembolism

Risk factors for thrombosis may include a personal history of VTE, known inherited or acquired thrombophilia, obesity, older maternal age, high parity, or prolonged immobilization. The optimal anticoagulation for pregnant women has not been established, although UFH and LMWH are used and have an advantage of not crossing the placenta. Compared to UFH, LMWH appears to have a lower risk for inducing osteoporosis and heparin-induced thrombocytopenia (28). Warfarin carries a risk of teratogenecity between 6 weeks and 12 weeks and bleeding after 36 weeks gestation. Heparin and warfarin can be given to mothers who are nursing because they do not appear in breast milk.

Tables 23-8 to 23-13 offer a guide to correlate clinical situations in pregnancy with management options. These tables are adapted from reference 29, which has a complete description of thrombotic conditions in pregnant women and appropriate treatments, including the antiphos-

TABLE. 23–8. *Single episode of prior venous thromboembolism associated with a transient risk factor*

Treatment during pregnancy	Treatment during postpartum period
Surveillance	Begin anticoagulation with UFH or LMWH and then overlap with warfarin. Warfarin daily for 4–6 weeks, adjust dose to maintain INR 2.0–3.0.

UFH, unfractionated heparin; LMWH, low molecular weight heparin; INR, International normalized ratio.

TABLE. 23–9. *Single episode of idiopathic venous thromboembolism in women not receiving long-term anticoagulation*

Treatment during pregnancy	Treatment during postpartum period

Surveillance
or
choice of either:
UFH: 5,000 U SQ every 12 hours (or
  dose adjusted to achieve a peak.
  anti-Xa level of 0.1–0.3 U/mL).
or
LMWH (enoxaparin): 40 mg SQ daily,
  or other LMWH (Anti-Xa level of
  0.2–0.6 U/mL should be achieved).
	Begin anticoagulation with UFH or LMWH and
	then overlap with warfarin. Warfarin daily for
	4–6 weeks, adjust dose to maintain INR
	2.0–3.0.

UFH, unfractionated heparin; LMWH, low molecular weight heparin; SQ, subcutaneously; INR, international normalized ratio.
*Level to be achieved with other LMWH should be measured 4 hours after injection.

pholipid syndrome. Our chapter focuses on commonly encountered clinical situations. Recommendations are also included for the postpartum period, when the risk for thrombosis is increased above that of pregnancy. LMWH and aspirin should be discontinued prior to placement of an epidural catheter or induction of labor. LMWH should be held 24 hours prior and aspirin should be stopped 7 days prior to such a provocation to bleeding; either agent may be resumed 24 hours after delivery once hemostasis has been achieved.

RECOGNITION AND MANAGEMENT OF PERIPHERAL VENOUS AND ARTERIAL DISEASE

The diagnosis and management of two common conditions, postphlebitic syndrome and peripheral arterial disease, are often overlooked by patients and physicians until the conditions

TABLE. 23–10. *Single episode of venous thromboembolism and thrombophilia (confirmed laboratory finding) in women not receiving long-term anticoagulation*

Treatment during pregnancy	Treatment during postpartum period

Surveillance
or
choice of either:
UFH: 5,000 U SQ every 12 hours (or
  dose adjusted to achieve a peak
  anti-Xa level of 0.1–0.3 U/mL).
or
LMWH (enoxaparin): 40 mg SQ daily
  or q 12 hours, or other LMWH
  (Anti-Xa level of 0.2–0.6 U/mL
  should be achieved).
	Begin anticoagulation with UFH or LMWH and
	then overlap with warfarin. Warfarin daily for
	4–6 weeks, adjust dose to maintain INR
	2.0–3.0.

UFH, unfractionated heparin; LMWH, low molecular weight heparin; SQ, subcutaneously; INR, international normalized ratio.
*Level to be achieved with other LMWH should be measured 4 hours after injection.

TABLE. 23–11. *Women with thrombophilia and with no prior venous thromboembolism***

Treatment during pregnancy	Treatment during postpartum period

Surveillance
or
choice of either:
UFH: 5,000 U SQ every 12 hours (no
  need to dose adjust in this situation),
  no laboratory monitoring needed.
or
LMWH (enoxaparin): 40 mg SQ daily,
  or other LMWH (Anti-Xa level of
  0.2–0.6 U/mL should be achieved).
	Begin anticoagulation with UFH or LMWH and
	then overlap with warfarin. Warfarin daily for
	4–6 weeks, adjust dose to maintain INR
	2.0–3.0.

UFH, unfractionated heparin; LMWH, low molecular weight heparin; SQ, subcutaneously; INR, international normalized ratio.

*Level to be achieved with other LMWH should be measured 4 hours after injection.

**Women who have antithrombin deficiency or are compound heterozygotes or homozygous for prothrombin gene mutation or factor V Leiden must have prophylaxis with UFH or LMWH. Surveillance is not a recommended option with these specified conditions.

are sufficiently severe to require the attention of the vascular surgeon. Early recognition and treatment of both conditions can greatly improve the quality of life for patients and delay disease progression.

POSTPHLEBITIC SYNDROME (POSTTHROMBOTIC SYNDROME OR VENOUS INSUFFICIENCY)

Hematologists and internists are well trained to diagnose and manage acute VTE; however, additional attention needs to be given to postphlebitic syndrome, which occurs in as many as 20% to 50% of patients within 1 to 2 years after an episode of DVT (30). Postphlebitic syndrome is due to venous hypertension, which results from obstruction and damage to the venous valves, usually caused by DVT. The syndrome manifests as chronic pain in the affected

TABLE. 23–12. *Multiple episodes of venous thromboembolism and/or women receiving long-term anticoagulation therapy*

Treatment during pregnancy	Treatment during postpartum period

Choice of either:
UFH: Dose adjust SQ every 12 hours to
  target a midinterval aPTT into therapeutic
  range
or
LMWH: LMWH adjusted to target a peak anti-
  Xa level of 0.2 to 0.6 U/mL or enoxaparin
  1 mg/kg every 12 hours
	Warfarin—resume long-term therapy with
	appropriate monitoring of INR.

UFH, unfractionated heparin; SQ, subcutaneous; aPTT, activated partial thromboplastin time; LMWH, low molecular weight heparin; INR, international normalized ratio.

TABLE. 23–13. *Treatment of venous thromboembolism during pregnancy*

Treatment during pregnancy	Treatment during postpartum period
Choice of either: LMWH (enoxaparin): 1 mg/kg every 12 hours, anti-Xa level of 0.5–1.2 U/mL, measured 4 hours after injection or IV UFH: Bolus followed by a continuous infusion to maintain the aPTT in the therapeutic range for at least 5 days, followed by adjusted-dose UFH for the remainder of the pregnancy. To avoid unwanted anticoagulant effect in women receiving adjusted-dose LMWH or UFH during the delivery, discontine heparin therapy 24 hours prior to elective induction of labor. If patient is high risk of recurrent VTE (e.g., proximal DVT within 2 weeks), therapeutic IV UFH therapy can be initiated and discontinued 4–6 hours prior to time of delivery.	Treatment depends on the time of thrombosis during pregnancy. LMWH can be used or warfarin can be initiated while the patient is receiving LMWH or UFH. Treatment in the postpartum period should be continued for at least 6–8 weeks.

[29]
LMWH, low molecular weight heparin; UFH, unfractionated heparin; aPTT, activated partial thromboplastin time; VTE, venous thromboembolism; DVT, deep venous thrombosis; IV, intravenous.

leg, as well as edema and hyperpigmentation of the skin, and painless ulcers on the medial malleolar area in severe cases. The diagnosis is primarily clinical; duplex scanning can be used if the symptoms increase in severity and if surgery is contemplated. More extensive testing is often requested by the vascular surgeon.

According to a recent report, the application of graduated compression stockings prevents or slows the progression of the postphlebitic syndrome (31). In the presence of arterial insufficiency, stockings may be advisable, and therefore patients who are elderly or have known atherosclerosis may need to be assessed to develop an appropriate treatment plan (discussed later).

Application of graduated compression stockings should be initiated within two to three weeks after the first DVT and continued for at least 2 years and for as long as 5 years. Because stockings lose elasticity they should be replaced every 6 months.

The degree of venous insufficiency can be classified according to the Clinical, Etiologic, Anatomic, Pathophysiologic system (CEAP), with the "C" category being the one primarily used.

This category is further subdivided into C0, no visible disease; C1, telangiectasis; C2, varicose veins; C3, edema; C4, skin changes without ulcers; C5, skin changes with healed ulcers; and C6, skin changes with active ulcers.

RECOMMENDATIONS FOR MANAGEMENT OF POSTPHLEBITIC SYNDROME

Minimal Symptoms

- Graduated stockings with moderate compression (15 to 20 mm Hg) or leg elevation at the end of the day.

Mild to Moderate Symptoms (Edema, Aching, or Heaviness of Legs)

- Graduated stockings with firm compression, 20 to 30 mm Hg; extra firm is also available (30 to 40 mm Hg) with or without nighttime pneumatic device.
- Patients who have had ulcer formation should wear stockings continuously throughout the day, every day, beginning in the morning and continuing throughout the day. Nonelastic stockings that are comprised of multiple layers attached by Velcro (CircAid) can also be used and may be easier to apply.

Consultation with Vascular Surgeons

Surgical procedures are available for patients with active ulcers that do not respond to therapy or who have varicose veins in addition to postphlebitic syndrome.

Peripheral Arterial Disease

Peripheral arterial disease (PAD) is present in approximately 20% of individuals over the age of 70 years and overall in 12% of the adult population (32). The presence of PAD indicates systemic atherosclerosis and is associated with carotid and coronary disease. Risk factors for PAD are as for atherosclerosis: smoking, hyperlipidemia, hypertension, diabetes, and advanced age. Clinically, the diagnosis of PAD should be suspected in patients who complain of intermittent claudication, which can increase in severity to chronic pain at rest. Pain from claudication usually involves one or both calves, develops with walking, and resolves within minutes of resting. The more severe manifestation of PAD, chronic limb ischemia, causes pain during the night at bed rest. The differential diagnosis of PAD includes diabetic neuropathy, reflex sympathetic dystrophy, and spinal stenosis, which can be inherited or acquired due to degenerative changes that cause narrowing of the lumbar spinal canal.

Evaluation of the patient includes, in addition to a careful history and physical examination, measurement of the systolic pressures in both lower legs compared to the upper extremities to calculate the ankle brachial index (ABI; Table 23-14).

TABLE. 23–14. *Measurement and interpretation of the ankle/brachial index*

Measurement can be made with a blood pressure cuff and hand-held Doppler
Systolic blood pressure is measured in both arms (brachial); the higher of the two arm pressures is used in the denominator of the ABI
Systolic blood pressure is then recorded for the right and left ankles, using the dorsalis pedis pulses (DP) and the posterior tibial pulses (PT).

Right ABI = $\dfrac{\text{higher \textbf{right} ankle pressure (DP or PT)}}{\text{Higher arm pressure}}$

Left ABI = $\dfrac{\text{higher \textbf{left} ankle pressure (DP or PT)}}{\text{Higher arm pressure}}$

Interpretation of results:
ABI 0.00–0.41—severe PAD (this range of values is measured in patients with critical limb ischemia)
ABI 0.41–0.90—mild to moderate PAD
ABI 0.91–1.30—normal (patient with complaints of leg pain on exertion could undergo repeat measurement of ABI after treadmill testing)
ABI >1.30—noncompressible vessel suggests calcification and other tests may be required

ABI, ankle/brachial index; PAD, peripheral arterial disease.

Treatment

Treatment of PAD addresses the underlying processes and include statins (with or without niacin) for management of hyperlipidemia and antihypertensive agents for control of blood pressure. No specific antihypertensive is specifically superior in PAD; however, β-blockers should be used with caution in chronic limb ischemia. For diabetics, management of hyperglycemia is essential, but intensive control of the blood glucose level does not confer benefit with respect to improvement in PAD symptoms. Patients who smoke should receive counseling and support for smoking cessation.

Aspirin at a dose of 81 to 325 mg per day may be effective in reducing the risk of other vascular events. Clopidogrel, an inhibitor of ADP-induced platelet aggregation, used at a dose of 75 mg daily may be even more effective than aspirin in preventing ischemic events in patients with PAD as described in the Clopidogrel versus Aspirin in Patients at Risk of Ischemic Events (CAPRIE) trial (32). Prescribing physicians should know that thrombotic thrombocytopenic purpura occurs, albeit rarely, in patients receiving clopidogrel.

Treatment for Relief of Claudication

Graded exercise therapy under the care of a nurse or trained technician reduces symptoms of claudication. Exercises are usually performed in one hour sessions on a treadmill.

Cilostazol (Pletal) was approved by the FDA in 1999 for treatment of patients with symptoms of claudication. This drug increases the intracellular concentration of cyclic adenosine monophosphate (cAMP) by inhibiting phosphodiesterase 3. Although cilostazol has multiple functions, such as inhibiting platelet aggregation and inducing vasodilatation, its mode of action in relieving symptoms in patients with PAD is not well understood. The usual dose is 100 mg orally twice daily; the most common side effect is headache. The drug should not be used in patients with congestive heart failure.

For arterial lesions requiring surgery, endovascular techniques are increasingly used and include laser-assisted angioplasty and balloon angioplasty, both reducing the morbidity of the procedures. For patients with acute arterial thrombosis, local thrombolytic therapy can be utilized, as well as rheolytic thrombectomy, in which a suction catheter removes the occlusive thrombus. Knowledge of the techniques available for the recognition and management of PAD and of options available to patients with chronic or acute arterial occlusion allows the hematologist to serve as a more effective consultant.

REFERENCES

1. Levine MN, Lee AY, Kakkar AK. From Trousseau to targeted therapy: new insights and innovations in thrombosis and cancer. *J Thromb Haemost* 2003;1:1456–1463.
2. Mismetti P, Laporte S, Darmon JY, et al. Meta-analysis of low molecular weight heparin in the prevention of venous thromboembolism in general surgery. *Br J Surg* 2001;88:913–930.
3. Bergqvist D, Agnelli G, Cohen AT, et al. Duration of prophylaxis against venous thromboembolism with enoxaparin after surgery for cancer. *N Engl J Med* 2002;346:975–980.
4. Rasmussen MS. Does prolonged thromboprophylaxis improve outcome in patients undergoing surgery? *Cancer Treat Rev* 2003;29(Suppl 2):15–17.
5. Efficacy and safety of enoxaparin versus unfractionated heparin for prevention of deep vein thrombosis in elective cancer surgery: a double-blind randomized multicentre trial with venographic assessment. ENOXACAN Study Group. *Br J Surg* 1997;84:1099–1103.
6. Geerts WH, Heit JA, Clagett GP, et al. Prevention of venous thromboembolism. *Chest* 2001;119 (1 Suppl):132S–175S.
7. Rickles F, Levine M. *Hemostatic and Thrombotic Disorders of Malignancy*. Philadelphia: W.B. Saunders Company, 2002.

8. Agnelli G, Piovella F, Buoncristiani P, et al. Enoxaparin plus compression stockings compared with compression stockings alone in the prevention of venous thromboembolism after elective neurosurgery. *N Engl J Med* 1998;339:80–85.

9. Goldhaber SZ, Dunn K, Gerhard-Herman M, et al. Low rate of venous thromboembolism after craniotomy for brain tumor using multimodality prophylaxis. *Chest* 2002;122:1933–1937.

10. Nurmohamed MT, van Riel AM, Henkens CM, et al. Low molecular weight heparin and compression stockings in the prevention of venous thromboembolism in neurosurgery. *Thromb Haemost* 1996; 75:233–238.

11. Levine M, Hirsh J, Gent M, et al. Double-blind randomised trial of a very-low-dose warfarin for prevention of thromboembolism in stage IV breast cancer. *Lancet* 1994;343:886–889.

12. Lee AY, Levine MN. Venous thromboembolism and cancer: risks and outcomes. *Circulation* 2003; 107(23 Suppl 1): I17–21.

13. Samama MM, Cohen AT, Darmon JY, et al. A comparison of enoxaparin with placebo for the prevention of venous thromboembolism in acutely ill medical patients. Prophylaxis in Medical Patients with Enoxaparin Study Group. *N Engl J Med* 1999;341:793–800.

14. Wen PY, Marks PW. Medical management of patients with brain tumors. *Curr Opin Oncol* 2002; 14:299–307.

15. Dickinson LD, Miller LD, Patel CP, et al. Enoxaparin increases the incidence of postoperative intracranial hemorrhage when initiated preoperatively for deep venous thrombosis prophylaxis in patients with brain tumors. *Neurosurgery* 1998;43:1074–1081.

16. O'Shea SI, Ortel TL. Issues in the utilization of low molecular weight heparins. Semin Hematol 2002;39:172–178.

17. Levine M, Gent M, Hirsh J, et al. A comparison of low-molecular-weight heparin administered primarily at home with unfractionated heparin administered in the hospital for proximal deep-vein thrombosis. *N Engl J Med* 1996;334:677–681.

18. Walsh-McMonagle D, Green D. Low-molecular-weight heparin in the management of Trousseau's syndrome. *Cancer* 1997;80:649–655.

19. Hirsch J, Warkentin T, Shaughnessy S, et al. Heparin and low-molecular weight heparin: mechanisms of action, pharmacokinetics, dosing, monitoring, efficacy, and safety. *Chest* 2001;119:64S–94S.

20. Ridker PM, Goldhaber SZ, Danielson E, et al. Long-term, low-intensity warfarin therapy for the prevention of recurrent venous thromboembolism. *N Engl J Med* 2003;348:1425–1434.

21. Jackson M. *Consultations on Patients with Venous or Arterial Diseases III. Interventional Approaches in the Mangement of Thrombosis.* Washington, DC: American Society of Hematology Educational Program Book, 2003:555.

22. Bern MM, Lokich JJ, Wallach SR, et al. Very low doses of warfarin can prevent thrombosis in central venous catheters. A randomized prospective trial. *Ann Intern Med* 1990;112:423–428.

23. Heaton DC, Han DY, Inder A. Minidose (1 mg) warfarin as prophylaxis for central vein catheter thrombosis. *Intern Med J* 2002;32:84–88.

24. Bona RD. Thrombotic complications of central venous catheters in cancer patients. Semin Thromb Hemost 1999;25:147–155.

25. Mandala M, Ferretti G, Cremonesi M, et al. Venous thromboembolism and cancer: new issues for an old topic. *Crit Rev Oncol Hematol* 2003;48:65–80.

26. Altepase [package insert]. Vacaville, CA: Genetech, Inc., 2001.

27. Konkle B. *Thrombotic Disorders: Diagnosis and Treatment III. Thrombosis: Diagnosis and Management Issues Before, During, and After Pregnancy.* Washington, DC: American Society of Hematology Educational Program Book. 2003:525–528.

28. Bates SM, Ginsberg JS. How we manage venous thromboembolism during pregnancy. *Blood* 2002; 100:3470–3478.

29. Bates S, Greer I, Hirsh J, et al. Use of antithrombotic agents during pregnancy. *Chest* 2004;126: 627S–644S.

30. Kahn SR, Ginserg J. Relationship between deep venous thrombosis and the postthrombotic syndrome. *Arch Intern Med* 2004;164:17–26.

31. Prandoni P, Lensing AWA, Prins MH, et al. Below-knee elastic compression stockings to prevent the post-thrombotic syndrome. *Ann Intern Med* 2004;141:249–256.

32. Hiatt WR. Medical treatment of peripheral arterial disease and claudication. *N Engl J Med* 2001; 344:1608–1621.

24

Blood Transfusion

Firoozeh Alvandi and Harvey G. Klein

BLOOD CELL ANTIGENS

Red blood cell (RBC) antigens have varying biochemical, phenotypic, and immunologic characteristics. Based on these characteristics, they have been assembled into group systems. The best known and most clinically important are ABO, Rh, Kell, Kidd, and Duffy:

- Naturally occurring antibodies such as anti-A and/or anti-B are present in the absence of prior sensitizing stimulus.
- Development of most other alloantibodies requires prior sensitization.

The *antiglobulin* or *Coombs' test* provides a method by which alloantibodies may be detected and compatible blood units identified. When a clinically important alloantibody is present in a recipient's serum, *antigen-negative blood* must be selected. If the alloantibody is against a very high frequency antigen (present in greater than 90% of individuals) or when multiple alloantibodies are present, procurement of compatible blood may be difficult or impossible. In some cases, the presence of red cell autoantibodies makes all units (including those of the patient) appear incompatible and masks the presence of alloantibodies.

ANTIGLOBULIN TEST

The antiglobulin test uses antibodies to human globulins to detect the presence of antibody (or complement) on the RBC surface or in a patient's serum.

The direct antiglobulin test (DAT), or the direct Coombs' test, detects antibody or complement that is coating RBC, and may be positive in:

- Hemolytic transfusion reactions (for which it is the single most important assay).
- Hemolytic disease of the newborn.
- Autoimmune hemolytic anemia, including with medications.
- After administration of immune globulins (passively acquired).
- Post-marrow or organ transplant (donor's lymphocytes producing antibody to red cells of the recipient).

A positive DAT does not necessarily indicate *in vivo* hemolysis or shortened RBC survival. False-positive results may occur with hypergammaglobulinemia when rouleaux formation may be mistaken for agglutination.

The indirect antiglobulin test (IAT), or indirect Coombs' test, is the method used in the antibody screen portion of a "type and screen" and in the serologic cross-match (patient serum and donor/reagent red cells). The IAT detects antibody present in the serum, but not bound to the RBC. When the IAT is positive, antibody specificity must be identified and the corresponding antigen always avoided in transfusions. A negative antibody screen (IAT) does not necessarily indicate absence of alloantibodies, because the titer of antibody may be below the level of detection or the antibody might be directed against a low incidence antigen (present in less than 10% of individuals) not present on reagent testing cells, but expressed on some patient cells. A negative IAT does not guarantee that blood is compatible, nor does a weak IAT indicate that hemolysis is likely to be mild. Regardless, a positive IAT demands further investigation.

In autoimmune hemolytic anemias, where the antibody may be present in the serum and on the RBC of the patient, both the DAT and IAT may be positive.

BLOOD COMPATIBILITY

In general, blood components that contain more than 2 mL of RBC must be compatible with the patient's plasma. Particular attention is paid to Rh type because less than 1 mL of RBC, a volume found in most platelet concentrates, is sufficient to sensitize an Rh-negative patient. Plasma-containing components, including platelet preparations, should be ABO compatible with the patient's RBC when possible, to prevent passive antibodies in the plasma from causing hemolysis in recipient red cells (Table 24-1).

The most basic practical application of blood group serology involves the selection of compatible blood. The absence or presence of blood cell antigens can have important biological and clinical implications. Compatible blood takes time to prepare.

- In an emergency, group O RBC may be released un–cross-matched with the consent of the requesting physician, although testing will be completed after release.
- Group-specific red cells (group A for group A patient, etc.) and an abbreviated cross-match can be prepared in 15 minutes.
- Fully tested red cells can be prepared in 45 to 60 minutes; cryopreserved RBC and fresh-frozen plasma (FFP) and may take even longer.

Alloimmunized patients pose a particular problem; patient blood specimens should be submitted well in advance of elective procedures for a "type and screen," which will identify most compatibility difficulties. After 3 days, a new sample will be needed to detect newly appearing antibodies, especially when the patient has been pregnant or transfused within the last 30 days.

ABO INCOMPATIBILITY IN TRANSPLANT SETTINGS

Hematopoietic stem cell (HSCT) transplantation relies on compatibility at the major histocompatibility locus, so that selection of the recipient-donor pair is determined by similarity of human leukocyte antigens (HLA) at the expense of ABO compatibility. Because HLA and

TABLE. 24–1. *Compatibility of recipient blood with donor blood components*

Patient ABO Group	Whole Blood	Red Blood Cells	Platelets	Plasma	Cryoprecipitate
O	O	O	Any (O preferred)	O, A, B, AB	N/A
A	A	A or O	Any (A preferred)	A or AB	N/A
B	B	B or O	Any (B preferred)	B or AB	N/A
AB	AB	AB, A, B, or O (in order of preference)	Any (AB preferred)	AB, A, or B	N/A

Modified from Brecher ME. *Technical Manual,* 14th ed. Bethesda, MD: AABB Press, 2003:454,467, with permission.

ABO genes are inherited independently, some (10% to 30%) of these transplants will be ABO incompatible.

While ABO incompatibility does not appear to impact graft failure, mismatches can cause immediate hemolysis, delayed RBC engraftment, or delayed hemolysis based on the nature of ABO incompatibility between the recipient and donor (1).

Minor Incompatibility

- *Donor's serum* contains antibodies against RBC antigens of the recipient (e.g., recipient group A, B, or AB and donor group O, etc.).
- Prior to infusion of the stem cell preparation, plasma containing anti-A and anti-B can be removed to prevent immediate postinfusion hemolysis of the recipient's RBC.
- Of minor ABO-incompatible transplant recipients, 10% to 15% may experience abrupt onset of hemolysis 7 to 10 days posttransplant when immune-competent B lymphocytes in the graft mount a response against the recipient RBC antigens.
- Hemolysis may be severe or even fatal unless recognized promptly.

Major Incompatibility

- *Recipient's serum* contains antibodies against the RBC antigens of the donor (e.g., recipient group O and donor group A, B, or AB; recipient group A or B and donor group AB).
- Hemolysis of RBC in the stem cell preparation upon infusion may occur if the graft is not processed to remove RBC prior to infusion.
- Posttransplant, the recipient may produce antibodies against donor red cell antigens for months, especially with nonmyeloablative regimens
- RBC engraftment and erythropoiesis may be delayed, resulting in red cell aplasia (2).

Minor and major (bidirectional) incompatibility between the donor and recipient occurs when each has antibodies against the ABO blood group antigens of the other (e.g., recipient's blood group is A and that of the donor is B, or vice versa). Table 24-2 describes appropriate transfusion management during transplantation. All transfusions must be irradiated.

Rh Incompatibility

Rh incompatibility occurs in 10% to 15% of stem cell transplants. Transfusion practice is analogous to that of major and minor ABO incompatibility, but the consequences are less severe.

For Rh-negative recipients of Rh-positive hematopoietic stem cell preparations:

- RBC from the donor should be removed to decrease risk of alloimmunization similar to ABO major incompatibility.

For Rh-positive recipient from Rh-negative donor previously alloimmunized to the Rh antigen:

- Monitor the patient for signs of delayed hemolysis (as in minor incompatibility).

BLOOD COMPONENTS AND DERIVATIVES

Blood Components and Transfusion Therapy

Blood components can be separated from whole blood by centrifugation or by apheresis. Twenty-nine million blood components (RBCs, platelets, plasma, cryoprecipitate; Table 24-3) are transfused annually in the United States.

TABLE. 24–2. *Transfusion in minor and major ABO incompatible transplants*

Minor Mismatch

	Phase I			Phase II		Phase III
Recipient	Donor	All components	RBC	Platelets	FFP	All components
A	O	Recipient group	O	A; *AB; B; O*	A; *AB*	Donor group
B	O	Recipient group	O	B; *AB; A; O*	B; *AB*	Donor group
AB	O	Recipient group	O	AB; *A; B; O*	AB	Donor group
AB	A	Recipient group	A	AB; *A; B; O*	AB	Donor group
AB	B	Recipient group	B	AB; *B; A; O*	AB	Donor group

Major Mismatch

	Phase I			Phase II		Phase III
Recipient	Donor	All components	RBC	Platelets	FFP	All components
O	A	Recipient group	O	A; *AB; B; O*	A; *AB*	Donor group
O	B	Recipient group	O	B; *AB; A; O*	B; *AB*	Donor group
O	AB	Recipient group	O	AB; *A; B; O*	AB	Donor group
A	AB	Recipient group	A	AB; *A; B; O*	AB	Donor group
B	AB	Recipient group	B	AB; *B; A; O*	AB	Donor group

Minor and Major and Mismatch

	Phase I			Phase II		Phase III
Recipient	Donor	All components	RBC	Platelets	FFP	All components
A	B	Recipient group	O	AB; *A; B; O*	AB	Donor group
B	A	Recipient group	O	AB; *B; A; O*	AB	Donor group

Phase I = From time patient is prepared for hematopoietic progenitor cell transplant.
Phase II = From initiation of myeloablative therapy from the time DAT is negative and isohemagglutinins against donor are no longer detectable (for RBC) or when recipient erythrocytes are no longer detectable.
Phase III = After the forward and reverse type of the patient are consistent with donor ABO group.
Italicized blood groups indicate next best choice in order of preference.
Modified from Brecher ME, ed. *Technical Manual*, 14th ed. Bethesda, MD: AABB Press, 2003:556, with permission; and from Friedberg RC. Transfusion therapy in hematopoietic stem cell transplantation. In: Mintz PD, ed. *Transfusion Therapy: Clinical Principles and Practice.* Bethesda, MD: AABB Press, 1999.

- Blood components should be infused through standard 170- to 260-μm infusion filters to remove any clots that form during storage.
- An approved infusion pump may be used for strict control of transfusion rate. *Nonapproved pumps may damage or hemolyze cells.*
- Bedside leukoreduction filters may be used when leukoreduction is indicated for whole blood, packed RBCs, and platelets that have not been leukocyte reduced prior to storage.
- *Hypotensive reactions* have been associated with bedside leukoreduction, especially in patients receiving angiotensin converting enzyme (ACE) inhibitors.
- Allow blood to filter by gravity.
- *Granulocyte concentrates must never be infused through leukoreduction filters—these filters are designed to remove white blood cells!*
- Whole blood and other cellular blood components may be infused with isotonic solutions: USP 0.9% NaCl (normal saline) and certain Food and Drug Administration (FDA)-approved electrolyte solutions.

TABLE. 24–3a. *Blood component administration per NIH practice*

	Whole Blood	Packed RBC	Granulocytes	Platelets	Plasma
ADULTS					
First 15 minutes	2 mL/min	2 mL/min	2 mL/min	2–5 mL/min	2–5 mL/min
Subsequently	100–230 mL/hr	100–230 mL/hr	75–100 mL/hr	200–300 mL/hr	200–300 mL/hr
CHILDREN					
First 15 minutes	N/A	N/A	N/A	5% of total volume* ordered for transfusion	5% of total volume* ordered for transfusion
First 15 minutes	5% of total volume* ordered for transfusion	5% of total volume* ordered for transfusion	5% of total volume ordered for transfusion	N/A	N/A
Subsequently	Variable (as tolerated)	2–5 mL/kg/hr	Over 2–3 hours (for a 200 mL product)	As tolerated	1–2 mL/min

*Volume ordered for pediatric transfusion should be based on the child's weight (10–15mL blood product/kg); excludes granulocyte transfusion.

- Cellular blood products must never be infused with hypertonic or hypotonic solutions; solutions containing glucose or calcium, such as D5W (5% dextrose in water); and lactated Ringer's. Hemolysis, clotting, or agglutination of RBC may result if cellular blood components are infused with hyper or hypotonic solutions.
- Medications should never be added to blood components.
- Never store blood components in unmonitored refrigerators in nursing units or surgical suites. The risk for administration of blood components to the wrong patient increases when blood is stored in satellite refrigerators. Return blood to storage (or bank) if transfusion is not started within 30 minutes of issue.
- Warming devices with internal monitors have been designed for blood to avoid transfusion of large volumes of cold fluid. Blood components should never be warmed in uncertified devices (e.g., microwave ovens or water baths). Hemolysis can be lethal.

Most adverse transfusion reactions occur in the first 15 minutes:

- Administration of blood products should start slowly under close observation.
- The time of transfusion should not exceed 4 hours.
- The risk of bacterial growth increases with time at room temperature. If transfusion is anticipated to take longer, the transfusion service can divide the unit into smaller aliquots. (see Table 24-3b for indications for additional modifications to blood components).

Storage conditions for different blood components vary and are designed to maximize preservation and effectiveness:

- Red cells are refrigerated for up to 42 days.
- Platelets are stored at room temperature and become outdated in 5 days.
- Plasma components are stored frozen for a year or more, but must be thawed before use and are often not immediately available.

As with any medical treatment, blood transfusion requires informed consent:

- Patients must be advised of the indications and common adverse events as well as any potential alternatives to transfusion.

TABLE 24-3b. *Indications for additional modifications of cellular blood components*

Leukoreduction	Irradiation (red blood cells, platelets, granulocytes)	Washing (plasma removal)	Volume reduction	Freezing-deglycerolization (red blood cells)
Description: Filtration of component after collection, at bedside, or removal of WBC during automated collection for a 3-log reduction (99.9%) of WBC; final WBC content ≤5 ×10^6.	**Description:** Gamma irradiation (cesium or cobalt) of component with 2500 cGy (centigrays) to inactivate viable lymphocyte proliferation in the component.	**Description:** Component washed with sterile normal saline to remove >98% of plasma proteins, electrolytes, and antibodies; WBC content 5×10^8.	**Description:** Removal of plasma from cellular components (mainly platelets; RBC concentrates have very little plasma).	**Description:** Addition of glycerol and freezing generally within 6 days of collection (depending on the additive solution used at the time of collection and glycerolization-freezing method used).
Purpose: Reduction of febrile nonhemolytic transfusion reactions (FNHTR); reduction of CMV transmission (CMV-safe); reduction of HLA alloimmunization.	**Purpose:** Prevention of transfusion-associated graft-versus-host disease.	**Purpose:** Prevention of allergic reactions; decrease risk of hyperkalemia.	**Purpose:** Reduction of circulatory overload; removal of antibodies.	**Purpose:** Long-term storage of autologous or allogeneic rare blood phenotypes.
Indications: Patients who have experienced an episode of FNHTR; alternative to CMV-negative components (from donor tested negative for CMV): neonates, transplant patients.	**Indications:** Recipients of allogeneic hematopoietic or solid organ transplants; recipients of transfusion from blood relatives; patients on immunosuppressive regimens; patients with congenital immunodeficiencies and with certain malignancies; premature infants (especially those undergoing extracorporeal membrane oxygenation).	**Indications:** Patients who experience recurrent severe allergic reactions (not responsive to premedication with antihistamines); IgA deficient patients when IgA-deficient component is not available; recipients at risk from hyperkalemia: newborns, intrauterine transfusions. May be effective when ABO identical blood is not available for patients with paroxysmal nocturnal hemoglobinuria (PNH).	**Indications:** Patients who are plasma volume expanded: normovolemic chronic anemia; thalassemia major; sickle cell disease; congestive heart failure; pediatric, elderly, and other patients susceptible to volume overload.	**Indications:** Patients with rare blood phenotypes or multiple alloantibodies.
Comments: Equivalent to CMV seronegative components; *Not* effective and *not* indicated for prevention of transfusion-associated graft-versus-host disease.	**Comments:** *Not* indicated for prevention of FNHTR and unnecessary for aplastic anemia patients (despite ATG therapy) or HIV patients in the absence of other indications for irradiation (above). RBC shelf-life is decreased to 28 days (if greater than the original expiration date) but platelet or granulocyte shelf-life is not affected.	**Comments:** Washing results in a 15–20% loss of red cells or platelets. *Not* equivalent to "leukoreduced." Red blood cells must be used within 24 hours and platelets must be used within 4 hours of washing (due to opening of the closed system).	**Comments:** *Not* equivalent to washing for prevention of allergic reactions. Results in a 4-hour post volume reduction expiration time due to the decreased plasma/volume needed for optimal platelet metabolism.	**Comments:** May *not* be feasible for red blood cells with certain abnormalities (such as Hgb S, hereditary spherocytosis, PNH). *Not* equivalent to "leukoreduced" *(may remove >95% of WBC)*. Depending on the method of glycerolization used (open or closed system), the postdeglycerolization shelf-life may be 24 hours or 2 weeks (respectively).

Whole Blood

Whole blood is rarely available and infrequently used:

Indications: acute hypovolemia with red cell loss, massive transfusion, and exchange transfusion.

Nonindications: chronic anemia (where blood volume is often increased). A unit of whole blood typically has a volume of 450 to 500 mL and a hematocrit of 35% to 45%.

Whole blood is not a source of functional platelets or granulocytes, which deteriorate in less than 24 hours at refrigerator temperatures.

Red Blood Cells

RBC (packed red cells) are separated from whole blood by centrifugations. A unit of RBC contains approximately 200 mL and a hematocrit of 60% to 80%. In general, 1 unit of packed RBC will increase the hemoglobin by 1 g/dL in an average-sized adult. In the average pediatric patient, transfusion of 8 to 10 mL/kg of RBC is expected to increase hemoglobin by 3 g/dL. Hemoglobin (Hb) determination is frequently used to determine the transfusion trigger. However, the decision to transfuse should be based on assessment of a patient's clinical symptoms, coexisting or underlying medical conditions, and the cause of the anemia. The single adequately powered prospective study (intensive care unit [ICU] patients) and numerous observational studies indicated that patients with cardiovascular disease are particularly sensitive to anemia and do better at a higher level (3).

Indications: Treatment of symptomatic anemia.

In general, clinicians transfuse if the Hb falls below 6 g/dL and rarely consider transfusion when it exceeds 10 g/dL. The interval between these values is the area of controversy. Practice guidelines support a Hb level of less than 7 g/dL as generally acceptable for the initiation of RBC transfusion in symptomatic patients (4).

Nonindications: RBC should not be transfused for volume expansion or nutritional purposes. Transfusion is rarely indicated in otherwise treatable anemias, including anemias associated with B_{12}, iron, or folate deficiency; if symptoms are severe; these patients may benefit from a single-unit transfusion.

Platelets

Platelets (Table 24-4) may be separated from whole blood shortly after collection (random donor or platelet concentrates) or collected by apheresis (single donor or apheresis platelets). A therapeutic dose of platelets for an average adult is 1 unit of platelets (5.5×10^{10} platelets) per 10 kg of body weight, which should increase the platelet count in an average-sized adult by approximately 5,000 per microliter. Each apheresis (single-donor) platelet product is expected to contain approximately 3×10^{11} platelets, roughly equivalent to 4 to 6 units of random-donor platelets. Indications for use are the same for both preparations, except for immunized refractory patients who may require single-donor HLA-matched and compatible platelets. Single-donor platelets offer the additional advantage of decreased donor exposure and a lower risk of bacterial sepsis.

Indications: Bleeding associated with thrombocytopenia, rapid decrease in platelet counts, qualitative platelet defects, or as prophylaxis for major bleeding in severely thrombocytopenic patients.

Nonindications: Bleeding unassociated with thrombocytopenia (except for the unusual patient with a clinically significant platelet function defect), other defects in hemostasis (such

TABLE. 24–4. *Guidelines for platelet transfusion per NIH practice*

Patient Population	Threshold
Stable Aplastic Anemia Patient	<10,000/uL or bleeding
General Oncology Patient	<10,000/uL
Stable Non-Oncology Patient	<10,000/uL
Post Hematopoietic Stem Cell Transplant	<10,000/uL
Aplastic Anemia Patient Receiving ATG	<20,000/uL
Patients Undergoing Invasive Procedures	<50,000/uL
Neurosurgery Patients	<100,000/uL

as factor deficiencies), or platelet dysfunction caused by many common medications (aspirin, penicillins, nonsteroidal anti-inflammatory drugs [NSAIDs]).

Platelets are usually contraindicated in thrombotic thrombocytopenic purpura (TTP), because most thrombosis is a greater risk than hemorrhage. (Patients with TTP who develop life-threatening hemorrhage may benefit from a cautious trial of platelets.)

The threshold for prophylactic platelet transfusion varies based on the patient's underlying condition and likelihood of hemorrhage:

- A threshold of 10,000 per microliter is effective in preventing morbidity and mortality from bleeding in stable oncology patients undergoing chemotherapy.
- A platelet count greater than 50,000 per microliter is desirable prior to invasive procedures and in the immediate postprocedure period; skin biopsy and marrow aspirate and biopsy are routinely accomplished at platelet counts lower than 50,000 per microliter.
- Platelet counts closer to 100,000 per microliter may be prudent for patients at high risk of intracranial hemorrhage, such as those with cerebral leukostasis, or when undergoing neurosurgical or ocular procedures.
- Stable chronically thrombocytopenic patients (such as those with aplastic anemia or myelodysplasia) may tolerate platelet counts as low as 5,000 per microliter in the absence of complicating factors such as fever, infection, and additional defects in hemostasis.

More aggressive support is indicated for patients who are unstable—febrile, infected, receiving multiple medications—especially if the platelet counts are decreasing (2,5).

Platelet transfusions should be monitored by a posttransfusion complete blood count (CBC; 1 to 24 hours) to assess response and guide subsequent transfusion therapy. A corrected count increment (CCI) may be used to determine the increase in platelet count in an individual postplatelet transfusion:

$$CCI = \frac{(\text{Posttransfusion platelet count* } - \text{ pretransfusion platelet count}) \times \text{body surface area**}}{\text{Number of platelets transfused***}}$$

* Posttransfusion platelet count is best obtained 15 minutes to 1 hour posttransfusion.

** Body surface area = the square root of [(height in cm $\times$ weight in kg)/3600].

***Expressed as multiples of 1×10^{11}.

An absolute posttransfusion increment of 10,000 per microliter or greater (2,000 per unit of random donor platelets) in an average-sized adult corresponds to a CCI of 5,000.

Platelet Refractoriness

Patients who respond poorly to repeated platelet infusions are considered refractory. Posttransfusion platelet counts (1 hour and 24 hour) are critical. Failure to achieve a CCI of 5,000 or greater is cause to suspect platelet refractoriness. Refractoriness may be immune- or nonimmune-mediated.

- *Nonimmune-mediated* causes of platelet refractoriness: fever, infection, splenomegaly, disseminated intravascular coagulation (DIC), massive bleeding, and medications that enhance platelet destruction.
- *Immune-mediated* causes of platelet refractoriness: repeated transfusions, especially with nonleukocyte-reduced platelets and multiparity (alloimmunization to HLA and human platelet antigens). Platelets and granulocytes also have antigens to which an antigen-negative individual may become alloimmunized.

In practice, the distinction between immune- and nonimmune-mediated platelet refractoriness is less clear. When immune-mediated platelet refractoriness is suspected and CCI is less than 5,000 after each of two platelet transfusions the following steps should be taken:

- ABO-compatible fresh (less than 72 hours in storage) platelets should be used for two subsequent transfusions.
- If CCI does not exceed 5,000: HLA antibody screen to detect alloantibodies or commercial platelet compatibility tests should be performed.
- If HLA antibodies are detected, HLA-compatible platelets should be tried.
- When alloantibodies with broad specificity are found (for HLA A and B loci), platelets from HLA matched donors are indicated.
- Cross-match compatible platelets may be beneficial when HLA antibody status of the recipient cannot be determined, HLA-matched platelets cannot be obtained, or when the patient is refractory to HLA-matched platelets (up to 40% to 50% of cases).
- Corticosteroids, washed platelets, or intravenous immunoglobulin (IVIG) have not proved useful in the treatment of refractoriness.

Granulocytes

Granulocytes are collected by apheresis for specific patients, from donors who are mobilized prior to collection with corticosteroids and/or cytokines (granulocyte colony-stimulating factor [G-CSF]) in order to enhance collection.

- Granulocytes can be stored at room temperature for only up to 24 hours postcollection.
- Granulocyte collections have a volume of 250 mL and contain plasma, approximately 30 mL RBC, and variable amounts of mononuclear leukocytes and platelets.
- Granulocyte concentrates should be ABO, Rh, and RBC cross-match compatible.
- The minimal therapeutic dose is greater than 1×10^{10} granulocytes. However, granulocyte increments are unlikely to be measured unless three to four times this number is infused.

Indications: Neutropenia in patients with expected marrow recovery who have an absolute neutrophil count (ANC) of less than 0.5×10^9/L, and documented infection not responding to appropriate antibiotic treatment for 24 to 48 hours, or defective granulocyte function despite normal counts (in chronic granulomatous disease).

A 1- to 6-hour posttransfusion CBC with differential for determination of ANC may help assess efficacy. The posttransfusion increment in ANC varies based on the granulocyte content of the transfused unit. Because granulocytes traffic to the lungs before equilibrating in peripheral blood, a 6-hour posttransfusion increment may be higher than a 1-hour posttransfusion ANC. If the patient's ANC fails to reach expected levels or if a reaction occurs, investigation, including an HLA antibody screen and tests for antibodies to human neutrophil antigens (HNA) is indicated.

Nonindications: Absence of above criteria.

Contraindicated in patients with prior severe pulmonary reactions to HLA or HNA or alloimmunization (serologic HLA or HNA incompatibility). Alloimmunized patients may develop chills, fever, rigors, shortness of breath, wheezing, pulmonary infiltrates, cyanosis, and hypotension (2,6).

- Pulmonary toxicity may be exacerbated when granulocytes and amphotericin B are administered in close temporal proximity (within 4 hours) (7).
- Rigors and fever may respond to intravenous meperidine (25 mg).

Granulocyte transfusion therapy should be evaluated after an initial course of four infusions and periodically thereafter.

Granulocyte concentrates may contain leukocyte-associated pathogens such as cytomegalovirus (CMV), which is a particular concern for immunosuppressed individuals such as stem cell transplant recipients, solid organ transplant recipients, neonates undergoing extracorporeal membrane oxygenation, and low birth weight and premature infants.

While granulocyte transfusions decrease the length of bacterial infection, proof that granulocyte transfusions decrease mortality in any situation has been elusive.

Fresh-Frozen Plasma

Plasma separated from whole blood or collected by apheresis and frozen within 8 hours is labeled FFP. FFP contains most plasma proteins at the time of thaw at about the same concentration as at the time of collection. A unit of plasma contains approximately 200 mL.

- By convention, 1 mL of FFP is expected to provide 1 unit of activity of all factors (except labile factors V and VIII). In practice, individual units may vary in content.
- To increase factor levels by 20%, the dose used in replacement of coagulation factors is approximately 10 to 20 mL/kg in adults (equivalent to approximately 4 to 6 units of FFP).

Indications: Correction of multiple clotting factor deficiencies in patients who are bleeding or scheduled for an invasive procedure, replacement of factors consumed in DIC, coagulation factor deficiencies caused by liver disease, coagulation factors diluted by replacement fluids during massive transfusion, replacement fluid in the treatment of TTP (plasma exchange), rapid reversal of warfarin (Coumadin) effect, replacement of congenital factor deficiencies when the specific factor concentrate is not available (i.e., replacement of factors II, V, X, XI).

- Concentrated or recombinant factor preparations are preferable as these have been treated to reduce the risk of viral transmission and are labeled for potency.
- An international normalized ratio (INR) greater than 1.6 or activated partial thromboplastin time (aPTT) greater than 1.5 times the upper range of normal (factor level activity less than 30%), is a guide to consider treatment (4,4a).

Nonindications: Volume expansion, protein replacement in nutritional deficiencies. Crystalloids and colloids, synthetic volume expanders, can be used for that purpose, without exposing the recipient to infectious disease risks.

Cryoprecipitate

Cryoprecipitate (cryo) is the cold-insoluble portion of plasma containing high molecular weight glycoproteins. Ordinarily stored frozen, cryoprecipitate can be kept at room temperature for up to 6 hours; on pooling it must be transfused within 4 hours.

- Compatibility testing is unnecessary.
- A unit of cryoprecipitate is usually less than 15 mL of plasma and contains more than 80 international units (IU) of factor VIII (antihemophilic factor), more than 150 mg of fibrinogen, and approximately 30% of the factor XIII of the original plasma. Cryoprecipitate also contains von Willebrand complex activity.
- One unit of cryoprecipitate can increase fibrinogen in an average adult by 5 to 10 mg/dL.
- A therapeutic dose for an adult is 80 to 150 mL of cryoprecipitate (8 to 10 units pooled).

Indications: Treatment of fibrinogen deficiency, dysfibrinogenemia, factor XIII deficiency, DIC, and urgent treatment of hemophilia A and von Willebrand disease in the absence of factor VIII concentrate or recombinant factor VIII. Cryoprecipitate has also been used to correct the platelet defect of uremic bleeding, although with variable success.

The dosage of cryoprecipitate depends on the underlying deficiency and on the plasma volume of the patient. To determine the number of bags of cryoprecipitate to replace fibrinogen:

$$\frac{(\text{Desired fibrinogen level mg/dL} - \text{initial fibrinogen level mg/dL}) \times \text{patient's plasma volume dL}}{250 \text{ mg (fibrinogen per cryo bag)}}$$

The plasma volume for an average adult $= (1\text{-HCT\%}/100) \times$ patient weight in kg $\times$ 70 mL/kg. For infants and children under 40 kg, the plasma volume $= (1\text{-HCT\%}/100) \times$ patient weight in kg $\times$ 80 to 85 mL/kg.

Nonindications: Absence of specific hemostatic abnormality for which it is indicated (see previous text) or for which specific factor concentrates/recombinant factor preparations (e.g., Factor VIII) are available.

Hematopoietic Stem and Progenitor Cells

Hematopoietic Stem and progenitor cells and umbilical cord blood are commonly collected and stored by blood banks. *Progenitor or stem cells* that were originally derived from bone marrow harvests are now more often collected from the peripheral blood (referred to as peripheral blood stem cells or PBSC) via apheresis for reconstitution of hematopoiesis and immune function in patients with a variety of malignancies and immune disorders.

The number of circulating progenitor cells is increased by mobilizing the donor with hematopoietic growth factors, most often G-CSF, or, in autologous transplants, a combination of chemotherapy and growth factors. The degree of mobilization and the probability of a successful collection are best predicted by measuring circulating cells that express the membrane glycoprotein CD34, a marker for committed PBSC. Where this assay is not available, total white blood cell (WBC) and mononuclear cell count have been used (8,9).

Standard collections of allogeneic PBSC involve 3 to 4 hours per apheresis procedure, during which approximately 10 L of blood are processed. Two to four collections are usual, but large volumes of 25 to 30 L are used increasingly to allow complete collections with a single procedure.

While PBSC apheresis collections are generally well tolerated, side effects associated with the several day administration of growth factor are common. Bone pain, headache, fatigue, insomnia, and gastrointestinal disturbances occur, usually respond to administration of acetaminophen or NSAIDs, and cease after the growth factor injections. Vascular complications and citrate toxicity are not unlike those experienced in other long apheresis procedures (see below). With cell mobilization, splenomegaly occurs frequently and splenic rupture has been reported as a rare complication; PBSC donors should be advised to refrain from contact sports for a few weeks after the last mobilization.

PBSC grafts are infused as fresh collections or stored frozen with the cryoprotectant dimethyl sulfoxide (DMSO) in liquid nitrogen. Thawed cells infused with DMSO may cause nausea, vomiting, fever, dyspnea, and anaphylaxis. Reactions are dose-dependent and may be lessened by prophylactic administration of antihistamines. As with other blood components, PBSC carry the risks of transfusion-transmitted infectious agents and are tested in the same manner as are other blood components. However, given their highly specialized use and their life-saving potential, exceptions are made to donor selection criteria normally used for allogeneic blood collections, with concurrence of the treating physician and the recipient.

Adequate cell dose for engraftment depends on whether the procedure is an autograft, a related allograft, or an unrelated transplant. Cell dose, cell source, and patient characteristics are all important variables. The dose of stem cells for unrelated donors (National Marrow Donor Program) is 2 to 4 $\times$ 10^6 CD34$^+$ cells per kilogram of recipient weight (2 to 4 $\times$

10^8 nucleated cells per kilogram of recipient weight) (10). Lower doses may be adequate in related donor settings, but engraftment of both leukocytes and platelets correlate with CD34 cell content.

Cord blood frozen in liquid nitrogen is obtained from the placenta during the third stage of delivery or postdelivery, with the consent of the mother, and stored in liquid nitrogen. The component volume is usually 50 to 100 mL and may be further reduced by removing nucleated red cells and plasma. HLA type is determined and used as a search criterion for cord blood. The estimated likelihood of using cord blood stored for a family member (related bank) is approximately 1 in 10,000. The small volumes and yields of $CD34^+$ progenitor cells currently make cord blood most suitable for children and smaller adults. PBSC stored in liquid nitrogen likely remain stable for many years, but maximum safe storage periods have not been determined.

Blood Derivatives

Derivatives or *blood products* are produced commercially by fractionation of plasma and include colloids such as albumin and plasma protein fraction, immune globulins, coagulation factor concentrates, and a variety of orphan proteins such as α-1-antitrypsin and antithrombin (Table 24-5).

Rh Immune Globulin

Rh immune globulin (RhIg) is available in intramuscular (IM) form and intravenous (IV) form.

Indications: Prevention of alloimmunization of Rh-negative recipients exposed to Rh-positive RBC.

- Prevention of development of anti-D by pregnant Rh-negative women with Rh-positive fetuses and subsequent hemolytic disease of the newborn.
- Greater than 90% success in preventing Rh alloimmunization in pregnancy. Failure is usually because of missed or insufficient injections.
- Treatment of immune thrombocytopenic purpura (ITP) in Rh-positive patients only (intravenous RhIg).

Intramuscular RhIg is used in Rh-negative subjects after exposure to small-volume Rh-positive RBC (with platelet transfusions or the accidental transfusion of an Rh-positive unit of RBC). RhIg IV is used for large volume exposures.

Use of RhIg in males and postmenopausal females depends on the magnitude of exposure, the possibility the individual may require transfusion in the future, and the likelihood that the individual will form antibody (anti-D). For large exposures requiring many doses of RhIg, treatment may not be feasible, especially if the patient is unlikely to become pregnant, form antibody (due to leukemia, solid tumors), or to be retransfused.

A full dose contains 300 μg of anti-D to cover an exposure of 15 mL of Rh-positive RBC.

- Pregnant or postpartum women: within 72 hours of delivery.
- After amniocentesis and chorionic villus sampling performed at more than 34 weeks of gestation.
- Minidose contains 50 μg anti-D to cover an exposure of 2.5 mL of Rh-positive RBC.
- Fetus delivered or aborted at less than 12 weeks of gestation.
- After amniocentesis and chorionic villus sampling at less than 34 weeks of gestation.

Erroneous transfusions:

- RhIg dose should be calculated based on the RBC volume transfused.

The half-life of RhIg is 21 days. Additional RhIg should be administered in the following situations:

- Expected ongoing risk of feto-maternal hemorrhage.

TABLE. 24–5. *Selected Blood Derivatives*

Derivative	Indications	Cautions	Derivation	Content
Albumin (Available as 5% or 25% solution)	Hypovolemia: volume expansion Acute liver failure: osmotic pressure, binds excess bilirubin Cardiopulmonary bypass surgery: hemodilution 25%: maintains plasma colloid osmotic pressure 24 hours after extensive burns treated initially with crystalloids Prior to exchange transfusion for hemolytic disease of the newborn: binds excess free bilirubin to decrease risk of kernicterus	Use with caution in patients at risk of hypervolemia Some Jehovah's Witnesses may not accept albumin	Pooled human plasma concentrated by fractionation and treated to reduce virus transmission 5%: osmotically and oncotically equivalent to plasma 25%: hyperoncotic	96% albumin and 4% globulin and other proteins 145 mEq/L sodium
PPF* (Available only as 5% solution)	Similar to albumin	Contraindication: Intra-arterial administration/ infusion in the setting of cardiopulmonary bypass Administration at greater than 10mL/min has been associated with hypotension, especially in patients taking angiotensin converting enzyme (ACE) inhibitors	Similar to albumin	Active ingredient: albumin 83% albumin 17% globulin and other proteins 145 mEq/L sodium

IVIG**

Passive immunity and passive antibody prophylaxis Replacement in primary immunodeficiencies Immunomodulation of some autoimmune disorders: refractory ITP Treatment of certain infectious disorders: thrombocytopenia related to HIV, pediatric HIV infection, CMV interstitial pneumonitis post-hematopoietic transplantation neurological disorders such as Guillain- Barre syndrome and chronic inflammatory demyelinating polyneuropathy Relative indications: post-transfusion purpura, neonatal alloimmune thrombocytopenia, refractory warm type autoimmune hemolytic anemia	Should not be administered in close temporal association with attenuated vaccines (3 months) Rapid administration IgA deficient patients must receive immune globulins from IgA deficient donors only Intramuscular immune globulins must never be administered intravenously	Fractionation of pooled human plasma treated to reduce virus transmission	90% IgG, trace IgM, trace IgA Immune globulin half-life in preparation: 18–32 days

* Plasma Protein Fraction
** Intravenous Immune Globulin

TABLE. 24–6. *Coagulation factor preparations*

Coagulation Factor	Content	Indication	Risks and Cautions
*Recombinant factor VIIa (rVIIa)**	Activated coagulation factor VII	Licensed use: refractory hemophilia A or B High factor VIII or IX inhibitor levels in hemophilia A or B Used successfully in: severe bleeding refractory to other therapy Glanzmann's thrombasthenia	Thrombosis in DIC, atherosclerotic cardiovascular disease Allergic reactions Hypertension
Factor VIII concentrate	Factor VIII Humate P has vWF	Factor VIII deficiency von Willebrand disease	Development of factor VIII inhibitor (10% of severely hemophilic patients) Viral transmission (small) Hemolysis (passive AB antibodies)
Recombinant factor VIII	Factor VIII No human albumin in ReFacto (B domain-deleted preparation)	Hemophilia A	Viral transmission potential (small) if not B domain deleted Allergic reactions
Factor IX complex (prothrombin complex)	Specified amount of concentrated Factor IX, and variable amounts of activated Factors II, VII, and X, and protein C	Hemophilia B Factor X deficiency (rare) Factor VII deficiency (rare)	Thrombosis in liver disease Viral transmission (small) Hemolysis (passive AB antibodies)
Coagulation factor IX	Purified factor IX and non-therapeutic amounts of factors II, VII, and X	Hemophilia B	Less thrombosis than factor IX concentrate Viral transmission (small) Hemolysis (passive AB antibodies)
Recombinant factor IX	Factor IX	Hemophilia B	Less thrombosis than with factor IX concentrate Allergic reactions

* Hemostatic agent

- Nonobstetric cases with additional transfusion of products containing Rh-positive RBC 21 days or more after the last dose of RhIg.

If RhIg has not been given within 72 hours of a sensitizing event, it should still be administered as soon as the need is recognized for up to 28 days. The mechanism of action is unknown (11).

Nonindications: Use in Rh-positive individuals, Rh-negative individuals who have developed anti-D from prior exposure, pregnancy in Rh-negative female with known Rh-negative fetus or newborn, or in Rh-negative patients with ITP.

Derivative and Recombinant Coagulation Factors

Recombinant and derivative coagulation factors provide a concentrated source of the desired coagulation factor in a fraction of the volume that would be necessary using FFP. Recombinant factors contain no other human products and no risk of viral disease transmission (Table 24-6).

Other plasma derivatives include antithrombin complex, protein C concentrate, C1-esterase inhibitor, α-1-proteinase inhibitor, and factor XIII, which are indicated for the corresponding specific deficiencies.

TRANSFUSION REACTIONS AND ADVERSE SEQUELAE

Any adverse response to blood-component transfusion is considered a transfusion reaction. Most transfusion reactions occur at the beginning or during transfusion. Others, including development of alloantibodies, iron overload, and some parasitic and viral infections, do not become apparent for months or years.

- Because most transfusion reactions occur within 15 minutes, early, close monitoring of vital signs and status may prevent more severe reactions.
- If a reaction is suspected, the infusion should be halted, the transfusion service notified, appropriate samples collected, and the patient continued to be monitored.

Transfusion reactions are generally classified as hemolytic versus nonhemolytic and acute versus delayed. Hemolytic reactions may be immune-mediated or nonimmune-mediated (Table 24-7).

TABLE. 24–7. *Transfusion reactions*

	Acute/Severe	Delayed/Potentially Severe	Other
Immunologic	Acute hemolytic transfusion reaction Sickle cell hemolytic transfusion syndrome Anaphylaxis Transfusion-related acute lung injury	Delayed hemolytic transfusion reaction (RBC antigen alloimmunization) Human leukocyte antigen alloimmunization Transfusion-associated graft-versus-host disease	Mild allergic/urticarial Posttransfusion purpura Febrile non-hemolytic transfusion reaction
Nonimmunologic	Bacterial sepsis Air embolism Circulatory overload	Viral transmission Parasitic infection Hemosiderosis	Angiotensin converting enzyme inhibitor-related hypotension

Acute Hemolytic Transfusion Reaction (Immune-Mediated)

Acute hemolytic transfusion reactions may be severe and fatal. Most result from ABO blood group incompatibility between patient plasma and donor RBC, and may involve mistransfusion of a unit (or several units) of blood intended for another patient.

Presentation: Fever, chills, flank/back pain, dyspnea, chest pain, anxiety, and in severe cases hypotension, renal failure, shock, and death

Mechanism: ABO incompatibility resulting from destruction of transfused RBC by preformed, naturally occurring isohemagglutinins (AB antibodies) of the immunoglobulin M (IgM) class in the recipient's plasma.

- Intravascular hemolysis caused by complement fixation by IgM and clearance of hemoglobin by the kidneys: patient plasma becomes pink and the urine may have a red-brown tinge.
- Severe hemolysis may result in anemia.
- Cytokine release contributes to renal failure, hypotension, shock and DIC.

Evaluation: Submit to the blood bank:

- The infusion set, the implicated unit, and any units transfused within 4 hours of the reaction.
- Blood specimens (repeat type and cross-match, DAT [should be positive], hematocrit [decreased], lactate dehydrogenase [increased], haptoglobin levels [decreased], bilirubin [increased within 6 to 12 hours] as indices of hemolysis) from the patient and the first posttransfusion voided urine.
- Transfusion reaction report detailing the events and documenting the patient's pre- and posttransfusion vital signs.

Management: Transfusion must be stopped and disconnected at the hub of the needle and intravenous access maintained with physiologic saline.

- Support of blood pressure and renal blood flow with fluids and pressors, and induction of diuresis to maintain urine output at greater than 100 mL/hr (2).
- Withhold further transfusion until the cause of the reaction is determined.
- Coagulation status should be monitored.

Prevention: Meticulous clerical check of the blood unit and patient identification. In case of error in patient identification, immediate steps must be taken to insure that a second patient does not receive the wrong unit.

Sickle Cell Hemolytic Transfusion Syndrome

Patients with sickle cell anemia are at increased risk from hemolytic transfusion reactions. More profound anemia may develop because of autologous red cell destruction in addition to the destruction of incompatible transfused RBC, and to suppression of erythropoiesis after transfusion (hyperhemolytic syndrome) (12). Transfusion-associated hemolysis may mimic a severe posttransfusion pain crisis and may be exacerbated by various factors such as decreasing hemoglobin, complement activation, and increased oxygen consumption with fever. Additional transfusion may result in exacerbation of the syndrome. In the United States, inherent differences in RBC antigen phenotypes between patients with sickle cell anemia (almost exclusively of African descent) and the majority of blood donors (primarily non-African), place patients with sickle cell anemia at increased risk of alloantibody formation and immune hemolysis. In addition, patients with sickle cell disease are often chronically and heavily transfused. Phenotyping of the red cells of patients with sickle cell anemia in the early stages of transfusion therapy helps to manage alloimmunization and suspected transfusion reactions.

Delayed Hemolytic Transfusion Reaction

Delayed hemolytic transfusion reactions (DHTR) occurs within days to weeks posttransfusion in patients who have been immunized previously (primary immunization) by transfusion or pregnancy. Because its manifestation may be mild and symptoms delayed in onset, DHTR may go unrecognized. The incidence of DHTR is estimated to be between 1 per 11,000 to 1 per 5,000 transfusions; it may be considerably underreported. Death is rare. The importance of recognizing these reactions is to document antibody formation and so prevent severe hemolysis from future transfusions (2).

Presentation: fever, chills, decreasing hematocrit, hyperbilirubinemia, and jaundice

- Subtle decrease in hemoglobin may be the only clinical manifestation.
- DAT is usually positive.
- Hemoglobinuria is rare because hemolysis is extravascular.

Mechanism: Repeat stimulation and accelerated (anamnestic) appearance of the antibody in a previously alloimmunized patient upon re-exposure to the offending antigen.

Management: Close monitoring of the patient's hemoglobin for evidence of continuing hemolysis and supportive therapy.

Prevention: Future transfusions must be antigen-negative for the implicated antibody even if antibody is no longer detectable.

- Notification of the patient to prevent future reactions (antibody card or bracelet).

Other Causes of Hemolysis

Other causes of hemolysis temporally associated with transfusion that may mimic hemolytic transfusion reactions include drug-induced hemolysis, mechanical and thermal hemolysis, and hemolysis related to bacterial contamination of the RBC unit.

- Drug-induced hemolysis may present with anemia, positive DAT, elevated LDH and bilirubin. Hemolysis may be either intravascular or extravascular, so that haptoglobin may be decreased and hemoglobinuria and hemoglobinemia present.
- Hemolysis may result from administration of blood with hypotonic solutions (D5W, hypotonic saline, distilled water) or medications.
- Mechanical hemolysis may result from prosthetic heart valves and other intravascular devices and transfusion through small-bore catheters
- Thermal hemolysis results from exposure of red cells to cold (ice, temperatures below 1°C to 6°C, use of unmonitored refrigerators) or to temperatures above 42°C (malfunction or blood warmers, or unmonitored unconventional blood warming methods). The DAT should be negative in these cases. Some of these reactions have been fatal.

Anaphylactic Transfusion Reactions

Anaphylactic transfusion reactions may occur after very small amounts of blood containing plasma are transfused. Although rare, anaphylactic reactions may be rapidly fatal.

Presentation: Sudden onset of flushing, chills, vomiting, diarrhea, initial hypertension followed by hypotension, generalized edema, coughing, stridor, laryngeal edema, and progression to respiratory distress and shock.

- Fever is not a feature of anaphylaxis.

Mechanism: IgE-mediated response to transfused proteins.

- Sensitized IgA-deficient patients are particularly susceptible to anaphylaxis on receiving plasma containing IgA.

Management:

- Discontinue transfusion and employ standard measures for anaphylaxis.
- Epinephrine, corticosteroids, circulatory support.
- Anti-IgA or antibody to a subspecies must be demonstrated to confirm the diagnosis.

Prevention: Usually not predictable or preventable. Subsequent transfusions to IgA deficient patients should come from IgA-deficient donors. If IgA-deficient blood components are not available, patients may benefit from receiving blood products that are depleted of plasma, such as washed RBC and platelets or frozen-deglycerolized RBC.

Transfusion-Related Acute Lung Injury

Transfusion-related acute lung injury (TRALI) is noncardiogenic pulmonary edema associated with transfusion of plasma containing blood components (13,14).

- Underreported
- Fatality rate of 5% to 8%

Presentation: Acute respiratory insufficiency, tachycardia, dyspnea, hypotension, oxygen desaturation, chills, rigors, fever with 1°C to 2°C temperature increase, and a bilateral pulmonary infiltration (white-out) by chest x-ray in the absence of heart failure or elevated central venous pressure.

- May occur during or within 6 hours (most commonly after 2 hours) of transfusion.
- Hypoxemia may require intubation (70% to 75% of cases).
- Symptoms subside rapidly; chest x-ray normal within 96 hours, clinical recovery in 48 to 96 hours.

Mechanism: Reaction of neutrophil antibodies and/or anti-HLA class I and II antibodies to the corresponding antigens between donors and recipients, occurring in the pulmonary vasculature.

- Transfused *donor* antibodies responsible in more than 85% of cases.
- Antibodies from the *recipient* against cells in the donor plasma implicated in approximately 5% of cases.
- In 10% of cases no donor or recipient antibodies are identified.

Management: Discontinue transfusion.

Prevention: A patient who has experienced TRALI is not necessarily at increased risk for development of TRALI with future transfusions, unless receiving blood from the same donor.

Circulatory Overload

The symptoms of circulatory overload or hypervolemia with blood product transfusion are similar to TRALI. However, unlike TRALI, circulatory overload is associated with central venous pressure elevation and cardiac failure. Pulmonary edema in circulatory overload is cardiogenic in origin and may result in the development of or exacerbation of preexisting congestive heart failure. In the absence of other complicating factors, circulatory overload is rarely fatal. Children, the elderly, those with cardiac or pulmonary function compromise, and patients in states of plasma volume expansion (normovolemic chronic anemia, thalessemia major, and sickle cell disease) are at particular risk (2,13).

Presentation: Cough, dyspnea, cyanosis, orthopnea, chest discomfort, rales, headache, distension of jugular veins, restlessness, and tachycardia.

Management: Discontinue transfusion and administer supportive care (oxygen, diuresis, phlebotomy) if necessary.

Prevention: At-risk patients should receive smaller aliquots of blood infused at slower rates (1 mL/kg per hour to 4 mL/kg per hour) (13).

Transfusion-Associated Graft-versus-Host Disease

Transfusion-associated graft-versus-host disease (GVHD) is a rare but severe adverse outcome of transfusion. Immunocompromised post-stem cell or organ transplant patients, those with congenital immune deficiencies, patients with some tumors (particularly lymphomas) and blood relatives (especially first degree) of donors are at particularly high risk of transfusion-associated GVHD. Absent of these indications, patients with acquired immune deficiency (such as HIV) and aplastic anemia patients do not need irradiated blood products (2,13).

Presentation: Rash, diarrhea, mucositis, and pancytopenia. Death is inevitable.

Mechanism: Lymphocytes from an immune-competent donor engraft, recognize the patient's antigens as foreign, and initiate an immune response.

Management: None.

Prevention: Irradiation of blood components.

- Gamma irradiation at 2500 cGy.
- Leukoreduction does not prevent TAGVHD.

Bacterial Contamination and Sepsis

The initial symptoms of bacterial contamination occur during or several hours posttransfusion and include chills and fever. Temperature increase is less marked in patients premedicated with antipyretics or receiving cortosteroids.

Mild septic reactions may be initially missed in the presence of underlying conditions that predispose the patient to fever or manifest similar signs and symptoms (2,13).

Presentation: Rigors and shaking chills, fever, nausea, vomiting, abdominal cramp, bloody diarrhea, hemolysis, hemoglobinuria, severe hypotension, and rapid progression to circulatory compromise, renal failure, shock, and DIC.

Not all contaminated blood products result in clinically detectible sepsis, and fewer yet are fatal.

Mechanism: Common sources of bacterial contamination are subclinical/unrecognized bacteremia in the donor or at the phlebotomy site (skin contaminants). The highest mortality is usually associated with blood components contaminated with endotoxin-producing gram-negative bacteria.

Commonly implicated bacteria in RBC bacteria that survive the cold storage conditions: *Yersinia, Pseudomonas.*

- Platelets are stored at room temperature and are therefore more susceptible to bacterial growth. Commonly implicated bacteria in platelets: *Staphylococcus* and *Propionibacteria* (skin flora); many species are not implicated in serious transfusion reactions (15,16).

Evaluation and management:

- Transfusion must be stopped.
- All transfusion units and blood component bags transfused within 4 hours should be returned to the blood bank for culture.
- Blood samples from both the blood component unit(s) and the patient should be sent for culture.

Prevention:

- Strict hygienic practice from collection to processing, storage, and administration of the component.
- Visual inspection and implementation of objective methods to determine safety of the product (culture or a surrogate method) prior to issuing of the unit (mainly platelets).
- Transfusion of blood components within the allotted 4 hours.

Mild Allergic/Urticarial Transfusion Reactions

Allergic transfusion reactions are relatively common, do not generally progress to anaphylaxis, are rarely lethal, and do not necessarily recur with subsequent transfusions.

Presentation: Localized erythema, pruritus, flushing, and urticaria, usually near the IV site.

- Severe urticaria and pruritus may be the initial signs.

Mechanism: Release of histamine and other anaphylotoxins.

Evaluation and management: Mild allergic reactions generally resolve when transfusion is temporarily stopped, and symptoms improve with administration of oral or parenteral antihistamines.

- *Mild allergic reactions* (hives only): transfusion with the same unit may be resumed, at a slower rate and with close monitoring of the patient.
- Transfusion reaction evaluation generally not necessary.

Prevention: Mild allergic reactions are considered atopic reactions and generally unpredictable.

- No method to prescreen for all possible offending antigens.
- Premedication with antihistamines ameliorates mild allergic reactions in patients with previous reactions.

Posttransfusion Purpura

Posttransfusion purpura (PTP) is a profound thrombocytopenia that may occur after transfusion with any blood component.

Presentation: Abrupt decline in the platelet count 1 to 3 weeks posttransfusion.

- Usually self-limited: resolves within 2 to 3 weeks without treatment.

Mechanism: Antibodies against platelet-specific antigens to which the patient may have become sensitized as a result of pregnancy or prior transfusion.

- Most commonly anti-human platelet antigen 1a (HPA-1a).

Management: Usually self-limited, but IVIG is effective.

- Transfusion with platelets negative for the implicated antigen is not beneficial during the PTP episode, but antigen-negative components will prevent recurrence.
- Family members provide a good source of donors if antigen-negative blood is otherwise not available.
- Severe PTP that does not resolve spontaneously and if refractory to high-dose IVIG may respond to plasmapheresis (13).

Hypotension Associated with Transfusion

Mechanism: Transient isolated hypotension that resolves after discontinuation of transfusion may be caused by activation of bradykinin and associated with use of bedside leukoreduction filters (17).

- Patients receiving ACE inhibitors are at particular risk.

Evaluation and Management: Anaphylaxis, acute hemolytic transfusion reaction, TRALI and bacterial contamination (sepsis) must be excluded.

Prevention: Avoid bedside leukoreduction (especially for patients taking ACE inhibitors).

Febrile Nonhemolytic Transfusion Reaction

Febrile nonhemolytic transfusion reactions (FNHTR) are defined by a greater than 1°C increase in temperature. FNHTR is a diagnosis of exclusion, made after consideration of acute hemolytic transfusion reaction, TRALI, and sepsis and determination that the symptoms are not related to the patient's underlying condition or medications. The incidence of FNHTR varies between patient populations and depends on the age and type of blood component and a variety of donor and recipient factors. Platelets are more likely to be implicated than are RBC or FFP, and older blood components more than fresh, leukocyte-reduced components (since cytokines accumulate during storage). The incidence is higher in multiply transfused patients (13).

Presentation: Chills, fever, rigors, tachycardia, tachypnea, headache, nausea, and general discomfort.

• Patients who sustain significant fever with transfusion are likely to have repeated reactions.

Mechanism: Antibodies in the recipient against donor leukocytes or platelets, cytokines accumulated in blood component bag during storage, and/or pyrogens passively transferred from the donor to the recipient in the blood component.

Evaluation and management: As with a hemolytic reaction.

• Antipyretics may be administered.

Prevention: Leukoreduction (especially prestorage leukoreduction), removal of plasma in extreme situations, and premedication with antipyretics.

Hemosiderosis

Hemosiderosis or iron overload occurs in patients who receive repeated (usually more than 50) RBC transfusions.

Presentation: Bronze skin, hepatic fibrosis and malfunction, diabetes and other endocrine gland dysfunction, and cardiac failure.

Mechanism: Accumulation of iron in the skin and internal organs.

• One unit of RBC typically contains 200 to 250 mg of iron.

Evaluation and management: Iron studies and iron chelation or phlebotomy when appropriate.

Prevention: Consider chelation for more than 50 unit red cell burden; red cell exchanges using apheresis help delay iron accumulation in patients with sickle cell disease (2).

Transfusion-Transmitted Viral Infections

Current testing of donor blood prior to release of blood components includes:

• *Antibodies* to: human immunodeficiency virus (HIV) types 1 and 2 (anti-HIV-1/2); hepatitis C virus (HCV) (anti-HCV), hepatitis B core antigen (anti-HBc); human lymphotrophic virus types I and II (anti-human T-cell leukemia virus [HTLV] I/II).
• *Surface antigen:* Hepatitis B surface antigen (HBsAg).
• *Nucleic acid testing (NAT)* for: HIV, HCV, West Nile virus (WNV).

With the current testing the estimated risk of transmission of viral infections per transfusion is reported in Table 24-8. Blood is also tested by *RPR* for the detection of *Treponema pallidum* bacterium.

TABLE. 24–8. *Estimated risk of transfusion transmission of viral disease*

Virus	Risk per transfusion
HIV 1 and 2	1 : 2,000,000–3,000,000
Hepatitis B	1 : 100,000–200,000
Hepatitis C	1 : 1,000,000–1 : 2,000,000
HTLV I and II	1 : 641,000 (cellular components)
Parvovirus B19	1 : 20,000 (most recipients immune)
West Nile virus	Range 1.46 : 10,000 to 12.33: 10,000 depending on region*

* Nebraska, Ohio, Illinois, Louisiana, Mississippi, and Michigan are among the more heavily affected states, with the highest incidence from late July to mid October; In some areas the risk of transfusion transmission was estimated to be as high as 21.32 in 10,000 during peak West Nile virus epidemic. See also reference 18.

Transfusion-Transmitted Parasitic Infections

Parasitic infections, not as common in the United States and Europe as in other parts of the world, include mainly malaria (*Plasmodium*), trypanosomiasis, and babesiosis. *Toxoplasma* is a protozoa that can be transmitted by transfusion, as reported in immunocompromised patients (15,19).

- *Malaria:* Three cases per year on average in the United States.
- *Babesia:* Thirty reported cases in the literature.
- *Trypanosoma cruzii:* Seven cases by transfusion in the United States and Canada.
- *Leishmaniasis:* Fifteen cases have been reported worldwide (none in the United States).

Prions

Prions are protein particles believed to be responsible for transmission of Creutzfeldt-Jakob disease (CJD) and its variant nonfamilial form (vCJD). Until recently, a theoretical association between transfusion and transmission of prions in humans was based on evidence from animal models. Recently, the first probable transfusion-transmitted case has been reported (20).

There is currently no screening test for detection of prions.

Alternatives to Allogeneic Blood Transfusion

Alternatives to the use of blood component therapy are available and may be particularly useful for bleeding patients who refuse allogeneic blood component or blood product transfusions (such as Jehovah's witnesses) or bleeding patients unresponsive to appropriate transfusion therapy.

Patients with religious concerns about blood transfusion must be informed of any human derived contents in any products that may be administered, allowing them to make an informed decision (21).

Examples of alternatives to allogeneic blood transfusion are listed in Table 24-9. Indications for use of some pharmaceutical hemostatic agents are summarized in Table 24-10.

Massive Transfusion

Massive transfusion is the administration of blood components over a 24-hour period in amounts that equal or exceed the total blood volume of the patient (10 or more units of whole

TABLE. 24–9. *Examples of alternatives to allogeneic blood transfusion*

Preoperative	Intraoperative	Postoperative
Autologous Blood Collection	Blood Salvaged from a Sterile Surgical Field ANVH	Blood Recovered from Drainage

Donor's HGb should meet or exceed 11 g/dL
Donor must be at no increased risk of bacterial infection
Donations up to every 5 days with last collection no later than 72 hours prior to procedure
Autologous blood subject to the same shelf-life limitations as allogeneic blood components
Unit may be frozen until used
Prevention of transmission of viral infections, red cell alloimmunization and some transfusion reactions
Risk of bacterial contamination and of clerical error leading to transfusion of ABO incompatible units not decreased significantly*
Increase preoperative hematocrit
   Erythropoietin
   Correction of nutritional anemias
	Use in oncologic procedures is controversial
	Gross contamination of the surgical field with malignant cells constitutes a relative contraindication
	Blood salvaged by devices that collect, centrifuge, wash, and concentrate red blood cells
	Blood may be stored at room temperature for 4 hours from the end of the collection and at 1–6°C for up to 24 hours if refrigeration began within 4 hours from initiation of collection**
	ANVH
	Whole blood is collected from patient and replaced with crystalloid or colloid and reinfused after cessation of major blood loss, or sooner if indicated. Blood collected in this manner may be kept at room temperature up to 8 hours or refrigerated at 1–6°C up to 24 hours after collection *,**
		Used primarily with cardiac and orthopedic surgery*
		Blood recovered is generally dilute (hematocrit of approximately 20%) and may be partially hemolyzed
		Transfusion should start within 6 hours of initiation of collection*,**

* See reference 2.
**See reference 22.
ANVH = Acute normovolemic hemodilution

blood or 20 units of packed RBC in an adult). After transfusion of one or more blood volumes, an abbreviated RBC cross-match (see general concepts) is performed to provide RBC more rapidly. Group O, Rh-negative, or Rh-positive blood, depending on the age and gender of patient, or ABO/Rh-specific blood are effective and relatively safe ways to obtain blood urgently.

- Adequate intravascular blood volume and blood pressure may be maintained initially with colloids (albumin, plasma protein fraction) or crystalloids (lactated Ringer's solution or normal saline).
- Transfusion of packed RBC may become necessary after a loss of more than 30% of the blood volume, depending on the rate of blood loss, tissue perfusion and oxygenation status of the patient (24).
- Transfusion of blood components based on fixed ratios or algorithms should be avoided.

TABLE. 24–10. *Pharmacologic hemostatic agents*

Agent	Indications and Monitoring	Non-Indications and Adverse Effects	Administartion and Preparations
Vitamin K	Vitamin K deficiency resulting in coagulopathy (factors II, VII, IX, X) Reversal of warfarin anticoagulation (when prolonged effectiveness is desired and simple discontinuation of warfarin is not feasible) INR to monitor effectiveness and determine dosing	Not effective emergently for urgent reversal of warfarin or correction of vitamin K-dependent factors	IV faster effect than SC, or PO Solution and tablet forms, 0.5–20 mg
Protamine	Neutralization of anticoagulation due to unfractionated heparin (displaces antithrombin III and complexes heparin) After cardiac bypass surgery in patients who have received unfractionated heparin Close monitoring of coagulation parameters (due to possible heparin rebound) Activated clotting time to monitor effectiveness and determine dosing	Possible heparin rebound (due to shorter half life of protamine compared to heparin) Dosing should not exceed 100 mg in 2 hours	Immediate onset of action; 2 hour half-life 1mg of protamine neutralizes 80–100 USP heparin
Conjugated Estrogens	Coagulopathy related to uremia, GI bleeding associated with angiodysplasia (Osler-Weber-Rendu syndrome), end stage renal disease, von Willebrand disease	Not useful when immediate hemostasis is required May be associated with gynecomastia, weight gain, and dyspepsia	Onset of effect within 6 hours and duration of up to 2 weeks Maximum effectiveness between 5–7 days Usual dosage: IV: 0.6 mg/kg Patch: 50–100 μg/ 24 hrs PO: 50 mg
DDAVP*	Bleeding associated with hemophilia A and von Willebrand disease Bernard-Soulier disease Aspirin ingestion Platelet hemostasis defects where other treatment options are not effective	Not useful in type 2B von Willebrand disease due to thrombocytopenia and increased affinity of vWF for platelets May be associated with hyponatremia when administered with hypotonic fluids	Usual dosage: IV: 0.3 μL/kg in 50 mL normal saline (adults) over 30 minutes 0.3 μL/kg in 10 mL normal saline (children weighing<10 kg) over 30 minutes

(continued)

TABLE. 24–10. *(continued)*

Agent	Indications and Monitoring	Non-Indications and Adverse Effects	Administration and Preparations
	Peak response iv is within 1 hour	Hypertension, facial flushing, nausea Increased risk of myocardial infarction in cardiac surgery patients	Intranasal: 300 μg (adults) Peak response: IV: within 1 hour SC: within 2 hours Intranasal: within 2 hours
AMCA[**]**/** **EACA**[***]	α2-antiplasmin deficiency. AMCA: Topical hemostatic in hemophilia A and B patients during dental procedures along with fibrin sealant and DDAVP May be used in GI and uterine bleeding where antifibrinolytic action is necessary, amegakaryocytic and peripheral immune mediated thrombocytopenia May be useful as irrigation in intractable bleeding from the bladder AMCA more potent than EACA	Contraindicated in thrombotic disorders with fibrinolysis (DIC) or active intravascular clotting Reduce dose in renal insufficiency EACA: May be associated with myonecrosis on prolonged usage	Usual Dosage: EACA: 4 g/3–4 hours 10–24 g in 24 hours AMCA:1 g/6–8 hours 3–4 g in 24 hours Half-life: 2–10 hours
Aprotinin	Antifibrinolytic and anticoagulant properties Intravenous preparations approved for use as a hemostatic in cardiac bypass surgery Off label use: Liver transplant	Anaphylaxis: 10,000 kallikrein inhibitory units IV test dose should be given prior to surgery	Dosage in adults ranges from 250,000–500,000 kallikrein inhibitory units/hr IV for cardiac bypass surgery 2 million units IV for liver transplant

*1-deamino-8-D-arginine vasopressin; **tranexamic acid; *** ε-aminocaproic acid
See also reference 23.

Adverse sequelae of massive transfusion:

• Dilution and/or consumption of hemostatic constituents of blood. Platelet count, prothrombin time (PT), PTT, and fibrinogen levels should be determined frequently.
• Generally a platelet count of greater than 50,000 per microliter (80,000 to 100,000/μL for neurologic surgery, ophthalmologic surgery, or cardiopulmonary bypass), PT or PTT of less than 1.5 times normal range, and a fibrinogen concentration of greater than 80 to 100 mg/dL are considered adequate for maintenance of hemostasis.
• Combinations of low values seen during massive transfusion may require replacement therapy (4,24,25).
• Hypothermia, acidosis, hypocalcemia, and other biochemical disturbances may occur and electrolytes, particularly potassium and calcium, should be monitored (25).
• Hypocalcemia secondary to citrate accumulation may occur when large volumes of blood are administered at rapid rates (more than 100 mL/min), especially in the presence of liver and renal dysfunction.

Disseminated Intravascular Coagulation

DIC probably complicates massive transfusion less often than suspected, although DIC is associated with shock, independent of blood loss or transfusion.

• Laboratory coagulation test results consistent with a consumptive coagulopathy.
• Transfusion management of DIC is supportive while the underlying cause is addressed.
• Administration of cryoprecipitate when fibrinogen levels are below 80 mg/dL.
• Other components, such as platelets may be necessary, especially if bleeding is severe.
• Usually massive transfusion, even in trauma settings, requires only replacement of platelets (26).
• If multiple factors are consumed, plasma factor levels of above 30% can be achieved with an FFP dose of 10 to 15 mL/kg.

IMMUNOHEMATOLOGIC DISORDERS

Hemolytic Disease of the Newborn

Hemolytic disease of the newborn (HDN) is the destruction of fetal RBC by maternal IgG antibodies that cross the placenta and react with a paternally derived antigen present on the fetal RBC. Although traditionally associated with Rh antibodies (anti-Rh$_0$D), other antibodies including anti-A, anti-B, and anti-Kell have been implicated and may cause significant HDN.

• *Mild cases:* The newborn is asymptomatic and laboratory findings of a positive DAT and mild bilirubinemia the only abnormalities.
• *Severe cases:* May result in intrauterine death (hydrops fetalis, erythroblastosis fetalis).
• High risk of *kernicterus* caused by high unconjugated bilirubin.

Treatment: Intrauterine RBC transfusion (in severe cases) using compatible (with the mother's antibody), irradiated, CMV-negative, sickle-negative RBC suspended in 5% albumin or FFP.

• Usually a two-blood-volume exchange removes approximately 25% of excess bilirubin, provides albumin to which excess bilirubin can bind, and removes antibody and approximately 70% of RBC coated with antibody.
• Additional exchange transfusions may be necessary if level of bilirubin continues to rise.

Neonatal Alloimmune Thrombocytopenia and Maternal Immune Thrombocytopenic Purpura

Neonatal Alloimmune Thrombocytopenia

Neonatal alloimmune thrombocytopenia (NAIT), the platelet equivalent of HDN, refers to the destruction of platelets that carry paternally derived antigens by maternal antibodies that cross the placenta. As with HDN, NAIT may vary in severity from very mild and asymptomatic thrombocytopenia to life-threatening bleeding, and may occur *in utero* or in the neonatal period. The vast majority of NAIT is associated with antibody (IgG) against the common platelet antigen HPA-1a (PL ^{A1}), especially in the presence of HLA DRw52a phenotype.

NAIT is usually self-limiting and resolves within 2 to 3 weeks. If NAIT is suspected, often as a result of a previous affected pregnancy, cordocentesis to determine platelet counts may be performed in conjunction with administration of compatible platelets (maternal platelets or platelets known to be negative for the implicated antigen).

- In utero NAIT: IVIG with or without steroid administration to the mother on a weekly basis (1 g/kg) until delivery.
- High risk of intracranial hemorrhage: platelet transfusion immediately prior to delivery.
- When compatible platelets are unavailable, high-dose IVIG has been administered to the neonate with variable effectiveness.
- An increase in platelet counts within 24 to 48 hours may be seen in patients who respond (2).

Maternal Immune Thrombocytopenic Purpura

In *maternal* ITP, antibodies related to maternal ITP such as IgG (as in NAIT) are implicated and have broad specificity.

- Degree of thrombocytopenia is milder than that associated with NAIT.
- Lower risk of fetal or neonatal intracranial hemorrhage.
- Maternal platelets and random donor platelets may be equally effective or ineffective.
- IVIG may also be beneficial.
- Usually resolves in days to weeks (upon clearance of maternal antibodies from the neonate's circulation.)

Autoimmune Hemolytic Anemias

Autoimmune hemolytic anemias (AIHA) are characterized by the presence of antibodies against the individual's own RBC antigens (autoantibodies), resulting in accelerated destruction of these RBC. AIHA may be associated with autoimmune disorders, infections, medications or malignancies, or may be primary. The laboratory hallmark is the positive DAT, indicating the presence of autoantibody directed against red cells. Antibody may also be present in the serum so that positive DAT and IAT may coexist, making identification of underlying alloantibodies and compatibility testing difficult (2).

Warm Autoimmune Hemolytic Anemia

Warm AIHA is approximately four times as common as hemolysis from cold-reacting antibodies. The implicated antibody is usually IgG and reacts with all cells, although occasionally a warm autoantibody will appear to have specificity against Rh antigens and several others. Patients with compensated warm AIHA require no specific treatment but should be investigated for an underlying condition such as systemic lupus erythematosus or a lymphoproliferative disorder. In children, viral illness may be accompanied by transient AIHA. Warm-reacting autoantibodies may be present only as a laboratory finding, or they may cause severe, even life-threatening hemolysis; these antibodies react optimally at 37°C in vitro. Patients are often totally asymptomatic, but some present with fatigue, jaundice, or mild anemia. Moderate splenomegaly occur in about one-third to one-half of the cases and hepatomegaly in one-third of the patients. Hemolysis is usually not severe and is mainly extravascular (27).

Laboratory findings include a positive DAT, spherocytes on the blood smear, elevated unconjugated bilirubin and LDH as indices of cell turnover, and high reticulocyte count. Rarely, reticulocytopenia may be seen, either because of inadequate bone marrow response or because the autoantibody reacts with red cell precursors as well as with mature cells.

Red cell alloantibodies developed as a result of previous transfusions or pregnancies, found in approximately one-third of patients with AIHA, are capable of causing severe hemolytic transfusion reactions. Broadly reactive autoantibody may mask underlying alloantibodies and make procurement of compatible blood difficult.

Occasionally hemolysis may result in severe anemia accompanied by changes in mental status and coma. This medical emergency requires immediate transfusion even when compatible blood cannot be obtained. The term "least incompatible" has not been adequately defined, does not correlate to clinical events, and would be best abolished (27).

Treatment with oral glucocorticoids (prednisone 60 mg per day) is effective in more than half of the cases and splenectomy is effective in approximately half of those who are refractory to steroids. Immunosuppressive regimens and IVIG (400 mg/kg per day for 5 days) may benefit selected patients (27).

Cold Agglutinin Syndrome

Cold-reacting antibodies are common and usually of no significance, but some cold agglutinins, especially those with very high titer at 4°C but broad thermal amplitude (reactivity up to 30°C) may result in cold agglutinin syndrome (cold hemagglutinin disease). IgM is the immune globulin classically implicated. Cold agglutinin syndrome may be primary (cause undetermined) or secondary to a viral infection or lymphoproliferative disorder. Acute cold agglutinin syndrome may be associated with Mycoplasma pneumonia and infectious mononucleosis, is seen mostly in children and young adults, and tends to be transient and self-limited. Chronic cold agglutinin syndrome may be associated with lymphoma, chronic lymphocytic leukemia, Waldenstrom's macroglobulinemia, and a high-titer monoclonal cold agglutinin. Patients may present with acrocyanosis and hematuria precipitated by cold, and/or severe pain in the nose, ears and distal extremities upon cold exposure. Severe anemia is rare in the chronic form.

Transfusion is rarely necessary, but, when performed, the typing specimen must be kept at body temperature from the time of phlebotomy through the testing procedure. Up to 50% of transfused cells may be destroyed by autoantibodies of the patient even when blood warmers are used.

Treatment with corticosteroids and splenectomy is not effective, and most patients do well by avoiding exposure to the cold. Rituximab, a monoclonal antibody targeted against the B lymphocyte CD20 antigen, has been useful, administered as four weekly infusions in a small number of patients (27).

Paroxysmal Cold Hemoglobinuria

Paroxysmal cold hemoglobinuria (PCH) is a rare autoimmune hemolytic anemia that results from a biphasic IgG antibody (Donath-Landsteiner antibody). Originally associated with untreated syphilis, it is now found most often with viral infections in children. The Donath-Landsteiner antibody binds to the RBC at cold temperatures and causes intravascular hemolysis as complement is fixed at warmer temperatures, accounting for the paroxysms of hemoglobinuria. Anemia associated with PCH is usually transient and self-limited over 2 to 3 weeks. If transfusion support becomes necessary, cross-match-compatible blood may be found if the antibody is not reactive at temperatures above 4°C. Unavailability of compatible RBC should not preclude transfusion in life-threatening anemia associated with hemolysis, despite shortened survival of the transfused RBC (2,27).

Therapeutic Apheresis in the Management of Immunohematologic Disorders

Apheresis is the process by which selected components or substances in blood are removed from the circulation and the remainder of the blood returned to the patient. Apheresis is used for routine blood component (platelets, plasma, stem cells) collection and therapeutic removal of undesirable components and substances from the circulation, achieved through automated machines.

- The kinetics of most intravascular substances indicate that exchange of 1 to 1.5 plasma volumes results in the highest efficiency removal with progressively decreased efficiency with each additional consecutive exchange.
- The volume of blood processed in order to attain the desired apheresis effect (for therapeutic component collection) depends on the nature of the component of interest, including its intravascular distribution and its concentration in the particular patient.
- The patient's total blood volume determines the safe extracorporeal blood volume (which should not exceed 15% of blood volume).
- Small patients may require that the machine be primed with saline or blood.

See Table 24-11 for the types of apheresis procedures.

Apheresis is generally safe, especially for normal component donors. Complications mainly relate to vascular access, hemodynamic changes (especially for patients with cardiovascular disease), and a variable loss of blood components. Risks associated with apheresis are usually associated with a patient's underlying disease.

- Plasma exchange may result in a 30% or more decrease in platelet counts (28).
- Platelet transfusion may be required for patients with low platelet counts and hemostatic problems.
- Cellular blood component counts return to normal after a few days and proteins and electrolytes reequilibrate within hours, although fibrinogen may remain below baseline levels after 72 hours (29).
- Hypotension may occur as a result of volume shifts and bradykinin activation from blood contact with plastic (2,30). Withhold ACE inhibitors, which potentiate this effect, from patients for 24 to 48 hours prior to an apheresis procedure.
- Plasma exchange may reduce blood levels of certain medications, especially those bound to plasma proteins or those with a long plasma half-life (30).
- Citrate is used to prevent coagulation of blood in the circuit and may result in *citrate toxicity:* binding of calcium and decreased levels of ionized calcium (30). Symptoms: Mild perioral tingling and discomfort, chest tightness, and tetany in severe cases. If symptoms do not subside with adjustment of citrate and whole blood flow rates, administration of oral calcium (as chewable tablets) or intravenous calcium chloride (for large volume apheresis procedures) help prevent hypocalcemia and the accompanying syndromes.

Therapeutic Apheresis (Cytapheresis and Plasmapheresis)

Thrombocytapheresis

Increased platelet counts, particularly in myeloproliferative disorders where the platelets are qualitatively abnormal as well, may be associated with bleeding or thrombosis.

TABLE. 24–11. *Recommendation for therapeutic apheresis in hematologic disorders*

Category I **Accepted as standard first line or primary therapy**
ABO-mismatched marrow transplant (red cell removal from marrow)
Cutaneous T-cell lymphoma (photopheresis)
Erythrocytosis or polycythemia vera (phlebotomy)
Leukocytosis/thrombocytosis (cytapheresis)
Posttransfusion purpura (plasma exchange)
Sickle cell disease (RBC exchange)
Thrombotic thrombocytopenic purpura (plasma exchange)

Category II **Generally accepted as adjunctive or supportive therapy**
ABO-mismatched marrow transplant (plasma exchange in recipient)
Erythrocytosis or polycythemia vera (erythrocytaphersis)
Coagulation factor inhibitors (plasma exchange)
Cryoglobulinemia (plasma exchange)
Cryoglobulinemia with polyneuropathy (plasma exchange)
Hyperviscosity (plasma exchange)
Idiopathic (autoimmune) thrombocytopenic purpura (immunoadsorption)
Myeloma, paraproteins, or hyperviscosity (plasma exchange)
Myeloma with acute renal failure (plasma exchange)
Polyneuropathy with IgM, with or without Waldenstrom's (plasma exchange)

Category III **No clear indication based on conflicting or insufficient evidence of efficacy or favorable risk-to-benefit ratio. Sometimes used as a last resort**
Aplastic anemia or pure RBC aplasia (plasma exchange)
Autoimmune hemolytic anemia (plasma exchange)
Cutaneous T-cell lymphoma (leukaphersis)
Hemolytic disease of the newborn (plasma exchange)
Hemolytic uremic syndrome (plasma exchange)
Platelet alloimmunization and refractoriness (plasma exchange or immunoadsorption)
Malaria or babesiosis (RBC exchange)
Multiple myeloma with polyneuropathy (plasma exchange)

Modified from Smith JW, Weinstein R, Hillye KL, et al. Therapeutic apheresis: a summary of current indication categories endorsed by the AABB and the American Society for Apheresis. *Transfusion* 2003;43:820–822.

Patients with elevated platelets who are symptomatic (from essential thrombocytosis or polycythemia rubra vera) or hemorrhage (chronic myelogenous leukemia, CML) may have immediate benefit from therapeutic cytapheresis. Generally plateletpheresis is a first-line therapy for thrombocytosis (platelet counts greater than 500,000 per microliter) in symptomatic patients.

- Each procedure will lower the count 30% to 50%.
- Cytoreductive chemotherapy should be initiated simultaneously, since plateletpheresis is not effective long term (30).

Leukocytapheresis (Leukapheresis)

Malignant leukocytosis or hyperleukocytosis (immature white blood cell counts of greater than 100,000 per microliter), in association with some leukemias, may result in leuko-stasis in the central nervous system, kidneys, and lungs. Symptoms may occur with rapidly rising blast cells at counts less than 100,000/μL, especially in acute myeloid leukemia (AML) and CML.

- Changes in mentation, dizziness, blurred vision, hypoxia, or respiratory symptoms constitute a medical emergency.
- Therapeutic leukapheresis can reduce the leukocyte count by 30% to 50% in hours.
- Symptoms may abate promptly.
- Reduction of the white cell count permits cytoreductive chemotherapy by abrogating fever, increased uric acid, renal failure, and electrolyte imbalances of the acute cytolysis syndrome.
- Chemotherapy with hydroxyurea or a similar agent should be initiated concurrently since repeated leukocytapheresis may not control hyperleukocytosis (30).

Erythrocytapheresis/Red Cell Exchange

Red cell exchange involves the removal of abnormal red cells.

- Patient's RBC are replaced with stored RBC.
- Erythrocytapheresis may be used to reduce red cell mass acutely in symptomatic (visual disturbances, confusion, lethargy, hemorrhage, threatened stroke, thrombosis of abdominal vasculature) patients with excessive polycythemia (30).
- Saline or colloid volume replacement is administered to maintain isovolemia.

Red Cell Exchange and Sickle Cell Anemia

Red cell exchange may be used acutely in the treatment of complications of sickle cell disease, including acute chest syndrome, stroke, retinal infarction, priapism, and hepatic crisis, or as protracted or chronic treatment for the prevention of recurrent complications such as stroke and severe painful crises, and for reduction of iron overload secondary to transfusion (30).

- In the perioperative setting, simple transfusion or a single red cell exchange has been shown to prevent morbidity associated with sickle cell disease.
- Goal is to achieve hemoglobin A of more than 50%.
- Transfusion and exchange have been used to treat sickle complications during pregnancy; routine use is unnecessary. Exchange transfusion can raise hemoglobin A to levels difficult to achieve with simple transfusion and may benefit patients in the third trimester for pree-clampsia, sepsis, and preoperative management (30).

Red Cell Exchange and Parasitemia

Red cell exchange has been used as antiparasitic treatment in malaria to decrease the circulating parasite load when it exceeds 5% (32) (Table 24-11).

Plasmapheresis

Plasmapheresis may be used to collect plasma for transfusion or manufacturing of plasma derivatives, or to remove undesirable substances from the circulation. Colloids or saline (plasma with TTP) are administered to maintain isovolemia. The indications for therapeutic plasma exchange (TPE) are listed in Tables 24-11 and 24-12.

Thrombotic Microangiopathies

Thrombotic thrombocytopenic purpura (TTP) and hemolytic uremic syndrome (HUS) belong to a spectrum of thrombotic microangiopathies. TTP may be associated with prominent

TABLE. 24–12. *Category I and II recommendations for therapeutic plasma exchange*

Category I	Category II
Acute inflammatory demyelinating polyradiculoneuropathy	ABO-mismatched marrow transplant (plasma exchange recipient)*
Antiglomerular basement membrane antibody disease	Acute central nervous system inflammatory demyelinating disease
Chronic inflammatory demyelinating polyradiculoneuropathy	Coagulation factor inhibitors
Demyelinating polyneuropathy with IgG and IgA	Cryoglobulinemia
	Cryoglobulinemia with polyneuropathy
	Hyperviscosity
Familial hypercholesterolemia (selective adsorption)	Idiopathic (autoimmune) thrombocytopenic purpura
Myasthenia gravis	Familial hypercholesterolemia
Posttransfusion purpura	Lambert-Eaton myasthenia syndrome
Phytanic acid storage disease	Myeloma, paraproteins, or hyperviscosity
Thrombotic thrombocytopenia purpura	Myeloma or acute renal failure
	Pediatric autoimmune neuropsychiatric disorders (PANDAS)
	Polyneuropathy with IgM (with or without Waldenstroms)
	Rapidly progressive glomerulonephritis
	Rheumatoid arthritis (lymphoplasmaphersis)
	Sydenham's chorea

* Removal of RBC from the marrow is the preferred method.
Modified from Smith JW, Weinstein R, Hillye KL, et al. Therapeutic apheresis: a summary of current indication categories endorsed by the AABB and the American Society for Apheresis. *Transfusion* 2003;43 : 820–822.

neurologic symptoms, HUS presents with a more prominent renal component. Characteristic findings of TTP include fever, renal impairment, neurologic symptoms such as change in mental status, seizures or coma, thrombocytopenia (platelet counts less than $30,000/\mu L$), and hemolytic anemia with schistocytes (2,30).

- TTP results from the accumulation of ultra-large von Willebrand factor multimers caused by immune mediated (IgG) interference with the serum protease ADAMS13.

  When TTP and HUS-like syndromes are associated with immunosuppressive agents (e.g., vinca alkaloids, mitomycin, bleomycin, BL22, cisplatin, tacrolimus, and cyclosporin A), they do not respond well to TPE.

- TPE is first-line therapy for the treatment of TTP and a last resort for HUS.
- TPE should be performed promptly after diagnosis of TTP.
- The effectiveness of TPE in TTP depends on the removal of ultra-large VWF multimers and reduction of the IgG antibodies against VWF-cleaving protease.
- Plasma (FFP) is the fluid replacement of choice in TPE for TTP and also replaces the VWF-cleaving protease.
- TPE is often done daily, then tapered until platelet counts stabilize at more than 100,000 per microliter for 2 consecutive days.
- Response can be monitored by clinical assessment and laboratory measurements (platelet count, LDH, extent of schistocytosis).

  Platelet transfusion is generally discouraged because patients suffer from thrombosis rather than bleeding. However, platelet transfusion may be necessary with life-threatening hemorrhage (2).

Immune (Autoimmune) Thrombocytopenic Purpura

ITP involves destruction of platelets by IgG autoantibodies. In its acute form, typically presenting in small children after a viral infection, ITP is usually self-limited. In adults, ITP is more chronic, and TPE has been used to treat severe cases, refractory to corticosteroids and high-dose IVIG (30).

- Anti-Rh immune globulin (WinRho) is effective in Rh-positive patients.
- Therapeutic plasmapheresis in combination with steroids may result in fewer relapses and decreased need for splenectomy (30).

Coagulation Factor Inhibitors

- TPE may be used to treat coagulation factor inhibitors (factor VIII, IX).

Plasmapheresis can lower inhibitor titers in patients who experience uncontrollable hemorrhage, or prevent bleeding from invasive procedures (30).

Dysproteinemias

Complications of paraproteinemias of multiple myeloma, Waldenstrom's macroglobulinemia, and cryoglobulinemia respond to TPE.

- Hyperviscosity syndrome with mental status changes, mucosal and gastrointestinal bleeding, retinopathy, and hypervolemia constitutes a medical emergency.
- Hyperviscosity responds to even small volume exchanges, but procedures need to be repeated until the paraprotein is controlled with chemotherapy (30).

REFERENCES

1. Mielcarek M, Leisenring W, Torok-Storb B, et al. Graft-versus-host disease and donor-directed hemagglutinin titers after ABO-mismatched related and unrelated marrow allografts: evidence for graft-versus-plasma cell effect. *Blood* 2000;96:1150–1156
2. Brecher ME, ed. *Technical Manual*, 14th ed. Bethesda, MD: AABB Press, 2002.
3. Hébert PC, Wells G, Blajchman MA, et al. A multicenter randomized, controlled clinical trial of transfusion requirements in critical care. *N Engl J Med* 1999;340:409–417.
4. Practice guidelines for blood component therapy: Report by American Society of Anesthesiologists Task Force on Blood Component Therapy. Anesthesiology 1996;84:732–747.
4a. Development Task Force of the College of American Pathologists. Practice parameter for the use of fresh frozen plasma, cryoprecipitate, and platelets. *JAMA* 1994;271:777–781.
5. Schiffer CA, Anderson KC, Bennett CL, et al. Platelet transfusion for patients with cancer: clinical practice guidelines of the American Society of Oncology. *J Clin Oncol* 2001;19:1519–1538.
6. Stroncek DF, Leonard K, Eiber G, et al. Alloimmunization after granulocyte transfusions. *Transfusion* 1996;36:1009–1015.
7. Hume H. Transfusion support of children with hematologic and oncologic disorders. In: Petz LD, Swisher SN, Kleinman S, et al., eds. *Clinical Practice of Transfusion Medicine*. 3rd ed. New York: Churchill Livingstone, 1996:711.
8. Haas R, Mohle R, Fruehauf S, et al. Patient characteristics associated with successful mobilizing and autografting of peripheral blood progenitor cells in malignant lymphoma. *Blood* 1994;83:3787–3794.
9. Fruehauf S, Haas R, Conradt C, et al. Peripheral blood progenitor cell (PBPC) counts during steady-state hematopoiesis allow to estimate the yield of mobilized PBPC after filgrastim (R-metHuG-CSF)-supported cytotoxic chemotherapy *Blood* 1995;85:2619–2626.
10. Snyder EL, Haley NR, eds. *Hematopoietic Progenitor Cells. A Primer for Medical Professionals.* Bethesda, MD: AABB Press, 2000.

11. ACOG Practice Bulletin. Prevention of Rh D alloimmunization. Number 4, May 1999 (replaces educational bulletin Number 147, October 1990). Clinical management guidelines for obstetrician-gynecologists. American College of Obstetrics and Gynecology. *Int J Gynecol Obstet* 1999; 66:63–70.

12. Davenport RD. Hemolytic transfusion reactions. In: Simon TL, Dzik WH, Snyder EL, et al. *Rossi's Principles of Transfusion Medicine.* 3rd ed. Philadelphia: Lippincott Williams and Wilkins, 2002:818.

13. Popovsky MA, ed. *Transfusion Reactions.* 2nd ed. Bethesda, MD: AABB Press, 2001.

14. Webert KE, Blajchman MA. Transfusion-related acute lung injury. *Transfus Med Rev* 2003;17: 252–262.

15. Goodnough LT, Shander A, Brecher ME. Transfusion medicine: looking to the future. *Lancet* 2003; 361:161–169.

16. Jacobs MR, Palavecino E, Yomtovian R. Don't bug me: the problem of bacterial contamination of blood components—challenges and solutions. *Transfusion* 2001;41:1331–1334.

17. Mair B, Leparc GF. Hypotensive reactions associated with platelet transfusions and angiotensin-converting enzyme inhibitors. *Vox Sang* 1998;74:27–30.

18. Biggerstaff BJ, Peterson LR. Estimated risk of transmission of the West Nile virus through blood transfusion in the US, 2002. *Transfusion* 2003;43:1007–1017.

19. Dodd RY. Transmission of parasites by blood transfusion. *Vox Sang* 1998;74(Suppl 2):161–163.

20. Llewelyn CA, Hewitt PE, Knight RS, et al. Possible transmission of variant Creutzfeldt-Jakob disease by blood transfusion. *Lancet* 2004;363:417–421.

21. Spence RK. Transfusion guidelines for cardiovascular surgery: lessons learned from operations in Jehovah's Witnesses. *J Vasc Surg* 1992;16:825–829; discussion 829–831.

22. Santrach P, ed. *Standards for Perioperative Autologous Blood Collection and Administration.* 1st ed. Bethesda, MD: AABB Press, 2001:14, Reference Standard 5R-A.

23. Bolan CD, Klein HG. Transfusion medicine and pharmacologic aspects of hemostasis. In: Kitchens C, Kessler C, Alving BM, eds. *Consultative Hemostasis and Thrombosis.* New York: Harcourt Health Sciences, 2002:395–418.

24. Mintz PD, ed. *Transfusion Therapy Clinical Principles and Practice.* Bethesda, MD: AABB Press, 1999:177–191.

25. Ray A, Hess JR. Treating coagulopathy in trauma patients. *Transfus Med Rev* 2003;17:223–231.

26. Counts RB, Haisch C, Simon TL, et al. Hemostasis in massively transfused trauma patients. *Ann Surg* 1979;190:91–99.

27. Petz LD, Garratty G, eds. *Immune Hemolytic Anemias.* 2nd ed. New York: Churchill Livingstone, 2003.

28. Rogers RL, Johnson H, Ludwig R, et al. Efficacy and safety of plateletpheresis by donors with low-normal platelet counts. *J Clin Apheresis* 1995;10:194–197.

29. Flaum MA, Cuneo RA, Appelbaum FR, et al. The hemostatic imbalance of plasma-exchange transfusion. *Blood.* 1979;54:694–702.

30. McLeod BC, ed. *Apheresis: Principles and Practice.* 2nd ed. Bethesda, MD: AABB Press, 2003.

31. Smith JW, Weinstein R, Hillyer KL, et al. Therapeutic apheresis: a summary of current indication categories endorsed by the AABB and the American Society for Apheresis. *Transfusion* 2003;43: 820–822.

32. White NJ. The treatment of malaria. *N Engl J Med* 1996;335:800–806.

25

Hemochromatosis

Susan F. Leitman and Charles D. Bolan

Hereditary hemochromatosis (HH) is an autosomal recessive disorder caused by inappropriate dietary absorption of iron and abnormal iron cycling. HH is characterized by progressive accumulation of iron in tissues, particularly the liver, pancreas, heart, endocrine organs, and skin, which may lead to end-stage organ damage during or after middle age (1–3). HH is one of the most common inherited disorders in whites of northern European descent, with an incidence of 1 in 200 and a carrier rate of 1 in 10 persons. However, although the homozygous hemochromatosis genotype is relatively common, the clinical penetrance of the disorder is highly variable, and only a minority of affected persons develop severe or life-threatening organ dysfunction (4,5).

GENETIC BASIS FOR HEREDITARY HEMOCHROMATOSIS: HFE MUTATIONS

- Mutations in HFE, a major histocompatibility complex (MHC) class I-like gene on chromosome 6, are found in nearly 90% of persons with the clinical phenotype and 100% of affected persons with a strong family history (6,7).
- Substitution of tyrosine for cysteine at amino acid 282 of the HFE gene product (C282Y) is the founder mutation; linkage disequilibrium studies are consistent with its origin within the past 2000 years. C282Y occurs with highest frequency in northwestern European populations, reaching 14% in areas of Great Britain (Table 25-1). Allele frequency decreases in a north-to-south and west-to-east direction across Europe, suggesting that the ancestral haplotype is of Viking or Celtic origin; it is extremely rare in African and Asian populations. Homozygosity for C282Y occurs in 64% to 96% of persons with clinical hemochromatosis.
- A second HFE mutation, replacement of histidine by aspartate at residue 63 of the HFE protein (H63D) is frequently found on the non-C282Y–containing chromosome of persons with clinical hemochromatosis who are heterozygous for C282Y (6). H63D is an older mutation with a wider population distribution, having an allele frequency of 5% to 14% throughout Europe and Asia. H63D is a genetic polymorphism without apparent clinical impact unless another genetic or environmental process is present. Compound heterozygosity for C282Y/H63D is seen in 4% to 7% of persons with a hemochromatosis phenotype.
- Seventeen additional polymorphisms in HFE have been described. Of these, only the S65C mutation appears to cause mild iron overload when present in a compound heterozygous state with C282Y or H63D.

PATHOPHYSIOLOGY

Because iron excretion in the gut is fixed at 1 mg per day, normal iron balance must be maintained by meticulous control of iron absorption in the intestine and iron release from macrophages. These are modulated in response to body iron stores and the erythropoietic demand for iron.

TABLE. 25–1. *Frequency of HFE genotypes in the U.S. white population*

Genotype	Frequency (percent)
C282Y/C282Y	1 in 200 (0.5%)
C282Y/wt	1 in 7 to 12 (8 to 14%)
H63D/H63D	1 in 40 (2.5%)
H63D/wt	1 in 4 (25%)
S65C/wt	1 in 25 (4%)

wt, wild-type.

Iron Homeostasis

The distribution of body iron is shown in Table 25-2, with a comparison of iron stores in the normal state and in subjects with hemochromatosis.

- *Excess iron and tissue injury.* When the capacity for iron storage is exceeded, excess tissue iron causes cellular damage by catalyzing the formation of oxyradicals (8). Oxidative damage to lipids, proteins, carbohydrates, and DNA may lead to widespread impairment in cell function and integrity. In particular, lipid peroxidation may result in impaired membrane-dependent mitochondrial and lysosomal function. Oxidative injury to DNA, particularly in hepatocytes, predisposes to mutagenesis and cancer.
- *Nontransferrin-bound iron (NTBI)* represents "free iron in serum." NTBI enters cells freely, independent of receptor-mediated uptake. NTBI levels are low or undetectable at a transferrin saturation below 40%, and increase linearly with transferrin saturation above 40% to 50%. NTBI and its intracellular labile iron counterpart may be the direct mediators of oxidant stress (8).

HFE Localization and Function

HFE is highly expressed in Kupffer cells of the liver and in tissue macrophages. In the gut, HFE is differentially expressed in duodenal crypt (precursor) versus apical (absorptive) cells (9). In its normal configuration, HFE binds to β_2-microglobulin (β_2m), allowing expression of HFE/β_2m on the cell surface (10). On the cell membrane, HFE forms a stable complex with the transferrin receptor (TfR), where it may modulate transport of iron from plasma into the cell through endocytosis of diferric transferrin bound to the HFE/β_2m/TfR complex. The

TABLE. 25–2. *Body iron distribution (g)*

	Men	Women
Hemoglobin (red cells)	3.0	2.4
Storage iron (liver)	1.0	0.4
Myoglobin and respiratory enzymes (muscle)	0.3	0.2
Total non-HH adult	4.4	3.1
Total HH adult	5–20	4–10

HH, hereditary hemochromatosis.

C282Y mutation prevents formation of a disulfide bond in HFE, disabling β_2m binding, and preventing cell surface expression. In contrast, the H63D mutation allows cell surface expression of HFE and complexing to TfR, but may impair HFE interaction with other proteins.

The exact mechanism by which the HFE/β_2m/TfR complex regulates intestinal iron absorption is unclear; two models have been proposed.

Crypt Programming Model

Dietary iron absorption occurs mainly in the duodenum. Duodenal crypt cells express HFE, but expression is lost as crypt cells migrate to the villus tip and differentiate into absorptive enterocytes. One model holds that HFE facilitates cellular uptake of plasma iron in duodenal crypt cells through the TfR-mediated pathway, modulating the regulatory iron pool in crypt cells, and affecting the translation and transcription of iron transport proteins such as the divalent metal transporter (DMT1) on the apical surface and ferroportin on the basolateral surface of the mature villus enterocyte (9). The HFE/TfR interaction thus serves as a sensing mechanism of body iron stores, capable of programming the absorptive capacity of villus enterocytes through its effect on the labile iron pool in undifferentiated crypt cells.

Hepcidin Model

Hepcidin is a peptide hormone made in the liver that acts predominately on mature villus enterocytes and reticuloendothelial macrophages to limit iron release. It acts in part by decreasing the expression of the major cell–surface iron export molecule, ferroportin. High hepcidin levels reduce intestinal iron absorption and macrophage iron release, and are associated causally in the anemia of chronic disease. Reduced hepcidin levels allow greater intestinal iron absorption and egress of iron from macrophages. Although hepcidin is ordinarily induced by dietary iron loading, its expression is inappropriately reduced in patients with HH (11). Patients homozygous for null mutations in HAMP, the gene encoding hepcidin, have a severe iron overload phenotype identical to that of patients with HH. HFE may exert its effects predominantly as an inducer of hepcidin expression in the liver, while hepcidin functions as a downstream effector, decreasing intestinal iron transport at the enterocyte level. Missense HFE mutations result in reduced hepcidin expression, leading to intestinal iron hyperabsorption and reticuloenbdothelial iron depletion, as seen in HH. In this model, it might be possible to treat hemochromatosis by hepcidin replacement. The allele frequency of the most prevalent HAMP mutation is 0.3%. Heterozygosity for hepcidin mutations can worsen iron overload and elicit a hemochromatosis phenotype in persons heterozygous for C282Y.

Classification of Iron Overload Disorders

Hemochromatosis related to HFE mutations is commonly referred to as classic, genetic, or HFE hemochromatosis, but there are other genetic forms of iron overload and secondary forms of hemochromatosis as well (Table 25-3). The most common form of secondary hemochromatosis is transfusional iron overload: 1 mL of red cells contains approximately 1 mg of iron. Inappropriate absorption of iron in the gut may also occur in association with ineffective erythropoiesis, worsening the iron overload that accompanies transfusions in these settings.

CLINICAL FEATURES AND DIAGNOSIS

Prior to the availability of biochemical and genetic screening tests, hemochromatosis was most commonly identified by damage to the liver, pancreas, heart, and joints, and diagnosed by demonstrating increased iron stores on liver biopsy. The classic triad of cirrhosis, diabetes, and skin pigmentation appeared in many publications and textbooks (1). Patients typically presented with:

TABLE. 25–3. *Classification of iron overload disorders*

Primary (genetic) hemochromatosis	Secondary hemochromatosis
Type 1: Classic/hereditary hemochromatosis (*HFE* gene)	1. Transfusional siderosis
Type 2: Juvenile hemochromatosis (severe phenotype) *2a:* Hemojuvelin mutations (HJV gene, 1q-linked) *2b:* Hepcidin mutations (HAMP gene)	2. Congenital anemia with ineffective erythropoiesis (thalassemia, red cell enzyme deficiencies)
Type 3: Transferrin receptor-2 deficiency (TFR2 gene)	3. Acquired sideroblastic and dyserythroblastic anemias
Type 4: Ferroportin deficiency (IREG-1 gene)	
Type 5: African iron overload	

- Severe liver disease resulting from hepatic fibrosis, cirrhosis, or cancer.
- Cardiac failure and refractory arrythmias.
- Polyendocrine failure: insulin-dependent diabetes and hypogonadotrophic hypogonadism.
- Debilitating symmetric polyarthritis.
- Grayish skin pigmentation.

It is now recognized that this severe clinical phenotype is relatively rare, and only develops in 1% to 4% of untreated C282Y homozygotes over their lifetime (4). Approximately 40% to 60% of C282Y homozygote males and 60% to 80% of homozygote females will remain asymptomatic or minimally symptomatic throughout their lives, and of the roughly 40% to 50% who do develop symptoms that affect quality of life, arthritis, fatigue, and sexual dysfunction are the most common complaints (Table 25-4) (12,13).

New Diagnostic Definition

In the current era of molecular testing, and with recognition of significant variability in clinical penetrance of the homozygous genotype, the diagnosis of hemochromatosis is now established by the detection of two mutated HFE alleles. This definition does not require active symptoms or signs of illness or the presence of iron overload. Four stages of the disorder are recognized (14):

1. Genetic predisposition with no other abnormality (age 0 to 20, 0 to 5 g of tissue iron storage).
2. Iron overload without symptoms (age older than 20, more than 5 g of iron storage).
3. Iron overload with early symptoms (age older than 30, more than 8 g of iron storage).
4. Iron overload with organ damage (age older than 40, 10 to 20 g of iron storage).

TABLE. 25–4. *Clinical Features of Hereditary Hemochromatosis: Historical versus Current*

Historical description	Current common presentation
Liver disease	Fatigue
Skin "bronzing"	Arthropathy
Diabetes	Impotence (men)

Common Clinical Presentation

The most common clinical presentation of HH is with nonspecific symptoms. Practitioners should have a low threshold for ordering serum transferrin saturation and ferritin studies in patients with unexplained chronic fatigue, arthralgia or arthritis, sexual dysfunction, hepatomegaly, or elevated liver function studies (alanine aminotransferase [ALT] and aspartate aminotransferase [AST]). Such symptoms are easily overlooked. The single most common event currently leading to a diagnosis of HH is the incidental detection of an abnormal laboratory test result, either an elevated transferrin saturation, serum ferritin, and/or ALT or AST.

Typical findings related to the most common clinical signs and symptoms of hemochromatosis are shown in Table 25-5. It is difficult to assign a frequency to these symptoms, because there is a continuum of increasing occurrence with age, and for male versus female gender (14).

TABLE. 25–5. *Clinical and Laboratory Features of Hereditary Hemochromatosis (C282Y Homozygotes)*

Sign/Symptom	Frequency	Features
Fatigue	30–50%	May be related to liver disease, endocrine dysfunction.
Arthritis	30–60%	Major feature affecting quality of life; symmetric, degenerative noninflammatory osteoarthritis; characteristic radiographic features: sclerosis of joint margins, narrowing of joint space, subchondral cysts, osteophytes, osteopenia. Chondrocalcinosis (pseudogout) and gout more common than in non-HH population. Disproportionate involvement of hands and feet, with MCP and MTP joints commonly affected. Hip replacement more common than in age-adjusted non-HH population.
Sexual dysfunction	30–50%	Excess iron deposited in anterior pituitary and testes. Reduced shaving, loss of libido, failure of ejaculation, impotence, gynecomastia in men. Low free testosterone levels, inappropriately low LH and FSH. Testosterone replacement therapy may restore libido and potency.
Skin changes	10–20%	Grayish or gray-brown hue; bronzing is rare. Portal
Hepatomegaly	10–20%	circulation leads directly from GI tract to liver; liver is first site of iron deposition; hepatic iron loading precedes other organs. 70% of all HH-related deaths are due to liver disease.
Hypothyroidism	10–15%	Primary hypothyroidism; thyroid gland fibrotic; elevated TSH
Elevated TS	>80%	TS >50% in 94% of men and 82% of women >age 40 years
Elevated ferritin	>60%	Ferritin >normal in 90% of men and 60% of women >age 40
Elevated ALT	10–25%	Influenced by other factors: alcohol, drugs, obesity

ALT, alanine transaminase; FSH, follicle-stimulating hormone; GI, gastrointestinal; HH, hereditary hemochromatosis; LH, lutenizing hormone; MCP, metacarpal-phalangeal joint; MTP, metatarsal-phalangeal joints; TS, transferrin saturation.

TABLE. 25–6. *Factors Influencing Clinical Penetrance*

Factors that accelerate iron overload and organ damage	Factors that lessen iron overload
Environmental/lifestyle	
Alcohol use	Blood donation
Oral iron supplementation	Multiparity/menorrhagia (women)
Dietary habits (meat-rich diet)	Dietary habits (vegetarian diet, tea)
Exogenous estrogen, vitamin C	
Genetic/Acquired Disorders	
Hepatitis B or C infection (HBV, HCV)	
Nonalcoholic steatohepatitis (NASH)	
Porphyria cutanea tarda (PCT)	
Alpha-1 anti-trypsin deficiency (AAT)	
Mutations in hepcidin, ferroportin, transferrin receptor, other genes	

The considerable variability in clinical penetrance of C282Y homozygosity, both in rate of accumulation of iron stores and appearance of organ dysfunction, may be the result of environmental, lifestyle, and genetic factors (Table 25-6).

LABORATORY TESTING

Once the clinical suspicion of hemochromatosis is raised, the diagnosis should be confirmed by laboratory testing, including:

1. Confirmatory laboratory tests

- *Serum iron, transferrin, and transferrin saturation:* transferrin is the major iron transport protein in plasma. Several assay methods for transferrin saturation exist: most accurate is direct colorimetric analysis of serum iron (SI) combined with nephelometric assay of transferrin, wherein transferrin saturation = molar concentration of iron divided by twice the molar concentration of transferrin. Less expensive but also less robust methods include chemical analyses of total serum iron binding capacity (TIBC) and unbound iron capacity (UIBC). Saturation of serum iron binding capacity is measured by dividing the serum iron by either TIBC (SI/TIBC) or by the sum of iron and UIBC [(SI)/(SI + UIBC)]. Normal range for transferrin saturation is 15% to 40%.
- *Serum ferritin:* major intracellular iron storage protein; measured immunologically. Estimates degree of iron overload and size of mobilizable iron stores (1 μg/L ferritin = 7 to 8 mg stored iron; e.g., 1,000 μg/L ferritin = 7,000 to 8,000 mg stored iron). Used to determine pace of initial phlebotomy therapy. Normal levels less than 300 μg/L in men, less than 200 μg/L in women.
- *HFE genotype:* definitive diagnostic test, assesses predisposition to serious illness, useful for family counseling.

2. Ancillary laboratory tests

- *Hepatic aminotransferase (ALT):* to assess degree of liver injury.
- *Blood counts:* obtain baseline hemoglobin and red cell mean corpuscular volume (MCV), which will be monitored during therapy (decrease in MCV is an accurate indicator of iron-limited erythropoiesis).

- *Blood glucose and electrolytes.*
- *Total and free testosterone:* as indicated by symptoms.
- *Thyroid function tests:* as indicated by symptoms.
- α-*Fetoprotein:* as baseline for subsequent surveillance monitoring for liver cancer.
- *Serologic tests for exposure to hepatitis B and C (HBsAg and anti-HCV):* active viral hepatitis worsens liver injury; useful to guide vaccine administration.

Role of Liver Biopsy

Liver biopsy, the historic gold standard, is generally not required for diagnosis. The diagnosis is now more safely and reliably made with use of the HFE genotype (14).

Indications for Biopsy

1. For prognosis, to confirm high clinical suspicion of cirrhosis:
   a. Ferritin greater than 3,000 μg/L.
   b. Hepatomegaly and/or signs of portal hypertension (large spleen, low platelets).
   c. ALT does not normalize with phlebotomy.
2. If concomitant hepatitis B virus (HBV) or hepatitis C virus (HCV) infection present.
3. In diagnostic evaluation of markedly elevated ferritin and ALT, with normal HFE genotype and absence of other genetic causes listed above.

Histologic Findings

1. Marked increase in hepatocellular iron, with relative sparing of Kupffer cells. Iron is distributed in a decreasing gradient from the periportal to the centrolobular areas.
2. With progressive damage, may see portal fibrous expansion, bridging fibrosis with piecemeal necrosis, and macro or micronodular cirrhosis.
3. Hepatic iron index (hepatic iron concentration/$56 \times$ age) greater than 1.9 (in the absence of transfusional siderosis) strongly suggests iron overload due to HH rather than other causes.

Radiographic and Other Tests

- *Skeletal x-rays:* performed to evaluate symptomatic joints.
- *Liver ultrasound:* useful in evaluation of non-HH causes of elevated ferritin; may show steatosis. Used in surveillance for liver cancer.
- *Computed tomography (CT) and/or magnetic resonance imaging (MRI) of liver:* not indicated diagnostically. Useful if liver cancer is suspected.
- *Superconducting quantum interference device (SQUID) assessment:* provides most sensitive noninvasive assessment of iron stores; limited availability.

POPULATION SCREENING

The clinical course of HH meets the definition of a disorder for which population screening should be performed (2,3):

1. High prevalence in selected populations.
2. Burden of disease (clinical penetrance) sufficient to warrant medical and public attention.
3. Prolonged presymptomatic phase, during which detection and treatment lead to reductions in morbidity and mortality (early detection prevents complications and improves outcomes).

4. Availability of reliable, accurate, easily available, and inexpensive screening tests.
5. Treatment is effective, safe, inexpensive, and easily accessible.

Thus, the costs of widespread testing and preventative treatment are considered favorable: screening is more effective and less expensive than delaying identification and therapy until the development of late symptoms. This is particularly true when early, presenting symptoms are nonspecific, often not recognized as being caused by HH, and associated with a 5 to 10 year delay until accurate diagnosis.

Laboratory Screening

- *Transferrin saturation:* The single best screening test is the serum transferrin saturation. It is inexpensive, widely available, and highly sensitive and specific for the presence of the C282Y HFE allele (15). The decision threshold at which confirmatory testing should be initiated ranges from transferrin saturation values of 45% to 62%, depending on whether sensitivity or specificity is preferred (Table 25-7). Because transferrin saturation is affected by dietary and diurnal variation, an elevated valued should be confirmed by a second transferrin saturation after an overnight fast, in the absence of oral iron supplements. Phenotype screening with transferrin saturation is not advised until age 20 to 30, because iron burdens are generally low below this age (14). An algorithm for evaluation of persons detected through screening programs is shown in Figure 25-1.
- *Ferritin screening:* Ferritin is an acute phase reactant; levels rise with inflammation, infection, non-HH liver disease, and hemolysis. The ferritin is neither sensitive nor specific enough to be used as a screening test.
- *Genotype screening:* A 1998 consensus conference decided against widespread population screening by genetic testing. The high cost of genetic tests and the variable clinical penetrance of HH, coupled with concerns over stigmatization, discrimination, and insurability, led to this conclusion (16).

Screening of Family Members of C282Y Homozygotes

- *Screening of children:* The most cost-effective test is HFE genotype; biochemical screening is also acceptable; testing should be delayed until age 20 to 30. If more than two children are involved, the best approach may be genotyping of the other parent (17).
- *Screening of siblings:* All siblings should be counseled to undergo either genetic or phenotypic screening. The most cost-effective test is HFE genotype, but phenotypic screening with combination of transferrin saturation and ferritin is also acceptable (17).

TABLE. 25-7. *Diagnostic Yield of Transferrin Saturation (TS) Screening*

Gender	TS Decision Threshold (%)	Sensitivity (Detection rate)	Specificity (False positive)
Male	≥50	94%	7%
	≥60	86%	1.5%
Female	≥50	82%	5%
	≥60	67%	0.6%

Further evaluation is recommended if transferrin saturation is greater than 55–62% in men and greater than 45–50% in women.

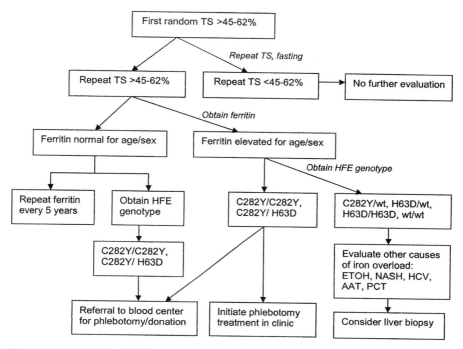

FIG. 25-1. Decision Tree for Hemochromatosis Population Screening. AAT, alpha-1 antitrypsin; HCV, hepatitis C virus; NASH, nonalcoholic steatohepatitis; PCT, porphyria cutanea tarda.

TREATMENT

Phlebotomy Therapy

- Phlebotomy: periodic removal of 1 unit (500 mL) of whole blood. Safe, inexpensive, standard of care for past 50 years (18). One unit of whole blood removes 200 to 250 mg of iron. Double red cell collection by apheresis removes 360 mL of packed red cells (400 to 420 mg of iron) and may be particularly useful in blood center setting.
- Controversy regarding treatment indications for subjects with modest iron burdens.
  - Patients generally desire treatment and are eager to be blood donors.
  - Therapy safe, accessible, prevents late organ damage.
  - Referral to blood center shifts argument in favor of treatment (double benefit to subject and to community).

Guidelines for Phlebotomy Therapy

Phase 1: Iron Depletion

- *Pace:* Initiate phlebotomy at 1 to 4 week intervals, depending on ferritin, hemoglobin, ALT, gender, and weight. As iron depletion approaches, decrease to monthly.
- *Target of "de-ironing" therapy:* several assays may be used.
  - Ferritin less than 30 μg/L.
  - Transferrin saturation less than 30%.
  - Decrease in red cell mean corpuscular volume (MCV) to 3% below prephlebotomy level (19).

- *Monitoring parameters*
  - Prephlebotomy fingerstick hemoglobin or hematocrit (with or without venous complete blood count [CBC]) at each visit.
  - Ferritin every 4 to 8 weeks initially, then ferritin and transferrin saturation every 1 to 2 treatments once ferritin is less than 100 μg/L.
- *Safety guide:* threshold hemoglobin for therapeutic bleed 12.5 g/dL or more (hematocrit 38% or higher). In general, do not bleed below this level; defer therapy for 1 to 4 weeks until hemoglobin recovers. Iron deficiency is not necessary; anemia should be avoided.
- *General guide:* for initial ferritin 500 to 1500, patients generally require between 15 to 30 phlebotomies to achieve iron depletion. If ferritin greater than 2,000 μg/dL, may require more than 50 bleeds.

Phase II: Preventing Reaccumulation (Maintenance)

- *Pace:* 500 mL removed every 8 to 26 weeks (mean, 10 to 12 weeks), depending on gender, weight, age, dietary habits. This is usually a lifelong requirement, although some subjects reaccumulate iron very slowly.
- *Goal of maintenance therapy*
  - Ferritin, 20 to 50 μg/L.
  - Transferrin saturation less than 45%.
  - Hemoglobin greater than 12.5 g/dL.
- *Monitoring parameters*
  - Prephlebotomy fingerstick hemoglobin or hematocrit (with or without venous CBC) at each visit, and transferrin saturation and/or ferritin every 1 to 2 treatments.

Evaluation of Anemia During Phlebotomy Therapy

Persistent hemoglobin less than 12.5 g/dL despite elevated ferritin levels may have an endocrine cause and should be evaluated with thyroid function studies and testosterone levels (in men). If concomitant disorders of erythroid production are present (thalassemia, renal insufficiency) and urgent need for phlebotomy exists, weekly erythropoietin may be helpful. Anemia may also be caused by the development of liver cancer.

Arthritis, Endocrine Replacement, Vaccinations, and Cancer Surveillance

- *Arthritis:* responds moderately well to nonsteroidal anti-inflammatory agents.
  - Joint aspiration to rule out gout or pseudogout in acutely inflamed joints.
  - Orthopedic evaluation for joint replacement for chronic, debilitating hip or knee pain.
- *Testosterone replacement:* consider in males with symptomatic sexual dysfunction and low testosterone levels.
- *Hepatitis A virus (HAV) and HBV vaccination:* should be given as prophylaxis against future hepatic injury in unexposed patients.
- α-*Fetoprotein and liver ultrasound:* surveillance for hepatocellular cancer. Repeat every 6 months if cirrhosis documented by biopsy.

Dietary and Lifestyle Counseling

- Avoid oral iron supplements.
- Limit alcohol intake.
- Red meat in moderation, but major change in dietary habits not required. Iron stores are most efficiently controlled by adjusting frequency of bleeds rather than reducing intake of iron-rich foods.
- Avoid raw shellfish until iron depletion achieved to prevent *vibrio vulnificus* infection.
- If ALT elevated:

• Discontinue alcohol intake until iron depletion completed and ALT normal.
• Consider discontinuation of medications with potential hepatic toxicity.

PROGNOSIS AND RESPONSE TO THERAPY

If cirrhosis is not present, long-term survival is unchanged from the non-HH population (20). If cirrhosis is present, risk of hepatic cancer is increased and persists for life; 18.5% of subjects with cirrhosis will develop liver cancer, which may not be detected until 5 to 10 years after iron depletion. Overall incidence of hepatic cancer is 100-fold greater in HH than non-HH subjects and accounts for 10% to 30% of HH-related deaths. Progression of cirrhosis due to HH is slower than in other types of cirrhosis (alcoholic, viral); however, HH subjects undergoing liver transplant for end stage liver disease or liver cancer have a higher peritransplant mortality.

The response to phlebotomy varies by tissue site (Table 25-8).

HEMOCHROMATOSIS SUBJECTS AS BLOOD DONORS

• *Regulatory issues.* FDA allows blood centers to obtain a variance from federal code to permit blood from HH subjects to be made available for transfusion into others, even if collected more frequently than 56 day-interval allowed for non-HH donors.
• *FDA requirements:* Phlebotomy must be performed under a physician's direction, without charge regardless of whether subjects qualify as donors, and with periodic laboratory monitoring.
• *Logistics and safety (19)*
  • Seventy-five percent of all HH subjects meet allogeneic donor eligibility criteria.
  • Fifty-five percent of HH subjects were blood donors prior to knowledge of their diagnosis.
  • Potential HH-donor contribution estimated at 1 to 2 million red cell units per year.
  • Recent rapid increase in number of U.S. blood centers with Food and Drug Administation (FDA)-approved variances to allow HH subjects to be blood donors (57 centers, May 2004).
  • HH subjects documented to be safe, reliable donors.
• *Advantages of phlebotomy care in the blood center*
  • Treatment is free, consistent, accessible, convenient.
  • Increased patient satisfaction: avoid frustration of knowing blood will be discarded.
  • Alleviate national blood shortages.

TABLE. 25–8. *Response to Phlebotomy Therapy in Hereditary Hemochromatosis*

Complication	Prevents	Reverses or Improves
Arthropathy	Unknown	Partly, if initiated early in course
Fatigue	Yes	Yes, to a variable degree
Skin greying	Yes	Yes
Liver fibrosis	Yes	Partly, if initiated early in course
Cirrhosis	Yes	No; but portal hypertension may improve
Cardiomyopathy	Yes	Partly, if initiated early in course
Diabetes	Yes	No
Hypogonadism	Yes	No
Hypothyroidism	Yes	No

FUTURE CHALLENGES

The process of molecular discovery is rapidly leading to a more comprehensive understanding of role of the HFE protein in iron homeostasis. At the same time, availability of a genetic test is focusing increased public and medical attention on hemochromatosis. Large population screening studies are currently in progress to more accurately determine clinical penetrance, both for early as well as late complications. Increased emphasis on educational campaigns to foster prompt recognition of early symptoms by primary care providers should complement or even alleviate the need for targeted screening programs. Better appreciation of the advantages of referral to the blood center should improve the quality and accessibility of care and also confer a benefit to the general public health.

REFERENCES

1. Bothwell TH, MacPhail AP. Hereditary hemochromatosis: etiologic, pathologic, and clinical aspects. *Semin Hematol* 1998;35:55–71.
2. Bomford A. Genetics of hemochromatosis. *Lancet* 2002;360:1673–1681.
3. Tavill AS. Diagnosis and management of hemochromatosis: AASLD practice guidelines. *Hepatology* 2001;33:1321–1328.
4. Beutler E. Penetrance in hereditary hemochromatosis. The HFE Cys282Tyr mutation as a necessary but not sufficient cause of clinical hereditary hemochromatosis. *Blood* 2003;101:3347–3350.
5. Ajioka R, Kushner JP. Clinical consequences of iron overload in hemochromatosis patients. *Blood* 2003;101:3351–3354.
6. Feder JN, Gnirke A, Thomas W, et al. A novel MHC class I-like gene is mutated in patients with hereditary haemochromatosis. *Nat Genet* 1996;13:399–408.
7. Jazwinska EC, Cullen LM, Busfiled F, et al. Haemochromatosis and HLA-H. *Nat Genet* 1996;14:249–251.
8. Brissot P, Loreal O. Role of non-transferrin bound iron in the pathogenesis of iron overload and toxicity. In: Hershko C, ed. *Iron Chelation Therapy*. New York: Kluwer Academic/Plenum Publishers, 2002:45–53.
9. Roy CN, Enns CA. Iron homeostasis: new tales from the crypt. *Blood* 2000;96:4020–4027.
10. Feder JN, Penny DM, Irrinki A, et al. The hemochromatosis gene product complexes with the transferrin receptor and lowers its affinity for ligand binding. *Proc Natl Acad Sci USA* 1998;95:1472–1477.
11. Bridle KR, Frazer DM, Wilkins SJ, et al. Disrupted hepcidin regulation in HFE-associated haemochromatosis and the liver as a regulator of body iron homeostasis. *Lancet* 2003;361:669–673.
12. Olynyk JK, Cullen DJ, Aquilia S, et al. A population-based study of the clinical expression of the hemochromatosis gene. *N Engl J Med* 1999;341:718–724.
13. Bulaj ZJ, Ajioka RS, Phillips JD, et al. Disease-related conditions in relatives of patients with hemochromatosis. *N Engl J Med* 2000;343:1529–1535.
14. Adams P. Brissot P, Powell LW. EASL International Consensus Conference on Haemochromatosis—Part II. Expert document. *J Hepatol* 2000;33:487–496.
15. Bradley LA, Haddow JE, Palomaki GE: Population screening for hemochromatosis: expectations based on a study of relatives of symptomatic probands. *J Med Screen* 1996;3:171–177.
16. Burke W, Thomson E, Khoury MJ, et al. Hereditary hemochromatosis. Gene discovery and its implications for population-based screening. *JAMA* 1998;280:172–178.
17. El-Serag HB, Inadomi JM, Kowdley KV. Screening for hereditary hemochromatosis in siblings and children of affected patients. *Ann Intern Med* 2000;132:261–269.
18. Barton JC, McDonnell SM, Adams PC, et al. Management of hemochromatosis. *Ann Intern Med* 1998;129:932–939.
19. Leitman SF, Browning JN, Yau YY, et al. Hemochromatosis subjects as allogeneic blood donors: a prospective study. *Transfusion* 2003;43:1538–1544.
20. Niederau C, Fischer R, Purschel A, et al. Long-term survival in patients with hereditary hemochromatosis. *Gastroenterology* 1996;110:1107–1119.

26

Consultative Hematology

Pierre Noel

HEMATOLOGIC COMPLICATIONS OF PREGNANCY

Anemia in Pregnancy

During normal pregnancies, plasma volume increases by 40% to 60% and red cell mass increases by 20% to 40% (1). The hematocrit typically decreases to 30% to 32%, the lower limit of normal for hemoglobin decreases to 11 g/dL in the first trimester and 10 g/dL in the second and third trimesters. The most common forms of anemia of pregnancy in North America are iron- and folate-deficiency anemias.

One thousand milligrams of additional iron are required during pregnancy. The normal 500-mg iron storage pool is insufficient and iron-deficiency anemia develops unless iron supplementation occurs throughout pregnancy (300 mg ferrous sulfate daily). Low values of serum iron and ferritin are reliable indicators of iron deficiency in pregnancy. The consequences of maternal iron deficiency on the neonate are controversial. Mild to moderate maternal iron deficiency anemia is not associated with significant anemia in the fetus.

Folate needs are increased during pregnancy. Folate deficiency is associated with anemia, neural tube defects, and cleft palate. Neural tube closure occurs during the fourth week of pregnancy; folate supplementation needs to be given prior to conception to prevent neural tube defects. Most prenatal vitamins contain both folate and iron.

Sickle Cell Disease in Pregnancy

Women with sickle cell anemia are part of the high-risk pregnancy group. With modern obstetric and perinatal care, maternal mortality is less than 1% and perinatal mortality is less than 15%.

Prophylactic red cell transfusions are associated with fewer maternal painful episodes but they have no impact on maternal morbidity, birth weight, gestational age, fetal distress, or perinatal mortality.

Maintenance transfusions should be given to women who are symptomatic of vaso-occlusive or anemia-related problems or when signs of fetal distress are present.

Thrombocytopenia in Pregnancy

The platelet count decreases by approximately 10% during pregnancy, most of this decrease occurs in the third trimester. The most common cause of thrombocytopenia is incidental thrombocytopenia of pregnancy (75%) (2), followed by thrombocytopenia complicating hypertensive disorders of pregnancy (20%), and finally immunologic disorders of pregnancy (5%).

Thrombocytopenia of less than 100,000 per microliter in the first trimester of pregnancy is most consistent of immune thrombocytopenic purpura. Thrombocytopenia of over 70,000 per microliter occurring late during the second trimester or during the third trimester in the absence of hypertension or proteinuria, most likely represents incidental thrombocytopenia of pregnancy. Platelet-associated immunoglobulin (Ig) G are elevated in both incidental thrombocytopenia of pregnancy and immune thrombocytopenic purpura.

It is important in any patient with thrombocytopenia to consider human immunodeficiency virus (HIV), systemic lupus erythematosus, and thrombocytopenia associated with antiphospholipd antibodies in the differential diagnosis.

Incidental Thrombocytopenia of Pregnancy

The platelet count in incidental thrombocytopenia usually remains above 100,000 per microliter. Incidental thrombocytopenia usually develops in the third trimester and is not associated with neonatal thrombocytopenia. The likelihood of a more serious cause of thrombocytopenia increases once the platelet count decreases below 70,000 per microliter. The pathogenesis of incidental thrombocytopenia is not clearly defined, but may involve a combination of hemodilution and decreased platelet half-life.

Incidental thrombocytopenia remains a diagnosis of exclusion. The diagnosis is made by observing no other physical or laboratory abnormality in patients with no antecedent history of immune thrombocytopenia. Women with incidental thrombocytopenia should receive standard obstetrical care.

Immune Thrombocytopenic Purpura

Immune thrombocytopenic purpura (ITP) is the most common cause of severe thrombocytopenia in the first trimester. An antecedent history of ITP or autoimmune disorder makes the diagnosis more likely. The nadir platelet count in ITP usually occurs in the third trimester.

Patients with platelet counts greater than 20,000 per microliter and no evidence of bruising or mucosal bleeding generally do not require treatment in the first two trimesters of pregnancy. A platelet count of greater than 50,000 per microliter is considered safe for normal vaginal delivery or cesarean section. Although there is no consensus, a platelet count of greater than 80,000 per microliter is felt to be sufficient for epidural anesthesia. The bleeding time is not an accurate predictor of risk of bleeding in these situations.

Optimal first-line therapy for ITP in pregnant patients is controversial. Corticosteroids are the least expensive option, but they have been associated with pregnancy-induced hypertension, gestational diabetes, osteoporosis, excessive weight gain, and premature rupture of fetal membranes. Ninety percent of the administered dose of prednisone is metabolized by the placenta; serious fetal side effects are unlikely. Prednisone is initiated at a dose of 1 mg/kg per day (based on the prepregnancy weight) and subsequently tapered to the minimum hemostatically effective dose. Intravenous immunoglobulin (IVIg) should be considered if the maintenance dose of prednisone is in excess of 10 mg per day. IVIg at a dose of 1 g/kg (based on prepregnancy weight) leads to a response in more than 60% of patients; the response lasts on average 1 month.

In patients refractory to corticosteroids and IVIg; splenectomy should be considered. Splenectomy is best performed in the second trimester of pregnancy. Splenectomy in the first trimester may induce labor and splenectomy in the third may be technically difficult. Splenectomy has been successfully performed laparoscopically during pregnancy. High-dose methylprednisolone and intravenous anti-D have been used in small series of refractory patients. Experience with immunosuppressive and cytotoxic agents during pregnancy is limited. Danazol and vinca alkaloids are best avoided. Interventions that elevate maternal platelet count are not effective in raising that of the fetus.

The use of nonsteroidal anti-inflammatory drugs should be avoided postpartum in patients with platelet counts less than 100,000 per microliter. Thromboprophylaxis should be considered in all women with a platelet count greater than 50,000 per microliter; if they have undergone surgical delivery, are immobilized for a prolonged amount of time or have acquired or congenital thrombophilia.

Neonatal mortality is less than 1% in ITP; 5% of neonates will have a platelet count of less than 20,000 per microliter. Most hemorrhagic events in neonates occur 24 to 48 hours after delivery at the nadir of the platelet count. There is no evidence that cesarean section is safer for the neonate than vaginal delivery. The mode of delivery should be decided on obstetric indications.

Maternal platelet count, maternal platelet antibody levels, or a history of maternal splenectomy for ITP are not accurate predictors of neonatal platelet counts. The most accurate predictor of fetal thrombocytopenia is a history of thrombocytopenia at delivery in a prior sibling. Fetal scalp blood sampling and cordocentesis have been abandoned.

A cord platelet count should be determined following delivery, in every neonate. Thrombocytopenic neonates should be followed closely following delivery, as the platelet count nadir may not occur before 2 to 5 days. Neonates presenting with clinical bleeding or a platelet count less than 20,000 per microliter should be managed with IVIg, 1 g/kg. Life-threatening bleeding can be treated with a combination of IVIg and platelet transfusions.

Preeclampsia and the HELLP Syndrome

Preeclampsia is defined as hypertension and proteinuria (greater than 300 mg of protein per 24 hours) occurring after 20 weeks of gestation. Preeclampsia occurs in 5% of all pregnancies, it accounts for 18% of maternal deaths in the United States, and is more frequent in nulliparous women or multiparous women with new partners. Thrombocytopenia develops in 50% of patients with preeclampsia. Endothelial damage and activation of the coagulation system with thrombin generation may be the pathophysiology. D-dimers and thrombin–antithrombin complexes are increased in patients with thrombocytopenia. Aspirin prophylaxis does not reduce the incidence of preeclampsia or HELLP.

The criteria for HELLP syndrome (*he*molysis, elevated *l*iver *e*nzymes, and *l*ow *p*latelets) include:

• Microangiopathic hemolytic anemia.
• Increased transaminases.
• Thrombocytopenia (less than 100,000 per microliter).

HELLP occurs in up to 10% of women with severe preeclampsia, usually occurs in white, multiparous women above the age of 25 years. Maternal mortality is 1% and fetal mortality is 10% to 20%. Fetal mortality is attributed to placental ischemia, abruption of the placenta, immaturity, and intrauterine asphyxia. Neonatal thrombocytopenia can occur in both preeclampsia and HELLP. The mechanism of neonatal thrombocytopenia remains unclear. There is a 3% risk of recurrence of HELLP in subsequent pregnancies.

The definitive treatment for eclampsia and HELLP is delivery of the fetus. Management focuses on stabilization of the patient and maturation of the fetal lung. The presence of multiorgan dysfunction, fetal distress, or a gestational age greater than 34 weeks warrants immediate delivery. Coagulopathy resulting from preeclampsia-associated disseminated intravascular coagulation (DIC) occurs in 20% of patients. The clinical manifestations of preeclampsia and HELLP resolve within a few days of delivery. Rarely HELLP syndrome can present postpartum. If the manifestations worsen or persist after 1 or 2 days, plasma exchange is indicated.

Acute fatty liver of pregnancy (AFLP) is associated with hypertension and proteinuria in 50% of patients. Microangiopathic hemolytic anemia and thrombocytopenia are not prominent in this syndrome. Patients usually have a prolonged prothrombin time and low fibrinogen and antithrombin levels.

Thrombotic thrombocytopenic Purpura and Hemolytic Uremic Syndrome

Thrombotic thrombocytopenic purpura (TTP) and hemolytic uremic syndrome (HUS) occurs in only 0.004% of pregnancies. The classic pentad of symptoms of TPP include:

- Microangiopathic hemolytic anemia
- Thrombocytopenia
- Neurologic abnormalities
- Fever
- Renal dysfunction

The classic pentad is present in only 40% of patients. Pregnancy is a precipitating factor for TTP. The mean time of onset of TTP is 23.5 weeks of pregnancy. Plasma therapy is recommended for the management of the pregnant TTP patient. Delivery is recommended only for patients who do not respond to plasma exchange, pregnancy termination is not considered therapeutic in TTP or HUS.

Ultralarge von Willebrand factor (vWF) multimers are found in TTP; this is thought to be secondary to the deficiency of a specific vWF-cleaving protease, identified as ADAMTS13. The deficiency can be congenital or acquired. All cases of idiopathic TTP to date have been associated with severe protease deficiency; secondary TTP can occur in the context of a normal protease. Idiopathic TTP is associated with an IgG inhibitory autoantibody directed against ADAMTS13 in 60% of cases.

Reduced vWF-cleaving protease is not specific for TTP; reduced levels are seen in the third trimester of pregnancy, uremia, acute inflammation, malignancy and diffuse intravascular coagulation.

The mean time of onset of HUS is 26 days after delivery. Patients with HUS present with microangiopathic hemolytic anemia and acute renal failure. The vWF levels are usually elevated while multimer analysis may or may not show ultralarge multimers. Deficiency of vWF-cleaving protease is usually not associated with this syndrome.

Several women with a familial history of pregnancy-associated HUS have developed their first episode of HUS during pregnancy, and HUS has occurred in such patients with the use of oral contraceptives. Postpartum HUS is associated with a poor prognosis; plasma therapy is less effective in reversing renal failure, but a trial of plasma exchange is indicated. Dialysis and other supportive care measures may also need to be initiated (Table 26-1).

TABLE. 26–1. *Pregnancy-associated microangiopathies*

Diagnosis	Preeclampsia	HELLP	PP-HUS	TTP
Time of onset	>20 weeks	>34 weeks	Postpartum (90%)	<24 weeks
MAHA	No	Yes	Yes	Yes
Thrombocytopenia	Yes	Yes	Yes	Yes
Coagulopathy	No	20%	No	No
Renal failure	Rare	Rare	Yes	Possible
Liver disease	No	Yes	No	No
Hypertension	Yes	Possible	Possible	Possible
Effect of delivery on disease	Yes	Yes	None	None

HELLP syndrome, hemolysis, elevated liver enzymes, and low platelets; PP-HUS, postpartum hemolytic uremic syndrome; TTP, thrombotic thrombocytopenic purpura; MAHA, microangiopathic hemolytic anemia.

TABLE. 26–2. Causes of obstetrical disseminated intravascular coagulation

Placental abruption
Fetal death syndrome
Aminiotic fluid embolism
HELLP syndrome
Clostridial sepsis
Sepsis
Major obstetrical hemorrhage

HELLP syndrome, hemolysis, elevated liver enzymes, and low platelets.

Disseminated Intravascular Coagulation

Placental abruption is the most common cause of DIC (Table 26-2). Placental abruption has an increased incidence in cocaine addicts. Amniotic fluid embolism is associated with cardiopulmonary collapse and a mortality of 85%. The incidence of DIC complicating placental abruption and fetal death syndrome has decreased with advances in ultrasonography and prenatal care.

Fetal death syndrome is recognized by ultrasonography; delivery of the dead fetus removes the source of tissue thromboplastin release. Blood component support and the use of antithrombin III have been useful in the management of the coagulopathy.

Placental abruption is managed with blood component support followed by delivery. Antithrombin III and activated protein C have been used with success in this disorder.

Transient DIC occurs in patients undergoing hypertonic saline abortions; the DIC usually resolves once the fetus is delivered. Clostridial sepsis after abortions is associated with DIC and poor clinical outcome.

VENOUS THROMBOEMBOLISM IN PREGNANCY

The incidence of venous thromboembolism (VTE) (4) is increased twofold to fourfold during pregnancy and is higher in patients undergoing cesarean delivery. Proven deep venous thrombosis (DVT) occurs with similar frequency in each of the three trimesters. Venous thrombi occur predominantly in the left leg, partly because of the compression of the left iliac vein by the right iliac artery as they cross. Hemodynamic changes causing venous stasis and hypercoagulabity, most likely play a role in the increased risk of VTE during pregnancy. Hypercoagulability is thought to be secondary to an increase in fibrinogen, factor VIII, vWF, as well as a decrease in protein S, the development of acquired protein C resistance, and reduced fibrinolytic activity.

Inherited thrombophilias and antiphospholipid antibodies increase the risk of VTE during pregnancy.

Diagnosis of Venous Thromboembolism in Prgnancy

The diagnosis of VTE during pregnancy is complicated by the potential fetal oncogenicity and teratogenicity associated with the use of ionizing radiation for diagnostic purposes (5).

Compression ultrasonography (CU) of the entire proximal venous system to the trifurcation should be performed as the initial test for suspected deep vein thrombosis in pregnancy. A normal CU does not exclude a calf DVT. The CU needs to be repeated at day 2 and day 7 to rule out an extending calf-vein thrombosis. A limited venogram with fetal shielding can be used in equivocal cases. When iliac DVT is suspected, pulsed Doppler should be used. If the results of pulsed Doppler are negative or equivocal, magnetic resonance venography (MRV) or venography should be considered.

In patients with suspected pulmonary emboli (PE) during pregnancy a ventilation/perfusion (V/Q) lung scan should be performed. If the results of the V/Q scan are equivocal, bilateral compression ultrasounds should be performed. In cases where the diagnosis cannot be established by V/Q scan and CU, pulmonary angiography should be considered. There is controversy regarding the use of spiral computed tomography (CT) in pregnancy.

D-dimer levels increase with gestational age and during preterm labor as well as with abruptio placenta and gestational hypertension: these characterisitics reduce the test's usefulness during pregnancy.

Treatment of Venous Thromboembolism in Pregnancy

Unfractionated heparin (UFH), low molecular weight heparin (LMWH), and danaparoid do not cross the placenta; therefore the risk of fetal bleeding or teratogenicity is not present. Heparin-induced thrombocytopenia, bleeding and heparin-induced osteoporosis are more common with UFH than with LMWH.

Direct thrombin inhibitors such as hirudin and pentasaccharide have not been evaluated during pregnancy. Hirudin crosses the placenta; there is published data suggesting that pentasaccharide does not cross the placenta. Coumarin derivatives cross the placenta and have been associated with fetal bleeding and teratogenicity. Central nervous system abnormalities have been associated with the use of coumarin derivatives in every trimester of pregnancy. Nasal hypoplasia and/or stippled epiphyses have been associated with the use of coumarin derivatives between the sixth and twelfth week of pregnancy.

The activated partial thromboplastin time (aPTT) response to UFH is blunted in pregnancy because of increased factor VIII levels and increased heparin-binding proteins. This blunted response may lead to heparin overdosing. Measuring anti-FXa levels may obviate this problem. LMWH have less nonspecific binding to heparin-binding proteins, hence they have a more predictable dose-response than UFH.

UFH and LMWH are not secreted in breast milk. Clinical evidence suggests that warfarin sodium is not excreted in breast milk and that it is safe to breast-feed while taking warfarin sodium.

The initial dose of LMWH is based on the patient weight. Because of variation of weight and glomerular filtration rate during pregnancy it is recommended to monitor anticoagulation by performing monthly anti-Fxa levels. LMWH should be discontinued 24 hours prior to elective induction of labor and neuroaxial anesthesia. Intravenous UFH can be initiated in patients at high risk for thrombosis and discontinued 4 to 6 hours prior to the time of expected delivery. LMWH can usually be restarted within 12 hours of delivery.

UFH is usually initiated by an intravenous bolus followed by a continuous infusion. The continuous infusion is usually continued for 5 days prior to transitioning to adjusted-dose subcutaneous UFH. The aPTT should be maintained within therapeutic range. Anti-FXa levels can be obtained to prevent overanticoagulation. Adjusted-dose subcutaneous UFH can be used for the remainder of pregnancy with weekly midinterval monitoring of the aPTT. The subcutaneous heparin should be discontinued 24 hours prior to elective induction of labor. Intravenous UFH can be used in patients at high risk for thrombosis and discontinued 4 to 6 hours prior to the time of expected delivery. UFH can usually be restarted within 12 hours of delivery.

UFH or LMWH should be continued for at least 4 days after initiation of Coumadin and until the international normalized ratio (INR) has been therapeutic at 2.0 or more for 2 consecutive days.

TABLE. 26–3. *Most common thrombophilias*

Inherited
    Factor V Leiden
    Prothrombin G20210A mutation
        4G/4G mutation of the plasminogen activator inhibitor
            gene (PAI-I)
        Thermolabile variant of methylenetetrahydrofolate reductase,
            the most common cause of homocysteinemia.
    Antithrombin III deficiency
    Protein C deficiency
    Protein S deciciency
Acquired
    Antiphospholipid antibody

Prophylactic Anticoagulation in Patients with a Previous History of Venous Thromboembolism

More than half of thromboembolic events in pregnancy are related to thrombophilias (Table 26-3). Intrauterine fetal growth retardation, stillbirth, abruption, and severe pereclampsia have also been linked to thrombophilias; there are conflicting reports on the association between thrombophilias and recurrent early abortions (less than 10 weeks).

Patients with idiopathic VTE who are pregnant or plan to become pregnant should undergo screening for thrombophilias. Patients with history of fetal loss, abruption, severe preeclampsia, and intrauterine fetal growth retardation should also be screened for thrombophilias.

Patients with thrombophilia and an idiopathic VTE (not associated with a temporary risk factor such as surgery, trauma, prolonged immobilization) should be prophylactically anticoagulated during pregnancy as well as postpartum. The management of the pregnant patient with thrombophilia without a previous VTE is controversial; the evidence for prophylaxis is more compelling in patients with antithrombin III deficiency and in patients with antiphospholipid antibodies.

Thrombophilias and Recurrent Miscarriage

Recurrent miscarriage is defined as three consecutive spontaneous abortions of an intrauterine pregnancy of less than 20 weeks' gestation. Anticardiolipin antibodies have been linked with recurrent miscarriage. There are insufficient data to include inherited thrombophilias in the evaluation of women with recurrent miscarriage (6).

Prednisone, low-dose aspirin, UFH, LMWH, and IVIg have been used in the management of this problem. Prednisone was found to be equally effective to low dose subcutaneous UFH in preventing pregnancy loss but was associated with an increased incidence of side effects. UFH and aspirin are superior to aspirin alone in preventing pregnancy loss. Low molecular weight heparin can be used instead of UFH. The optimal dosage of UFH and LMWH remains to be defined.

HEMATOLOGIC MANIFESTATIONS OF TROPICAL DISEASE

Malaria

Anemia is a serious complication of malaria, especially *Plasmodium falciparum* infection. The prevalence and degree of anemia depends on the nutritional and immune status of the patient. Anemia cannot be explained entirely by intravascular rupture of parasitized red cells

TABLE. 26–4. *Causes of anemia in malaria*

Intravascular rupture of parasitized red cells
Hypersplenism
Autoimmune hemolysis (50% of patients have a
  positive direct Coombs')
Reticulocytopenia (anemia of chronic disease)
Dyserythropoiesis (cytokine-mediated)
Secondary bacterial, fungal or viral infections.
Nutritional anemias

(Table 26-4). *P. vivax,* and *P. ovale* invade only reticulocytes, *P. malaria* invades only mature red cells and *P. falciparum* invades red cells of all ages. The proportion of cells parasitized in *P. vivax* malaria rarely exceeds 1%, whereas as many as 50% of red cells may be parasitized in *P. falciparum* infections (7–9).

P. vivax uses the Duffy antigen as a receptor for junction formation during invasion. Sialic acid residues of glycophorin A and B serve as invasion receptors for *P. falciparum.* Certain inherited defects confer resistance to parasitization by malarial organisms (Table 26-5).

There are two major clinical patterns in malaria: (i) acute malaria in the nonimmune and (ii) recurrent malaria. Acute malaria is associated with a rapid decrease in hemoglobin. Recurrent malaria is associated with splenomegaly, less severe anemia, and only scanty asexual forms and some gametocytes in the peripheral blood smear (Table 26-6). In tropical areas, anemia tends to be more prevalent and most severe in children from 1 to 5 years of age and during pregnancy. Pregnant women who are nonimmune to *P. falciparum* develop severe malaria with high rates of abortion, premature delivery, and perinatal and maternal mortality. In women who are immune, extravascular hemolysis and secondary folic acid deficiency plays a major role in the pathogenesis of anemia. The extravascular hemolysis in immune women peaks during the second trimester and is associated with progressive splenomegaly.

Hyperreactive malarial splenomegaly (HMS) is characterized by splenomegaly, hypersplenism, a polyclonal B-lymphocyte proliferation, high IgM levels, and elevated titers of antibodies against the predominant species of malaria. Sickle cell trait is protective against HMS. Patients with HMS have a persistence of malaria-induced IgM lymphocytotoxic anti-

TABLE. 26–5. *Protective genetic alterations*

Southeast Asian ovalocytosis (autosomal dominant, 27 base pair deletion in the band 3 gene).
Heterozygotus β-thalassemias (protection against *Plasmodium falciparum*)
Hemoglobin E, hemoglobin S
Hereditary persistence of fetal hemoglobin
Glucose-6-phosphate dehydrogenase deficiency
Duffy-null phenotype (Duffy antigen receptor for chemokines serves as a receptor for red cell invasion by *P. vivax*; individuals who are Duffy-null are resistant to vivax malaria.)
Glycophorin A-deficient phenotypes [En(a-), M^k] (Glycophorins are important ligands for the attachment and invasion of *P. falciparum* merozoites)
Glycophorin B-deficient phenotypes [S-s-U-]
CD35 (Knops antigen) variants (CD35 is involved in the resetting of *P. falciparum*-infected red cells with uninfected cells).

TABLE. 26–6. *Hematologic manifestations of malaria*

	Acute malaria (nonimmune)	Recurrent malaria
Decreased hemoglobin	Decline in Hct within 24–48 hours of onset of symptoms	Chronic
Severity of anemia	Hemoglobin can decrease to 2 g/dL	2 g/dL lower than noninfected controls
Neutrophils	Neutrophilia in the first 2 days, followed by neutropenia for 1 to 2 weeks, followed by neutrophilia	May be decreased because of hypersplenism
Monocytes	Monocytosis	Variable
Lymphocytes	Lymphocytosis	Variable
Platelets	Thrombocytopenia	May be decreased because of hypersplenism
Hypersplenism	No	Yes

Hct, hematocrit.

bodies, which reduce the numbers of T-suppressor lymphocytes and permit the proliferation of B-lymphocytes. HMS has been associated with the development of splenic lymphoma with villous lymphocytes. Fifteen percent of patients with HMS will develop significant lymphocytosis, which may be mistaken for chronic lymphocytic leukemia.

Visceral Leishmaniasis

Visceral leishmaniasis. (VL), (Kala-azar) is caused buy one of three species of *Leishmania donovani* complex. *L. donovani* is transmitted by phlebotomine sandflies. VL can also be transmitted through sexual contact, blood transfusions, and congenital transmission.

L. donovani infects macrophages throughout the reticuloendothelial system. Patients develop irregular fever, weight loss, hepatosplenomegaly, pancytopenia and hypergammaglobulinemia. The pancytopenia is secondary to hypersplenism and is worsened by folic acid deficiency. Monocytosis and lymphocytosis are typically present.

Chronic VL infection can be associated with marrow hypoplasia, gelatinous transformation, dyserythropoiesis, and myelofibrosis.

African Trypanosomiasis (Sleeping Sickness)

African trypanosomiasis (AT or sleeping sickness) is endemic in sub-Saharan Africa. *Trypanosoma brucei gambiense* and *Trypanosoma brucei rhodiense* are the etiologic agents; the tsetse fly is the vector. Infection is associated with proliferation of macrophages and lymphocytes. Patients typically develop splenomegaly, pancytopenia secondary to hypersplenism, polyclonal hypergammaglobulinemia, monocytosis, and lymphocytosis.

Helminth Infections

Eosinophilia is present during the invasive migrating phase of hookworms, Strongyloides and Ascaris. Hookworm is second only to malaria as an infectious cause of anemia. The daily loss of blood in the gut is 0.03 to 0.05 mL for each *Necator americanus* worm and 0.15 to 0.23 mLfor each *A.* duodenale worm. The development of iron deficiency is related to the

TABLE. 26–7. *Iron deficiency associated with Helminth infections*

Helminth	Site of blood loss
Trichuriasis (whipworm)	Intestinal bleeding
Urinary schistosomiasis	Bladder
Intestinal schistosomiasis	Colon

dietary intake of iron, the size of the iron stores, and the hookworm load. Iron depletion is more common in women, during pregnancy and in children. Less frequent causes of iron deficiency are outlined in Table 26-7.

CLONAL EOSINOPHILIC DISORDERS

Blood eosinophilia (10) is defined as an eosinophil count superior to 450 per microliter. Eosinophils are much more abundant in tissues than in the peripheral blood. Sustained eosinophilia is associated with end organ damage in a minority of patients (Table 26-8).

Interleukin (IL)-5, IL-3, and granulocyte macrophage colony-stimulating factor (GM-CSF) both stimulate eosinophil production and inhibit eosinophil apoptosis. Eotaxin-1 and eotaxin-2, are regulated on activation, normal T-cell expressed, and secreted RANTES are chemotactic

TABLE. 26–8. *End-organ damage associated with hypereosinophilia*

End-organ	Eosinophil granule proteins	Clinico-pathologic manifestations
Heart	Peroxidases, eosinophil major basic protein, eosinophil cationic protein	Constrictive pericarditis, fibroplastic endocarditis, endomyocardial fibrosis, myocarditis, intramural thrombus formation, mitral and tricuspid regurgitation, coronary arterial thrombi
Nervous system	Eosinophil-derived neurotoxin	Mononeuritis multiplex, paraparesis, central nervous system dysfunction, cerebellar involvement, recurrent subacute encephalopathy, cerebral infarction, seizures, eosinophilic meningitis
Lungs		Infiltrates, fibrosis, pleural effusions, pulmonary nodules.
Skin		Angioedema, urticaria, papulonodular lesions, mucosal ulcerations (buccal and genital)
Eyes		Retinal vasculitis, microthrombi
Gastrointestinal/ hepatic		Ascites, diarrhea, gastritis, colitis, pancreatitis, hepatitis, hepatic nodules.
Muscle/joints		Destructive arthritis, effusions, arthralgia, myositis

TABLE. 26–9. *Diseases commonly associated with eosinophilia*

1. Infectious (helminth, protozoa, fungi, HIV, HTLV-1)
2. Allergic diseases (asthma, atopic dermatitis, allergic rhinitis, urticarias, allergic drug reactions)
3. Respiratory tract disorders (hypersensitivity pneumonitis, Loeffler's syndrome, allergic bronchopulmonary aspergillosis, tropical pulmonary eosinophilia)
4. Endocrinologic disorders (Addison's disease)
5. Gastrointestinal disorders (inflammatory bowel disease, eosinophilic gastroenteritis)
6. Cutaneous and subcutaneous disorders (atopic dermatitis, eosinophilic cellulitis, scabies, episodic angioedema with eosinophilia, chronic idiopathic urticaria, recurrent granulomatous dermatitis, eosinophilic fasciitis)
7. Immunodeficiency syndromes
8. Connective tissue disease (Churg-Strauss and cutaneous necrotizing eosinophilic vasculitis).
9. Neoplastic (Lymphomas, T-ALL, T-cell lymphoproliferative disorders, solid tumors)
10. Myeloid leukemias and myeloproliferative disorders (acute eosinophilic leukemia, myelomonocytic leukemia with eosinophilia, chronic myelomonocytic leukemia with eosinophilia, chronic myeloid leukemia).
11. Idiopathic hypereosinophilic syndrome.
12. Cytokines (IL-2, GM-CSF)
13. L-tryptophan and toxic oil syndrome

HIV, human immunodeficiency virus; HTLV-1, human T-cell leukemia virus; T-ALL, T-cell acute lymphoblastic leukemia; IL-2, interleukin 2; GM-CSF, granulocyte macrophage colony-stimulating factor.

cytokines, causing eosinophils to migrate into tissues. Eosinophils are the source of multiple cytokines (IL-2, IL-3, IL-4, IL-5, IL-7, IL-13, IL-16, tumor necrosis factor [TNF]-α, transforming growth factor [TGF]-β) and RANTES. Eosinophils are also the source of cationic proteins such as eosinophil cationic protein, eosinophil peroxidase, major basic protein, eosinophil-derived neurotoxin, and Charcot-Leyden crystal lysophospholipase.

When the blood eosinophil count is greater than 1,500 per microliter for a period of 6 months, and end-organ damage can be demonstrated in the absence of a clonal abnormality or a reactive cause, the term idiopathic hypereosinophilic syndrome can be applied.

Helminthic infections are the most common cause of eosinophilia worldwide, atopic disorders are the most common cause in industrialized countries. Clonal eosinophilic disorders account for only a small proportion of all esosinophilia cases (Table 26-9).

Sustained hypereosinophilia, whether reactive or clonal, can lead to end-organ damage. The factors playing a role in determining who will develop end-organ damage are unclear.

The evaluation of a patient with eosinophilia is influenced by the patient's geographical origin and travel history. Serial stool examinations for ova and parasites, may need to be supplemented by endemically relevant serologies and occasionally tissue biopsies.

A clonal eosinophilic disorder needs to be investigated in patients without evidence of infectious or reactive causes of eosinophilia. Clonal eosinophilic disorders can be subdivided into (i) clonal T-cell disorders, (ii) clonal myeloid disorders, (iii) cases in which clonality is suspected but cannot be proven (idiopathic hypereosinophilic syndrome [IHES]). The number of patients classified as having IHES is decreasing as diagnostic tools improve (Table 26-10).

Clonality of eosinophils can be demonstrated by the expression of a single alloenzyme of glucose-6-phosphate dehydrogenase in purified eosinophils from female heterozygotes. Polymerase chain reaction amplification of the human androgen receptor gene locus (HUMARA) can also document clonality in female patients. Analysis of Wilm's tumor gene

TABLE. 26–10. *Clonal hypereosinophilic disorders*

Clonal T-cell disorders
  T-ALL
  T cell lymphomas
  Aberrant T cell clones ([CD3$^+$, CD4+, CD8$^-$], [CD3$^+$, CD4$^-$, CD8+], [CD3+, CD4$^-$, CD8$^-$], [CD3$^-$, CD4+]
Clonal myeloid disorders
  Acute leukemias (M2 AML with eosinophilia, M4 Eo AML with inv(16) (p13;q22), t(16;16) (p13;q22)
  Chronic myelomonocytic leukemias with eosinophilia
  Myeloproliferative disorders with eosinophilia (Polycythemia vera, chronic myelogenous leukemia, essential thrombocytosis, agnogeneic myeloid metaplasia)
  Systemic mast cell disease with eosinophilia
  FIP1L1-PDGFR-α hypereosinophilic disorders
Clonal hypereosinophilic disorders
The evaluation of patients with suspected clonal hypereosinophilic disorders should include:
  CBC differential and peripheral blood smear
  Chemistry group
Serum IgE
  B12
  Serum tryptase (Increased in mast cell disease with eosinophilia and the myeloproliferative variant of FIP1L1-PDGFR-α hypereosinophilic disorders)
  Peripheral blood flow cytometry (used to identify an aberrant population of T-lymphocytes)
  T-cell receptor gene (β) or (γ) rearrangement studies
HIV serology
  CT scans of the chest, abdomen and pelvis.
  Bone marrow aspirate and biopsy (with reticulin and tryptase staining of the biopsy)
  Bone marrow cytogenetics
  PCR for FIP1L1-PDGFR-α fusion gene

T-ALL, T-cell acute lymphoblastic leukemia; AML, acute myeloid leukemia; CBC, complete blood count; IgE, immunoglobulin E; HIV, human immunodeficiency virus; PCR, polymerase chain reaction.

expression has been used to differentiate clonal form reactive eosinophilic disorders in both males and females.

T-Cell Clonal Disorders

IL-5 overproduction by T_H2 lymphocytes has been demonstrated in both clonal and reactive hypereosinophilic disorders. Aberrant clones of T-lymphocytes are present in 25% of patients with clonal hypereosinophilic disorders. The aberrant phenotypes are heterogeneous ([CD3$^+$, CD4$^+$, CD8$^-$], [CD3$^+$, CD4$^-$, CD8$^+$], [CD3$^+$, CD4$^-$, CD8$^-$], [CD3$^-$, CD4$^+$]). An activated T-cell phenotype is usually present with expression of CD25 and HLA-DR. In 50% of cases, clonal rearrangement of the T-cell receptor gene (β) or (γ) can be found. T-cell lymphomas develop in a proportion of patients. Patients with aberrant CD4$^+$, CD3$^-$ T cells producing high levels of IL-5, IL-4, and IL-13, typically present with skin manifestations, lack severe end-organ involvement, and have elevated IgE levels and polyclonal hypergammaglobulinemia.

Optimal treatment of patients with aberrant T-cell clones remains unclear. Corticosteroids have been associated with some responses. Interferon-alpha has *in vitro* antiapoptotic effects on the clonal CD4$^+$CD3$^-$ population and may increase the risk of lymphomatous transformation. Cyclosporine and chlorodeoxyadenosine in these disorders are being evaluated.

Acute Leukemias

Acute eosinophilic leukemia is rare. Cyanide-resistant peroxidase can identify eosinophilic blasts. In M2 acute myeloid leukemia (AML) with eosinophilia, eosinophils have a normal appearance. Myelomonocytic leukemia (M4-Eo) with eosinophilia is associated with inv (16) (p13;q22) and t(16;16) (p13;q22). The core binding factor-β, a transcription factor, is located at 16q22 and the smooth muscle myosin heavy chain is located at 16p13. Eosinophils in M4-Eo frequently have a dysplastic appearance.

Chronic Myelomonocytic Leukemia with Eosinophilia

The two predominant subtypes of chronic myelomonocytic leukemia with eosinophilia (CMML-Eo) involve, respectively, platelet derived growth factor receptor-β (PDGFR-β) and fibroblast growth factor receptor 1 (FGFR1). In both subtypes fusion oncoproteins are constitutively activated and activate downstream stimulatory and antiapoptotic pathways.

Chronic Myelomonocytic Leukemia with Eosinophilia Subtypes

Platelet-derived growth factor receptor-β subtype

- Age 50 to 60
- Male predominance (more than 90%)
- Monocytosis, eosinophilia, splenomegaly
- Imatinib-responsive
- t(5;12) (q33;p13) ETV6-PDGFR-β, t(5;7) (q33;q11.2) HIP1-PDGFR-β, t(5;10) (q33;q21) H4/D10S170-PDGFR-β, t(5;17) (q33;p13) Rabaptin 5- PDGFR-β

Fibroblast growth factor receptor 1 subtype

- Median age, 32
- Male to female ratio, 1.5:1
- Associated with lymphoblastic lymphoma transformation (B and T)
- Not responsive to imatinib.
- t(8;13) (p11;p12) ZNF198-FGFR1, t(8;9) (p12;q32-34) FAN-FGFR1, t(6;8) (q27;p12) FOP-FGFR1

FIP1L1-PDGFR-α Hypereosinophilic Disorders

FIP1L1-PDGFR-α is a constitutively activated tyrosine kinase that was first described in a patient with hypereosinophilic syndrome with an interstitial deletion on chromosome 4q12 (11,12). The FIP1L1-PDGFR-α in hypereosinophilic disorders is inhibited by imatinib and is more sensitive to inhibition (100 mg per day) than BCR-ABL in CML (300 to 400 mg per day). The large majority of patients with the FIP1L1-PDGFR-α obtain clinical remission with imatinib within 3 weeks of initiating therapy. Long-term evaluation of these patients is not yet available. The optimal dosage and duration of treatment remain to be defined. Resistance to imatinib is associated with a T6741 mutation in PDGFR-α: this mutation occurs in the adenosine triphosphate (ATP)-binding region of PDGFR-α at the same position as the T3151 mutation in BCR-ABL.

The myeloproliferative variant of hypereosinophilic syndrome associated with the FIPL1-PDGFR-α fusion tyrosine kinase is characterized by elevated serum tryptase levels, increase atypical mast cells in the bone marrow, and tissue fibrosis. Clinical improvement, resolution of eosinophilia, reversal of bone marrow fibrosis and hypercellularity, and disappearance of spindle-shaped marrow mast cells are seen in all patients treated with imatinib (300 to 400 mg per day) within 4 to 8 weeks of initiation of therapy. Molecular remission occurs in the majority. Cardiac dysfunction is not altered by therapy: early treatment may be desirable.

Treatment of Clonal Hypereosinophilic Disorders

Treatment of hypereosinophilia is aimed at reducing the eosinophil count and preventing end-organ damage. Imatinib is the treatment of choice in hypereosinophilic disorders associated with the FIP1L1-PDGFR-α fusion protein as well as CMML-Eo associated with PDGFR-β fusion proteins. Interferon-α is used in corticosteroidresistant patients with idiopathic hypereosinophilic syndrome, but may increase the incidence of lymphomatous transformation in clonal T-cell disorders.

In patients with idiopathic hypereosinophilia, in whom a constitutively activated tyrosine kinase cannot be found, corticosteroids represent the first-line therapy. Both corticosteroids and cyclosporine will inhibit IL-2 gene transcription factors NF-AT and AP-1 and inhibit IL-5 production by peripheral lymphocytes. Cyclosporine and chlorodeoxyadenosine (2-CDA) can minimize the toxicities of long-term steroid therapy. Hydroxyurea and interferon-alpha have been used in steroid-resistant patients. The role of imatinib as front-line therapy in patients without FIP1L1-PDGFR-α fusion proteins remains unclear. Allogeneic stem cell transplantation has been employed in treatment-resistant patients with progressive disease.

EVALUATION OF NEUTROPENIA

Neutropenia is defined as a decrease in neutrophils below 1,500 per microliter (13,14). Severe neutropenia is defined as a decrease in neutrophils below 500 per microliter. In patients of African origin, the neutrophil count may normally be as low as 1,000 per microliter.

Neutropenias can be divided into intrinsic disorders of the hematopoietic system and secondary forms. The secondary forms are caused by extrinsic factors such as immune causes, hypersplenism, infections and drugs (Table 26-11).

Intrinsic Disorders

Congenital Neutropenias

Congenital neutropenias (15) include Kostmann syndrome, cyclic neutropenia, congenital immunodeficiency syndromes, as well as several other rare syndromes that are not discussed in this chapter.

Kostmann syndrome is an autosomal-dominant disorder presenting in the newborn. Characterisitic findings include: neutrophils below 200 per microliter, monocytosis, anemia, throm-

TABLE. 26–11. *Neutropenia classification*

Intrinsic disorders
  Congenital
  Acquired
Extrinsic disorders
  Immune neutropenias
  Neutropenia associated with autoimmune disorders
  Neutropenia associated with large granular lymphocytes
  Hypersplenism
  Neutropenia associated with infectious diseases.
  Drug related neutropenias.
  Nutritional deficiencies (B$_{12}$, folate, copper)

bocytosis, splenomegaly and evidence of maturation arrest in the marrow at the promyelocyte level. Accelerated apoptosis of neutrophilic precursors is secondary to a mutation of neutrophil elastase. 90% of children with Kostmann syndrome respond to granulocyte colony-stimulating factor (G-CSF). Evolution to myelodysplasia and acute leukemia occurs in some patients. It is unclear if G-CSF increases the risk of leukemic transformation.

Cyclic neutropenias can be congenital (autosomal-dominant congenital disorder) or acquired in association with clonal large granular lymphocyte syndrome. Congenital cyclic neutropenia are associated with mutations of the neutrophil elastase gene at the enzyme active site, which leads to accelerated apoptosis of neutrophils. Characteristically, patients present with cycles of neutropenia every 21 days. The neutropenia can be severe and last 3 to 6 days. Fever, mucosal ulcers and lymphadenopathy occur during the nadir of cycles. G-CSF is useful in the management of cyclic neutropenia.

Congenital immunodeficiency syndromes frequently associated with neutropenia, include: X-linked agammaglobulinemia, X-linked hyperimmunoglobulin M syndrome, and reticular dysgenesis.

Acquired Intrinsic Disorders

Acquired intrinsic disorders include leukemias, myelodysplastic syndromes, lymphoproliferative disorders, aplastic anemia, neutropenia of prematurity, and chronic idiopathic neutropenia.

Chronic idiopathic neutropenia occurs in both children and adults. The neutropenia in some can be severe. Patients have negative antineutrophil antibodies, normal marrow cytogenetics, and either normocellular marrows or marrows showing decreased postmitotic cells. The prognosis is excellent; patients do not progress to myelodysplasia or leukemia. A proportion of these patients may have autoimmune neutropenia with undetectable antineutrophil antibodies. G-CSF is effective in increasing the neutrophil count.

Extrinsic Disorders

Immune Neutropenias

Alloimmune neonatal neutropenia occurs when maternal antibodies cross the placenta and react with the infant's neutrophils. In isoimmune neutropenia, the mother produces an antibody to the paternal CD16 isotype that is different from her own.

Autoimmune neutropenia is diagnosed in patients with isolated neutropenia who have detectable antineutrophil antibodies.

Neutropenias Associated with Autoimmune Disorders

In systemic lupus erythematosus, neutrophils have increased amounts of IgG and immune complexes on their surface, leading to their rapid turnover. Marrow cellularity and granulocytic maturation are usually normal.

Patients with Felty's syndrome have deforming rheumatoid arthritis, splenomegaly, and elevated rheumatoid factor titers. Neutropenia in Felty's is thought to be antibody mediated, in a proportion neutropenia is secondary to the presence of clonal large granular lymphocytes.

Neutropenia Associated with Large Granular Lymphocyte Syndrome

Large granular lymphocyte (LGL) syndrome is caused in the majority of cases by an expansion of either T-lymphocytes or natural killer (NK) cells. The NK-cell subtype is more aggressive and accounts for 15% of cases. Forty percent of LGL cases are associated with other diseases, such as rheumatoid arthritis.

TABLE. 26–12. *Mechanisms of drug induced isolated neutropenia*

Dose-dependent inhibition of granulopoiesis
β-lactam antibiotics, carbamazepine, valproic acid
Immune-mediated destruction of neutrophils and neutrophil precursors.
Agent acts an hapten to induce antibody formation, complement fixation and neutrophil destruction: Penicillin, gold, cephalosporins, antithyroid drugs
Immune complex related: Quinidine
Direct toxic effect on marrow granulocytic precursors
Sulfasalazine, captopril, phenothiazines, clozapine
Chemotherapy drugs seldom cause isolated neutropenia

The T-cells in clonal large granular lymphocyte syndrome express the CD3-TCR complex and rearrange TCR genes. These cells are thought to represent *in vivo* activated cytotoxic T cells. Clonal LGLs express high levels of Fas ligand. Normal neutrophil survival is regulated by the Fas-Fas ligand apoptotic system. The neutropenia in clonal LGL syndrome is mediated by dysregulated expression of Fas ligand.

Neutropenia Associated with Infectious Diseases

The most common cause of acquired neutropenia is infection. Gram-negative septicemia, *Staphylococcus aureus,* typhoid fever, paratyphoid fever, tularemia, and brucellosis can cause neutropenia. Infectious hepatitis, influenza, measles, Colorado tick fever, mononucleosis, cytomegalovirus, Kawasaki disease, HIV, and parvovirus B19 can also cause neutropenia.

Parvovirus B19 is frequently associated with transient neutropenia and can cause protracted leucopenia in immunosuppressed patients. Neutropenia is seen in more than 70% of patients with acquired immunodeficiency syndrome and can be associated with hypersplenism and the presence of antineutrophil antibodies.

Drug-Induced Neutropenias

The second most common cause of neutropenia is medication exposure. Approximately 70% of agranulocytosis cases in the United States are attributed to medications. Procainamide, antithyroid drugs, and sulphasalazine are most commonly implicated.

Three pathogenetic mechanisms for isolated neutropenia include: dose-dependent inhibition of granulopoiesis, immune-mediated destruction of neutrophils and their precursors, and direct toxic effect on marrow granulocytic precursors (Table 26-12).

The onset of neutropenia is rapid (1 to 2 days) in immune-mediated destruction of neutrophils and variable with agents causing either direct toxic effect or dose-dependent inhibition. Immune-mediated destruction of neutrophils and their precursors occurs by two mechanisms. In the hapten-mediated mechanism, the agent acts as an hapten to induce antibody formation and needs to be present for neutropenia to occur. In the immune complex mechanism, once the immune complex is formed it does not require continued drug presence for neutrophil destruction.

REFERENCES

1. Burrows RF. Haematological problems in pregnancy. *Curr Opin Obstet Gynecol* 2003;15:85–90.
2. McCrae K. Thrombocytopenia in pregnancy: differential diagnosis, pathogenesis, and management. *Blood Rev* 2003;17:7–14.

3. Allford SL, Hunt BJ, Rose P, et al. Guidelines on the diagnosis and management of the thrombotic microangiopathic haemolytic anaemias, Br J Haematol 2003;120:556–573.

4. Ginsberg JS, Bates SM. Management of venous thromboembolism during pregnancy. *J Thromb Haemostas* 2003;1:1435–1442.

5. Bates SM, Ginsberg JS. How we manage venous thromboembolism during pregnancy. *Blood* 2002; 100:347–3478.

6. Lockwood CJ. Inherited thrombophilias in pregnant patients: detection and treatment paradigm. *Obstet Gynecol* 2002;99:333–340.

7. Fleming AF. Hematologic diseases. In: Strickland GT, ed. *Hunter's Tropical Medicine and Emerging Infectious Diseases.* 8th ed. Philadelphia: WB Saunders, 2000.

8. Wickramasinghe SN, Abdalla SH. Blood and bone marrow changes in malaria. *Baillieres Best Pract Res Clin Haematol* 2000;13:277–299.

9. Chitnis CE. Molecular insights into receptors used by malaria parasites for erythrocyte invasion. *Curr Opin Hematol* 2001;8:85–91.

10. Brito-Babapulle F. The eosinophilias, including the idiopathic hypereosinophilic syndrome. *Br J Haematol* 2003;121:203–223.

11. Cools J, DeAngelo DJ, Gotlib J, et al. A tyrosine kinase created by fusion of the PDGFRA and FIP1L1 genes as a therapeutic target of imatinib in idiopathic hypereosinophilic syndrome. N *Engl J Med* 2003;348:1201–1214.

12. Klion AD, Noel P, Akin C, et al. Elevated serum tryptase levels identify a subset of patients with a myeloproliferative variant of idiopathic hypereosinophilic syndrome with tissue fibrosis, poor prognosis and imatinib responsiveness. *Blood* 2003;101:4660–4666.

13. Boxer L, Dale DC. Neutropenia: causes and consequences. *Semin Hematol* 2002;39:75–81.

14. Palmblad J, Papadaki HA, Eliopoulos G. Acute and chronic neutropenias. What is new? *J Intern Med* 2001;250:476–491.

15. Ancliff PJ. Congenital neutropenia. *Blood Review* 2003;17:209–216.

27

Interpretation of Standard Hematologic Tests

Roger Kurlander and Geraldine P. Schechter

AUTOMATED COMPLETE BLOOD COUNT

The complete blood count (CBC) is a critical tool in clinical evaluation of hematopoiesis, hemostasis, and host immunity. The informed hematologist should have at least a general understanding of how contemporary, high-volume automated counters make their measurements, and familiarity with the more common preanalytic and analytic problems, which can cause errors in this measurement.

PREANALYTIC ARTIFACTS

The automated instruments designed to perform the CBC are extremely accurate and reproducible in assaying properly collected normal specimens. However, reliability can be compromised by problems during sample collection or storage.

Artifacts Associated with Blood Collection

The CBC requires anticoagulated whole blood, and even minimal blood coagulation during collection can markedly affect the results. Clots consume platelets and trap other cell types, depressing the reported values. Most counters contain a clot detector, but some clots elude detection by this device. Samples collected from indwelling catheters are particularly prone to clotting and to inadvertent dilution with intravenous fluids. Incomplete filling of ethylenediaminetetraacetic acid (EDTA) or citrate tubes with blood can also cause artifacts by exposing cells to toxic quantities of anticoagulant and excessively hypertonic conditions.

Storage Artifacts

Measurements of white blood cell, red blood cell, and platelet counts and the hemoglobin concentration are relatively stable for at least 3 days in EDTA-treated samples stored at room temperature (1). However, EDTA increases the mean platelet volume (2) and alters fine detail of white cell morphology on a blood film within 2 to 3 hours. Mean corpuscular volume (MCV) and red cell distribution width (RDW) are affected within 4 to 8 hours and the accuracy of automated WBC differentials after approximately 24 hours (2,3). While these time intervals do not pose a problem for samples analyzed on site, the accuracy of some parameters can be compromised by delays in processing mailed specimens.

Anticoagulant-Associated Artifacts

EDTA, the anticoagulant normally used for CBC samples, causes platelet clumping or platelet-leukocyte satellite formation in approximately 0.1% of normal samples. Either of these artifacts will falsely depress the automated platelet count and may elevate the white cell count. In some published studies, 15% of patients referred for low platelets were found to have this pseudothrombocytopenia (4).

Whenever unexpected thrombocytopenia is encountered, the tube should be inspected for evidence of clotting and a blood film should be examined for platelet agglutination or adherence to leukocytes. If clumping is absent, a manual estimate of the platelet count should also be made from the peripheral blood film and compared to the automated counts (see below). In most institutions, this sequence is triggered automatically by the clinical pathology laboratory when new thrombocytopenia is recognized.

Despite these efforts, clotting or agglutination artifacts can be difficult to detect. Clinically suspicious results should be repeated, preferably in duplicate in tubes containing EDTA and sodium citrate, an anticoagulant that usually does not cause rapid platelet agglutination. Platelet counts obtained from citrate tubes must be corrected for dilution by the liquid anticoagulant. A normal platelet count from the citrate anticoagulated specimen establishes the diagnosis of EDTA-associated pseudothrombocytopenia. However some patients' platelets will also clump in citrate tubes. In such cases, an accurate count can only be obtained if blood is added directly into the platelet-diluting fluid and counted immediately; occasionally, even this method fails.

INTERPRETATION OF THE AUTOMATED COMPLETE BLOOD COUNT

The basic methods used to generate an automated CBC were developed almost 50 years ago, but new technologic tools are being continuously incorporated into each new generation of counters to improve reliability. The following discussion reviews generally how the elements in the CBC are measured and how results may be influenced by interfering factors. It must be stressed, however, that each specific instrument uses its own proprietary methods of analysis. Consequently, performance characteristics vary substantially (5). Hematologists should become familiar with the specific strengths and limitations of the instruments used by the clinical laboratories at their institution as well as the local laboratory policies for evaluating abnormal samples.

- *Red cell parameters:* Automated counters measure hemoglobin concentration, red blood cell concentration (RBC count), and MCV directly from patient samples. Automated counters usually derive other parameters by mathematical manipulation of these primary values.
- *Hemoglobin concentration* is measured spectrophometrically after the red cells are osmotically or chemically lysed and the released hemoglobin is modified (using cyanide or newer agents) to assure quantitative measurement. While this method is usually extremely reliable, any condition that alters plasma turbidity or color can artifactually increase hemoglobin values (Table 27-1). Such interference also causes telltale elevations in the mean corpuscular hemoglobin concentration (MCHC) (see later). The laboratory often can compensate for interference using spun plasma to adjust the baseline, but it is prudent to use the RBC count or hematocrit in lieu of hemoglobin to monitor red cell status in this setting.
- *The RBC count* is obtained either by measuring pulses of electrical impedance produced by the passage of cells between precisely positioned electrodes within an aperture, and/or by measuring the absorption or scatter of light by cells passing through an optical cell. Each brand of automated counters has its own protocol for distinguishing red cells from leukocytes and platelets, based on size, resistance to osmotic lysis, and other factors. Because automated counters sample large numbers of cells, RBC counts are usually much more accurate and sensitive than are manual counts, but instruments are vulnerable to the following problems:
  - Red cell agglutination within the test tube caused by cold or warm antibodies can artifactually reduce the red cell count because clumped cells cannot be properly identified and counted.
  - In many counters, white blood cells (WBC) are routinely included along with erythrocytes in the RBC count. Extreme leukocytosis therefore can falsely increase the (RBC) count.

TABLE. 27–1. *Sources of potential artifact in red cell parameters of the complete blood count*

RBC Count
 Extreme leukocytosis with WBC >100,000 per microliter (particularly small lymphocytes) increases values
 Autoagglutination and cold agglutinins decrease values
Hemoglobin
 Each of the following may falsely increase the level:
  High lipids (more than 700 mg/dL)
  Plasma hemoglobin due to in vivo hemolysis
  Extreme leukocyosis (usually WBC >50,000 per microliter)
  Hyperbilirubinemia (greater than 30 mg/dL)
MCV
 Factors which may alter the MCV include:
  Leukocytosis (WBC >50,000 per microliter)
  Auto-agglutinins or cold agglutinins
  Clinical conditions altering plasma osmolality change MCV by swelling or dehydrating red cells
Hematocrit
 Factors interfering with the MCV and RBC count will affect the hematocrit
MCH
 Factors interfering with the RBC count and hemoglobin will affect the MCH
MCHC
 Factors interfering with the hemoglobin and hematocrit will affect the MCHC

RBC, red blood cell; WBC, white blood cell; MCV, mean corpuscular volume; MCH, mean corpuscular hemoglobin; MCHC, mean corpuscular hemoglobin concentration.

- Because red cells are detected in part based on size, RBC counts in patients with extremely small or fragmented red cells may be artifactually low.
- *Hematocrit:* In the past, when the CBC was performed manually, the spun hematocrit was the most direct technique for monitoring the erythroid component in blood. The automated counter, however, computes the hematocrit indirectly by multiplying the MCV (see below) by the RBC count. While less direct than measurement of blood hemoglobin concentration, the hematocrit is usually reliable. The hematocrit can be distorted (Table 27-1); the clinical laboratory usually can identify and correct for such interference before reporting, but a major deviation from the "rule of 3" (hemoglobin in g/dL $\times$ 3 = hematocrit in %) should raise suspicion of an undetected interference with the MCV or the RBC.
- *Red cell indices* were developed to help recognize deviations in the size and hemoglobin content of erythrocytes. The MCV is measured either electronically by analyzing the shape of the impedance spike produced during cell counting, or optically by monitoring light scattering by individual cells. While usually an accurate measure of mean red cell size, the MCV is relatively insensitive to the presence of small numbers of abnormal cells found during the early stages of a microcytic or macrocytic anemia. The mean corpuscular hemoglobin (MCH), calculated by dividing the hemoglobin concentration by the RBC count, provides similar information. Because the MCV, the red blood cell count, and the hemoglobin concentration are all vulnerable to artifact (Table 27-1), in some situations one or even both indices may be invalid.
- The automated MCHC, the hemoglobin concentration divided by the hematocrit, has more limited clinical utility. In part because of balanced technical artifacts, in most machines it is slow to deviate from the normal range, even in patients with iron deficiency anemia, until erythropoiesis is severely affected. High values of the MCHC are usually artifactual

(Table 27-1), but levels greater than 36 fmol are characteristic of spherocytosis and should prompt examination of the blood film.

- *RDW* is a measure of the variability in size within the red cell population. The precise mathematical equation used for calculation varies with the specific instrument, but in all cases elevated values indicate anisocytosis. For casual observers, the RDW is more reliable than inspection of the blood film for detecting this characteristic (6). Although nonspecific, an elevated RDW is valuable for alerting the clinician and laboratory to abnormalities in red cell morphology. When markedly increased, inspection of the blood film is essential, because findings with different implications (for example anisocytosis and red cell fragmentation) can cause equivalent elevations.

- Because the RDW is sensitive to the presence of small subpopulations of large or small cells, it is more useful than the MCV for the early detection of nutritional deficiencies of iron, cobalamin, or folate. On the other hand, the RDW usually remains normal in thalassemia. The combination of a high or normal RBC count, a low MCV, and a normal RDW suggests thalassemia trait (7). However, a high RDW does not exclude the diagnosis, since some thalassemia variants commonly elevate this parameter. Attempts to use the RDW in conjunction with the MCV to classify anemias have not been widely accepted because they tend to be unreliable in complex anemias.

WHITE BLOOD CELL PARAMETERS

White Blood Cell Counts

The white blood cell (WBC) count is measured using the same impedance and optical methods used to count red cells and platelets. Because there are approximately 1,000-fold more red cells and 40-fold more platelets than white cells, it is essential for the automated counter to distinguish between cell types. To facilitate the process, red cells are usually destroyed by osmotic lysis before white cell counting. Residual red cells or platelets are excluded from the count by selective gating based on size and granularity. Automated counting is faster, more reproducible, and usually more accurate than the older manual methods, particularly in counting leukopenic samples. In the absence of interference (see below) counters can quantitate WBC counts as low as 100 cells per microliter. However, hematologists should be aware of several potential sources of interference which may influence automated WBC counts measured by older or smaller automated counters (Table 27-2).

TABLE. 27–2. *Artifacts affecting white blood cell and platelet counting*

Factors that may increase the white blood cell count
Nucleated red blood cells
Lysis-resistant red cells
Platelet clumps
Cryoglobulins
Factors that may increase the platelet count
WBC fragmentation
Extreme red cell microcytosis
RBC fragments
Cryoglobulinemia
Factors that decrease the platelet count
Platelet clumps
Platelet satellitism

WBC, white blood cell; RBC, red blood cell.

Automated Leukocyte Differentials

Subclassifying leukocytes is more difficult than simply counting them. To distinguish the different types of peripheral blood leukocytes, each manufacturer has developed its own proprietary combination of impedence-based, optical, and/or histochemical methods. Depending on the sophistication of the counter, a three-part, a five-part (neutrophil, lymphocyte, monocyte, eosinophil, and basophil), or more than five-part differential count may be generated. These are quite accurate in characterizing white cells from normal controls or patients with qualitatively normal white cell morphology.

In patients with hematologic disease or qualitative leukocyte abnormalities, automated differentials may still be accurate, but reliability can no longer be assumed. One of the most important tasks for the instrument is to identify and flag abnormalities in leukocyte size, granularity, and other features for morphologic review. Because neither automated counters nor laboratory technologists are infallible, the hematologist should personally review the white cell differential of new patients with complex clinical findings and not rely on reported laboratory values.

Automated calculation of the absolute granulocyte counts plays an extremely important role in grading chemotherapy induced toxicity. Fortunately, chemotherapy usually does not cause changes that interfere with neutrophil recognition by the sophisticated automated instruments used in central laboratories. With only occasional exceptions, which can be identified based on machine flags, the absolute granulocyte counts obtained are sufficiently accurate for making clinical decisions.

PLATELET MONITORING

Similar to the RBC and WBC counts, the platelet count is measured by impedance- and/or optical-based techniques. Platelets are distinguished from red cells by size and in some cases by resistance to osmotic lysis. As noted earlier, clumping is a frequent cause of error in the platelet counting, and sometimes falsely elevates the WBC count. Conversely, small white or red cell fragments, or protein precipitates may artifactually increase the platelet count (Table 27-2).

Automated counters are more accurate than older manual counting methods in monitoring thrombocytopenia, and they can accurately count less than 10,000 platelets per microliter. On occasion, it may be difficult even with advanced optical techniques to distinguish true platelets from debris derived from precipitated proteins, or cell fragments. One manufacturer has developed a fluorescently labeled anti-CD61 (platelet-specific) monoclonal antibody reagent for use with their instrument to improve the accuracy of the platelet count in samples with extensive interference.

Mean Platelet Volume

The mean platelet volume (MPV) is routinely measured by automated analyzers. The MPV may have modest value as a measure of increased platelet turnover and/or activation. However, the MPV may increase rapidly during the first 2 hours after collection because of shape changes and swelling in EDTA, and there are not well developed reference standards for comparing values from different institutions (2). Consequently, the "casual" MPV included in the routine CBC is of limited utility.

THE PERIPHERAL BLOOD FILM

Verification of Automated Results in the Clinical Pathology Laboratory

When an automated counter flags one or more CBC parameters it implies some aspect of the measurement(s) is atypical, but not necessarily invalid. For some flags, inspection of the blood film is sufficient to verify that the value of the parameter in question was measured correctly. For example, when thrombocytopenia is newly noted, a laboratory technologist will scan a blood film for evidence of platelet clumping before releasing the results. When the WBC or platelet count are flagged, the automated value will be compared to a manual estimate obtained by counting the average number of platelets present in 5 to 10 high-power (1,000×) fields (hpf) and/or the number of leukocytes in a similar number of low (100×) power fields (lpf). The selected fields are chosen from representative regions, away from the edge of the film containing an even monolayer of cells.

The platelet count and leukocyte count are estimated by using the formulas:

$$\text{Platelet count (platelets/mm}^3) \ = \ \text{average platelets per hpf} \times 15,000 \qquad [1]$$

$$\text{Leukocyte count (cells/mm}^3) \ = \ \text{average leukocytes per lpf} \times 250 \qquad [2]$$

Manual counts have limited precision, but when a source of machine interference can be identified or the automated result deviates from manual estimates beyond the laboratory's acceptable limits, the manual count will be reported in place of the automated result.

This process of manual verification remains an important and time-consuming laboratory responsibility. Depending on the criteria used and the disease severity of the patient population, up to 30% of CBCs may require some form of review before final reporting (5). When there is a clear discrepancy between platelet or leukocyte frequencies on a blood film and the automated value, the possibility of undetected machine error must always be considered.

Evaluation of Red Cell Abnormalities

Blood film inspection by a skilled observer may permit the detection of abnormal cells in the early stages of macrocytic anemia and iron deficiency before red cell indices and RDW become abnormal. In practice, however, serum iron, cobalamin and folate levels are far more valuable than inspection of the blood film in the diagnosis of uncomplicated mild deficiency states.

The film plays a more important role in the evaluation of other types of anemia. While detection of anisocytosis, poikilocytosis, or polychromasia often does not lead to a specific diagnosis, their severity indicates the seriousness of the disorder. More important is the recognition of characteristic abnormalities such as sickled cells, dacryocytes, spherocytes, schistocytes, ecchinocytes, acanthocytes, or intracellular parasites. These can critically influence the direction of an anemia evaluation and in some cases the finding itself is diagnostic.

Evaluation of White Cell Disorders

Automated cell counters are proficient in detecting the presence of large immature myeloid and lymphoid cells, but the blood film remains one of the most important tools in diagnosing hematologic malignancies. Morphologic findings alone may be sufficient to make a diagnosis in some patients with myeloproliferative, myelodysplastic, or lymphoproliferative disorders. In other cases, the peripheral blood findings must be supplemented with ancillary data obtained from flow cytometric, cytogenetic, and histochemical studies.

Automated counters are unlikely to identify small malignant lymphoid cells that would be readily recognizable by a skilled observer based on the presence of nuclear clefts or irregularities in nuclear contour. In the absence of lymphocytosis, samples containing such cells may not be flagged at all. Automated counters are also not useful in detecting qualitative findings such as granulocyte hypogranularity, a shift to the left in granulocytic maturation, Pelger-Huet cells, toxic granulation, or Döhle bodies. Inspection of the film remains essential in patients with high clinical suspicion of a leukocyte abnormality or hematologic malignancy, even if the automated differential is reported as normal.

Quantitation of Bands

A shift to the left in the myeloid series—an increased proportion of young forms—is a common finding during the early response to stress. The band count historically has been used to quantitate this phenomenon. The band count is performed manually by grading 1,000 neutrophils on a Romanowsky-stained peripheral blood film and the result is expressed in percent or as an absolute number. From a technical viewpoint the band count is an imprecise, poorly reproducible assay because of high interobserver differences in band identification and inadequate sample of cells counted (8,9). Despite these flaws, the band count is still occasionally used in trying to identify the early stages of acute bacterial infection, particularly in infants. Its usefulness in this role is at best controversial, and its employment in clinical decision making has been discouraged (8,9).

Evaluation of Platelet Disorders

Routine inspection of platelet morphology is indicated in evaluating thrombocytopenia or suspected platelet function disorders. The role of the film in detecting platelet clumping has been described above, but abnormalities in platelet morphology can also be helpful. The presence of large platelets suggests accelerated platelet turnover. Giant platelets (larger than a red cell) may indicate an inherited syndrome (Bernard-Soulier disesase, Alport's syndrome, May-Hegglin anomaly), or an acquired myelodysplasia or myeloproliferative syndrome. Hypogranular platelets suggest the congenital gray platelet syndrome or a myelodysplastic syndrome.

THE RETICULOCYTE COUNT

Erythrocytes newly released from the bone marrow contain intracellular RNA that usually disappears within 1 day. These cells are designated reticulocytes based on the presence of RNA-containing reticulum recognizable microscopically after supravital staining with appropriate dyes. The reticulocyte count plays an important role in the evaluation of anemia because it is a noninvasive indicator of new red cell production by the bone marrow.

Counting Methods

Reticulocytes historically have been counted microscopically by scoring 1,000 new methylene blue-stained red cells. Automated optical and fluorescent methods that detect the uptake of an RNA-binding dyes by red cells have largely replaced the manual reticulocyte count. Both methods generate similar values (approximately 1% of red cells from normal individuals are reticulocytes) but the automated technique with its standardized criteria and larger sample is more precise.

Both methods are vulnerable to interference from intracellular organisms, basophilic stippling, and other artifacts (Table 27-3). These artifacts are often flagged by the automated counter or noted during the course of manual counting. Nonetheless, whenever a reticulocyte count seems inappropriately high for the clinical context, microscopic inspection of a standard blood film, and/or of a reticulocyte preparation is warranted to identify potentially relevant causes for interference.

TABLE. 27–3. *Factors that can artifactually increase the reticulocyte count*

Howell-Jolly bodies
Basophilic stippling
Red cell parasites including malaria, babesiosis
Giant platelets

Interpretation of the Reticulocyte Count

The significance of the reticulocyte percentage is highly dependent on the red cell count of the patient. To provide a more quantitative picture of new red blood cell production, reticulocyte levels are now commonly expressed as an absolute count by using the expression: Absolute reticulocyte count = % reticulocytes × RBC count/100.

The relationship between the absolute reticulocyte count and bone marrow production is not linear in patients who have severe anemia or who are receiving erythropoietin treatment. A highly stimulated marrow not only makes more new cells but also releases them more quickly. The resulting stress reticulocytes (10), which are larger, more polychromatophilic, and more RNA-rich than normal steady state forms, may stain with supravital dyes for up to 3 days. Because these cells survive longer, the absolute reticulocyte count will overestimate the true rate of reticulocyte production. Attempts to take into consideration the impact of prolonged reticulocyte survival by calculating a corrected reticulocyte production index have not been validated rigorously or used widely in clinical practice. While the relationship between reticulocytosis and marrow production cannot be defined precisely, the implication is that a modestly elevated absolute reticulocyte count may still represent an inadequate marrow red cell response in a patient with severe anemia and high numbers of stress erythrocytes.

Immature Reticulocyte Fraction

With automated reticulocyte counters, it has become possible to measure not only the number of reticulocytes but also the amount of RNA per cell. This information allows the machine to distinguish normal reticulocytes from the more RNA-rich stress forms. At least two distinct subpopulations containing intermediate and high amount of RNA have been identified and comprise the immature reticulocyte fraction (IRF) (11).

The IRF clearly provides previously unrecognized data about reticulocyte heterogeneity, particularly during the early phases of the marrow erythroid response to growth factors, but it has not been widely used in the diagnosis of anemia, in part due to lack of a uniform reference method or standard. Despite attempts to develop guidelines (12), it is not yet clear how the IRF should be used to supplement the reticulocyte count in evaluating red cell production. The best documented role for the IRF in clinical practice is in monitoring early red cell responses to erythropoietin (13) and in detecting the early phases of marrow recovery after chemotherapy or bone marrow transplantation (14). In the latter setting, elevations in the IRF may precede early myeloid recovery by at least 1 day.

BONE MARROW ASPIRATE/BIOPSY

Indications for the Aspirate and Biopsy

The hematologist, unlike many subspecialists in internal medicine, can safely biopsy the organ of interest in an outpatient setting. The procedure, however, involves some expense and discomfort for the patient, and should be reserved for situations where the findings may influence clinical care. Common indications for the aspiration and biopsy are considered below.

Evaluation of Neutropenia, Thrombocytopenia, or Pancytopenia

In the evaluation of unexplained persistent or severe thrombocytopenia and granulocytopenia, bone marrow aspirate and biopsy may establish or exclude diagnoses such as aplastic anemia, myelodysplasia, marrow replacement by nonhematopoietic cells, or hemophagocytosis. Bone marrow studies are sometimes also obtained in the evaluation of prolonged pancytopenia after intensive chemotherapy for cancer to determine simultaneously early evidence of marrow recovery or marrow replacement by malignancy as the cause for delayed recovery.

There is no clear consensus as to the role of bone marrow evaluation in patients with isolated thrombocytopenia or granulocytopenia suggestive of an autoimmune or drug-induced process. Since the findings are usually nonspecific, the study is sometimes omitted in patients with classic clinical features of autoimmune disease. On the other hand, it is of definite value when the picture is atypical and potentially compatible with another diagnosis.

Evaluation of Patients with Anemia in the Absence of Thrombocytopenia or Neutropenia

The bone marrow study has a limited role in the evaluation of isolated anemia. Most patients with iron, cobalamin or folate deficiency, hemoglobinopathy, anemia of inflammation, renal insufficiency, gastrointestinal blood loss, thyroid disease, or hemolytic anemia can be diagnosed using the clinical examination and blood tests without a marrow examination. In patients with unexplained anemia, particularly those requiring transfusions, a bone marrow study is appropriate. The yield of new diagnoses in patients with persistent anemia and multifactorial chronic disease is low, but the study does occasionally reveal an unexpected treatable diagnosis.

The assessment of iron stores in patients with chronic inflammation represents a common and difficult problem. Serum-based assays to define iron status are often confusing (see below), and as a last resort Prussian blue stainable marrow iron stores are often used as a gold standard. This approach may not resolve the uncertainty. In a recent study, the authors reviewed the findings from 108 patients who were diagnosed as iron-depleted based on the absence of stainable iron on bone marrow. A reevaluation of the marrow films and sections revealed 19 cases with technically inadequate iron stains, usually because of hypocellularity. In a more detailed assessment of 37 of the remaining 89 patients who had full clinical data and adequate serum iron studies available, 18 (48%) had other clinical and laboratory data, arguing strongly against the original diagnosis of iron deficiency (15).

When stainable marrow iron is demonstrated, tissue iron stores can be assumed to be adequate unless the patient has had previous parenteral iron supplementation, which may be associated with residual nonmobilizable macrophage iron. The presence of these stores does not assure that iron is being mobilized properly for new blood formation *in vivo*, especially in the patient with chronic inflammation. Absent stainable iron in a technically adequate specimen is consistent with iron deficiency but may underestimate available body iron stores.

Detection of Marrow Infiltration with Neoplasm, Infectious Organisms, Fibrosis, or Other Processes

Marrow aspiration and biopsy are extremely valuable in staging and serially monitoring patients with malignancies such as multiple myeloma, lymphoma, and aleukemic leukemia, which diffusely invade the bone marrow compartment. Marrow studies may also be valuable in screening for metastatic spread of nonhematologic malignancies, such as small cell carcinoma of the lung, which diffusely metastasize to bone marrow early in the course of disease. However, given the focal nature of the lesions in most nonhematologic cancers, radiologic or nuclear medicine techniques are more sensitive and reliable tools for detecting metastatic disease.

Bone marrow studies can also identify infectious agents, especially mycobacteria and fungi. Occasionally, metabolic disorders such as Gaucher's disease and infiltrative disorders such as amyloidosis may also be discovered, but biochemical tests or less invasive biopsies are preferable.

Methodology

Choice of Sites

In adults, the posterior iliac crest is the site of choice for marrow aspiration and biopsy. The anterior iliac crest is a reasonable alternative when obesity, local irradiation, or local skin conditions preclude a posterior approach. Aspiration from the sternum can also be performed safely by experienced operators, but it is less well accepted by patients and more vulnerable to local complications because major vessels and thoracic structures lie nearby. Sternal aspiration may be justified when an iliac approach is not possible.

Bone Marrow Aspiration

The aspiration is performed, after appropriate local anesthesia, by advancing a specially designed 14- to 16-gauge needle fitted with an obturator through the cortex into the medullary space. After the obturator is removed, marrow is aspirated using a syringe and negative pressure. Individual marrow particles are spread on a glass slide and stained with Romanowsky stains. The final product, similar to a peripheral blood film, is particularly useful in identifying abnormalities in cellular morphology. The cell suspensions obtained are also valuable for cytogenetic, molecular, and flow cytometric analyses.

At the time of aspiration, unused marrow particles (or the aspirate clot itself) can also be fixed in a standard preservative to prepare an aspirate (or clot) section, which is stained with hematoxylin and eosin, or other stains in the same way as a bone marrow biopsy (see below).

The major limitation of the marrow aspirate is its vulnerability to sampling error. Marrow may be inaspirable because of hypercellularity, hypocellularity, or the presence of reticulum or collagen fibrosis. Aspirates are less reliable than marrow biopsies in detecting involvement with malignancy and not useful to detect myelofibrosis or granulomas.

Bone Marrow Biopsy

This procedure is performed using a larger needle (a Jamshidi needle), which can cut a cylinder of bone from the medullary space. In practice, after administering local anesthesia, the needle is advanced through the skin and bone cortex with the obturator in place to prevent unwanted material from entering the needle bore. Once the tip has entered the medullary space, the obturator is removed and the needle advanced until the desired length of specimen (usually 1 to 2 cm) is captured. The needle is rotated extensively to release the captured sample and then withdrawn. The sample is ejected from the needle by using a metal probe, fixed, decalcified, sectioned, and stained with hematoxylin and eosin, histochemical stains (for reticulum, collagen, iron), or a wide variety of immunohistochemical stains. Because of the required decalcification process iron stains and some immunohistochemical stains may be falsely negative.

It is almost always possible to obtain a biopsy specimen, even when hematopoietic cells have been totally replaced by fibrous tissue or tumor. Hematoxylin and eosin-stained biopsy sections show less cytoplasmic and nuclear detail than do Romanowsky-stained aspirate films, but they provide other essential information about marrow architecture and cellularity.

Risks and Contraindications of Marrow Aspiration and Biopsy

Hemorrhage

Hemorrhage is the most frequent serious complication of the procedure and fortunately is rare. In a British survey of complications from 54,890 biopsies, there were 14 instances of serious hemorrhage with one death, and 6 instances requiring transfusion (16). This may underestimate the risk, since cases with complications may go unreported.

Thrombocytopenia is common in patients requiring bone marrow aspirate/biopsy and the procedure is routinely done in patients with platelet counts below 50,000 per microliter without incident. Platelet function defects (such as those associated with aspirin administration, myelo-proliferative disorders or disseminated intravascular coagulation) may increase the risk of local bleeding in severely thrombocytopenic patients. Prolonged local pressure to the puncture site may be sufficient to attain hemostasis, but platelet transfusion or desmopressin acetate may be necessary if bleeding after the procedure is persistent.

Risks are much greater in patients with major bleeding disorders such as hemophilia or active fibrinolysis associated with severe liver disease. In these instances, factor replacement and meticulous local care after the procedure are essential. Anticoagulation poses an intermediate level of risk. Where practical, anticoagulation should be reversed before bone marrow procedures are performed. With heparin or enoxaparin, reversal can be accomplished by withholding the drug for 6 and 12 hours, respectively. If the procedure cannot be delayed, warfarin-treated patients with an internation normalized ratio (INR) in excess of 2 should receive fresh-frozen plasma at the time of the procedure, or failing this, should be carefully monitored postprocedure to ensure adequate hemostasis.

Other Complications

Local infection is usually preventable by use of sterile technique and proper local care after the procedure. There are rare reports of broken needles sometimes requiring surgical removal (16). Traumatic fracture of the sternum with damage to underlying structures is a rare but serious complication and is of particular concern when there is underlying structural damage secondary to malignancy. Sternal aspirates should be avoided in patients with multiple myeloma.

Interpretation of the Aspirate and Biopsy

In reporting results the interpreter should always indicate the site of acquisition and methodically review at least the following elements:

Marrow Cellularity

Estimates of cellularity are best obtained by inspection of a marrow biopsy. Because it can vary focally, larger specimens are particularly valuable in this regard. Marrow cellularity decreases with age; an approximate rule is that the normal percent cellularity can be estimated by subtracting patient age from 100. Inappropriately low cellularity suggests marrow damage, and high cellularity is consistent with a proliferative disorder, reaction to stress, or the use of growth factors.

Rough estimates of cellularity can sometimes be obtained from an aspirate but may be misleading, particularly when the marrow is inaspirable (a "dry tap"). Failure to obtain an aspirate may reflect a packed marrow or myelofibrosis, but dry taps are sometimes encountered in the absence of obvious hematologic disorder, presumably because of unappreciated technical problems.

Megakaryocytes

Normocellular biopsy or aspirate specimens should contain multiple megakaryocytes per low-power ($100 \times$) field. An increase in megakaryocytes is consistent with increased turnover secondary to peripheral destruction, a response to inflammation, or myeloproliferative/myelodysplastic disorders. Reduced megakaryocytes may reflect a primary marrow disease such as aplastic anemia, amegakaryocytic thrombocytopenia, or suppression secondary to chemotherapy.

Normal megakaryocytes are large cells containing multilobated (three or more) attached nuclei. The presence of substantial numbers of smaller cells or megakaryocytes with less than three lobes suggests either a shift to the left in megakaryocyte maturity because of increased platelet turnover, or dysplasia. The presence of normal or large megakaryocytes with a single nucleus or with multiple small separated nuclei is particularly suggestive of myelodysplasia.

Myeloid to Erythroid Ratio

This distribution can be estimated by inspection of an aspirate or biopsy specimen and quantitated more precisely by counting 300 to 500 cells from a marrow aspirate sample. There are often substantial local variations in myeloid to erythroid (M:E) ratio, hence it is important to sample multiple areas within the sample. In normal adults the M:E ratio varies from 1:1 to approximately 3:1. A ratio below 1:1 implies too much erythroid or too little myeloid activity; levels above 4:1 suggest the opposite. The implications of the M:E ratio must always be judged in the context of the overall cellularity, the qualitative appearance of the affected cells, and the clinical setting.

- Marked erythroid hyperplasia, a low M:E ratio in a cellular marrow, suggests an erythroid response to anemia (particularly to hemolysis), megaloblastic anemia, myelodysplasia or erythropoietin administration.
- Marked erythroid hypoplasia with rare giant erythroblasts suggests parvovirus-induced pure red cell aplasia.
- Myeloid hyperplasia may reflect a host response to physiologic stress, exogenous growth factors, or a myeloproliferative disorder.
- Myeloid hypoplasia with a "maturation arrest" (an absence of myeloid precursors beyond the promyelocyte or myelocyte stage) may reflect drug-induced or autoimmune agranulocytosis.

Myeloid and Erythroid Morphology

The disruption of the normal maturation sequence (with a complete maturation arrest or a marked shift to the left), the presence of excess numbers of blasts, or dysplastic changes affecting at least two of the three major hematopoietic cells suggests a serious hematologic disorder such as leukemia, myelodysplasia, or megalobastosis. Other changes such as a mild shift to the left or mild megaloblastic changes are more nonspecific.

Lymphocytes and Plasma Cells

There is substantial normal variation in the number of lymphocytes encountered in a marrow specimen, and these elements may be distributed diffusely or in well-defined lymphoid aggregates. Paratrabecular lymphoid collections (collections immediately adjacent to bony trabeculae) are of greatest concern because they are common in follicular lymphoma. When immunohistochemical stains are performed, benign lymphoid collections typically contain more T cells than B cells. Monotonous B cell-rich lymphoid collections are more likely the result of clonal B cell lymphoproliferative disorders. The diagnosis of lymphoid malignancies from marrow specimens is frequently possible, particularly when aided by immunohistochemical techniques, but peripheral lymph node biopsy is often necessary for definitive diagnosis.

Plasma cells usually constitute less than 2% of marrow cells, but increases are seen in a variety of inflammatory diseases, benign monoclonal gammopathy, and multiple myeloma. It is may be difficult to distinguish reactive from neoplastic plasma cells in a routine aspirate film. Extensive multinuclearity, and the presence of plasma cell collections of greater than 5 to 10 cells, are all features suspicious, if not diagnostic, of malignancy. The percentage of plasma cells in patients with reactive plasmacytosis caused by inflammation or liver disease may reach 20% to 30%, and hypocellular marrows are often relatively rich in plasma cells. To diagnose myeloma with confidence from the routine aspirate, it is helpful to see marked atypia of plasma cell morphology, including conspicuous variation in cell size and immature nuclei with nucleoli. These features are easier to appreciate in the marrow aspirate than in the biopsy. Immunohistochemical staining for intracellular kappa and lambda chains within plasma cells, and/or electrophoresis or immunofixation studies of serum and urine are needed to establish the presence of a monoclonal disorder (see later). Once clonality is established, distinguishing between benign monoclonal gammmopathy and multiple myeloma may require additional clinical and laboratory data (see Chapter 17). The presence of concentrated collections of plasmacytoid lymphocytes suggests Waldenstrom's macroglobulinemia.

Malignant cells of epithelial or mesenchymal origin adhere tightly together and aspirate poorly, forming tightly clumped groups of unusually large cells with a very high nuclear-cytoplasmic ratio. Such clumps may be rare, and, when screening an aspirate for malignant cells, the whole slide should be scanned at low power, including the leading edge of the film. Tumor cells are can also be readily identified in marrow biopsies and specialized immunohistochemical stains can sometimes help identify the site of origin.

Iron Stores

When marrow iron is markedly increased, yellow granules of hemosiderin may be seen in Romanowsky and hematoxylin and eosin preparations. Prussian blue, which specifically stains iron, is necessary to appreciate lesser iron stores and the iron granules in erythroid cells. Macrophage iron is most easily recognized within marrow particles, while the few small iron granules in normal maturing erythroid precursors are best appreciated where the cells are separated from the particles. Ringed sideroblasts are erythroid precursors bearing coarse iron granules immediately surrounding at least half the circumference of the nucleus, due to accumulation of iron within mitochondria. They are always abnormal, implying anomalous porphyrin synthesis. Sideroblastic anemias may be caused by a congenital abnormality, nutritional deficiency of pyridoxine, exposure to a toxin (especially lead and alcohol) or medication, or myelodysplasia.

SERUM TESTS TO EVALUATE NUTRITIONAL AND HYPOPROLIFERATIVE ANEMIAS
Serum Iron and Total Binding Capacity Assays

Serum iron is measured by automated chemical assays following dissociation from transferrin (17,18). Total iron binding capacity (TIBC), which is mainly attributable to transferrin, is usually assayed by the addition of excess iron to the sample. Unbound iron is removed by absorption, and the iron bound to protein is again dissociated and measured by the serum iron assay. In some institutions transferrin levels may be measured directly. Measurement of serum iron can be falsely elevated in specimens containing hemoglobin (hemolyzed specimens). The percent saturation of transferrin by iron is calculated by dividing the serum iron by the TIBC X 100. Iron deficiency is associated with low serum iron and elevated serum TIBC and therefore low iron saturation of transferrin. Although TIBC falls in patients with anemia of inflammation/chronic disease, the levels of serum iron and the percent iron saturation in patients with severe chronic inflammation/chronic disease and those with iron deficiency anemia frequently overlap. High TIBC levels (greater than 300 μg/dL) in patients with uncomplicated iron deficiency are helpful in distinguishing the two entities, but when they coexist the TIBC is frequently low (see later). Elevated serum iron levels occur in multiple conditions, including hemolysis, megaloblastic and sideroblastic anemias, pure red cell aplasia, and iron overload states caused by genetic hemochromatosis, transfusion hemosiderosis, chronic liver disease, and chronic alcoholism. A rise in the serum iron into the normal range 1 to 2 hours after ingestion of 325 mg of ferrous sulfate indicates appropriate bioavailability and normal small bowel absorption (19).

Soluble Transferrin Receptor

A truncated form of tissue transferrin receptor, soluble transferrin receptor is measured by a sandwich-type enzyme-linked immunoassay. Serum transferrin receptor levels are elevated in states of increased erythropoiesis, such as hemolytic anemias, megaloblastic anemia, thalassemia, and also in iron deficiency anemia. Transferrin receptor levels are decreased when erythropoiesis is reduced as in aplastic anemia and renal insufficiency. The assay can distinguish iron deficiency from the anemia of chronic inflammation/disease (20,21). The ratio of the serum transferrin receptor level to the ferritin level or to the log ferritin level may be more useful in distinguishing the two entities (20). Elevated transferrin receptor levels observed in some patients with anemia of inflammation may reflect the availability of iron for erythropoiesis rather than the actual iron stores (22,23).

Serum Ferritin

The ferritin assay is most useful clinically at extremes; low values (less than 20 ng/mL) reflect storage iron depletion and high levels may indicate iron overload states resulting from genetic hemochromatosis, liver disease, or transfusion hemosiderosis. Because ferritin is an acute-phase reactant, even high levels above 5,000 ng/mL may be seen with severe inflammatory states (such as disseminated fungal disease) as well as in iron overload. Patients with both iron deficiency and inflammation or liver disease often have normal serum ferritin levels, usually not exceeding 100 ng/mL (21). In the presence of concurrent inflammation or liver disease, ferritin levels may not accurately gauge the response to iron chelation therapy in transfusion hemosiderosis.

Serum Vitamin B_{12} (Cobalamin)

Serum vitamin B_{12} (cobalamin) is generally assayed by an enzyme-linked immunoassay most frequently based on binding to intrinsic factor (17,18). Serum levels below 100 pg/mL are almost invariably associated with cellular cobalamin deficiency, as reflected by elevated serum methylmalonic acid levels (see below) (24). Fifty percent of patients with cobalamin levels of 100 and 200 pg/mL and up to 10% of patients between 200 and 300 pg/mL have elevated methylmalonic acid levels, indicating cellular deficiency. Above 300 pg/mL, only 0.1% have tissue cobalamin deficiency. Low cobalamin levels in patients without evidence of tissue deficiency presumably indicate early depletion of cobalamin stores or reduced levels of transcobalamin I binding protein (the major B_{12}-binding protein in the plasma). Clinical conditions where myeloid cells, the major producer of transcobalamin I, are severely depleted, such as aplastic anemia, may result in low serum cobalamin levels. Patients with myeloma and human immunodeficiency virus (HIV) infection frequently have unexplained low levels of cobalamin, which also may reflect reduced myeloid mass. Elevated levels are seen after treatment with parenteral vitamin B_{12}, in patients with hepatic necrosis, or because of increases in B_{12}-binding proteins associated with myeloproliferative disorders, particularly chronic myelogenous leukemia. Heterophil antibodies and human anti-mouse antibodies may interfere with the assay.

Serum Methylmalonic Acid

Methylmalonyl dehydrogenase is a cobalamin-dependent enzyme required for transformation of methylmalonate into succinate in mammalian cells. Methylmalonic acid is assayed by gas-liquid chromatography or mass spectrometry (18). Serum and urine methylmalonic acid increase in more than 95% of patients with cellular cobalamin deficiency. Some patients with low serum cobalamin and normal serum methylmalonic acid levels presumably have depleted stores without frank B_{12} deficiency. In renal insufficiency, reduced methylmalonic acid excretion can lead to elevated serum levels in the absence of cellular cobalamin deficiency. A diagnosis of cellular cobalamin deficiency can be confirmed by demonstrating a decrease in serum methylmalonic acid levels after initation of cobalamin treatment.

Serum Homocysteine

Folic acid and cobalamin deficiencies prevent the methylation of homocysteine to form methionine and lead to increased serum homocysteine levels, which can be measured by ion exchange chromatography (18). Cellular cobalamin deficiency usually causes elevated levels of both methylmalonic acid and serum homocysteine, but in 5% of cobalamin-deficient patients only serum homocysteine will be elevated. In usual practice, it is not cost effective to use homocysteine to confirm cellular deficiency of cobalamin or folate. Indeed, homocyteine levels are more often obtained for the clinical evaluation of arterial or venous hypercoagulability (see Chapter 2). Other causes of elevated levels of homocysteine include renal insufficiency and inherited abnormalities in the enzymes required for the folic acid cycle and sulfur amino acid metabolism.

Serum Intrinsic Factor Antibody Assay

A positive result in this assay is highly specific for a diagnosis of malabsorption of cobalamin caused by autoimmune depletion of intrinsic factor (pernicious anemia), but the sensitivity of the serum assay is less than 50%.

Serum and Red Cell Folate Assays

These levels are determined by a competitive receptor binding assay (18). Serum folate levels reflect recent dietary intake while red cell folate levels reflect body folate stores at the time that the red cell was formed. Because cobalamin is required for cellular uptake of folate, reduced red cell folate levels are found with either folate or cobalamin deficiency; therefore, a serum cobalamin level is always required to interpret a low red cell folate level. Red cell folate is measured from a hemolysate prepared from whole blood and elevated levels of serum folate may therefore affect the red cell folate value. Elevated serum folate is found in cobalamin deficiency states and following treatment with folic acid. The assessment of folic acid deficiency with serum and red cell folate assays is not cost effective because it is common in nutritionally deficient individuals and easily treated. Cobalamin levels, however, are essential in the evaluation of patients with presumed folate deficiency, because folic acid replacement may improve the anemia but not the potentially irreversible neurologic complications of B_{12} deficiency.

Serum Erythropoietin

In patients with refractory anemia caused by marrow failure, markedly elevated erythropoietin levels (greater than 1000 U/mL) usually predict failure of recombinant erythropoietin therapy. It is not worthwhile to assay erythropoietin levels in anemic patients with renal insufficiency, malignancy, or inflammation because erythropoietin levels in these conditions are invariably low (under 100 U/mL). The assay is useful in distinguishing polycythemia vera from other causes of erythrocytosis. Patients with polycythemia vera have levels below the normal range, indicating autonomous erythroid proliferation. Erythropoietin levels in patients with secondary polycythemia may be elevated but are often normal.

TESTS TO EVALUATE ABNORMAL HEMOGLOBINS AND HEMOLYTIC ANEMIAS

Hemoglobin Electrophoresis

Methods used to differentiate and quantitate abnormal hemoglobins and the minor hemoglobins include alkaline electrophoresis on cellulose acetate membranes, acid citrate agar gel electrophoresis, isoelectric focusing (IEF), and high-performance liquid chromatography (HPLC) (25). Clinical laboratories traditionally have used cellulose acetate electrophoresis at pH 8.6 to screen patient samples and to identify the common hemoglobins A, S, and C. When aberrant hemoglobins are observed, levels are quantified by densitometry (Fig. 27-1); minor hemoglobins F and A_2 are separated by this method but their levels in adults cannot be measured accurately. Because a number of common G and D hemoglobins comigrate with Hb S, a solubility test is routinely used to confirm the presence of S (see below). Acid citrate agar electrophoresis (which also separates hemoglobins A, S, C and F) is routinely used for secondary confirmation since (unlike cellulose acetate) it can distinguish Hb D (with mutated beta globin chains) and Hb G (with mutated alpha globin chains) from Hb S. Citrate agar electrophoresis can also distinguish Hb C from Hb E and Hb O Arab, variants that comigrate with Hb C on alkaline electrophoresis.

Cellulose acetate alkaline electrophoresis is not useful for neonatal screening since it does not clearly separate Hb F from Hb A. IEF and HPLC are used in neonatal screening programs because they are superior to cellulose acetate or acid agar electrophoresis in screening for atypical variant hemoglobins. These methods, however, are more expensive and require greater expertise.

Sickle Solubility Test

The insolubility of deoxygenated Hb S in a concentrated phosphate buffer can be exploited to confirm that a hemoglobin with the appropriate electrophoretic mobility is actually Hb S. This solubility test cannot distinguish between sickle trait and sickle cell disease and, therefore, is not a useful clinical test to diagnose sickle cell disease.

Sickle Cell Preparation

Red cells from sickle cell trait or homozygous S individuals will take on the sickle shape when deoxygenated. This test has been replaced by the sickle cell solubility test to confirm the presence of Hb S and does not distinguish sickle cell trait from disease.

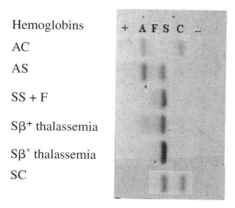

FIG. 27-1. Hemoglobin electrophoresis, cellulose acetate, pH 8.6.

Hb A$_2$ Quantitation

HPLC is the method of choice for these measurements (25). Column chromatography is also frequently used to measure Hb A$_2$, but is unreliable in the presence of Hb S. Elevated levels of Hb A$_2$ above 3.5% will generally confirm a diagnosis of β thalassemia trait; the clinician should be aware that iron deficiency will reduce Hb A$_2$ level. Patients with α and δβ thalassemia trait have normal levels of Hb A$_2$.

Hb F Quantitation

Many clinical laboratories continue to use the alkali-denaturation test to quantitate the percentage of Hb F. The test exploits the persistent solubility of Hb F under alkaline conditions, which precipitate most other hemoglobins. After treatment with alkali, the residual Hb F can be separated by filtration and quantified spectrophotometrically. The assay is accurate with samples containing as much as 10% to 15% hemoglobin F but will often underestimate higher levels for which HPLC-based methods are more accurate.

Hb F cells

Hb F can also be measured immunologically to determine the amount of Hb F in red cells and to distinguish high Hb F-containing cells (F cells) from red cells containing low levels of Hb F (see Chapter 4).

Tests for Unstable Hemoglobins

Unstable hemoglobins such as Hb Zurich and Hb Koln can be recognized by their propensity to precipitate when hemolysates are exposed to heat (50°C) or to 17% isopropanol. Unstable hemoglobins may also be detected by the formation of Heinz bodies (denatured hemoglobin) in intact red blood cells after exposure to oxidizing conditions. These purple inclusions, located near the red cell membrane, are detected microscopically after incubating red cells with supravital stains such as brilliant cresyl blue or new methylene blue (see Chapter 3).

Glucose-6-Phosphate Dehydrogenase

Both qualitative and quantitative tests are used in clinical laboratories to detect glucose-6-phosphate dehydrogenase (G6PD) deficiency. These tests depend on the generation of NADPH from NADP. Reticulocytes from individuals with the most common variant of G6PD deficiency seen in the United States (G6PD A-) have much higher quantities of enzyme in mature red cells. Deficiency can be missed if reticulocytosis has developed in response to hemolysis produced by an oxidant chemical or drug. Heinz bodies (denatured hemoglobin, see above) can also appear in G6PD deficiency.

Serum Haptoglobin

This hemoglobin-binding protein can be assayed by nephelometric or electrophoretic methods. Haptoglobin is an acute phase reactant, but its utility is that very low levels are an indicator of acute or chronic hemolysis. Free hemoglobin bound to haptoglobin is cleared by the reticuloendothelial system in less than 30 minutes. The *in vivo* hemolysis of as little as 50 mL of red blood cells will deplete the blood of haptoglobin. In the absence of continuing hemolysis, 5 days are required to regenerate to normal levels. The normal range varies widely due to genetic differences in the α chains. Occasional patients have low haptoglobin levels on a genetic basis. Severe liver disease decreases haptoglobin because of failure of hepatic synthesis.

Urine Hemosiderin

In patients with chronic intravasular hemolysis, such as paroxysmal nocturnal hemoglobinuria or cardiac valve hemolysis, renal excretion of hemoglobin leads to uptake of heme with subsequent accumulation of hemosiderin in the renal tubular cells. After staining the urine sediment for hemosiderin with Prussian blue, microscopic evaluation of the sediment will demonstrate blue-stained renal casts.

HEMOSTASIS AND COAGULATION ASSAYS

Activated Partial Thromboplastin Time

This assay measures the time required to initiate clotting after citrated plasma is incubated with calcium, a partial thromboplastin (a lipid source devoid of tissue factor), and a surface activating agent. Automated instruments detect clot initiation mechanically or based on turbidometric changes. The activated partial thromboplastin time (aPTT) is particularly sensitive to deficiencies of factors VIII and IX but will also be prolonged because of deficiencies of factors XII, XI, X, V, and II and fibrinogen. Mild reductions in factor VIII (levels above 30% to 50%) and fibrinogen (over 100 mg%) may not be detected by this assay (26). The aPTT is prolonged by anticoagulants (antithrombins such as heparin, hirudin, argatroban, bivalirudin, melagatran), factor-specific antibodies (most commonly against factor VIII) and lupus anticoagulants. Persistence of a prolonged aPTT in 1:1 mixing studies (50% patient plasma mixed with 50% normal plasma) suggests the presence of an antibody. Detection of antibodies against factor VIII may require incubation of the 1:1 mix with normal plasma for 1 hour at 37°C to allow antibody to bind to factor VIII. The presence of lupus anticoagulants can be confirmed by demonstrating correction of a prolonged aPTT by addition of phospholipid.

Unfractionated heparin therapy is monitored using the aPTT to avoid subtherapeutic or supratherapeutic levels. Although the sensitivity of the many available partial thromboplastins to heparin (as well as the instruments used) vary, an aPTT test to control ratio of 2.0 to 3.0 is a good target range for therapeutic heparin levels (27). The aPTT is not sensitive to low molecular weight heparins (LMWH). When monitoring of LMWH is indicated (as in patients with renal insufficiency, obesity, or pregnancy), an anti-Xa assay for the specific LMWH must be used.

Spurious results of the aPTT are usually due to poorly filled tubes, high hematocrits (low plasma to citrate ratio), delays in delivery of sample to the laboratory, or contamination with intravenous fluids or heparin.

Prothrombin Time

The prothrombin time (PT) is sensitive to deficiencies of factors VII, V, X, II, and fibrinogen (26), and therefore it is valuable in assessing liver function and monitoring warfarin therapy. Inherited deficiencies of these factors are uncommon and autoantibodies are rare. Some lupus anticoagulants may affect the PT as well as the aPTT. Rarely, exposure to bovine thrombin will trigger the development of anti-thrombin and anti-factor V antibodies. The international normalized ratio (INR) has been useful in standardizing the control of warfarin therapy. The INR is the ratio of the patient PT to the control PT raised to the power of the international sensitivity index (ISI). Commercial thromboplastins are calibrated and given an ISI value, which reflects their sensitivity to warfarinized plasma. It may be misleading to use the INR to describe the prolongation of the PT in a patient not receiving warfarin. The PT is vulnerable to the same preanalytic artifacts described above for the aPTT assay.

Activated Clotting Times

Activated clotting times (ACT) are used on site in cardiac surgery and cardiac catheterization procedures.

Thrombin Time

The thrombin time is prolonged by low fibrinogen levels or the presence of heparin, paraproteins, dysfibrinogens, or fibrin(ogen) split products (26). The reptilase time is prolonged by similar molecules but is insensitive to heparin.

Specific Factor Assays

Specific factor assays are based on the ability of patient plasma to correct clotting times of specific factor-deficient plasma in partial thromboplastin time (PTT) or PT-based assays (see Chapter 20).

Euglobulin Clot Lysis

Euglobulin, a plasma precipitate containing fibrinogen, plasminogen, and plasminogen inhibitor without most fibrinolysis inhibitors, is prepared from the patient sample, and clotted with thrombin; the time required for clot lysis is then determined. Because the euglobulins fraction lacks inhibitors, clot lysis normally occurs rapidly (within 90 to 300 minutes). Abnormally short lysis times occur in states of hyperfibrinolysis such as severe liver disease, but may also simply reflect poor clot formation due to hypofibrinogenemia.

D-Dimer

This immunologic assay detects cross-linked fibrin split products resulting from the action of thrombin and factor XIIIa. Elevated levels indicate extensive local clotting (deep vein thrombosis or pulmonary emboli) or disseminated intravascular coagulation. The value of a positive value in predicting localized thrombosis is poor; a negative study (depending on the sensitivity of the assay) is more helpful in excluding thrombosis.

Fibrinogen

Fibrinogen levels are routinely determined by a thrombin time-based assay but chemical or immunologic methods may also be used (26). Fibrinogen is an acute phase reactant and levels are frequently raised in patients with inflammation and malignancy. Decreased fibrinogen is found with disseminated intravascular coagulation, the hemophagocytic syndrome, advanced liver disease, treatment with asparaginase, or rarely as an inherited condition.

Bleeding Time

This in vivo test of platelet function is useful in evaluation of patients with normal platelet counts and suspected platelet dysfunction. In the modified Ivy technique, a template is used to make two incisions on the volar surface of the forearm parallel to the antecubital fold, while a blood pressure cuff applied to the upper arm is inflated to 40 mm Hg. Blood is gently removed from the incisions every 30 seconds. The bleeding time is not useful in evaluating patients with thrombocytopenia; they will have long bleeding times. The bleeding time is affected by the skill of the technologist and the depth of the incision. Because it is not reproducible and not a reliable predictor of hemorrhagic risk, it is not valuable as a general screening test. Its use should be limited to the evaluation of patients requiring an invasive procedure who are suspected to have inherited platelet function defects, such as von Willebrand disease, or significant acquired disorders that affect platelet function, such as severe renal insufficiency, myeloproliferative disorders, or drug-induced platelet dysfunction (26). Recently an automated *in vitro* instrument has been developed (Platelet Function Analyzer) that can be used as a screening test for platelet function abnormalities.

TESTS FOR HYPERCOAGULABILITY

Antithrombin III, Protein C, and Protein S

Functional tests of these proteins are more sensitive to deficiency than are antigen-based assays. Low levels are associated with inherited venous hypercoagulability. Acquired deficiency of antithrombin III occurs in disseminated intravascular coagulation, liver disease, heparin therapy and extensive thrombosis. Acquired deficiency of protein C and S occurs with vitamin K deficiency, warfarin therapy and extensive thrombosis. Free protein S deficiency occurs in patients with increased C4b binding protein secondary to inflammation. These assays should not be performed in the setting of acute venous thromboembolism.

Activated Protein C Resistance

Abnormality of this aPTT-based assay is mainly associated with the inherited polymorphism factor V Leiden.

Lupus Anticoagulants

These acquired antibodies to β_2 glycoprotein I (which has a high affinity to phospholipid) are associated with both arterial and venous hypercoagulability. Positive assays are frequently seen in otherwise healthy individuals and may be transient. The functional assays (dilute Russell viper venom test, platelet neutralization test) may be more sensitive to thrombosis risk than are serologic tests for anticardiolipin antibodies (see Chapter 22).

Factor V Leiden and Prothrombin G 20210A

These assays are DNA-based and mutations can be detected even in the setting of acute venous thromboembolism.

TESTS FOR EVALUATION OF PATIENTS WITH HEMATOLOGIC MALIGNANCIES

Serum Protein Electrophoresis

Electrophoresis separates proteins mainly on the basis of electric charge. When normal plasma proteins are electrophoresed on cellulose acetate or now more commonly on agar film and stained with a protein binding dye, five zones appear: albumin, α_1, α_2, and β globulins appear as discrete bands, and γ globulins migrate as a more diffuse, electrophoretically heterogeneous band (Fig. 27-2 and Table 27-4). Monoclonal immunoglobulins (M paraproteins) are recognized because they form discrete bands (spikes) in the β or γ globulin regions. The concentration of the proteins in normal or paraprotein bands can be determined by densitometry.

Protein electrophoresis is essential in detecting hyperglobulinemic states and in distinguishing between reactive polyclonal and monoclonal processes (Fig. 27-3). When a putative monoclonal band is noted in an electrophoretic pattern, immunofixation studies are required to confirm that the product is truly a monoclonal immunoglobulin with a single heavy chain and, more important, a single light chain. A monoclonal immunoglobulin is consistent with a plasma cell or lymphoid malignancy or light chain-related amyloidosis, but it is not diagnostic. Most monoclonal proteins of concentrations below 2 g/dL in serum are not associated with clinical or pathologic evidence of malignancy; they are referred to as monoclonal gammopathy of unknown significance (MGUS) because of the potential for malignant transformation. Occasional individuals exhibit two monoclonal proteins (diclonal gammopathy) either representing the products of two separate clones, or, if both bands contain the same heavy and light chain, two products of a single clone with differing electrophoretic mobilities, possibly due to multimer formation. Patients with marked polyclonal gammopathy, for exam-

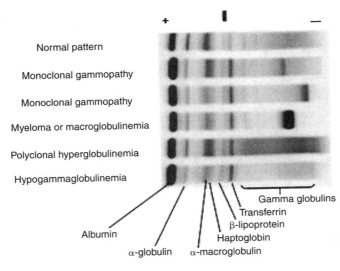

FIG. 27-2. Serum protein electrophoresis.

ple caused by HIV or liver disease, may have multiple small discrete bands termed oligoclonal gammopathy; the majority of the gamma globulin in these individuals is polyclonal.

M paraproteins of greater than 3.0 g/dL usually reflect the presence of a plasma cell dyscrasia. The concentration of M protein in the plasma (or urine) is a marker of tumor burden in myeloma patients, and serial monitoring by electrophoresis is important in assessing response to therapy. M paraproteins must be quantitated separately from polyclonal immuno-globulins.

TABLE. 27–4. Plasma protein migration patterns on standard protein electrophoresis

Albumin Zone
  Albumin
α^1 **Zone**
  α^1-antitrypsin
  α^1-lipoproteins (high-density lipoproteins [HDL])
α^2 **Zone**
  α^2-macroglobulin
  Haptoglobin
  β-Lipoprotein (low density lipoprotein [LDL])
β-**Zone**
  Transferrin
  C3 (complement)
γ **Zone**
  Fibrinogen (in incompletely clotted specimens)
  IgA
  IgM
  IgG

Ig, immunoglobulin.

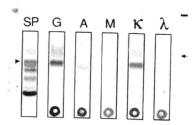

FIG. 27-3. Immunofixation illustrating an immunoglobulin IgG κ monoclonal protein. The arrowhead points to the putative monoclonal band in the SP lane stained with a protein binding dye. Staining in the remaining lanes indicates the presence of products reacting with specific antibodies directed against IgG (G), IgA (A), IgM (M), Ig κ (κ) λ chains (λ). Small arrow on the right indicates origin.

Urine Protein Electrophoresis

Light chain excretion must be examined in patients with hypogammaglobulinemia or other findings suspicious of a plasma cell dyscrasia. Approximately 15% of myeloma patients excrete monoclonal light chains in the urine (Bence-Jones proteinuria) in the absence of any detectable M protein in the serum. For screening, a random urine specimen is concentrated 25-fold and electrophoresed on cellulose acetate or agar films. Discrete bands are then assayed by immunofixation to confirm that they represent intact monoclonal immunoglobulins or free light chains. If a paraprotein is found, serial 24-hour urine collections are useful in monitoring tumor burden and response to therapy.

Immunofixation

Immunofixation has replaced immunoelectrophoresis to confirm monoclonality of discrete bands noted in the beta or gamma globulin regions of the electrophoresis. Antibodies against immunoglobulin IgG, IgA, IgM, and κ and λ are layered on membranes containing the electrophoresed sample. A monoclonal immunoglobulin will form immunofixation bands with antibodies against one heavy chain class and/or one light chain type (κ or λ) (Fig. 27–3). IgM and IgA proteins are more likely to be found close to the β globulin region; IgG proteins may be found in any area of the beta and gamma globulin zone. Free light chains are seen on serum protein electrophoresis only in myeloma with severe renal failure or in instances where the light chains form spontaneous tetramers too large for renal clearance. The uncommon IgD and rare IgE myelomas should be suspected when a serum paraprotein binds only to an anti-light chain antibody.

Serum Free Light Chain Assay

A nephelometric automated immunoassay has recently been devised to measure free light chains in the serum. This assay depends on the use of an antibody to light chain that reacts with epitopes that are hidden in intact monoclonal immunoglobulins but exposed in the free light chain. Because of its superior sensitivity compared to urine protein electrophoresis, this method can be used to monitor response to treatment of light chain myeloma and amyloidosis (28,29).

Quantitative Serum Immunoglobulins

Quantitative serum immunoglobulins are measured with an automated nephelometric immunoassay; this assay is most useful for quantitating normal immunoglobulins rather than

M paraproteins. Because this measurement depends on molecular weight, M proteins which form multimers or IgM monoclonal pentamers that disassociate into smaller molecular weight species can produce erroneous results.

Serum Cryoglobulins

The most critical step in this test is the treatment of the specimen before it reaches the laboratory. The blood should be drawn into a preheated syringe or warm tube, transported to the laboratory at 37°C and kept at this temperature until the serum is separated from the clot. The serum is then refrigerated at 4°C and examined after 24 hours. A precipitate that dissolves when the tube is rewarmed to 37°C indicates a serum cryoglobulin. Electrrophoresis and immunofixation of the separated and redissolved cryoprecipate will reveal the immunoglobulins involved in the cryoglobulin formation. Cryoglobulins may be (i) a monoclonal immunoglobulin, usually IgM, (ii) a monoclonal IgM that binds to polyclonal IgG (has rheumatoid factor activity), or (iii) polyclonal IgM bound to polyclonal IgG.

Serum Viscosity

The Ostwald viscosimeter measures viscosity by comparing the time required for serum and water to flow through a capillary tube at 37°C. Normal serum is 1.4 to 1.8 times more viscous than water. Symptoms resulting from hyperviscosity generally occur when the relative viscosity exceeds 6 but may occur with a relative viscosity as low as 3 or 4.

Serum β_2-Microglobulin

Serum β_2-microglobulin is a small protein noncovalently linked with class I human leukocyte antigen (HLA) molecules. Serum levels are measured by nephelometric immunoassay. Elevated levels may be found in inflammatory conditions, renal failure (due to failure of excretion), and in lymphoid and plasma cell malignancies. High serum β_2-microglobulin is an important prognostic feature indicating advanced disease and poor response to therapy in myeloma and certain lymphomas. In myeloma, elevated β_2-microglobulin predicts early relapse after autologous transplantation, but levels are not useful to follow chemotherapy responsiveness in myeloma because of lack of specificity.

Serum Lactic Dehydrogenase

This protein is measured by an automated enzyme activity-based assay. The normal range varies depending on the type of assay. Elevated serum levels reflect necrosis of cells rich in the enzyme. The most marked elevations (more than 5 times normal) usually are noted in severe megaloblastic anemia or with intravascular hemolysis. Similar levels can be seen in acute leukemia and lymphomas, often as harbingers of tumor lysis syndrome. An elevated serum level is a risk factor in the International Prognostic Index for non-Hodgkin's lymphoma. Distinguishing the five isoenzymes of lactic dehydrogenase is not helpful in hematologic diagnosis.

Serum Uric Acid

Serum uric acid is measured by an automated chemical or enzyme assay. Elevated serum levels, particularly over 10 mg/dL in patients with hematologic malignancies should raise concern for increased cell turnover (tumor lysis syndrome) and incipient renal compromise caused by uric acid precipitation. Hypouricemia may occur in Hodgkin's disease, for unknown reasons, and in Fanconi syndrome associated with interstitial renal disease caused by Bence-Jones proteinuria.

NEUTROPHIL EVALUATION

Marrow Granulocyte Reserve

Marrow granulocyte reserve may be assessed by the hydrocortisone stimulation test (30) or by the response to filgrastim (31). In the hydrocortisone stimulation test, the absolute neutrophil concentration is measured before administering 200 mg of hydrocortisone intravenously and again 3, 4, and 5 hours later. Failure of neutrophils to increase by at least 1,600 neutrophils per cubic millimeter indicates poor marrow granulocyte reserve. Similarly an absolute granulocyte level below 5000 per microliter 24 hours after a subcutaneous injection of 5 µg/kg filgrastim indicates increased risk for chemotherapy-induced febrile neutropenia.

Leukocyte Alkaline Phosphatase

This assay is an inexpensive cytochemical test of peripheral blood neutrophils used to screen patients with leukocytosis. The assay depends on the enzyme's ability to cleave a dye that then stains the cells. Individual neutrophils are scored by the intensity of staining as 0 to 4 +, and the sum of the scores of 100 cells are tallied. Neutrophils from patients with chronic myelogenous leukemia or paroxysmal nocturnal hemoglobinuria have low levels of leukocyte alkaline phosphatase (less than 10 Kaplow units). Neutrophils from patients with reactive leukocytosis and polycythemia vera have elevated scores (more than 80 Kaplow units). Patients with other myeloproliferative disorders may have normal, low, or high levels.

REFERENCES

1. Gulati GL, Hyland LJ, Kocher W, et al. Changes in automated complete blood cell count and differential leukocyte count results induced by storage of blood at room temperature. *Arch Pathol Lab Med* 2002;126:336–342.
2. Thompson CB, Diaz DD, Quinn PG, et al. The role of anticoagulation in the measurement of platelet volumes. *Am J Clin Pathol* 1983;80:327–332.
3. Narayanan S Preanalytical Issues in Hematology. *Laboratoriums Medizin* 2003;27:243–248.
4. Silvestri F, Virgolini L, Savignano C, et al., Incidence and diagnosis of EDTA-dependent pseudo-thrombocytopenia in a consecutive outpatient population referred for isolated thrombocytopenia. *Vox Sang* 1995;68:35–39.
5. Ward PC. The CBC at the turn of the millennium: an overview. *Clin Chem* 2000;46(8 Pt 2):1215–1220.
6. Simel DL, DeLong ER, Feussner JR, et al., Erythrocyte anisocytosis. Visual inspection of blood films vs automated analysis of red blood cell distribution width. *Arch Intern Med* 1988;148:822–824.
7. Bessman JD, Feinstein DI. Quantitative anisocytosis as a discriminant between iron deficiency and thalassemia minor. *Blood* 1979;53:288–293.
8. Cornbleet PJ. Clinical utility of the band count. *Clin Lab Med* 2002;22:101–136.
9. Ardron MJ, Westengard JC, Dutcher TF. Band neutrophil counts are unnecessary for the diagnosis of infection in patients with normal total leukocyte counts. *Am J Clin Pathol* 1994;102:646–649.
10. Crouch JY, Kaplow LS. Relationship of reticulocyte age to polychromasia, shift cells, and shift reticulocytes. *Arch Pathol Lab Med* 1985;109:325–329.
11. Davis BH, Ornvold K, Bigelow NC. Flow cytometric reticulocyte maturity index: a useful laboratory parameter of erythropoietic activity in anemia. *Cytometry* 1995;22:35–39.
12. Chang CC, Kass L. Clinical significance of immature reticulocyte fraction determined by automated reticulocyte counting. *Am J Clin Pathol* 1997;108:69–73.
13. Chuang CL, Liu RS, Wei YH, et al. Early prediction of response to intravenous iron supplementation by reticulocyte haemoglobin content and high-fluorescence reticulocyte count in haemodialysis patients. *Nephrol Dial Transplant* 2003;18:370–377.
14. Torres A, Sanchez J, Lakomsky D, et al. Assessment of hematologic progenitor engraftment by complete reticulocyte maturation parameters after autologous and allogeneic hematopoietic stem cell transplantation. *Haematologica* 2001;86:24–29.
15. Barron BA, Hoyer JD, Tefferi A. A bone marrow report of absent stainable iron is not diagnostic of iron deficiency. *Ann Hematol* 2001;80:166–169.

16. Bain BJ. Bone marrow biopsy morbidity and mortality. *Br J Haematol* 2003;121:949–951.
17. Henry JB. *Clinical Diagnosis and Management by Laboratory Methods*. 20th ed. Philadelphia: WB Saunders, 2001.
18. Tietz NW. *Clinical Guide to Laboratory Tests*. Philadelphia: WB Saunders, 1995.
19. Cook JD. Iron deficicency and overload. *Curr Ther Hematol Oncol* 1994;3:9.
20. Punnonen K, Irjala K, Rajamaki A. Serum transferrin receptor and its ratio to serum ferritin in the diagnosis of iron deficiency. *Blood* 1997;89:1052–1057.
21. Beutler E, Hoffbrand AV, Cook JD. Iron deficiency and overload. *Hematology (Am Soc Hematol Educ Program)* 2003:40–61.
22. Siebert S, Williams BD, Henley R, et al. Single value of serum transferrin receptor is not diagnostic for the absence of iron stores in anaemic patients with rheumatoid arthritis. *Clin Lab Haematol* 2003; 25:155–160.
23. Brugnara C. Iron deficiency and erythropoiesis: new diagnostic approaches. *Clin Chem* 2003;49: 1573–1578.
24. Stabler SP, Allen RH, Savage DG, et al. Clinical spectrum and diagnosis of cobalamin deficiency. *Blood* 1990;76:871–881.
25. Steinberg MH, Adams JGI. Laboratory detection of hemoglobinopathies and thalassemias. In: Hoffman R, ed. *Hematology: Basic Principles and Practice*. New York: Churchill Livingstone, 2000: 2481–2490.
26. Santoro SA, Eby CS. Laboratory evaluation of hemostatic disorders. In: Hoffman R, ed. *Hematology: Basic Principles and Practices*. New York: Churchill Livingstone, 2000:1841–1850.
27. Bates SM, Weitz JI, Johnston M, et al. Use of a fixed activated partial thromboplastin time ratio to establish a therapeutic range for unfractionated heparin. *Arch Intern Med* 2001;161:385–391.
28. Bradwell AR, Carr-Smith HD, Mead GP, et al. Serum test for assessment of patients with Bence Jones myeloma. *Lancet* 2003;361:489–491.
29. Bradwell AR, Carr-Smith HD, Mead GP, et al. Highly sensitive, automated immunoassay for immunoglobulin free light chains in serum and urine. *Clin Chem* 2001;47:673–680.
30. Mason BA, Lessin L, Schechter GP. Marrow granulocyte reserves in black Americans. Hydrocortisone-induced granulocytosis in the "benign" neutropenia of the black. *Am J Med* 1979;67:201–205.
31. Hansen PB, Johnsen HE, Ralfkiaer E, et al. Blood neutrophil increment after a single injection of rhG-CSF or rhGM-CSF correlates with marrow cellularity and may predict the grade of neutropenia after chemotherapy. *Br J Haematol* 1993;84:581–585.

28

Basic Principles and Clinical Applications of Flow Cytometry

Thomas A. Fleisher

Flow cytometry is a technology that has moved from a research tool to a standard method in most hematology laboratories. Its entry into the mainstream of clinical laboratory analysis has been aided by the ever-increasing availability of monoclonal antibody reagents linked to defining the distribution and biologic significance of the cell surface proteins targeted by these antibodies. Instrument design advances yielded benchtop cytometers with fixed optics and new developments in fluorochrome chemistry. Thus, the operational demands of flow cytometry have been simplified, while its strength in providing multiple measurements (multiparameters) on large numbers of individual cells makes it ideal for the clinical evaluation of circulating blood elements. Flow cytometric studies have extended our understanding of hematopoietic cell development, differentiation, activation and apoptosis. They have also provided important information in hematologic malignancies, insight into reconstitution after stem cell transplantation and understanding of cell defects causing immune deficiencies. Flow cytometry has helped to define characteristic features of a number of hematologic disorders.

The basic design of a flow cytometer involves four major elements: optics, fluidics, electronics, and computer (1,2). The optical system involves one or more light sources that typically involve a laser(s) producing monochromatic light that serves as the excitation beam(s). The other side of the optical bench involves collecting light generated from the cells that intersect the excitation beam. Filters and dichroic mirrors set in fixed locations linked to photodetectors allow quantitation of specific wavelength light. To ensure that all cells analyzed experience consistent exposure to the excitation beam, the fluidic system utilizes hydrodynamic focusing of the cells under evaluation. The cell suspension is injected into a flowing stream of sheath fluid, generating an inner stream of cells within the outer sheath fluid stream (1,2). Consistent and stable intersection of these cells with the excitation light beam(s) results in characteristic and cell-specific (nonfluorescent) light scatter signals plus fluorescent signals produced by the binding of specific reagents conjugated with fluorochromes. Cell-derived and light signals (parameters) are collected. Two reagent-independent parameters are typically collected for each cell: forward angle light scatter as an index of cell size/refractile index and side angle light scatter as an index of cellular regularity/granularity. The combination of these two parameters allows for the discrimination between the three major types of leukocytes as well as evaluation of red blood cells and platelets in whole blood samples without the use of additional reagents (3).

The fluorescent data collected by a flow cytometer require either cell surface or intracellular binding of specific reagents, either conjugated to fluorochromes or detected with secondary reagents conjugated to fluorochromes, as well as reagents that are inherently fluorescent. Fluorochromes absorb light of a defined wavelength and then, in response to this excitation, emit light of lower energy (longer wavelength). There are currently many different fluorochromes used in clinical flow cytometry including fluorescein isothyacyanate (FITC), phycoerythrin (PE), peridin chloryphyl protein (PercCP), and allophycocyanin (Table 28-1). More recently, combinations of two fluorochromes linked to each other have been developed that depend on the trans-

TABLE. 28–1. *Fluorochromes used commonly in clinical flow cytometry*

Flurochrome	Excitation (nm)	Flow cytometer Excitation (nm)	Emission (nm)
Fluoroscein isothyocyanate (FITC)	490	488	525
Phycoerythrin (PE)	480–565	488	578
Peridin chlorophyll protein (PerCP)	488	488	677
Allophycocyanin (APC)	650	633	660
CY5	649	633	674
PE-CY5[a]	480–565	488	674
PE-CY7[a]	480–565	488	784
PE-Texas Red[a]	480–565	488	620

[a]dual (tandem) fluorochrome—first of pair excites the second fluorochrome.

fer of energy from the first fluorochrome to excite the second fluorochrome (Table 28-1). These tandem fluorochromes extend the range of emission wavelengths available from one excitation beam. The availability of multiple fluorochromes that absorb light of the same wavelength but emit light at different wavelengths means that multiple reagents can be used simultaneously to yield a multicolor study. A second light source is present in most current clinical instruments to facilitate additional colors extending the range of multicolor studies. Research flow cytometers and the availability of a host of new fluorochromes have pushed multicolor limits. Instruments exist that allow 12 or more different fluorochromes (colors) to be evaluated simultaneously. Cells can be divided into multiple subpopulations (10 different conjugated reagents in one tube would generate 2^{10} or 1,024 different cell subpopulations). There are major demands related to color compensation and computer data management, and interpretation is also extremely complex, because conceptualization of any data beyond three dimensions is challenging and requires sequential evaluation.

The clinical application of flow cytometry saw its earliest use as a supplement to the morphologic classification of leukemias and lymphomas as well as a prognosticator in human immunodeficiency virus (HIV) infection (absolute CD4 T cell numbers) (4–7). More recently, flow cytometry has been an important tool in characterizing hematopoietic stem cells, defining immune deficiencies and certain red blood cell-related disorders, evaluating platelets, and assessing the cell cycle and apoptosis (8–14). Flow cytometry also can be used to look inside the cell as well as at the cell surface. Fixation and permeabilization facilitate intracellular entry of reagents to determine the presence of specific proteins and to assess functional characteristics (15). This chapter is directed at basic concepts of flow cytometric data presentation and interpretation followed by a brief review of applications for hematologists.

DATA PRESENTATION AND INTERPRETATION

Modern flow cytometers provide a variety of options for data generation. Generally, these are based on graphic display of the cell frequency versus the light intensity for one or more parameters. Figure 28-1, shows a single parameter histogram that reflects the quantitative distribution of cells (y-axis) versus signal strength (light intensity) of a single parameter (x-axis). Alternatively, the signal intensity of two parameters can be plotted versus cell frequency, using either a dot plot (Fig. 28-2A) or a contour plot (Fig. 28-2B). When evaluating multiple parameters (colors) the data are typically arranged in a sequence of two color displays, each reflecting a further subdivision of one or more specific cell populations or subpopulations defined by the prior data set. Typically, 10,000 to 20,000 collected events are needed to provide sufficient numbers of cells to generate meaningful data for cell population and subpopulation of interest. Where the cell of interest is in low abundance, such as for the presence

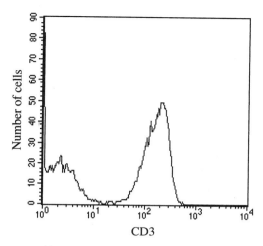

FIG. 28-1. Single parameter histogram, a distribution plot of CD3 fluorescence intensity (x-axis) versus number of events/cells (y-axis) evaluating lymphocytes.

of (CD34$^+$) hematopoietic stem cells in peripheral blood or to detect minimum residual disease, larger total numbers of cells must be collected ($\geq$100,000) (9).

Markers are typically set by the operator to distinguish cell populations or subpopulations, usually based on background signals from either unstained (no monoclonal antibody added) cells or cells that have been incubated with fluorochrome-conjugated but irrelevant antibody. Convention is to set the marker to include either 99% or 98% of all cells under the above background conditions; cells that emit a signal above this marker (cursor) following the addition of specific, conjugated monoclonal reagents are considered to be positive. Some circumstances may require modification or alternative interpretation, and not all positive cells

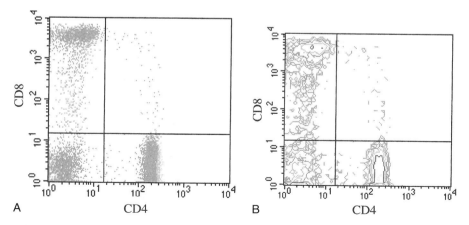

FIG. 28-2. **(A)** Dot plot of two-color (CD4 and CD8) staining evaluating lymphocytes. Frequency of events is reflected by the number of dots. **(B)** Contour plot of two-color (CD4 and CD8) staining evaluating lymphocytes. Frequency of events is reflected by the contour levels.

for a specific marker may be of the same cell population or subpopulation, reflecting the heterogeneity of cell surface protein expression.

The data generated by the computer are only as good as the instrument settings, reagents, and cell preparation. In flow cytometry, "garbage in–garbage out" means that results can be generated even though they are totally unreliable. To prevent reporting of data that are not valid, certain standards must be met in any flow cytometric study. First, optimal instrument performance is part of a quality control program utilizing manufacturer's software and methods. The use of validated reagents also depends on good laboratory practices, while the quality of cell preparations can be assessed for each study using the nonfluorescent parameters, forward angle light scatter and side angle light scatter, to confirm the presence of the population of interest. Each major blood cell type has distinctive features in this scatter plot. Platelets are obviously smaller than all other blood cells and heterogeneous in size, characteristics that can be confirmed when compared to red blood cells. Erythrocytes have a characteristic appearance based on forward angle light scatter and side angle light scatter (Fig. 28-3A). As a result of the distribution

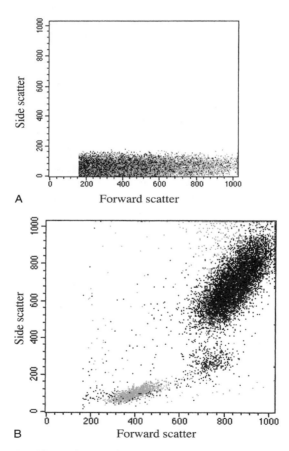

FIG. 28-3. **(A)** Dot plot of forward scatter (x-axis) versus side scatter (y-axis) on nonlysed whole blood sample **(B)** dot plot of forward scatter (x-axis) versus side scatter (y-axis) on lysed whole blood sample demonstrating a three-part leukocyte differential. L, lymphocytes; M, monocytes; G, granulocytes.

difference between erythrocytes and leukocytes, there is in a practical sense no real concern for the presence of scatter comparable leukocytes (lymphocytes) contaminating erythrocytes (collecting 10,000 erythrocytes would include less than 20 leukocytes under normal circumstances). The presence of significant erythrocytes, however, makes evaluation of lymphocytes virtually impossible, as their scatter properties overlap. Consequently, the study of leukocytes in a whole blood sample typically involves a red blood cell lysis step to eliminate the erythrocytes (Fig. 28-3B). A three-part differential emerges with normal lymphocytes representing the smallest (forward angle light scatter) and most regular/agranular (side angle scatter) cells, while granulocytes are slightly larger (forward angle scatter) and show substantial granularity (side angle scatter), and monocytes fall between these two cell types (Fig. 28–3B). The two less prevalent granulocytes differ in their location on a scatter plot with eosinophils falling within the granulocyte population while basophils overlap with lymphocytes. Hematopoietic stem cells are typically found in the lymphocyte part of the scatter plot. These scatter relationships are based on normal cells. Standard practice is to confirm the accuracy of the three-part differential using the pan-leukocyte monoclonal antibody, CD45, in combination with the myelomonocytic specific antibody CD14 (16). Alternatively, CD45 has been included in each staining combination as a specific lymphocyte identifier in certain clinical circumstances (17). On malignant cells, the staining characteristics of CD45 may be grossly altered (4–6).

The interpretation of fluorescent data based on monoclonal antibody binding is a reflection of the biology of that particular cell surface protein. When the monoclonal reagent identifies exclusively one cell population, data interpretation is unambiguous as for the pan-T-cell marker CD3 shown in Figure 28-1. In this example in which the evaluation is confined to lymphocytes based on the scatter plot, there clearly are two populations, CD3$^-$ cells that include B and natural killer (NK) cells and CD3$^+$ T cells. In other situations, biologic variability in protein expression must be taken into account; examples are shown in Figures 28-4 and 28-5. In both histograms there are at least three cell populations: cells negative for the antibody, cells showing intermediate fluorescence and cells that are brightly fluorescent. In Figure 28-4, the intermediate cells are predominantly NK cells while the bright staining cells are primarily CD8$^+$ T cells. In Figure 28-5A, the intermediate staining cells are monocytes while the bright staining cells are CD4$^+$ T cells, with the former being present only in very small numbers with proper gating on lymphocytes (Fig. 28-5B). The finding of low-density CD4 expression on monocytes explains HIV entry into this lineage.

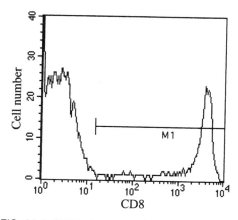

FIG. 28-4. CD8 histogram evaluating lymphocytes.

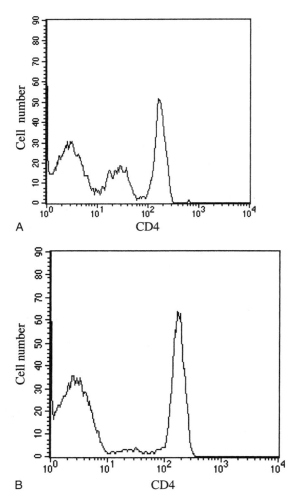

FIG. 28-5. **(A)** CD4 histogram evaluating mononuclear cells (lymphocytes and monocytes). **(B)** CD4 histogram evaluating only lymphocytes.

A host of monoclonal antibodies, individually or in combination, serve to distinguish cells of a specific lineage (Table 28-2), and characteristic binding features direct a flow study to a specific cell population of interest. Nonfluorescent parameters of forward angle and side angle scatter help distinguish grossly among lymphocytes, monocytes, granulocytes, and platelets. Within the granulocyte population, neutrophils and eosinophils are discriminated by the differential expression of the complement receptor CD16. Cells of the erythroid lineage can be identified based on the expression of glycophorin. Within the lymphocyte population, lineage specific antibodies differentiate various populations and subpopulations. Hematopoietic stem cells can be identified by the expression of the cell surface protein, CD34. This marker has enabled evaluation and *ex vivo* isolation of bone marrow or mobilized stem cells for transplantation.

TABLE. 28–2. *Commonly used leukocyte antigens used in clinical flow cytometry based on cluster of differentiation designation*

CD1a: Cortical thymocytes, dendritic cells, langerhan cells
CD2; T cells, thymocytes, NK cells subset
CD3: T cells, thymocytes
CD4: T-cell subset, thymocyte subset, monocytes/macrophages
CD5: T cells, B cell subset
CD7: Thymocytes, T cells, NK cells, early myeloid cells
CD8: T-cell subset, thymocyte subset, NK cell subset
CD10: Early B cell, neutrophils, bone marrow stromal cells
CD11b: Monocytes, granulocytes, NK cells
CD11c: Myeloid cells, monocytes
CD13: Myelomonocytic cells
CD14: Monocytes, myelomonocytic cells
CD15: Granulocytes, monocytes, endothelial cells
CD16: NK cells, granulocytes, macrophages
CD19: B cells (from pre–B cell stage)
CD20: B cells
CD21: Mature B cells, follicular dendritic cells
CD22: Mature B cells
CD23: Activated B cells
CD25: Activated T cells, activated B cells
CD33: Myeloid cells, myeloid progenitor cells, monocytes
CD34: Hematopoietic precursor cells, capillary endothelium
CD36: Platelets, monocytes/macrophages
CD41: Megakaryocytes, platelets
CD42b: megakaryocytes, platelets
CD45: Leukocytes
CD45RA: T-cell (naïve) subsets, B cells, monocytes
CD45RO: T cell (memory) subsets, B cell subsets, monocytes/macrophages
CD56: NK cells, NK T cells
CD57: NK cells, T cell subsets, B cells, monocytes
CD61: Megakaryocyte platelets, megakaryocytes, macrophages
CD79a: B cells
CD103: Intestinal epithelial lymphocytes
CD117: Myeloid blast cells, mast cells
Glycophorin: erythrocytes, erythrocyte precursors

CD, cluster of differentiation; NK, natural killer.

Many of the monoclonal reagents used to evaluate hematopoietic elements are not exclusively expressed on one specific cell type, and interpretation of data must incorporate knowledge of different expression patterns. A combination of additional antibodies often clarifies the relative expression of a specific surface protein. The expression of many surface proteins is altered under different circumstances of a cell's life cycle, preferentially expressed early and/or late during differentiation, or expressed in response to cell activation and in various states of cell function. Protein upregulation implies a range of expression from cells that are negative to clearly positive. The α chain of the interleukin (IL)-2 receptor (CD25) shows such an expression pattern on T cells (Fig. 28-6). When the interpretation of positive and negative is less clear, consistent criteria must be used for all studies involving such a reagent. In some circumstances isoforms of a specific protein are differentially expressed, and cells may express one or the other isoform or both (Fig. 28-7). Sometimes the use of percent positive for a specific marker is misleading, as shown in Figure 28-8, the histogram for the unstained cells overlaps significantly with that of stained cells; the overlay demonstrates that

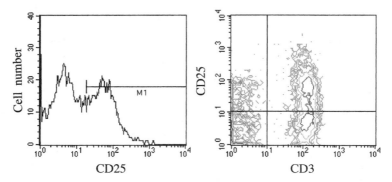

FIG. 28-6. Single parameter histogram of CD25 expression on lymphocytes (*left panel*) and contour plot of CD25 (y-axis) and CD3 (x-axis) expression.

there is a shift in the stained cells that would not be adequately reflected by simply scoring cells as positive versus negative. Our laboratory typically notes the geometric mean channel (GMC) fluorescence of the unstained and stained cells and then reports the cells to be 100% positive for the specific marker with an increased fluorescence of x-fold over background (based on the quotient of the GMC-stained cells divided by the GMC of unstained cells). These considerations are particularly relevant to many markers used in evaluating malignant cells.

Flow cytometry has been applied to investigate intracellular characteristics and, specifically, for the presence of intracellular proteins, both proteins that are ultimately expressed on the cell surface as well as proteins that are only expressed intracellularly. In addition, there are a series of reagents that bind to DNA and/or RNA that allow assessment of cell cycle status. More recently, intracellular flow cytometry has been applied to functional properties of cells, including intracellular cytokines following cell stimulation and the capacity to detect cell activation specific processes such as calcium flux, pH changes and phosphorylation of intracellular signaling proteins.

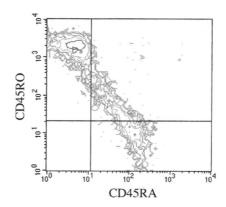

FIG. 28-7. Contour plot of CD45RA and CD45RO expression on CD4+ T cells.

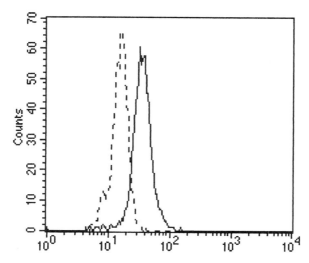

FIG. 28-8. Overlapping control and positively stained histograms

APPLICATIONS OF FLOW CYTOMETRY IN HEMATOLOGY

Characterization of lymphocytes by flow cytometry in nonmalignant states is one of the most common applications in the clinical laboratory (10). Flow cytometry remains a critical tool in monitoring disease progression and therapy in HIV infection (7). There are specific lymphocyte findings that characterize most primary immune deficiency disorders. Assessment of specific lymphocyte populations and subpopulations is being studied in a variety of disorders characterized by inflammation, with particular attention to expression of activation markers. Reconstitution of the immune system can be monitored by flow cytometry following intensive chemotherapy and stem cell transplantation (8), now more significant, due to recent focus on immunotherapy and vaccines, in experimental treatment protocols for malignancies.

Assessment of leukocytes other than lymphocytes is less common in the clinical laboratory. Monocytes are evaluated by flow cytometry to define deficiencies associated with defective monocyte surface receptor expression. The expression of critical adhesion molecules and the capacity to generate reactive oxygen species can be assessed on granulocytes (15). Granulo-cyte-specific autoantibodies can be detected using flow cytometry. Flow cytometric methods can now consistently identify and characterize eosinophils in settings of increased production (18), and basophils have been studied for intracellular cytokine production.

Hematopoietic stem cell identification and isolation are dependent on flow cytometry. Specific methods are now recommended to consistently quantitate $CD34^+$ stem cells (8,9). Additional markers have been studied in attempts to identify the the pluripotent stem cell. Separation techniques to purify stem cells from either bone marrow or peripheral blood typically utilize CD34 selection methods, and patients are followed by flow cytometry to assess engraftment and chimerism.

The evaluation of erythrocytes by flow cytometry has been applied to autoantibodies in hemolytic anemia and the detection of F-cells in fetomaternal hemorrhage and sickle cell anemia (11). The detection of glycosylphosphatidylinositol-anchored proteins on erythrocytes and leukocytes by flow cytometry is now the optimal method to diagnose paroxysmal noctur-nal hemoglobinuria.

Flow cytometric evaluation of platelets is an evolving application that provides a major advantage by allowing study of whole blood, thus eliminating the need for platelet isolation and minimizing cell manipulation (12,13). This approach allows for the detection of reticulated platelets, assessment for states of platelet activation and aggregation, and detection of platelet associated immunoglobulin.

SUMMARY

Flow cytometry has been integral in the laboratory assessment of many hematologic disorders. This technology provides a powerful tool to assess many cell surface and intracellular characteristics. The increasing range of reagents and expanded understanding of cell biology mean that flow cytometry will play an even larger role in the study of blood cells.

REFERENCES

1. Givan AL. *Flow Cytometry: First Principles.* 2nd ed. New York: Wiley-Liss, 2001.
2. McCoy JP. Basic principles of flow cytometry. *Hematol Oncol Clin North Am* 2002;16:229–243.
3. Loken MR, Brosnan JM, Bach BA, et al. Establishing optimal lymphocyte gates for immunophenotyping by flow cytyometry. *Cytometry* 1990;11:453–459.
4. Riley RS, Massey D, Jackson-Cook C, et al. Immunophenotypic analysis of acute lymphocytic leukemia. *Hematol Oncol Clin North Am* 2002;16:245–299.
5. Weir EG, Borowitz MJ. Flow cytometry in the diagnosis of acute leukemia. *Semin Hematol* 2001; 38:124–138.
6. Stetler-Stevenson M, Braylan R. Flow cytometric analysis of lymphomas and lymphoproliferative disorders. *Semin Hematol* 2001;38:111–123.
7. Mandy F, Nicholson J, Autran B, et al. T-cell subset counting and the fight agains AIDS: reflections over a 20-year struggle. *Cytometry* 2002;50:39–45.
8. Lamb LS. Hematopoietic cellular therapy: implications for the flow cytometry laboratory. *Hematol Oncol Clin North Am* 2002;16:455–476.
9. Gratama JW, Sutherland DR, Keeney M. Flow cytometridc enumeration and immunophenotyping of hematopoietic stem and progenitor cells. *Semin Hematol* 2001;38:139–147.
10. Bleesing JJH, Fleisher TA. Immunophenotyping. *Semin Hematol* 2001;38:100–110.
11. Davis BH. Diagnostic advances in defining erythopoietic abnormalities and red blood cell diseases. *Semin Hematol* 2001;38:148–159.
12. Hickerson DH, Bode AP. Flow cytometry of platelets for clinical analysis. *Hematol Oncol Clin North Am* 2002;16:421–454.
13. Ault KA. The clinical utility of flow cytometry in the study of platelets. *Semin Hematol* 2001;38: 160–169.
14. Darzynkiewiewicz Z, Bedner E, Smolewski P. Flow cytometry in analysis of cell cycle and apoptosis. *Semin Hematol* 2001;38:179–193.
15. Bleesing JJH, Fleisher TA. Cell function-based flow cytometry. *Semin Hematol* 2001;38:169–178.
16. Stelzer GT, Shults KE, Loken MR. CD45 gating for routine flow cytometric analysis of human blone marrow specimens. *Ann NY Acad Sci* 1993;677:265–280.
17. Schnizlein-Bick CT, Mandy FF, O-Gorman MRG, et al. Use of CD45 gating in three and four-color flow cytometric immunophenotyping: guidelines from the National Institute of Allergy and Infectious Diseases, Division of AIDS. *Cytometry* 2002;50:46–52.
18. Gopinath R, Nutman TB. Identification of eosinophils in lysed whole blood using side scatter and CD16 negativity. *Cytometry* 1997;30:313–316.

29

Molecular Diagnostics in Hematology

Jaroslaw P. Maciejewski, Carmine Selleri, and Antonio M. Risitano

The application of molecular biology and genetic techniques has greatly contributed to recent advances in hematology. Many new technologies have found utility in the clinical routine. This chapter illustrates the application of molecular techniques in the diagnosis of hematologic diseases and explains the principles and details of the most commonly used tests. The individual techniques are described in the context of specific applications; many of the methods are applied in variety of diseases described in specific chapters of this handbook.

Introduction of the polymerase chain reaction (PCR) revolutionized molecular diagnostics in hematology; various modifications of this technique exist. Both DNA and RNA reverse transcribed into cDNA can be used as a template. In the presence of forward and reverse DNA primers that bind to the sequence-specific regions of the target DNA, Taq polymerase extends both strands of the DNA. Repeated cycles of annealing, extension, and denaturation lead to the exponential amplification of the targeted DNA sequence with the specificity provided by the DNA primers (Fig. 29-1).

DETECTION OF GERM-LINE GENE MUTATIONS

Precise diagnosis of many hematologic diseases or detection of susceptibility to develop complications depends on the identification of mutated genes. Clinically applicable methods mostly involve detection of defined mutations occurring at specific sites within the genes. Currently, most protocols use PCR to amplify the involved gene fragments. For the identification of the presence of individual mutations various methods can be used (Fig. 29-2).

Molecular techniques described in the following are currently used for the routine diagnosis of a number of genetic hematologic diseases including thalassemia and other hemoglobinopathies, hereditary familial hemochromatosis (HFE) gene mutations such as C282Y and H63D, factor V Leiden, prothrombin gene mutations G20210A, and thermolabile C677T 5,10-methylenetatrahydrofolate reductase (1,2). Clearly, similar methods can be applied for the detection of other clinically relevant mutations or polymorphisms.

Restriction Fragment Length Polymorphism Analysis

Prior to the advent of PCR technology, traditional Southern blotting of genomic DNA followed by probe hybridization was used to detect changes in the endonuclease restriction patterns. Currently, restriction fragment length polymorphism (RFLP) analysis is used in conjunction with PCR amplification. Restriction digest can be performed either prior to or after amplification. If a mutation affects the restriction endonuclease digestion patterns, its presence can be easily demonstrated using RFLP analysis. After PCR amplification of a relevant gene fragment that carries a specific mutation, the resulting amplicons are subjected to restriction endonuclease cleavage. Using gel electrophoresis changes in the fragment size can be demonstrated. Through comparison with a wild-type form, heterozygote and homozygote patterns can be easily distinguished. When a fluorochrome labeled primer is used

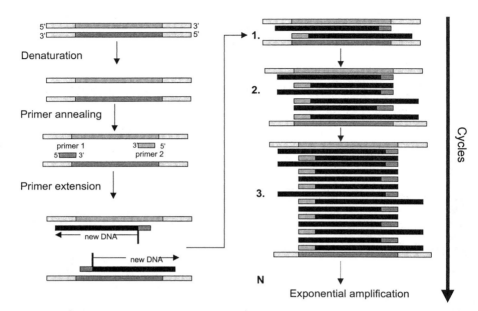

FIG. 29-1. Principle of polymerase chain reaction. Template consists of either DNA or cDNA generated by revrse transcription of mRNA. In the presence of forward and reverse DNA primers that bind to the sequence-specific region of the target DNA, Taq polymerase extends both strands of the DNA such that repeated cycles of annealing, primer extension, and denaturation lead to amplification and accumulation of the targeted newly synthesized DNA sequence with the specificity provided by DNA primers.

(e.g., 6-carboxyfluorescein; 6-FAM), capillary gel electrophoresis can be applied allowing for high sensitivity and throughput. Detection of HFE mutations by RFLP of PCR products serves as an example for this technique.

Melting Curve Analysis of Polymerase Chain Reaction Products

More recently, a light-cycler PCR method combined with melting curve analysis has been used for the detection of gene mutations allowing for a reduction in the workload and enabling automation. Melting curve analysis exploits the fact that even a single nucleotide mismatch between the labeled probe and the targeted sequence significantly reduces the melting temperature. Consequently, amplicon/probe mismatches will melt off at lower temperatures different than that of matched target DNA.

PCR amplification of specific gene fragments is performed in the presence of a fluorescent DNA probe or probes (anchor and sensor probe) that release light on hybridization to the internal portion of the amplicon containing the potential mutation. After completion of the reaction, the hybridized fragments are denatured; the release of the probe decreases the amount of the emitted fluorescence, a process recorded in the form of a melting curve. The shape of the melting curves identifies the presence of two normal alleles (singular curve), or heterozygotes (two peaks). For mutation homozygotes the curve is shifted, producing a singular characteristic peak. If multiple mutations are present in a gene, specific probes and primers must be applied to detect heterozygotes, homozygotes, and compound heterozygotes.

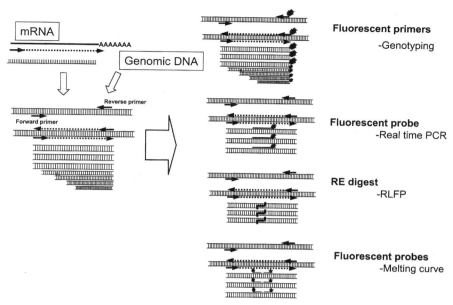

FIG. 29-2. Application of PCR technology for the detection of a gene mutation. Various techniques based on PCR can be used for specific applications in hematology. Fluorescent primers can be used for determining the small differences in the size of the amplified product, a technique called genotyping. Fluorescent probes can also be selected to hybridize between the primer sequences of the template allowing design of real-time PCR. DNA amplicons generated in the process of PCR reactions can be used for restriction endonuclease digestion. If restriction sites for specific enzymes within the amplicon contain a mutation, restriction endonuclease digestion of the PCR product will result in fragments of different sizes, which can be resolved on either capillary or agarose gel electrophoresis. Finally, using specific flourescent probes that hybridize to the amplified sequences, melting curves can be recorded to distinguish individual alleles. The presence of sequence differences between he probe and template results in different melting curves; these curves are recorded based on the emission of light induced by melting off the flourescent probes from the template.

Direct Polymerase Chain Reaction-Based Sequencing

Alternative methods of mutation analysis include direct sequencing of PCR products. Both alleles can be easily identified, and the direct sequencing method has the advantage that it does not target a specific mutation and that all possible sequence differences can be detected.

MOLECULAR DIAGNOSIS OF HEMOGLOBINOPATHIES

Hemoglobinopathies constitute a large group of inherited autosomal recessive hematologic disorders. While routine laboratory tests and clinical presentation are often sufficient for a proper diagnosis, molecular analysis is mandatory for the confirmation of the defect and precise characterization of the abnormal hemoglobin (3). For example, combinations of specific mutations may greatly affect the phenotype expected in the progeny. Thus, molecular diagnosis may have significant consequences for counseling affected patients, asymptomatic carriers, and prenatal diagnostics.

Traditionally, Southern blotting was used, but, recently, PCR-based methods are preferred. Allele-specific oligonucleotide (ASO) hybridization and allele-specific priming are the most commonly applied techniques. The first method relies on hybridization of ASO probes (wild-type and mutant) to PCR-amplified genomic DNA. In the dot-blot assay, ASO is labeled, while the reverse dot-blot technique utilizes labeled amplified DNA, allowing for simultaneous screening of multiple mutations. Allele-specific priming is based on the principle that a perfectly matched primer pair amplifies target DNA more efficiently than a mismatched pair. In the amplification refractory mutation system (ARMS), genomic DNA is challenged with both wild-type and mutant primer sets. Multiple mutations may be simultaneously screened in a multiplex PCR assay using fluorescently labeled ARMS primers, producing products of different length that can be detected using an automated DNA analyzer. Large deletions of both the α and β globin gene may be screened using the gap-PCR, with primers complementary to the breakpoint sequences. However, for some deletion mutants, Southern blotting is still standard.

Combining all these approaches in the context of the ethnic- and region-specific distribution of globin mutations, successful molecular identification is possible in more than 90% of cases. Mutations remaining unknown after standard molecular screening may be investigated further by denaturing gradient gel electrophoresis (DGGE) or heteroduplex analysis; nevertheless, complete sequencing of the globin gene represents the best option to identify rare or unknown mutations.

CHROMOSOME DIAGNOSTICS

Metaphase Karyotyping

Traditional cytogenetics, utilizing banding techniques, is performed on chromosomal metaphase spreads. Because mitotic activity is required, metaphase karyotyping is performed after cell culture in the presence of mitogens. For myeloid disorders, either lymphocyte-conditioned media or hematopoietic growth factors are most commonly used, while, for lymphoid malignancies, lectins are added. Various banding methods have been utilized for chromosome identification and resolution of individual chromosomal fragments, but G-banding is usual in clinical diagnostics. Characteristic bands result from the biochemical properties of chromatin such as AT and GC content (4–8).

Cellularity and mitotic activity affect the diagnostic yield of the procedure, and the proportion of noninformative spreads varies from disease to disease. In myelofibrosis, marrow is often not aspirable. In aplastic anemia and myelodysplasia, noninformative results are frequent due to the lack of progenitor cells. In such cases, cytogenetic analysis may be also performed on blood specimens.

Approximately 330 chromosomal bands can be distinguished by routine karyotyping and each band may contain as much as 10^7 base pairs (bp) and a multitude of genes. Classic karyotyping can identify defects of approximately 5 Mb; thus, smaller defects and their locations may remain undetected (resolution). The sensitivity level depends on the number of analyzed cells; routinely 20 cells are counted with a detailed analysis of at least 2 cells. Analysis may be more complicated if several clones, each harboring a distinct defect, are present. Depending on the nature of the identified defect, the sensitivity limit is approximately 10% (i.e., identification of 2 abnormal cells) in 20 cells tested.

Both balanced and unbalanced translocations can be identified, but some defects may require a more intricate analysis. Some of the balanced translocations are highly diagnostic; examples are t(9;22) in chronic myelogenous leukemia (CML), t(15;17), inv 16 and t(8;21) in acute myeloid lymphoma (AML), t(15;17) in acute promyelocytic leukemia (APL), t(9;22) and t(12;21) in acute lymphoblasic leukemia (ALL), as well as t(14;18), t(11;14), t(11;18) in lymphomas. Once a specific defect is identified, metaphase karyotyping can be used for monitoring of therapy response (cytogenetic remission); however, the sensitivity of this method is limited (5–8).

Fluorescence In Situ Hybridization

For the targeted detection of specific abnormalities, fluorescence in situ hybridization (FISH) is the most commonly applied method particularly helpful in the characterization of structural chromosomal abnormalities and identification of chromosomes of uncertain origin. However, FISH is not suitable for screening for unknown defects unless a high clinical suspicion exists. FISH does not require cell division and consequently cell culture and is more sensitive than traditional cytogenetics. FISH provides a more accurate measure for the true frequency of abnormal cells and can be used for the monitoring of minimal residual disease. Identification of the donor versus recipient origin of the blood cell production following hematopoietic stem cell transplantation is another application of this technology (see below). The technique can be applied to blood, marrow, body fluids, tissue touch preparations as well as to paraffin-embedded tissues (5,9).

In FISH, specific fluorescent-labeled single stranded DNA probes are hybridized to the nuclei of metaphase or interphase cells attached to glass slides. The use of probes labeled with different dyes allows for multicolor FISH on a single slide. Probes can also be designed to identify a specific chromosomal structure, hybridize to multiple chromosomal sequences, and to identify unique DNA sequences. Probes recognizing α-satellite sequences are chromosome specific; in diploid cells both chromosomes are labeled. Chromosome painting probes are derived from whole chromosomes (see also spectral karyotyping [SKY], discussed next). Probes can be derived from unique sequences cloned from specific regions of the genome. Finally, telomeric probes can be used to determine the telomere length based on the intensity of the hybridization.

For balanced translocations, probes spanning individual breakpoints are used. Dual-color/dual-fusion probes or single-fusion/dual-color FISH probes target sequences located at opposite ends of two breakpoints. In addition, two-color break-apart probes, recognizing DNA sequences from the 3′ and 5′ ends of a single gene, can be applied. These probes yield combined yellow signal in the normal germ line configuration while two colors are seen when target sequences are separated because of translocation. FISH is more reliable for the detection of duplication of chromosome fragments than deletions. In general, FISH is less sensitive than PCR, with detection limits of 1 of 100 cells. As a result of the false-positive rate, it is not clear whether sensitivity can be increased through routine counting of a higher number of cells.

FISH techniques have been widely applied for the detection of lymphoma-specific translocations, in the diagnosis of CML, myelodysplastic syndrome (MDS), and T-cell acute lymphoblastic leukemia (T-ALL) and B-cell acute lymphoblastic leukemia (B-ALL) (Table 29-1) (6,8–10). In addition, FISH is frequently used for intracellular detection of Epstein-Barr virus (EBV) in certain non-Hodgkin's lymphomas, Hodgkin's disease and aggressive natural killer (NK) cell lymphomas (see later).

Spectral Karyotyping

SKY allows for the visualization of all 24 chromosomes and analysis of their structure based on hybridization with multicolor painting probes (11). These probes are derived from individual chromosomes using degenerate primer-based PCR and differentially labeled with fluorochromes. After hybridization to metaphase spreads, a digital camera is used to record the complete emission spectra. As a result, each chromosome-specific probe is distinctively labeled and easily identified. SKY has a much higher precision than traditional cytogenetics and allows for identification of new, previously unidentified reciprocal translocations and defects that cannot be resolved by traditional banding. In one study, SKY allowed detection

TABLE. 29–1. *Translocations and deletions commonly detected by fluorescence in situ hybridization*

Disease	Chromosomal abnormality
CLL/SLL	del13q14, del11q22
LPL	t(9:14)
MZL	t(11:14), t(1:14), t(14:18)
FL	t(14:18)
MCL	t(11:14)
DLBCL	del3q27, t(14:18)
BL	t(8:14), t(2:8), t(8:22)
ALL	t(12:21), t(11q23), t(9:22)
AML	t(11q23), t(8:21), inv(16),
CML	t(9:22)
APL	c(15, 17)

CCL, chronic leukemia/lymphoma; SLL, small lymphocytic lymphoma; LPL, lymphoplasmacytoid lymphoma; MZL, marginal zone lymphoma; FL, follicular lymphoma; MCL, mantle cell lymphoma; DLBCL, diffuse large B-cell lymphoma; BL, Burkitt lymphoma; ALL, acute lymphocytic leukemia; AML, acute myeloid leukemia; CML, chronic myelogenous leukemia

of new translocations in 35% of cases and resulted in confirmation of the previously known defects and refinement of 35% of diagnoses.

Array-Based Comparative Genomic Hybridization

Array-based comparative genomic hybridization (A-CGH) is a new and efficient method that could be applied to facilitate cytogenetic diagnosis in MDS and AML. In this technique, the genomic DNA from malignant cells is labeled with a fluorescent dye in one color while a normal reference DNA sample is labeled in a different color. The labeled samples are then cohybridized to a substrate. Chromosomal imbalances across the genome in the tumor DNA are then quantified and positionally defined by analyzing the ratio of fluorescence of the two different colors along the target metaphase chromosomes. Initially, this analysis was performed on metaphase chromosome preparations (M-CGH). However, the resolution of CGH as applied to metaphase spreads is limited by the standard cytogenetic resolution of approximately 5 Mb, and considerable cytogenetic expertise is required to accomplish such analysis. Therefore, M-CGH has never become a widely utilized technique, and remained limited to specialist research applications.

Recently, the advent of bacterial artificial chromosome (BAC) array technology has focused attention to the applicability of CGH to the study of genomic alterations in human disease. BACs are large-insert DNA clones that have been cytogenetically and physically mapped to the human genome. This resource affords the opportunity to generate an ordered array of DNA segments at a high genomic resolution and circumvents the considerable limitations associated with the use of metaphase preparations as the hybridization template. The fluorescence ratio of the two colors can be compared between different spots representing different genomic regions, providing a genome-wide molecular profile of the sample with respect to regions of the genome that are deleted or amplified (Fig. 29-3). The resolution is dependent on a combination of the number, size, and map positions of the DNA elements within the array.

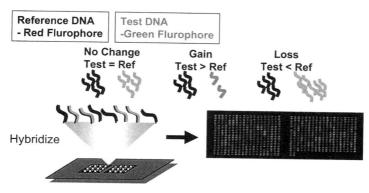

FIG. 29-3. Array-based comparative genomic hybridization (A-CGH). A-CGH consists of hybridization of tester and reference DNA samples that have been differentially labeled with fluorochromes to arrays of sequences corresponding to specific portions of chromosomes. Unbalanced translocations, such as deletion or duplication of individual genes (or portions of chromosomes) can be detected based on the disparity between flourescent spectra emitted by the tester vs. reference DNA. Consequently, depending on the number of probes, a very intricate analysis of chromosomes can be performed with regard to the presence or absence of specific DNA segments.

Because of the high resolution of this method and the convenient microarray format, this method will likely be introduced into the clinical routine, especially for diseases in which unbalanced translocations are expected (12).

DETECTION AND QUANTITATION OF SOMATIC MUTATIONS AND TRANSLOCATIONS

Polymerase Chain Reaction-Based Analysis of Translocations

PCR has found a wide application to the diagnosis of malignant disorders associated with specific translocations of genetic material (5,7,8). The main advantage of PCR is high specificity and sensitivity, but there is need for immaculate technique to avoid contamination. DNA primers are designed to flank the specific translocated region, producing a PCR product with a characteristic size, while in the absence of the specific translocation the amplification product is not generated. Appropriate controls can be incorporated into the reaction. Because of the higher template copy number per cell, reverse transcriptase real-time PCR may be a more sensitive modification of this technique. In real-time PCR, mRNA of the abnormal transcript is reverse transcribed and cDNA serves as template for the amplification reaction (Fig. 29-4). Sensitivity and specificity can be further improved by an additional round of amplification with a pair of internal primers, termed nested PCR. The sensitivity of this method approaches 1 malignant cell per 10^6 normal cells, allowing for the assessment of minimal residual disease (MRD) in various conditions (5).

Recently, introduction of the real-time light cycler PCR assay (Fig. 29-4) has led to quantification of the numbers of cell up to one malignant cells per 10^5 normal cells. The reference standard includes a single-copy gene. The principle of real-time PCR consists of target sequence amplification in the presence of fluorochrome-labeled probes. Such probes are designed to target the sequences between the forward and reverse primers. The probe is labeled at the 5′ end with a reporter fluorochrome (6-FAM) and a quencher fluorochrome (6-carboxytetramethyl-rhodamine [TAMRA]) at the 3′ end and are designed to have a higher

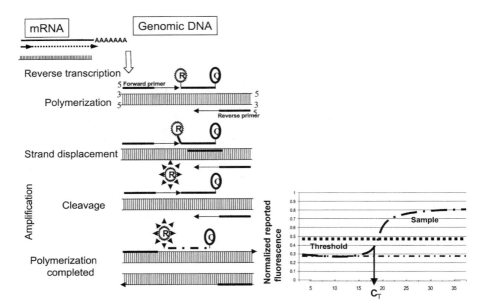

FIG. 29-4. Real-time quantitative PCR. Either cDNA generated from mRNA or DNA can be used as a template. The principle of real-time PCR consists of target sequence amplification in the presence of flurochrome-labeled probes. Such probes are designed to target the sequences between the forward and reverse primer that hybridize to the PCR product accumulated during amplification. The probes are usually labeled with a reporter fluorochrome at the 5′ and a quencher fluorochrome with the 3′ end. Probes are designed to have a higher melting temperature than the extension primer. As long as both fluorochromes are connected through the DNA sequence, no light is emitted. However, the 5′ to 3′ exonuclease activity of Taq polymerase degrades the probe and releases the fluorochromes. Consequently, progression of the reaction can be monitored by the detection of the fluorescent signal generated during the exponential phase of the reaction and the cycle number at which the reporter dye intensity rises above the background noise. This value, also referred to as the threshold number, is inversely related to the copy number of the target template.

melting temperature than the extension primers. As long as both fluorochromes are connected through the DNA sequence, no light is emitted. However, the 5′ to 3′ exonuclease activity of Taq polymerase degrades the probe and releases the fluorochromes. Consequently, progression of the reaction can be monitored by the detection of the fluorescent signal generated during the exponential phase of the reaction, and the cycle number at which the reporter dye intensity rises above the background noise. This threshold number is inversely related to the copy number of the target template. Measurement of the frequency of abnormal cells is based on standard curves and generated with dilution of control cells or DNA/cDNA containing the targeted mutation. The results can be expressed as copy numbers of fusion transcripts per microgram of RNA or as the frequency of abnormal cells. Ubiquitously expressed housekeeping transcripts/genes are commonly incorporated, and the PCR cycle threshold number of the fusion gene is normalized to the value of the housekeeping gene (5).

PCR technology, including quantitative PCR, in clinical practice has proven predictive of therapy response and relapse. For certain hematologic malignancies with translocations coding for specific targets, cytogenetic and molecular remissions have been defined as specific end points of therapy. Risks of relapse associated with molecular versus cytogenetic remission have been determined. The most common applications of PCR in the detection of disease-defining translocations are for CML (bcr/abl), APL (PML/RARA), mantle cell and follicular lymphomas (cycD1/IgH and IgH/bcl2, respectively) and B-cell lymphoblastic leukemia (bcr/abl, rearranged IgH) (Table 29-2).

Clearly, separate screening for all described abnormalities is too expensive and time consuming to be applied as a global diagnostic battery. Multiple attempts have been made to adapt PCR technology for precise molecular diagnosis associated with individual leukemias and lymphomas. In multiplex PCR, multiple primer pairs are combined to enable detection of several translocations in a single PCR reaction. For example, primer mixtures have been designed to allow for the detection of 28 different translocations, including 80 breakpoints and splice variants, using a limited number of PCR reactions. The introduction of such technologies in clinical practice is hampered by the need for positive controls and limited sensitivity. However, the potential value of more comprehensive screening techniques has been demonstrated in cases that showed PCR positivity for PML/RARA transcripts despite M3 morphology or the cytogenetic presence of t(15:17), and cryptic translocations such as t(12:21) or t(4;11) in ALL, and in AML.

Detection of Somatic Gene Mutations

Acquired mutations of individual genes can lead to the acquisition of a malignant phenotype and their presence or absence may have clinical significance (5). The principle of PCR-based detection of such mutations is similar to that used for germ line mutations. Methods include direct DNA PCR, if the mutation results in a length difference between the amplified fragments (e.g., internal tandem duplication of the FTL-3 gene [13]). Wild-type and mutated amplicons

TABLE. 29–2. *Common translocations diagnosed by polymerase chain reaction*

Translocation	Fusion product	Disease
t(9 : 22)	bcr/abl P190	CML
	bcr/abl P210	ALL
	bcr/abl P230	CNL
t(15 : 17)	PML/RAR-A	AML-M3
t(8 : 21)	AML/ETO	AML-M2
inv16	CBF-B/MYH11	AML-M4eo
t(5 : 12)	TEL/PDGF-R	CMML
t(1 : 19)	E2A/PBX1	ALL
t(4 : 11)	MLL/AF4	ALL
t(12 : 21)	TEL/AML1	ALL
t(14 : 18)	IgH/bcl2	FL
t(11 : 14)	bcl1/IgH	MCL
t(11 : 18)	API2/MLT	MZL
t(2 : 5)	NPM/ALK	ALCL
t(8 : 22)	c-myc/Igλ	BL
t(8 : 14)	c-myc/IgH	BL
t(2 : 8)	c-myc/Igκ	BL

CML, chronic myelogenous leukemia; ALL, acute lymphocytic leukemia; CNL, chronic neutrophilic leukemia; AML, acute myeloid lymphoma; CMML, chronic myelomonocytic leukemia; FL, follicular lymphoma; MCL, mantle cell lymphoma; MZL, marginal zone lymphoma; ALCL, anaplastic large cell lymphoma; BL, Burkitt lymphoma.

can be clearly identified by electrophoresis. When a labeled primer is used for amplification, even small size differences can be resolved by capillary gel electrophoresis. Single nucleotide changes can also be identified when the mutation produces a new or abolishes an existing restriction site. Consequently, after amplification, PCR products are digested with appropriate restriction endonucleases and subjected to electrophoresis to identify the presence of the mutation. Again, genotyping with a fluorochrome-labeled primer can be applied. In contrast to the detection of germ line mutations, the proportion of mutated cells in the sample may affect the results of the test: even if 100% of cells carry the mutation, only 50% of the alleles will be affected. The current detection limits of PCR-based techniques can reach 10% of cells carrying the mutation. These methods can be used for known invariant mutations. In contrast, if a gene can be affected by several mutations at various positions, sequencing may be required. Examples of clinically relevant somatic DNA alterations include internal tandem duplication of the FLT-3 gene, D835 FLT-3 mutation, p53, and Ras gene mutations.

CLONALITY STUDIES

Where acquired defects (point mutations, translocations) have been identified, they can serve as a suitable marker. However, in many clinical situations such a marker is not available. Consequently, a number of clonality assays have been developed that allow for the diagnosis of oligoclonal or skewed hematopoietic function.

X Chromosome Inactivation Pattern Analysis

X chromosome inactivation pattern (XCIP) analysis is particularly useful in the analysis of disorders without a disease-specific clonality marker (14). XCIP clonality analysis can be informative in a large proportion of female patients. Clearly, clonal/oligoclonal XCIP does not secure the diagnosis of malignancy but may be complementary with other clinical signs and laboratory results.

XCIP is based on the inactivation of one X chromosome in female mammalian cells (14). The inactivation pattern is random, laid down early in embryogenesis and stably inherited by all daughter cells. The inactivation mechanism includes methylation of certain portions of the DNA. Based on the single cell theory of malignant disorders, XCIP representation should change in the affected tissue, most significantly in blood. Consequently, the distinction between the two chromosomes made by using a polymorphic marker gene located on X chromosome and differentiation between the active and inactive X chromosomes underlie XCIP clonality analysis. While a disease-specific marker is not required, the pathologic change can be extrapolated from the expected pattern. The most commonly used polymorphic markers include human androgen receptors (HUMARA), phosphoglycerate kinase (PGK), or the fragile X (FRM1) genes. The heterozygosity rate for HUMARA is approximately 90%. Modern XCIP analysis techniques utilize PCR technology.

In the HUMARA assay, DNA is digested with a methylation-sensitive restriction endonuclease, amplified, and the electrophoretic pattern of the amplicons compared to the undigested amplicons. *Hpa*II digests the unmethylated allele and leaves methylated allele available for amplification. Comparison of the intensity of the bands allows extrapolation as to the skewing of the normally equally distributed amplicons of the methylated and unmethylated gene fragment.

In other common assays, single-base or short tandem repeat (STR) polymorphisms in the coding sequences of X chromosomal genes distinguish between the usage of the inactive or active chromosome by RNA based techniques. Reverse transcriptase (RT)-PCR is followed by RFLP of the amplicons.

Interpretation of the results of the XCIP analysis must account for age-rated skewing of inactivation and also for a nonrandom pattern among normal cells that may be encountered in up to 25% of women.

ANALYSIS OF T-CELL RECEPTOR AND IMMUNOGLOBULIN REARRANGEMENT

During T- and B-cell ontogeny, rearrangement of VDJ genes of heavy (H) and light (L) Ig chains and α (A) and β (B) or δ [D] and γ [G] chains of T-cell receptor (TCR), respectively, provides the molecular basis for the heterogeneity of B-and T-cell recognition repertoire (15–17).

For immunoglobulin (Ig) H-chain, there are at least 40 functional variable (VH) gene fragments, 27 diversity (DH) fragments, 6 functional junctional (JH) fragments, and several constant (CH) gene segments. The Igκ gene complex consists of 35 Vκ gene segments, 5 Jκ, and a single Cκ gene. Igλ gene is generated through recombination 30 Vλ segments and 4 Cλ segments all preceded by a Jλ region.

The TCR is a homodimer consisting either of TCR α and β or TCR δ and γ chains. Similar to Ig genes, α and δ chains are encoded by recombined VDJ fragments (65 VB segments, 7 JB fragments, and 2 CB segments, each preceded by a DB region for β chain and 8 VD, 3 DD and 4 JD gene segments, as well as a single CD region). TCR α and γ chain are generated through recombination of V and J regions. TCR α-chain gene complex consists of more than 50 VA, 61JA, and 1 CA gene segments. The TCR γ gene complex consists of 6 VG and 2 CG segments, each preceded by 2 or 3 JG1 or JG2 gene segments.

During recombination, Ig and TCR gene complexes rearrange and a specific combination VDJ segment is generated. This process is imprecise and nucleotides may be added or lost from the germ line VD and DJ junctions, a mechanism that further adds to the diversity of the TCR and Ig. Addition of nucleotides is mediated by the TdT enzyme. This junctional diversity is responsible for the variability of the complementarity determining region 3 (CDR3) of the IgH and TCRB chain. Because of the triple reading frame, 2 of 3 joinings will be out of frame and translation of a functional protein cannot occur. Indeed, a majority of B cells have rearranged both IgG, and T cells have a biallelic rearrangement of their TCR β and α chains. Postgerminal center B cells also have an additional mechanism of diversity in somatic hypermutation of the Ig V genes. Technically, detection of complete VH-JH rearrangement (as by PCR amplification) may fail to identify clonality, and assessment of incomplete DH-JH rearrangement may be required.

During B-cell development, the IgH chain rearranges first, followed by the recombination of Igκ and, if nonproductive, Igλ. As a result, all B cells harbor the IgH rearrangement and likely also Igκ rearrangement. The κde is a genetic element included in the Igκ locus and involved in its inactivation. Consequently, virtually all B cells harbor Igκ rearrangement, which is productive in Igκ+ cells, or nonfunctional in Igλ+ B cells, in which it likely involves Kde rearrangement.

During T-cell development, TCR δ genes rearrange first, followed by TCR γ. TCR β genes rearrange before TCR α. Because δ genes are located within the α locus, TCR α rearrangement results in the deletion of the entire δ locus. This process results in circular excision products, also called TCR excision circle (TREC). TREC are can serve as markers of recent thymic output and may be helpful in certain clinical conditions, such as immune reconstitution after transplantation. Virtually all mature A/B T cells have rearranged TCR γ genes (generally biallelic) but not δ genes, while G/D lymphocytes harbor functional rearrangement of both γ and δ genes, and often incomplete β rearrangement as well.

Ig and TCR rearrangements are not lineage-restricted: B and T cells may contain complete or incomplete cross-lineage rearrangements that can be used for assessment of clonality.

Clonal expansion results in overrepresentation of the specifically rearranged Ig or TCR configuration, a property of lymphocytes exploited for the diagnosis of T- and B-cell malignancies.

Southern blotting and PCR-based techniques can be used to detect overrepresented, specifically rearranged Ig and TCR genes.

Immunoglobulin and T-Cell Receptor Gene Southern Blotting

Southern blotting detects deleted and translocated gene segments based on changes in the distances between the cleavage sites of restriction enzymes (18). The method takes advantage of combinatorial diversity. DNA from experimental samples is digested with restriction enzymes, separated by electrophoresis and blotted. Specific bands appear after hybridization with labeled probes corresponding to Ig or TCR gene segments. Optimally designed probes will recognize sequences downstream of the rearranging segments. In a clonal process, specifically rearranged Ig or TCR genes are at high concentration, and the detected bands will differ from the normal germ line configuration. In contrast, polyclonal proliferations containing many different rearrangements produce a background pattern visible as a smear of multiple bands.

The sensitivity of Southern blotting is above 10% to 15% of clonal cells present in a polyclonal background. However, the technique is time consuming, requires longer amounts of DNA than PCR, and often is not be feasible, as in tissue biopsies. When DNA probes and restriction enzymes are appropriately selected, Southern blotting may reveal clonal rearrangements that remain undetected by PCR, as some of the V chains may not be included in the consensus Vβ primer mixture used for PCR (see later).

Immunoglobulin and T-Cell Receptor Junctional Region Polymerase Chain Reaction

PCR analysis of Ig and TCR gene segments is based on selective amplification of junctional regions. Amplification is only possible when the Ig or TCR gene are juxtaposed through rearrangement, because the distance between these gene segments in the normal germ line configuration is too large for PCR amplification. In contrast to the Southern blot, PCR relies on both the combinatorial and the junctional diversity of the appropriate rearrangements. PCR can be easily applied to blood and tissue specimens including lymph nodes and skin (particularly helpful in the diagnosis of cutaneous T cell lymphoma). For both IgH and TCR amplification, sets of consensus primers covering the full spectrum of the V regions combined with sets of JB primers are used in multiplex PCR. For B-cell populations, analysis of the IgH rearrangement is most informative, as the IgH locus rearranges first; a complete VH-JH rearrangement is usually investigated. However, as somatic hypermutation within the IgV gene hampers annealing and amplification, analysis of incomplete DH-JH rearrangement may also be helpful in identifying non-productive partial rearrangement in some immature B cells. Additionally, comprehensive Ig clonality assessment may include analysis of IgL chain, especially the Igκ locus. As discussed above, given the hierarchical rearrangement of IgL, all mature B cells have either a productive or a nonproductive Igκ rearrangement (generally involving the κde element) if cells are Igλ +. Further analysis of the IgL genes may be added to increase the sensitivity of clonality assessment.

For T-cell clonality, analysis of the γ TCR locus has been the paradigm; the main advantage is that the rearrangement of the γ chain occurs early and is present in both α/β and δ/γ cells, and in some B cells. Furthermore, the number of primers required for all the possible combinations is small, and junctional diversity is limited compared to other TCR loci. Rearrangement of β genes is a very powerful tool for detection of α/β clonality; even considering the extreme combinatorial diversity, amplification of almost the entire repertoire may be obtained using a relatively limited number of reactions containing appropriate sets of primers. Both complete VB-JB and incomplete DB-JB rearrangements may be studied, increasing the sensitivity of the method; the extreme junctional diversity of the B locus gives high sensitivity to β TCR clonality, even if sophisticated analysis of the PCR product may be required (see below). Analysis of the D locus is relatively easy and may add information on immature T cells and G/D populations, but is usually not informative for A/B cells. In contrast, α genes are not too helpful given the extreme complexity of gene segments, and concomitant rearrangement of β locus.

Two modifications of PCR are currently used for the detection of clonality: heteroduplex electrophoresis (19) and genescan analysis. In both methods, PCR amplicons are analyzed for fine discrimination and identification of identical products, utilizing different biologic properties of DNA.

Genotyping of rearranged TCR or Ig genes relies on the amplification of the gene fragments with primers that are labeled with a fluorochrome and detection of the labeled products using capillary gel electrophoresis (20). Most capillary electrophoresis-based automated gene sequencers can be adopted for this technique, which allows for resolution of PCR products that usually vary in size by multiples of 3 bp. Under normal circumstances, the amplification products are polyclonal, showing a large number of distinct peaks on capillary electrophoresis tracing. Best results are seen with IgH and TCR B loci, which both have a high frequency of in-frame V-J rearrangements, while for other loci the spacing between peaks is not preserved because of out-of-frame (nonproductive) or incomplete rearrangements. If a monoclonal population is present, a distinct singular peak is present that corresponds to the immunodominant clone. An equivalent technique can be used for the identification of Ig rearrangement. The sensitivity of genotyping is around 5% of malignant (clonal) cells in a cell mixture. As with heteroduplex analysis, frequently a biallelic rearrangement can be detected.

As discussed previously, Ig and TCR clonality can be assessed regardless of the lineage restriction of a putatively clonal population; however, a classic genescan pattern with triplet spacing of peaks is limited to functional in-frame rearrangements. In this case, representation of productive rearrangements may be also obtained by RT-PCR starting from RNA.

Rearranged dominant junctional CDR3 sequences can be sequenced and used for the design of clonotypic PCR primers that uniquely amplify only the malignant clone. Using nested PCR and variable and J primers, further rounds of amplification with a clonotype specific primer (such as an internal J primer) can be added. Such an approach may increase the sensitivity and specificity of detection, especially if utilized in the context of loci with extreme junctional diversity such as TCR β.

The application of TCR and Ig rearrangement analysis include determinations of B and T cell clonality in blood, marrow, lymph nodes and skin lesions for the diagnosis of T-ALL, B-ALL, multiple myeloma, lymphomas, large granular lymphocyte (LGL) leukemia, and chronic leukemia/lymphoma (CLL). In CLL, Ig rearrangement analysis is a major prognostic marker [see also Chapter 14]. Detailed sequencing of clonal IgH may reveal homology to the germ line IgV gene. Somatic hypermutations of the IgV gene usually occurs after antigen priming and, consequently, the IgV mutation status allows for distinction between pre- and postgerminal center CLL, entities with different clinical behavior.

MOLECULAR DIAGNOSIS OF INFECTIONS IN HEMATOLOGY

Molecular methods are increasingly supplementing serologic and histochemical methods in microbiology (21). Precise detection, localization, and quantitation of the nucleic acids of pathogenic viruses allows for better distinction of individual disease entities and are often used for therapeutic decisions. For instance, detection of EBV activation is essential for early diagnosis and therapy of posttransplant lymphoproliferative disorder. For DNA viruses such as herpesviruses, detection of mRNA transcripts by means of RT-PCR allows diagnosis of active infections, while DNA PCR is positive even when only latent virus in present. Molecular techniques are most often used for the diagnosis to EBV, cytomegalovirus (CMV), human herpes virus-6 (HHV-6), as well as retroviruses such as human T-cell leukemia virus (HTLV-1; Table 29-3) (22,23).

Epstein-Barr Virus

Both PCR and FISH can detect EBV in lymphoid neoplasms (Table 29-3). FISH probes complementary to EBV localize the virus to the malignant cells. Because of its sensitivity and lack of quantitation, DNA PCR may provide positive results without clinical relevance due to the frequency of latent EBV infection in the community. In contrast, quantitative light-cycler PCR assays provide highly precise copy numbers, but they are less sensitive methods. Both Taqman probes (single-stranded DNA probes that release light on degradation by Taq polymerase; see previous discussion) and beacon probes (DNA probes that release light on conformational change after hybridization to the internal segment of the amplicons) are used. TaqMan PCR is performed as described above for the detection of translocations. Sensitivity levels can be as low as 1 viral copy per 1 to 2×10^5 cells (24). Virus is always cell-associated and DNA for analysis is extracted from blood leukocytes.

FISH performed with probes detecting EBV-encoded RNA (EBER) is the most commonly applied test for the detection of virus in malignant cells. The sensitivity of this method is related to the high copy number of these transcripts and the ability to detect EBV genome in its latent state (EBER transcription is not dependent on induction of a productive rival life cycle).

Cytomegalovius

Molecular methods have a wide application in the diagnosis of CMV disease and compete with traditional culture and histochemistry-based techniques. DNA PCR can be used for the detection of the CMV genome, but because of its high sensitivity, results may not be informa-

TABLE. 29–3. *Viral pathogens in hematologic maligancies*

Disease	Pathogen
Diffuse large B cell lymphoma	EBV frequent in immunodeficiency, SV40 proposed
Plasmablastic B cell lymphoma	EBV
Primary effusion lymphoma	HHV-8, invariant occasional EBV
Diffuse T-cell lymphoma	EBV frequent
Burkitt lymphomas	EBV
Lymphomatoid granulomatosis	EBV occasional
Aggressive NK cell leukemia	EBV invariant
Extranodal NK/T cell lymphoma	EBV occasional
Angioimmunoblastic T cell lymphoma	EBV occasional
Lymphoplasmacytic lymphoma	HCV
Hodgkin's lymphoma	EBV certain forms
Posttransplant lymphoproliferative disorder	EBV 90%
Primary CNS lymphoma	EBV 100%
Follicular dendritic sarcoma	EBV occasional
Adult T cell leukemia	HTLV-1

EBV, Epstein-Barr virus; HHV-8, human herpesvirus 8; NK, natural killer; CNS, central nervous system; SV40, simian virus 40; HCV, hepatitis C virus; HTLV-1, human T-cell leukemia virus 1.

tive in seropositive individuals. CMV is strictly cell-associated and blood leukocytes are used as a source for DNA. Quantitative PCR utilizing the light cycler technology is the usual method for detection of CMV viremia and titer quantitation. Both beacon and Taqman probes have been developed (as described for EBV). Based on standard curves with calibrated positive controls, the number of viral genome copies can be precisely calculated (25). CMV can be detected at levels as low as one and as high as 5×10^5 copies per milliliter, correlating well with the antigenemia measured per 2×10^5 leukocytes.

B19 Parvovirus

Serologic methods are informative only in a minority of circumstances. Similar to CMV, B19 PCR may provide a high positivity rate that does not reflect clinically relevant viremia. Because of the extremely high copy number of virions during active infection, B19 can be detected and quantitated in serum using DNA hybridization methods without amplification. Dot-blot hybridization is most suitable to provide quantitation by serial dilution of positive sera with defined B19 genome copy numbers. Viral titer can be determined by comparison to the dilution standards (21).

Other Viruses

In theory, all viruses of known nucleic acid sequence can be detected using PCR. In some clinical circumstances, viral detection may have diagnostic consequences (Table 29-3). For example, herpes virus-6 may be identified in primary effusion lymphomas; presence of adenovirus (type 11) and polyomavirus (BK, JC) DNA may be helpful for diagnosis of hemorrhagic cystitis after bone marrow transplantation.

MOLECULAR DETECTION OF DONOR/RECIPIENT CHIMERISM AFTER STEM CELL TRANSPLANTATION

Determination of the contribution of host versus recipient blood cell production after allogeneic stem cell transplantation has become a standard laboratory test with clinically relevant implications. Several techniques have been devised, including short-tandem repeat (STR) analysis, RFPL or FISH for X or Y chromosomes. Selection of various cell types for analysis allows for the separate determination of chimerism in individual hematopoietic lineages.

Polymerase Chain Reaction-Based Short-Tandem Repeat Analysis

Highly polymorphic microsatellite STR exist for a large number of human loci. STR sequences show great variability in the number of repeats, their length is inherited, and their pattern may be individually specific (26–29). Examples of such loci include FGA, VWA, TH01, F13A1, and D21S11. A large number of primer pairs allow for amplification of STR from several loci that show biallelic deletion/insertion polymorphisms. Their size patterns enable forensic identity determination and paternity testing.

For bone marrow transplantation, STR for several loci can be amplified in a donor and recipient. Informative loci can be selected for the highest resolution of size differences between the donor and recipient pair. After transplantation, blood is sampled and DNA extracted. Following amplification of informative STR, gel electrophoresis is used to determine the presence of donor and/or recipient bands. When fluorochrome-labeled primers are used, PCR amplicons can be genotyped using capillary gel electrophoresis to precisely resolve the amplified products by size. The areas under the informative peaks are measured and the percentage of donor chimerism is calculated by the division of donor's peak area by the sum of the areas of the recipient and donor. This calculation can be performed for several informative loci and averaged. The sensitivity of this type of STR analysis permits the detection of 5% of donor/recipient cells for all loci and around 1% for all patients and selected loci. Combining this method with techniques of cell separation allows determination of chimerism within lymphoid or myeloid cells compartments, adding useful information in the setting of nonmyeloblative transplantation.

Short-Tandem Repeat Analysis by Real-Time (Quantitative) Polymerase Chain Reaction

Real-time PCR STR analysis is a more sensitive and highly quantitative method (30–32). Two primer pairs, each specific for the donor and recipient STR alleles, are selected. STR suitable for this analysis have biallelic polymorphism, with both alleles varying by at least two consecutive bases and showing a high level of heterozygosity. The sensitivity of this method can be as low as 0.1%, but there is need for a large selection of labeled primers and probes for identification of the most informative loci.

Restriction Fragment Length Polymorphism Analysis

Many loci within the human genome show significant allelic polymorphism, resulting in changes in endonuclease restriction sites. After enzyme digestion, DNA is electrophoresed. The resulting Southern blot is hybridized with tagged DNA probes derived from the polymorphic loci, resulting in the appearance of donor- and recipient-specific bands if there are allelic differences at the locus.

Fluorescence In Situ hybridization Analysis of Sex Chromosomes

Centromeric X and Y chromosome probes can be used for the detection and quantitation of donor and recipient cells. The assay is informative only in sex-mismatched transplants.

MOLECULAR HUMAN LEUKOCYTE ANTIGEN TYPING

Traditional serologic testing is increasingly replaced by molecular testing that allows for a higher precision and resolution of HLA alleles and polymorphisms (33,34). Molecular analysis of human leukocyte antigen (HLA) loci resulted in the identification of a large number of new alleles, with new polymorphisms still being added. PCR-based methods and primers have been developed for intermediate resolution (IR) and high-resolution (HR) level typing. Serologic testing continues to be performed in many institutions for class I and II alleles, but elsewhere serologic testing has been abandoned for class II alleles (35). Serologic testing retains some role, especially for the confirmation of null alleles after molecular testing.

Polymerase Chain Reaction-Based Human Leukocyte Antigen Testing

Two methods have dominated modern HLA testing technology: PCR amplification with sequence-specific primers (SSP) and hybridization with a sequence-specific oligonucleotide probe (SSOP). Allele- or group-level typing is commonly performed using SSP. Group- and locus specific primers can be used in the first stage of testing followed by allele specific primers. Standardized primer sets have been developed for both IR and HR testing (35).

SSOP testing can be used for the identification of individual alleles or for the detection of single nucleotide polymorphisms (SNPs). In general, SSOP analysis includes differential hybridization of amplicons to specific probes that are designed to match nucleotide sequences at all polymorphic sites of exons 2 and 3. Standardized probe sets have been developed.

Several modifications of SSOP hybridization are possible, including membrane- and bead-based fluorometric techniques. For flow cytometric approaches, such as using luminex technology, PCR amplification is performed in the presence of a fluorescently-labeled primer pair. The probes are immobilized to polystyrene beads tagged with fluorochromes that can be characterized by a flow cytometric technology using their orange-red emission profile combined with the counterfluorescence of the tagged amplicons. The presence of specific alleles can be identified based on a specific double-fluorescence profile of beads that carry a probe complementary to the amplicon. This assay can be multiplexed to allow a wide screening for many alleles.

SNPs within individual HLA alleles can also be detected using sets of primers designed to investigate polymorphism. This method, also referred to as single nucleotide extension (SNE), can also multiplexed, similar to SOP.

Finally, for greatest resolution and detection of previously unknown or new polymorphisms, individual region of HLA genes can be PCR amplified and directly sequenced.

REFERENCES

1. Lillicrap D. Molecular diagnosis of inherited bleeding disorders and thrombophilia. *Semin Hematol* 1999;36:340–351.
2. Arcasoy MO, Gallagher PG. Molecular diagnosis of hemoglobinopathies and other red blood cell disorders. *Semin Hematol* 1999;36:328–339.
3. Old JM. Screening and genetic diagnosis of haemoglobin disorders. *Blood Rev* 2003;17:43–53.
4. Spowart G. Mitotic metaphase chromosome preparation from peripheral blood for high resolution. In: Gosden JR, ed. *Methods in Molecular Biology Chromosome Analysis Protocols.* Vol. 29. Totowa, NJ: Humana Press, 1994:1–10.
5. Hokland P, Pallisgaard N. Integration of molecular methods for detection of balanced translocations in the diagnosis and follow-up of patients with leukemia. Semin Hematol. 2000;37:358–367.
6. Rowley JD. Cytogenetic analysis in leukemia and lymphoma: an introduction. *Semin Hematol* 2000; 37:315–319.
7. Bernard OA, Berger R. Location and function of critical genes in leukemogenesis inferred from cytogenetic abnormalities in hematologic malignancies. *Semin Hematol* 2000;37:412–419.
8. Ferrando AA, Look AT. Clinical implications of recurring chromosomal and associated molecular abnormalities in acute lymphoblastic leukemia. *Semin Hematol* 2000;37:381–395.
9. Gozzetti A, Le Beau MM. Fluorescence in situ hybridization: uses and limitations. *Semin Hematol.* 2000;37:320–333.
10. Kirsch IR, Ried T. Integration of cytogenetic data with genome maps and available probes: present status and future promise. *Semin Hematol* 2000;37:420–428.
11. Schrock E, Padilla-Nash H. Spectral karyotyping and multicolor fluorescence in situ hybridization reveal new tumor-specific chromosomal aberrations. *Semin Hematol* 2000;37:334–347.
12. Lichter P, Joos S, Bentz M, Lampel S. Comparative genomic hybridization: uses and limitations. *Semin Hematol* 2000;37:348–357.
13. Murphy KM, Levis M, Hafez MJ, et al. Detection of FLT3 internal tandem duplication and D835 mutations by a multiplex polymerase chain reaction and capillary electrophoresis assay. *J Mol Diagn* 2003;5:96–102.
14. Gale RE. Evaluation of clonality in myeloid stem-cell disorders. *Semin Hematol* 1999;36:361–372.
15. Arstila TP, Casrouge A, Baron V, et al. Diversity of human alpha beta T cell receptors. *Science* 2000;288:1135.
16. Macintyre EA, Delabesse E. Molecular approaches to the diagnosis and evaluation of lymphoid malignancies. *Semin Hematol* 1999;36:373–389.
17. Butler JE. Immunoglobulin gene organization and the mechanism of repertoire development. *Scand J Immunol* 1997;45:455–462.
18. Beishuizen A, Verhoeven MA, Mol EJ, et al. Detection of immunoglobulin kappa light-chain gene rearrangement patterns by Southern blot analysis. *Leukemia* 1994;8:2228–2236.
19. Langerak AW, Szczepanski T, Van Der BM, et al. Heteroduplex PCR analysis of rearranged T cell receptor genes for clonality assessment in suspect T cell proliferations. *Leukemia* 1997;11: 2192–2199.

20. Plasilova M, Risitano A, Maciejewski JP. Application of the molecular analysis of the T cell receptor repertoire in the study of immune-mediated hematologic disease. *Hematol J* 2003;8:173–181.
21. Brown KE. Molecular diagnosis of viral disease in hematology patients. *Semin Hematol* 1999;36: 352–360.
22. Precursor B-cell and T-cell neoplasms. In: Jaffe ES, Harris NL, Stein H, et al., eds. World Health Organization Classification of Tumours. Pathology and Genetics of Tumours of Haematopoietic and Lymphoid Tissues. Lyon: IARC Press, 2001:109–117.
23. Mature B-cell neoplasms. In: Jaffe ES, Harris NL, Stein H, et al. World Health Organization Classification of Tumours. Pathology and Genetics of Tumours of Haematopoietic and Lymphoid Tissue. Lyon: IARCPress, 2001:119–187.
24. Jebbink J, Bai X, Rogers BB, et al. Development of real-time PCR assays for the quantitative detection of Epstein-Barr virus and cytomegalovirus, comparison of TaqMan probes, and molecular beacons. *J Mol Diagn* 2003;5:15–20.
25. Li H, Dummer JS, Estes WR, et al. Measurement of human cytomegalovirus loads by quantitative real-time PCR for monitoring clinical intervention in transplant recipients. *J Clin Microbiol* 2003; 41:187–191.
26. Brouha PC, Ildstad ST. Mixed allogeneic chimerism. Past, present, and prospects for the future. *Transplantation* 2001;72:S36–S42.
27. Kreyenberg H, Holle W, Mohrle S, et al. Quantitative analysis of chimerism after allogeneic stem cell transplantation by PCR amplification of microsatellite markers and capillary electrophoresis with fluorescence detection: the Tuebingen experience. *Leukemia* 2003;17:237–240.
28. Leclair B, Fregeau CJ, Aye MT, et al. DNA typing for bone marrow engraftment follow-up after allogeneic transplant: a comparative study of current technologies. *Bone Marrow Transplant* 1995; 16:43–55.
29. Monaco AP. Chimerism in organ transplantation: conflicting experiments and clinical observations. *Transplantation* 2003;75:13S–16S.
30. Fernandez-Aviles F, Urbano-Ispizua A, Aymerich M, et al. Serial quantification of lymphoid and myeloid mixed chimerism using multiplex PCR amplification of short tandem repeat-markers predicts graft rejection and relapse, respectively, after allogeneic transplantation of CD34 + selected cells from peripheral blood. *Leukemia* 2003;17:613–620.
31. Nuckols JD, Rasheed BK, McGlennen RC, et al. Evaluation of an automated technique for assessment of marrow engraftment after allogeneic bone marrow transplantation using a commercially available kit. *Am J Clin Pathol* 2000;113:135–140.
32. Alizadeh M, Bernard M, Danic B, et al. Quantitative assessment of hematopoietic chimerism after bone marrow transplantation by real-time quantitative polymerase chain reaction. *Blood* 2002;99: 4618–4625.
33. Klein J, Sato A. The HLA system. First of two parts. *N Engl J Med* 2000;343:702–709.
34. Klein J, Sato A. The HLA system. Second of two parts. N Engl J Med. 2000;343:782–786.
35. Cao K, Chopek M, Fernandez-Vina MA. High and intermediate resolution DNA typing systems for class I HLA-A, B, C genes by hybridization with sequence-specific oligonucleotide probes (SSOP). *Rev Immunogenet* 1999;1:177–208.

30

Interpretation of Functional Genomics

Adrian Wiestner and Louis M. Staudt

The genome project has yielded a comprehensive list of genes encoded in our DNA and most of these genes fulfill functions in some cell types, during specific time points of development or under specific circumstances. Genes required for cell survival and function are transcribed into messenger RNA (mRNA), which can then be translated into protein. Not all genes are expressed in all cells at all times: thus the transcriptome, the genes that are expressed in a given cell at a given time, is only a fraction of the genome. This transcriptome is in large part determined by cell lineage, cell function, activity of regulatory pathways and response to external signals. Several genomic technologies have been developed to comprehensively view gene expression. Gene expression profiling on DNA microarrays has been particularly successful in analyzing expression of thousands of genes in parallel (1). Here we focus on this technology and briefly review principles of data collection and analysis and discuss some clinical applications of this method.

GENE EXPRESSION PROFILING ON DNA MICROARRAYS

DNA microarrays consist of solid supports onto which probes have been attached that detect the presence of a specific mRNA. Each array consists of thousands of such probes and each probe will specifically hybridize to one distinct mRNA. To measure gene expression, mRNA is extracted from the sample of interest and labeled with a fluorescent dye. The labeled mRNA is then placed onto the array where pairing between mRNA strands and their complementary probes takes place. After this hybridization step, unbound mRNAs are washed off and the level of gene expression in the specimen can be determined by quantifying the fluorescent signal bound to a given probe. The method is highly quantitative and accurately detects changes in gene expression over a 1,000-fold range.

One commonly used microarray technology utilizes oligonucleotide probes that are synthesized directly on the solid support. These oligonucleotide arrays contain sequence specific oligonucleotide probes to detect a distinct mRNA and corresponding oligonucleotides that contain a mismatch to control for nonspecific binding. Samples are labeled with a fluorescent dye and hybridized to the array, which yields an absolute measure of mRNA abundance. Affymetrix GeneChip arrays are commercially available oligonucleotide arrays that in the most recent generation (Human Genome U133 Plus 2.0) contain more than 54,000 probe sets able to measure the expression levels of approximately 24,547 human genes—the majority of genes encoded in the human genome.

Custom-made spotted microarrays are also widely used. These arrays often have cDNA sequences of several hundred base pairs, amplified by polymerase chain reaction (PCR) and then robotically spotted onto the solid support. The template for these arrays is usually a cDNA library derived from the tissue of interest, with or without the addition of selected named genes. Alternatively, presynthesized oligonucleotides complementary to an mRNA can be spotted. Spotted DNA microarrays typically use two fluorescent channels: one channel is dedicated to the sample of interest (often labeled with the Cy5 dye; red signal) while the second channel serves to analyze a comparator sample (often labeled with the Cy3 dye; green signal). The comparator mRNA can be derived from normal cells, a pool of cell lines, or a relevant control cell type. The comparator mRNA serves as a control for the performance of the hybridization as a whole and for the quality of the array probes. One example of a custom spotted DNA microarray is the Lymphochip, which was developed to study B-cell malignancies (2). This array contains roughly 15,000 cDNA spots representing about 8,000 genes. cDNAs for the Lymphochip have been selected from libraries representing different stages of normal B-cell development and different forms of B-cell malignancies with the addition of genes known to be important in cell growth or oncogenesis.

GENE EXPRESSION SIGNATURES IN MOLECULAR DIAGNOSIS AND OUTCOME PREDICTION

Microarray experiments typically yield several thousand data points per sample. The amount of data generated in such studies can easily overwhelm researcher and statistician alike and makes "by the eye" analysis of the data virtually impossible. Analytical techniques have been developed to aid in the interpretation of microarray data (3,4); they fall into two categories (Fig. 30-1). In a so-called unsupervised analysis, statistical methods are used to visualize patterns of shared gene expression and to identify distinct groups of samples. This approach is not hypothesis-driven and is independent of external data. In contrast, supervised approaches rely on statistical tests to relate gene expression characteristics to known biologic or clinical characteristics.

Unsupervised Analysis: Hierarchical Clustering Discovers Patterns and Defines Gene Expression Signatures

One commonly used unsupervised strategy is called hierarchical clustering (3). This analysis identifies genes that share a similar expression pattern across all samples. For example, hierarchical clustering will group genes together that are highly expressed in one group of samples and expressed at low levels in a second group (Fig. 30-1A). Clusters of coordinately expressed genes are frequently involved in the same cellular function and thus constitute a gene expression signature of a particular biologic process (5). To proliferate, for instance, a cell simultaneously expresses a set of genes involved in cell cycle progression, DNA replication, and metabolism that can be visualized as a proliferation signature by hierarchical clustering. Gene expression signatures relate to a variety of biologic characteristics including cell type, differentiation state, and activity of signaling pathways. Gene expression signatures provide a framework in which the complexity of microarray data can be related to the biology of the study sample. They provide a preliminary roadmap of the active biologic processes in a sample, stimulate the generation of testable hypotheses, and focus further investigations.

The hierarchical clustering algorithm can also be used to group samples that share a common pattern of gene expression. The result of hierarchical clustering of samples is highly dependent on the set of genes chosen. In some cases, the grouping of samples by hierarchical clustering may be dominated by a few genes with a high degree of variability between samples (such as immunoglobulin genes in B-cell malignancies) or by a large set of coordinately expressed genes. For example, hundreds of genes may be differentially regulated in cells with different proliferation rates, and these proliferation signature genes may dominate hierarchical clustering and obscure other interesting biologic differences between the samples. Therefore, it may be beneficial to narrow the list of genes considered in hierarchical clustering. With these caveats, hierarchical clustering can identify unexpected heterogeneity among tumor samples of clinical and biological importance (2).

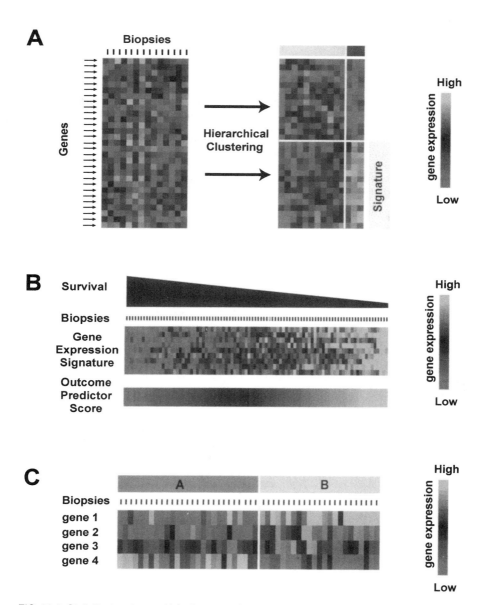

FIG. 30-1. Statistical analyses aid the interpretation of microarray data. **(A)** Hierarchical clustering discovers patterns of gene expression. The *left panel* shows the result of a microarray experiment. Samples are shown in columns and genes in rows. The relative gene expression level is visualized on a gray scale. Lines are introduced to highlight the subgroups identified by the algorithm. **(B)** A supervised approach can identify a gene expression signature predicting survival. Samples are arranged from left to right by decreasing survival. **(C)** A supervised approach to build a molecular diagnosis.

Supervised Analysis: Building Molecular Predictors of Diagnosis, Prognosis, and Treatment Response

Supervised analytical methods use biologic or clinical data to search for gene expression differences that are diagnostically or prognostically most informative. To derive a molecular predictor of survival one can, for example, use the Cox proportional hazard method to identify gene expression characteristics associated with a distinct outcome (Fig. 30-1B). This initial step may yield several hundred genes, depending on the sample size and significance cutoffs chosen. To organize these data further, hierarchical clustering can be used to identify specific gene expression signatures that reflect those biologic processes that may influence survival. The nature of gene expression signatures represented by a molecular outcome predictor and the optimal number of genes vary among different diseases and with analytical techniques. In a large study of diffuse large-B–cell lymphomas, 17 genes representing several signatures related to differentiation, tumor proliferation, and tumor host interactions were combined to form the best prognostic score (6). In contrast, chronic lymphocytic leukemia expression of a single gene, ZAP-70, was sufficient to distinguish biologic and prognostically distinct subtypes of the disease (7).

One important goal of gene expression profiling is to use molecular characteristics to define homogeneous disease entities. Within a homogeneous disease category, all samples could be expected to share common characteristics relating to cell of origin, pathogenesis, activity of signaling pathways, and sensitivity to toxins. Various methods have been devised to distinguish two cancer types by gene expression profiling (4,8,9). A classification strategy based on Bayesian statistics assigns to a given sample a probability of belonging to one of two disease entities (8). The algorithm starts by identifying the most differentially expressed genes between two disease categories by a supervised analysis (Fig. 30-1C). The gene expression measurements of the most informative genes are combined to form a linear predictor score (LPS) for each sample. The LPS is the sum of the gene expression measurements of the individual genes, multiplied by a scaling factor that depends on the degree to which each gene discriminates the subgroups. The LPS for each subgroup follows an approximately normal distribution that may be partially overlapping (Fig. 30-2). A new case can be classified

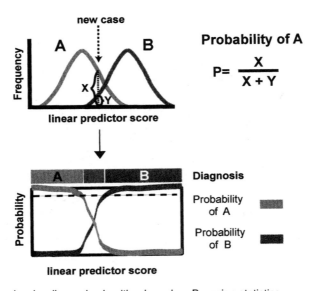

FIG. 30-2. A molecular diagnosis algorithm based on Bayesian statistics.

by calculating its LPS and estimating the probability of it belonging to one or the other group by applying Bayes' rule. In addition, some cases that do not fit well into a particular classification scheme and have an intermediate probability in the Bayesian predictor can remain unclassified. The stringency of the diagnostic method can be varied by altering the probability cutoff for assigning a case to one or the other group or to leave it unclassified. This Bayesian approach has made comparisons of gene expression studies performed using different microarray platforms possible (8) and has proven valuable in deriving and validating molecular diagnostic definitions in diffuse large B–cell lymphomas and mantle cell lymphoma (8,10).

Data Reproducibility: The Value of Training and Validation Sets

The wealth of data derived from gene expression studies using DNA microarrays increases the likelihood of finding chance associations between clinical variables and gene expression. A model can fit the data set from which it was derived yet not perform well in an independent data set. One approach against such overfitting problems is to randomly assign the cases in a study to two independent sets: the training set is used to derive the model while the validation set is used to test the general applicability of the model. Because this method requires a large number of samples, a less rigorous modification, termed "leave one out cross-validation," is often used. In this method, the model is derived from all samples within the study except one and then is applied to categorize the sample left out. This procedure is repeated for each sample, and the performance of the model is assessed by the number of samples that are correctly assigned.

CLINICAL APPLICATION OF GENE EXPRESSION PROFILING

Gene expression profiling is in rapid transition from research test to clinical application. Because of tissue availability, most clinical gene expression studies to date have been performed in malignancies (11–15). Gene expression profiling is redefining classification of hematologic malignancies on a molecular basis and has yielded prognostic scores of unprecedented power (Table 30-1). However, all these studies have been retrospective in nature and prospective studies have only been initiated recently.

Obtaining Gene Expression Profiling for Individual Patients

Gene expression profiling has been performed in large studies, often incorporating hundreds of patients. A specific sample may thus be viewed in the context of the whole study, and a given patient may be assigned accurately to a prognostic group with a well-defined survival probability. The interpretation of a single patient's gene expression profile obtained outside of a study and possibly done on a different experimental platform is a challenging problem, which nevertheless is likely to be solvable as algorithms for molecular diagnosis improve. Importantly, the molecular predictor of survival following treatment with a novel therapeutic agent may be different from the survival predictor developed in retrospective studies. Therefore, patients should be enrolled in prospective clinical trials that incorporate gene expression profiling in order to derive prognostic markers of responses to novel therapies and to understand which biologic features of a tumor influence therapeutic response.

Critical Interpretation of Studies Incorporating Gene Expression Profiling

When reading a publication reporting gene expression profiling studies, it is important to ask the following questions:

- How have the study samples been selected and/or purified prior to gene expression profiling?
- Is the number of samples in the study sufficient to address the hypothesis?

TABLE. 30–1. *Select gene expression profiling studies in hematologic malignancies*

Diagnosis, platform	Major findings and conclusions	Year, Reference
B-ALL, Affymetrix	Identified distinct GESs for each of the cytogenetically-defined prognostic subgroups of B-ALL in 360 pediatric cases and derived a molecular predictor that accurately classified patients into subgroups. Identified a novel subset of B-ALL not characterized by a diagnostic cytogenetic abnormality.	2002, (9)
T-ALL, Affymetrix	Showed that aberrant expression of key transcription factors is a central pathogenetic mechanism in 59 cases of T-ALL. Correlated GESs associated with over-expression of HOX11, TAL1 and LYL1 to distinct stages of T-cell differentiation and identified a distinct prognostic subgroup within T-ALL with high HOX11 expression.	2002, (16)
CLL, Lymphochip	Provided evidence that CLL can be viewed as a single disease characterized by a common GES. Two CLL subtypes, defined by Ig-genotype differentially expressed several hundred genes between subtypes, including ZAP-70.	2001, (17)
CLL, Lymphochip	Confirmed ZAP-70 as the most differentially expressed gene between subtypes defined by Ig-genotype in 107 patients and derived tests for its use as a prognostic marker in CLL.	2003, (7)
DLBCL, Lymphochip	Identified two molecularly and clinically distinct diseases within DLBCL that differentially express GESs associated with different stages of B-cell differentiation. One subgroup termed Germinal Centre B-cell like DLBC (GCB DLBCL) had a favorable 5-year survival and expressed genes characteristic of germinal center B cells while the second subgroup termed Activated B-cell like DLBCL (ABC DLBCL) expressed genes typically induced during mitogenic activation of blood B-cells.	2000, (2)
DLBCL, Affymetrix	Used supervised algorithm to define a molecular outcome predictor for 58 patients undergoing CHOP chemotherapy and identify two groups with 5-year survival rates of 70% versus 12%. Differences between microarray platforms hampered identification of DLBCL subgroups identified by Alizadeh et al. (2)	2002, (18)
DLBCL, Lymphochip	Reproduced earlier finding of distinct subgroups in 240 patients with DLBCL and demonstrated that these subgroups have distinct oncogenic events. Derived an outcome predictor that integrates 17 genes and confers prognostic information independent of IPI-scores with overall 5-year survival rates of 73% in the best quartile versus 15% in the lowest quartile.	2002, (6)
DLBCL, Lymphochip & Affymetrix	Described a diagnostic algorithm for the classification of cancers by gene expression based on Bayesian statistics. Identified GCB DLBCL and ABC DLBCL subgroups in a set of 274 patients analyzed on the Lymphochip and in 58 independent patients profiled on Affymetrix arrays by Shipp et al. (18)	2003, (8)

(continued)

TABLE. 30–1. *Continued*

Diagnosis, platform	Major findings and conclusions	Year, Reference
MCL, Lymphochip	Described a molecular diagnosis of MCL and defined a MCL subset lacking Cyclin D1 expression. Derived a molecular measurement of tumor proliferation based on gene expression. Identified one quartile of patients with a 6.7 year median survival and another quartile with a median survival of 0.8 years. Described MCL as a disease of cell cycle dysregulation with cooperating pathogenic events.	2003, (10)
MM, Affymetrix	Identified four MM subtypes in 79 patients based on characteristic GESs. Correlated GESs of MM subtypes with distinct stages of plasma cell differentiation.	2002, 2003 (19, 20)
PMBL, Lymphochip	Identified PMBL as a molecularly distinct subgroup of DLBCL with a favorable prognosis and defined a molecular diagnosis of PMBL based on the expression of 46 genes. Provided evidence of a relationship between PMBL and Hodgkin lymphoma.	2003 (21)

ALL, acute lymphocytic leukemia; CLL, chronic lymphocytic leukemia; DLBCL, diffuse large B-cell lymphoma; MCL, mantle cell lymphoma; MM, multiple myeloma; GES, gene expression signature; Ig, immunoglobulin gene; IPI, international prognostic index.

- Is the analysis unsupervised or supervised and what statistical approach is used?
- Has the statistical model derived from the study been validated in an independent data set?
- Do the reported findings reveal new insights into the biologic or molecular processes that influence the disease being studied?
- Are the major findings validated by independent methods or supported by observations from other studies?

OUTLOOK

DNA microarrays will soon be used routinely in the clinical laboratory. While it is possible to translate some of the insights gained from gene expression profiling into tests such as immunohistochemistry or flow cytometry, the number of genes necessary for the best molecular classification is rapidly expanding, making these other diagnostic techniques a temporary measure. Such conventional methods are semiquantitative, while gene expression profiling is highly quantitative, capable of making precise molecular diagnoses and prognoses. Besides providing an unprecedented amount of information, the use of arrays in the clinical laboratory could simplify and standardize diagnostic testing on a single technical platform to yield information currently obtained only from several different techniques. In addition microarrays provide a digital fingerprint of a specimen that can be analyzed by computer-based diagnostic algorithms and easily stored. Such data will certainly accelerate the transition to a molecular diagnosis of cancer.

REFERENCES

1. Staudt LM. Molecular diagnosis of the hematological cancers. *N Engl J Med* 2003;348:1777–1785.
2. Alizadeh AA, Eisen MB, Davis RE, et al. Distinct types of diffuse large B-cell lymphoma identified by gene expression profiling. *Nature* 2000;403:503–511.

3. Eisen MB, Spellman PT, Brown PO, et al. Cluster analysis and display of genome-wide expression patterns. *Proc Natl Acad Sci USA* 1998;5:14863–8.
4. Golub TR, Slonim DK, Tamayo P, et al. Molecular classification of cancer: class discovery and class prediction by gene expression monitoring. *Science* 1999; 286:531–537.
5. Shaffer AL, Rosenwald A, Hurt EM, et al. Signatures of the immune response. *Immunity* 2001;15: 375–385.
6. Rosenwald A, Wright G, Chan WC, et al. The use of molecular profiling to predict survival after chemotherapy for diffuse large-B-cell lymphoma. *N Engl J Med* 2002;346:1937–1947.
7. Wiestner A, Rosenwald A, Barry TS, et al. ZAP-70 expression identifies a chronic lymphocytic leukemia subtype with unmutated immunoglobulin genes, inferior clinical outcome, and distinct gene expression profile. *Blood* 2003;101:4944–4951.
8. Wright G, Tan B, Rosenwald A, et al. A gene expression-based method to diagnose clinically distinct subgroups of diffuse large B cell lymphoma. *Proc Natl Acad Sci USA* 2003;100:9991–9996.
9. Yeoh E-J, Ross ME, Shurtleff SA, et al. Classification, subtype discovery and prediction of outcome in pediatric acute lymphblastic leukemia by gene expression profiling. *Cancer Cell* 2002;1:133–143.
10. Rosenwald A, Wright G, Wiestner A, et al. The proliferation gene expression signature is a quantitative integrator of oncogenic events that predicts survival in mantle cell lymphoma. *Cancer Cell* 2003; 3:185–197.
11. Armstrong SA, Golub TR, Korsmeyer SJ. MLL-rearranged leukemias: insights from gene expression profiling. *Semin Hematol* 2003;40:268–273.
12. Ferrando AA, Look AT. Gene expression profiling in T-cell acute lymphoblastic leukemia. *Semin Hematol* 2003;40:274–280.
13. Haferlach T, Kohlmann A, Kern W, et al. Gene expression profiling as a tool for the diagnosis of acute leukemias. *Semin Hematol* 2003;40:281–295.
14. Wiestner A, Staudt LM. Towards molecular diagnosis and targeted therapy of lymphoid malignancies. *Semin Hematol* 2003;40:296–307.
15. Zhan F, Barlogie B, Shaughnessy J, Jr. Toward the identification of distinct molecular and clinical entities of multiple myeloma using global gene expression profiling. *Semin Hematol* 2003;40: 308–320.
16. Ferrando AA, Neuberg DS, Staunton J, et al. Gene expression signatures define novel oncogenic pathways in T cell acute lymphoblastic leukemia. *Cancer Cell* 2002;1:75–87.
17. Rosenwald A, Alizadeh AA, Widhopf G, et al. Relation of gene expression phenotype to immunoglobulin mutation genotype in B cell chronic lymphocytic leukemia. *J Exp Med* 2001;194:1639–1648.
18. Shipp MA, Ross KN, Tamayo P, et al. Diffuse large-B-cell lymphoma outcome prediction by gene-expression profiling and supervised machine learning. *Nat Med* 2002;8:68–74.
19. Zhan F, Hardin J, Kordsmeier B, et al. Global gene expression profiling of multiple myeloma, monoclonal gammopathy of undetermined significance, and normal bone marrow plasma cells. *Blood* 2002;99:1745–1757.
20. Zhan F, Tian E, Bumm K, et al. Gene expression profiling of human plasma cell differentiation and classification of multiple myeloma based on similarities to distinct stages of late-stage B-cell development. *Blood* 2003;101:1128–1140.
21. Rosenwald A, Wright G, Leroy K, et al. Molecular diagnosis of primary mediastinal B cell lymphoma identifies a clinically favorable subgroup of diffuse large B cell lymphoma related to Hodgkin lymphoma. *J Exp Med* 2003;198:851–862.

Appendix: Cytokines Approved for Clinical Use

ERYTHROPOIETIN (EPOIETIN ALFA, PROCRIT, EPOGEN)

Epoetin alfa has a half-life of 5 to 8 hours in the plasma. When administered subcutaneously therapeutic levels persist for several days compared to 18 to 24 hours for the intravenous route.

Epoietin alfa Indications

- Anemia in chronic renal failure patients (dialysis [+] or dialysis [-]).
- Anemia in zidovudine-treated human immunodeficiency virus (HIV)-infected patients.
- Anemia in patients with cancer undergoing chemotherapy.
- Reduction of allogeneic blood transfusion in surgical patients.

In anemia of chronic renal failure, doses of 50 to 150 IU/kg subcutaneously three times weekly are required to maintain a hematocrit in the mid- to high 30s. In zidovudine-treated patients with HIV, the recommended starting dose is 100 IU/kg subcutaneously three times per week. Benefit is significant if the pretreatment serum erythropoietin is below 500 mU/mL. In patients with cancer, 150 to 300 IU/kg subcutaneousl three times per week is required to maintain an hematocrit in the high 30s. It is possible to use once a week dosing at a dose of 600 IU/kg subcutaneously, and titrate subsequent dosing to maintain the desired hemoglobin level. In surgical patients, the reduction of allogeneic transfusions is achieved with an erythropoietin (EPO) dose of 300 IU/kg/day subcutaneously for 10 days prior to surgery, on the day of surgery, and for 4 days after surgery. All patients should receive iron supplementation. The pre-operative hemoglobin should be between 10 and 13 g/dL.

Prior to and during treatment with EPO, the patient's iron stores should be evaluated. Most patients require iron supplemetation during therapy with EPO.

Allergic reactions and antibody mediated pure red cell aplasia have been associated with the use of epoietin alfa. Other adverse reactions are discussed in conjunction with darbopoietin alfa.

DARBEPOIETIN ALFA (ARANESP)

Darbepoietin alfa differs from recombinant human EPO by having increased sialylated carbohydrate content increasing the molecular weight, prolonging its half-life and increases its biologic in vivo activity.

Darbepoietin alfa is indicated for the treatment of anemia associated with renal failure. The recommended starting dose in patients with chronic renal failure is 0.45 µg/kg administered intravenously or subcutaneously once per week. The dose should be titrated to not exceed target hemoglobin of 12 g/dL.

Epoeitin alfa and darbepoietin alfa have been associated with an increased risk of cardiovascular events in patients with chronic renal failure. The risk of cardiovascular events is higher in patients with chronic renal failure who have target hemoglobin of 14 g/dL compared to patients who have target hemoglobin of 10 g/dL. The target hemoglobin in chronic renal failure patients should not exceed 12 g/dL.

Blood pressure may rise during treatment of anemia with epoietin alfa and darbepoietin alfa; hypertension should be controlled before initiation of therapy.

Seizures have been reported in patients with chronic renal failure who had a rapid rate of increase of hemoglobin; the dose of epoietin alfa or darbepoietin alfa should be decreased if the hemoglobin increase exceeds 1.0 g/dL in any 2-week period.

Darbepoietin alfa is supplied in two formulations: one containing polysorbate 80 and another containing albumin. Albumin contains a small risk of transmitting viral diseases.

GRANULOCYTE COLONY-STIMULATING FACTOR (FILGRASTIM, NEUPOGEN)

Filgrastim regulates the production of neutrophils within the bone marrow and also impacts on their function.

Granulocyte Colony-Stimulating Factor Indications

- Nonmyeloid malignancies undergoing myelosuppressive chemotherapy with an expected risk of severe neutropenia with fever.
- Acute myeloid leukemia, following induction or consolidation chemotherapy.
- Nonmyeloid malignancies undergoing myeloablative chemotherapy followed by marrow transplantation.
- Mobilization of peripheral blood hematopoietic stem cells.
- Severe chronic neutropenia.

Granulocyte colony-stimulating factor (G-CSF) can be administered subcutaneously or intravenously, the usual dose is 5 μg/kg per day.

Patients treated with G-CSF have experienced allergic-type reactions, severe sickle cell crises, bone pain, splenomegaly, and splenic rupture. G-CSF has the potential of stimulating the proliferation of myeloid leukemic cells.

PEGYLATED GRANULOCYTE COLONY-STIMULATING FACTOR (PEGFILGRASTIM, NEULASTA)

Pegfilgrastim is produced by covalently conjugating a 20-kd polyethylene glycol molecule to the N-terminus of filgrastim. The pegfilgrastim molecule is larger than the threshold for renal clearance, prolonging its half-life in circulation.

Pegfilgrastim is indicated to decrease the incidence of febrile neutropenia, in patients with nonmyeloid malignancies receiving myelosuppressive chemotherapy associated with a clinically significant incidence of febrile neutropenia. The adult recommended dosage of pegfilgrastim is 6 mg administered subcutaneously once per chemotherapy cycle.

Splenic rupture, adult respiratory distress syndrome, allergic reactions, severe sickle cell crises, and proliferation of myeloid leukemic cells have been described in patients treated with filgrastim, which is the parent compound of pegfilgrastim.

Granulocyte-Macrophage Colony-Stimulating Factor (Sargramostim, Leukine)

Sargramostim induces a dose-dependant increase in neutrophils and to a lesser extent monocytes and eosinophils. When granulocyte macrophage colony-stimulating factor (GM-CSF) is discontinued, the leukocyte counts decrease to pretreatment levels over 3 to 5 days.

Granulocyte-Macrophage Colony-Stimulating Factor Indications

- After induction chemotherapy in patients with acute myeloid leukemia over the age of 55.
- Mobilization of peripheral blood hematopoietic progenitor cells.
- Myeloid reconstitution after autologous bone marrow transplantation for non-Hodgkins's lymphoma, Hodgkin's lymphoma, and acute lymphoblastic leukemia.
- Myeloid reconstitution after allogeneic marrow transplantation.
- Allogeneic and autologous bone marrow transplantation failure or engraftment delay.

GM-CSF can be administered subcutaneously or intravenously. The usual daily dose of GM-CSF is 250 $\mu g/m^2$.

The use of GM-CSF is potentially associated with fluid retention, capillary leak syndrome, pleural and pericardial effusions, sequestration of granulocytes in the pulmonary circulation, supraventricular arrhythmias, and renal and hepatic dysfunction. GM-CSF has the potential to stimulate the proliferation of myeloid leukemic cells.

Interleukin-11 (Oprelvekin, Neumega)

Oprelvekin is a thrombopoietic growth factor that stimulates the proliferation of megakaryocytic progenitors and induces megakaryocyte maturation.

Oprelvekin also promotes the integrity of gastrointestinal mucosal epithelial cells.

Interleukin (IL)-11 stimulates platelet production in a dose-dependent manner with peak platelet counts at 14 to 21 days after IL-11 treatment.

IL-11 is indicated for the prevention of severe thrombocytopenia in patients with non-myeloid malignancies undergoing myelosuppressive chemotherapy. IL-11 is not used after myeloablative chemotherapy.

The usual recommended dosage of IL-11 is 50 $\mu g/kg$ given once daily subcutaneously. The use of Oprelvekin has been associated with fluid retention, edema, pleural effusions and electrolyte imbalances.

Index

M